Livestock Production and Management

NIPA® GENX ELECTRONIC RESOURCES & SOLUTIONS P. LTD.
New Delhi-110 034

About the Editor

Dr. Tanmoy Rana obtained his Bachelor of Veterinary Sciences and Animal Husbandry degree (B.V.Sc. & A.H.) and Masters (M.V.Sc) in Veterinary Medicine, Ethics & Jurisprudence from West Bengal University of Animal and Fishery Sciences, Kolkata, India. He secured his Doctor of Philosophy (Ph.D.) in Veterinary Science from the University of Calcutta, Kolkata, India. He works currently as an Assistant Professor of the Veterinary Clinical Complex at West Bengal University of Animal and Fishery Sciences, Kolkata, India. Previously he has also worked as a Veterinary Officer, Animal Resources Development Department, Government of West Bengal, India. He is actively engaged in teaching and clinical practices in veterinary medicine and research related to animal health, production, and disease monitoring regimes. His research interests involve arsenic toxicity, molecular diagnosis, molecular toxicology and medicine, oxidative stress, immunopathology, nanoparticles, Echinococcosis, and microbes. He has published several research articles in reputed international and national journals along with review articles in international journals. He is an editorial board member (especially BMC Veterinary Research, Associate Editor of Frontier in Veterinary Science), and a reviewer of international and national journals. He is a member of many international scientific societies and organizations importantly the West Bengal Veterinary Council (WBVC), The Indian Society for Veterinary Medicine (ISVM), the Association of Public Health Veterinarians, and The Indian Science Congress Association (ISCA). He is also an associate of the West Bengal Academy of Science & Technology, West Bengal, India. He is an editor and author of so many national and international books.

Livestock Production and Management

Tanmoy Rana, Ph.D. AFWAST, FVASc.
Assistant Professor
Veterinary Clinical Complex
(Veterinary Medicine, Ethics & Jurisprudence)
Department of Veterinary Clinical Complex
West Bengal University of Animal & Fishery Sciences
Kolkata-700037, West Bengal, India

NIPA® GENX ELECTRONIC RESOURCES & SOLUTIONS P. LTD.
New Delhi-110 034

NIPA® GENX ELECTRONIC RESOURCES & SOLUTIONS P. LTD.

101,103, Vikas Surya Plaza, CU Block
L.S.C. Market, Pitam Pura, New Delhi-110 034
Ph : +91-11-43860225, Mob.: +91 9717133558, 9540816132
E-mail: newindiapublishingagency@gmail.com
Website: www.nipaersources.com

Print ISBN: 978-93-58878-28-8
ebook ISBN: 978-93-58878-53-0

Composed and Designed by NIPA®.

Preface

This book -"MCQ: Livestock Production and Management", a multiple choice questions (MCQs) book is well organized and structured for the essentials of students, academicians and job aspirants prepared for any competitive examination in the streams of Livestock Production and Management. The book magnifies fully MCQ questions with answer keys for the better understanding of the academic Excellency of the undergraduate, postgraduate students and postdoctoral fellows interested in higher studies in the field of Livestock Production and Management Science. This book has MCQ questions of 39 chapters dealing with all aspects of livestock production and its management aspect. Various authors are well experienced and acquainted with the basic as well as advanced aspect of livestock production science from the reputed Universities of the Country, and foreign also. The book also describes the latest information about the management, production, economy and marketing. Each chapter starts with a brief introduction about the chapter that helps the reader for the better understanding of the readership. The questions are unambiguous, analytical and comprehensive in nature. All chapters of this book are carefully edited to keep the book more interesting, focusing, and lucrative and easy grasping. The book is especially prepared for students appearing for various competitive examinations such as Junior Research Fellowship (JRF), Senior Research Fellowship (SRF), National Eligibility Test (NET), and other competitive examinations. Therefore, the book is a quick supplement/guide for students, and job aspirants for providing them an easy, elegant, and quick, approach to prepare for different competitive examinations. Furthermore, the MCQ book provides useful information about the Livestock Production and Management.

Dr. Tanmoy Rana
Department of Veterinary Clinical Complex
West Bengal University of Animal & Fishery Sciences
Kolkata, India

Acknowledgement

I would like to convey my sincere gratitude to the Hon'ble Vice Chancellor, West Bengal University of Animal & Fishery Sciences, Kolkata, India for providing me the opportunity to edit the MCQ book of Livestock Production and Management. I am also thankful to my all contributors who wholeheartedly help me by sending respective MCQ chapter within the scheduled time. I am also indebted to my colleagues for their active guidance, immense help and motivation for the completion of book project. I am thankful to all members of Publisher for giving me a wonderful platform to edit the MCQ book. Last but not the least, I would also like to thank my family for providing great support and time to finalize the book.

Dr. Tanmoy Rana
Department of Veterinary Clinical Complex
West Bengal University of Animal & Fishery Sciences
Kolkata, India

Contents

1

General Introduction and History About Livestock Production

Utkarsh Kumar Tripathi[1], Anshuman Kumar[1], Anuradha Kumari[1], Manish Kumar[1], and Tanmoy Rana[2]

[1]*Faculty of Veterinary and Animal Sciences, IAS, RGSC, BHU, India*

[2]*Department of Veterinary Clinical Complex, West Bengal University of Animal & Fishery Sciences, Kolkata, India*

Introduction

India's animal husbandry sector plays a vital role in the country's economy and food security. It provides livelihood to millions of people, contributes significantly to the agricultural gross domestic product (GDP), and meets the nutritional needs of the population. The sector encompasses various aspects of livestock production, including dairy farming, poultry farming, sheep rearing, goat rearing, and piggery.

Milk Production

India is the world's largest milk producer, with an annual production of 230.58 million tonnes in 2022-23. This represents an impressive growth rate of 3.83% over the previous year. The top five milk-producing states are Uttar Pradesh, Rajasthan, Madhya Pradesh, Gujarat, and Andhra Pradesh.

Egg Production

India is also the third-largest egg producer in the world, with an annual production of 138.38 billion eggs in 2022-23. Egg production has grown by 6.77% in the last year. The top five egg-producing states are Andhra Pradesh, Tamil Nadu, Telangana, West Bengal, and Karnataka.

Meat Production

India's meat production in 2022-23 was 9.77 million tonnes, with an annual growth rate of 5.13%. The top five meat-producing states are Maharashtra, Uttar Pradesh, West Bengal, Andhra Pradesh, and Telangana.

Wool Production

India's wool production in 2021-22 was 33.61 thousand tonnes, a increase of 2.12% compared to the previous year. The top five wool-producing states are Rajasthan, Jammu and Kashmir, Gujarat, Maharashtra, and Himachal Pradesh.

Livestock Population

The total livestock population in India is 535.78 million. Cattle are the most numerous livestock species, with a population of 192.49 million. Buffaloes, sheep, goats, and pigs also constitute significant portions of the livestock population.

Milch animals' average production

Exotic/ Cross bred is 8.55 Kg/day/animal and Indigenous/ non-descript 3.44 Kg/day/ animal.

Species wise contribution in total national milk yield (2022-23)

Indigenous Buffalo (31.94%) > Cross bred cattle (29.81%) > Non-Descript buffalo (12.87%) > Indigenous cattle (10.73%) > Non-Descript cattle (9.51%) > Goat (3.3%) > Exotic Cow (1.86%)

Per Capita Availability of Milk and Eggs

The per capita availability of milk in India has increased by 13 grams per day to 459 grams per day in 2022-23. The per capita availability of eggs has also increased by 6 eggs per annum to 101 eggs per annum in 2022-23. In year 2022-23 per capita meat consumption is 7.10 Kg/annum. The history of veterinary education in India dates back to the 19th century. The first veterinary school was established in Babugarh (Hapur), Uttar Pradesh in 1877, with the primary objective of training Indians to serve as assistants in remount depots and on military farms1. The first veterinary college was started in Lahore (now in Pakistan) in 1882.

The Bombay Veterinary College was founded in 18861. With the expansion of the activities of civil veterinary departments in several states, veterinary colleges arose in different centers. For example, Calcutta in 1893 and Madras in 1903. These veterinary colleges awarded a diploma based on the adoption of the program of study developed by the Royal College of Veterinary Surgeons, London. The curriculum was based primarily on equine practice1.In 1928, the Royal Commission on Agriculture in the Indian Subcontinent recommended a fourfold increase in the employment of veterinary assistant surgeons to cope with the enormous animal disease problems.The Madras Veterinary College took the lead, and in 1936, with the concurrence of Madras University, the Bachelor of Veterinary Science degree program began. Subsequently, veterinary degree programs were started in other states, including at Patna, Mathura, Bangalore, Trichur, Hyderabad, Tirupati, Ludhiana, and Anand

Reference for the data

Basic Animal Husbandry Statistics - 2022-23

1. What was the first animal domesticated by the human

   a) Dog b) Goat

   c) Cattle d) Horse

2. What was the first ruminant animal domesticated by the human

   a) Dog b) Goat

   c) Cattle d) Horse

3. Who was the first person to elaborate the scientific explanation of livestock domestication and its various aspect
   a) Lush (1945) b) Hermanns (1952)
   c) Zeder (2008) d) Payne & Hodges (1997)
4 Capture and care method is related with
   a) Selection and culling b) Isolation of animals
   c) Domestication method d) Identification ways
5. Imprinting is also known as
   a) Isolation and treatment b) Hunger sympathy
   c) Social dominance d) Capture and care
6. Hunger sympathy method is related with
   a) Selection and culling b) Isolation of animals
   c) Identification ways d) Domestication method
7. The development of breeds by the selective breeding by the mankind was started as early as
   a) 8000 BC b) 300 BC
   c) 30000 BC d) 5000 BC
8. Evolutionary changes responsible for altering gene frequencies is due to the major forces except
   a) Mutation b) Migration
   c) Adaptation d) Selection
9. The effect of domestication on production traits of animals
   a) Decreased b) Increased
   c) No changes observed d) Unpredictable
10. The animal which has escaped from a domestic or captive status and is living more or less as a wild animal is known as
   a) Culled b) Wild
   c) Feral d) Nomadic
11. Framework for classification where different categories of living being are placed in a logical sequence
   a) Taxonomy b) Hierarchy
   c) Lineage d) Heredity
12. Suborder Pecora include families except
   a) Cervidae b) Giraffidae
   c) Camelidae d) Bovidae
13. The work of biological taxonomy was started first by
   a) Linnaeus b) Aristotle
   c) Whittekar d) Herodotus
14. Father of taxonomy is referred to
   a) Linnaeus b) Aristotle
   c) Whittekar d) Herodotus

15. Interspecies cross of yak and cattle produce offspring as
    a) Sterile female offspring and fertile male offspring
    b) Sterile male offspring and fertile female offspring
    c) Both male and female sterile as the rule of species hybridization
    d) Both male and female fertile as the rule of species hybridization
16. In which year was the first veterinary school established in India?
    a) 1862 b) 1877
    c) 1882 d) 1886
17. Where was the first civil veterinary school in India established?
    a) Pune b) Babugarh, Uttar Pradesh
    c) Lahore, Pakistan d) Calcutta
18. What was the name of the first veterinary college in undivided India?
    a) Bombay Veterinary College b) Madras Veterinary College
    c) Calcutta Veterinary College d) Lahore Veterinary College
19. Which ancient Indian treatise is considered the foundation of veterinary science in India?
    a) Rigveda b) Arthashastra
    c) Shalihotra Samhita d) SushrutaSamhita
20. What was the primary purpose of the early veterinary schools in India?
    a) To train veterinarians for the army
    b) To improve animal husbandry practices
    c) To control epidemics of livestock diseases
    d) To promote animal welfare
21. What was the role of King Ashoka in the development of veterinary science in India?
    a) He established the first veterinary hospital in India
    b) He promoted Buddhism, which emphasized non-violence towards animals.
    c) He appointed veterinarians to his army.
    d) He commissioned the writing of the ShalihotraSamhita.
22. Which year did the Indian Veterinary Research Institute (IVRI) established?
    a) 1889 b) 1903
    c) 1928 d) 1948
23. What is the name of the statutory body responsible for regulating veterinary education in India?
    a) Indian Council of Agricultural Research (ICAR)
    b) Veterinary Council of India (VCI)
    c) Indian Veterinary Association (IVA)
    d) Animal Welfare Board of India (AWBI)

24. What is the minimum qualification required to practice veterinary medicine in India?
    a) Bachelor of Veterinary Science and Animal Husbandry (BVSc & AH) degree
    b) Master of Veterinary Science (MVSc) degree
    c) Doctor of Veterinary Medicine (DVM) degree
    d) Doctor of Philosophy (Phd) in Veterinary Science
25. What is the significance of the livestock sector in India's economy?
    a) It contributes about 4% to India's GDP.
    b) It provides employment to over 100 million people.
    c) It is a source of food and nutrition for over 1.3 billion people
    d) All of the above.
26. What are the major challenges faced by animal husbandry and veterinary science in India?
    a) Animal diseases and parasites
    b) Inadequate infrastructure and facilities
    c) Shortage of qualified veterinarians
    d) All of the above.
27. What are the recent initiatives taken by the Indian government to improve animal husbandry and veterinary science?
    a) Launch of the National Livestock Mission
    b) Establishment of veterinary colleges and hospitals
    c) Introduction of livestock insurance schemes
    d) All of the above.
28. What are the future prospects of animal husbandry and veterinary science in India?
    a) Growing demand for animal products
    b) Increasing importance of animal welfare
    c) Advancement of veterinary science and technology
    d) All of the above
29. Which of the following is NOT a traditional animal used for husbandry in India?
    a) Cow   b) Buffalo
    c) Elephant   d) Sheep
30. What is the name of the Indian agricultural university that is not considered the premier institution for animal husbandry and veterinary science education?
    a) Indian Veterinary Research Institute (IVRI)
    b) National Dairy Research Institute (NDRI)
    c) Jawaharlal Nehru University (JNU)
    d) Guru Nanak Dev Veterinary and Animal Sciences University (GADVASU)
31. Which of the following is NOT a major animal disease that affects cattle in India?
    a) Rinderpest   b) Foot-and-mouth disease
    c) Bovine tuberculosis   d) Avian influenza

32. What is the name of the Indian government agency responsible for promoting animal wellbeing and the issue related to it?
    a) Animal Welfare Board of India (AWBI)
    b) Central Bureau of Animal Husbandry and Dairying (CBAD)
    c) Livestock Development Board (LDB)
    d) Department of Animal Husbandry, Dairying & Fisheries (DAHDF)
33. What is the significance of the Livestock Census conducted every 5 years in India?
    a) To assess the population and distribution of livestock
    b) To identify livestock demography
    c) To plan and implement livestock development programs
    d) All of the above
34. What is the role of veterinary extension education in promoting animal husbandry practices?
    a) To train farmers in animal care and management
    b) To provide information on animal health and disease prevention
    c) To promote the adoption of new technologies in animal husbandry
    d) All of the above
35. What is the importance of veterinary research in improving animal health and productivity?
    a) To develop new vaccines and diagnostic tests for animal diseases
    b) To improve breeding and nutrition practices for livestock
    c) To develop new technologies for animal production and processing
    d) All of the above
36. What is the ethical responsibility of veterinarians in animal husbandry practices?
    a) To ensure the welfare of animals under their care
    b) To practice veterinary medicine in a responsible and ethical manner
    c) To educate the public about animal welfare
    d) All of the above
37. World milk production is having the contribution of different livestock in the relation of
    a) Buffalo > Cattle > Goat   b) Cattle > Buffalo > Goat
    c) Buffalo = Cattle > Goat   d) Buffalo < Cattle=Goat
38. World milk production is having the contribution of cattle in the year 2021-22 recorded roughly as
    a) 80%   b) 50%
    c) 60%   d) 70%
39. India is the largest producer of milk globally with the percent share in total milk productionin the world.
    a) 32.67%   b) 23.67%
    c) 42.67%   d) 16.67%

40. In India dairy is the assumed as the largestagricultural commodity contributing around what percent of the Indian national economy
    a) 2% b) 3%
    c) 5% d) 7%
41. India is standing at first position in the world for the following parameters except
    a) Total Livestock Population b) Total Buffalo Population
    c) Total Cattle Population d) Total Bovine Population
42. Per capita availability of milk in India in the year of 2021-22 was
    a) 208G/day b) 280G/day
    c) 232G/day d) 444G/day
43. Total milk production of milk in India in the year of 2021-22 was(in MT, milliontons)
    a) 221.06 MT b) 198.06 MT
    c) 201.06 MT d) 191.06 MT
44. Per capita availability of egg in India in the year of 2021-22 was
    a) 182 eggs/year b) 95 eggs/year
    c) 129 eggs/year d) 81 eggs/year
45. The recommended per capita availability from the Indian Council of Medical Research (ICMR) for the meat in India in the year of 2021-22 was
    a) 7 kg/year b) 18 kg/year
    c) 35 kg/year d) 11 kg/year
46. In the year of 2021-22, the milk production has registered an annual growth rate of
    a) 4.32% b) 5.29%
    c) 6.27% d) 7.35%
47. In the year of 2021-22,Increase in egg production compared to previous year was recorded as
    a) 5.29% b) 6.19%
    c) 6.97% d) 7.32%
48. The recorded increase in meat production in the year of 2021-22 as compared to the previous year was
    a) 5.62% b) 6.19%
    c) 7.32% d) 13.53%
49. In the year of 2021-22,the change was recorded in wool production compared to previous year as
    a) Increase of 10.30% b) Decrease of 10.30%
    c) Increase of 6.30% d) Decrease of 6.30%
50. The average Yield per In-Milk indigenous cattle in 2021-22 was recorded as
    a) 8.52 kg/day b) 3.36 kg/day
    c) 2.96 kg/day d) 5.96 kg/day
51. The average Yield per In-Milk indigenous buffaloin 2021-22 was recorded as
    a) 8.52 kg/day b) 3.36 kg/day
    c) 2.96 kg/day d) 5.96 kg/day

52. The average Yield per In-Milk indigenous goatin 2021-22 was recorded as
   a) 1.52 kg/day b) 0.36 kg/day
   c) 0.96 kg/day d) 0.47 kg/day
53. The average Yield per In-Milk indigenous exotic/cross bred cattle in 2021-22 was recorded as
   a) 8.52 kg/day b) 3.36 kg/day
   c) 5.96 kg/day d) 4.47 kg/day
54. The number of APEDA registered Integrated Abattoirs cum Meat Processing Plants in India is
   a) 52 b) 62
   c) 72 d) 82
55. The major export destinations of buffalo meat products in 2021-22 is as following except
   a) Egypt b) Vietnam
   c) Malaysia d) Bangladesh
56. Number of animals slaughtered for meat production in 2021-22 is as in order of
   a) Cattle>Buffalo >Sheep >Goat b) Buffalo >Cattle >Sheep >Goat
   c) Sheep>Buffalo >Cattle >Goat d) Goat >Buffalo >Cattle >Sheep
57. Which is the state with largest livestock population
   a) Rajasthan b) Madhya Pradesh
   c) Gujrat d) Uttar Pradesh
58. Which is the state with largest poultry population
   a) Tamil Nadu b) Andhra Pardesh
   c) Telangana d) Haryana
59. Highest milk producing state in India is
   a) Gujarat b) Rajasthan
   c) Madhya Pradesh d) Uttar Pradesh
60. State with highest per capita availability of milk
   a) Gujrat b) Haryana
   c) Punjab (1271 g) d) Uttar Pradesh
61. State with highest per capita availability of eggs
   a) Tamil Nadu b) Telangana
   c) Andhra Pradesh d) Karnataka
62. The state with the largest share in Total Meat Production in India is:
   a) Uttar Pradesh b) Maharashtra
   c) Kerala d) Tamil Nadu
63. The state with the largest Share in Total Wool Production in India:
   a) Rajasthan b) Gujarat
   c) Jammu Kashmir d) Bihar

64. The sector of animal husbandry for which the value output from Livestock Rearing in 2020-21 was found highest was
 a) Meat and Meat Products
 b) Milk and Milk Products
 c) Eggs
 d) Wool (carpet and apparel) and hairs

65. The contribution of Milk and Milk Productssector in the value output from Livestock Rearing in 2020-21 was found highest as
 a) 23.66% b) 65.88%
 c) 52.85% d) 42.85%

66. First livestock census in India was conducted as Dairy Cattle Census in the year.
 a) 1912 b) 1919
 c) 1947 d) 1965

67. Livestock Census which was 20th Livestock Census was conducted in the year.
 a) 2000 b) 2012
 c) 2019 d) 2023

68. Livestock Census takes place in India as in the span of ()
 a) Annual b) Biennial
 c) Quinquennial d) Decennial

69. Total livestockpopulation recorded as per 20th Livestock Census (2019) is
 a) 193.46 million b) 303.76 million
 c) 536.76 million d) 851.81 million

70. The percentage proportion of livestock type in India as per 20th Livestock Census (2019) is
 a) Cattle>Buffalo >Sheep >Goat b) Cattle>Goat>Buffalo>Sheep
 c) Cattle >Sheep>Buffalo>Goat d) Goat >Buffalo >Cattle >Sheep

71. Species wise egg contribution to total egg production in India in 2021-22 was
 a) Improved fowl>Desi fowl>Desi duck>Improved duck
 b) Improved fowl>Improved duck<Desi duck<Desi fowl
 c) Improved fowl>Desi fowl > Improved duck>Desi duck
 d) Desi fowl <Improved fowl <Desi duck <Improved duck

72. Species wise meat contribution to total meat production in India in 2021-22 was
 a) Goat>Poultry >Buffalo >Sheep b) Poultry>Buffalo>Sheep>Goat
 c) Poultry>Buffalo Goat Sheep d) Poultry >Goat >Sheep>Buffalo

73. Category wise contribution to total wool production in India in 2021-22 was
 a) Ewe =Ram =Lamb b) Ewe =Ram >Lamb
 c) Ram>Ewe >Lamb d) Ewe >Ram >Lamb

74. Demographic dependence on livestock tells that livestock sector employs what percentage of total Indian Workforce
 a) 6 b) 8
 c) 10 d) 12

75. The country which is keeping maximum number of cattle population is
   a) India b) China
   c) Brazil d) USA
76. The National Dairy Research Institute (NDRI) was established by the British government to cater to the needs of the Indian dairy industry in the year
   a) 1912 b) 1919
   c) 1923 d) 1947
77. The dwarf cattle breed of India is
   a) Vechur b) Bachaur
   c) Punganur d) All of the above
78. What is the percentage of buffalo of the total World Livestock is present in India
   a) 43.84% b) 53.84%
   c) 33.84% d) 63.84%
79. Which states are the top five egg producers in India?
   a) Andhra Pradesh, Tamil Nadu and Telangana
   b) Andhra Pradesh, West Bengal, and Karnataka
   c) Andhra Pradesh, Maharashtra, and Madhya Pradesh
   d) Andhra Pradesh, Uttar Pradesh and Karnataka
80. The first cattle crossbreeding in India was initiated in
   a) 1875 b) 1902
   c) 1912 d) 1919
81. The first cattle cross bred developed was
   a) Jersindh b) Karan Swiss
   c) Taylor d) Karan Fries
82. Tyalor breed was created by crossing
   a) Shorthorn cattle with local cows b) Jersy cattle cattle with local cows
   c) Ayrshire cattle with local cows d) HF cattle with local cows
83. Which is the first veterinary university of India
   a) Tamil Nadu Veterinary and Animal Sciences University, Chennai (TANUVAS)
   b) Rajasthan University of Veterinary and Animal Sciences, Bikaner (RAJUVAS)
   c) Pt. DeenDayalUpadhyay Veterinary & Animal Science University, Mathura (DUVASU)
   d) Guru Angad Dev Veterinary and Animal Sciences University (GADVASU)
84. The first known veterinarian in the world, Shalihotra, was an expert in
   a) Cattle b) Horses
   c) Elephant d) Camel
85. Among the ancient veterinarian of India the expert one in the Elephant for their treatment and management was
   a) Shalihotra b) Jaydautt
   c) Palkapya d) Nakul

86. Who is treated as the "father of veterinary medicine" is
   a) Bernhard LauritzFrederik Bang
   b) Peter C. Doherty
   c) Claude Bourgelat,
   d) Harold William Bennetts
87. Which is the world's oldest modern veterinary college
   a) Royal Veterinary College (London, UK)
   b) Lyon Veterinary College, France
   c) University of Veterinary Medicine Vienna (Vienna, AT)
   d) Royal (Dick) School of Veterinary Studies
88. Mithun is domesticated form of which animal?
   a) Banteng
   b) Gaur
   c) Yak
   d) Bison
89. Which buffalo has never been domesticated?
   a) Tamaraw buffalo
   b) Anoa buffalo
   c) Syncerus buffalo
   d) Carabao buffalo
90. The most ancient representative of genus *Bos*(cattle) found in the Siwalik hills were
   a) Bos acutifrons
   b) Bos nomadicus
   c) *Bos javanicus*
   d) *Bos bfrontalis*
91. The earliest evidence of animal domestication at Indus valley civilization comes from
   a) Mehrgarh
   b) Allahdino
   c) Chanhu Daro
   d) Mohenjo Daro
92. Which of the following domesticated animal were rarely used during early Indus Valley civilization?
   a) Dog
   b) Goat
   c) Cattle
   d) Horse
93. Dogs were domesticated following which pathway?
   a) Commensal pathway
   b) Prey pathway
   c) Directed pathway
   d) Commensal or prey pathway
94. Cats were domesticated following which pathway?
   a) Commensal pathway
   b) Prey pathway
   c) Direct pathway
   d) Commensal or prey pathway
95. Chicken were domesticated following which pathway?
   a) Commensal pathway
   b) Prey pathway
   c) Direct pathway
   d) Commensal or prey pathway
96. Sheep were domesticated following which pathway?
   a) Commensal pathway
   b) Prey pathway
   c) Direct pathway
   d) Commensal or prey pathway
97. Goats were domesticated following which pathway?
   a) Commensal pathway
   b) Prey pathway
   c) Directed pathway
   d) Commensal or prey pathway

98. Cattle were domesticated following which pathway?
   a) Commensal pathway b) Prey pathway
   c) Directed pathway d) Commensal or prey pathway
99. Camels were domesticated following which pathway?
   a) Commensal pathway b) Prey pathway
   c) Directed pathway d) Commensal or prey pathway
100. Horses were domesticated following which pathway?
   a) Commensal pathway b) Prey pathway
   c) Directed pathway d) Commensal or prey pathway
101. Water buffaloes were domesticated following which pathway
   a) Commensal pathway b) Prey pathway
   c) Directed pathway d) Commensal or prey pathway
102. Domestication of which of the following species of animal did not take place at fertile crescent region of Western Asia?
   a) Sheep b) Horse
   c) Cattle d) Goat
103. The skeletal remains of horse were found at which site of Indus valley civilization
   a) Mehrgarh b) Allahdino
   c) RanaGhundai d) Mohenjo Daro
104. Who wrote the *Haya Ayurveda* which describes the horse husbandry and its care and treatment?
   a) Shalihotra b) Palakapya
   c) Jayadatta d) Sushruta
105. Who wrote the *Hastyayurveda* which describes the elephant husbandry and its care and treatment?
   a) Shalihotra b) Palakapya
   c) Jayadatta d) Charak
106. Which Vedic literature referred Cow as *'Aghanya'* i.enot to be killed?
   a) Atharva Veda b) Rig Veda
   c) Yajur Veda d) Sama Veda
107. Which Vedic literature mentions the treatment of cows ailments through the use of animal ayurveda?
   a) Atharva Veda b) Rig Veda
   c) Yajur Veda d) Sama Veda
108. Domestication of animals started during which period?
   a) Mesolithic period b) Neolithic period
   c) Palaeolithic period d) Chalcolithic period
109. Domestication of cattle began during which period?
   a) Mesolithic period b) Neolithic period
   c) Palaeolithic period d) Chalcolithic period

110. Where did the domestication of taurine (*Bostaurus*) cattle take place?
   a) North-east Africa b) Indus valley in South Asia
   c) Fertile Crescent in Middle east d) Southern Europe

111. Where did the domestication of zebu (*Bosindicus*) cattle take place?
   a) North east Africa b) Indus valley in South Asia
   c) Fertile Crescent in Western Asia d) Anatolian Plateau in Middle East

112. The wild ancestor of domestic cattle is
   a) *Bosprimigenius* b) Bosnomadicus
   c) Bosjavanicus d) Bosfrontalis

113. The wild ancestor of domestic pigs is
   a) *Sus scrofa* b) Sus scrofa
   c) Sus celebensis d) Sus barbatus

114. The wild ancestor of domestic goat is
   a) *Capra falconeri* b) Capra nubiana
   c) Capra aegagrus d) Capra ibex

115. The wild ancestor of horse is
   a) *Equusferus* b) Equusprzewalski
   c) Equusasinus d) Equusquagga

116. The wild ancestors of the domesticated sheep of India are
   a) *Ovisorientalis* b) Ovismusimon
   c) Ovisaries d) Ovisnivicola

117. Which Indian goat breed resembles the ancestral wild goat (Bezoar) from which present day goats have descended?
   a) Changthangi b) Jamunapari
   c) Gaddi d) Bhakarwali

118. The wild ancestor of Indian cattle is
   a) *Bosprimigenius* b) Bosnomadicus
   c) Bosbrachyceros d) Bosmutus

119. In which country the last animal of aurochs (*Bosprimigenius)* died in 1927
   a) Poland b) Iran
   c) Turkey d) Egypt

120. According to archaeological data when did the taurine (*Bostaurus*) cattle have been domesticated?
   a) 8500 years ago b) 6000 years ago
   c) 10500 years ago d) 12500 years ago

121. According to archaeological data when did the taurine (*Bostaurus*) cattle have been domesticated?
   a) 8500 years ago b) 6000 years ago
   c) 10500 years ago d) 12500 years ago

122. Which Indian breed was used *to* evolve*Guzerá*cattleofBrazil was evolved by importing which Indian breed?

a) Gir b) Ongole
c) Kankrej d) Red Sindhi

123. *Nelore* ofBrazil were originated from which Indian breed?

a) Gir b) Ongole
c) Kankrej d) Red Sindhi

124. Which of the following is correct regarding order of domestication of animals?

a) Cattle>Goat>Horse>Pig b) Dog>Goat>Cattle>Horse
c) Dog>Pig>Goat>Sheep d) Dog>Horse>Sheep>Pig

125. Which of the following species of animal is not believed to be domesticated in India?

a) Mithun b) Chicken
c) River buffalo d) Camel

126. The wild ancestor of dog is

a) *Canisaureus* *b) Canis lupus*
c) Canisrufus *d) Canisf*amiliaris

127. The wild ancestor of water buffalo is

a) *Bubalusmindorensis* b) Bubalusarnee
c) Bubalusquarlesi d) Bubalusdepressicornis

128. Bezoar are considered the wild ancestor of which species of animal?

a) Sheep b) Goat
c) Cattle d) Horse

129. Mouflon are considered the wild ancestor of which species of animal?

a) Sheep b) Goat
c) Cattle d) Horse

130. Aurochs are considered the wild ancestor of which species of animal?

a) Sheep b) Goat
c) Cattle d) Horse

131. Which animal is called the "Cattle of Mountain"?

a) Yak b) Mithun
c) Buffalo d) Bison

132. Which Buddhist literature describes cattle as a giver of food, beauty and happiness

a) Kathavatthu b) Mahavamsa
c) Suttanipata d) Nettipakarana

133. Horse are supposed to be first domesticated in

a) Africa b) South East Asia
c) Central Asia d) Southern Europe

134. The wild ancestor of domestic chicken is
   a) *Gallus gallus* b) *Gallus sonneratii*
   c) *Gallus lafayetti* d) *Gallus domesticus*
135. When were the goats domesticated?
   a) 8500 years ago b) 15000 years ago
   c) 10000 years ago d) 11500 years ago
136. When did the domestication of dogs take place?
   a) 8500 years ago b) 15000 years ago
   c) 10000 years ago d) 11500 years ago
137. The wild ancestor of swamp buffalo is
   a) *Bubalusmindorensis* b) Bubalusarnee
   c) Bubalusquarlesi d) Bubalusdepressicornis
138. When did the domestication of pigs take place?
   a) 8000 years ago b) 15000 years ago
   c) 9500 years ago d) 11500 years ago
139. When did the domestication of horse take place?
   a) 8500 years ago b) 5500 years ago
   c) 10000 years ago d) 7000 years ago
140. When did the domestication of camel take place?
   a) 8500 years ago b) 4500 years ago
   c) 10000 years ago d) 7000 years ago
141. Total number of indigenous cattle breeds registered by National Bureau of Animal Genetic Resourcesin India so far is
   a) 212 b) 192
   c) 202 d) 205
142. Postal stamp of indigenous breeds released by Government of India
   a) Sahiwal, Hallikar, Kangayam, AmritMahal
   b) Gir, Hallikar, Kangayam, Kankrej
   c) Gir, Sahiwal, Kangayam, Kankraj
   d) Gir, Red Sindhi, Sahiwal, Kankraj
143. First organized plan to improve rural cattle in India
   a) Operation Flood b) White revolution
   c) Key Village Scheme d) Integrated cattle development
144. Under whose chairmanship, the first attempt to form the dairy cooperatives by rural milk producers for milk procurement without middleman
   a) Lal Bahadur Shastri b) Sardar Vallabh Bhai Patel
   c) Tribhuvandas Patel d) Balwantrai Mehta
145. All India Coordinated research project in buffalo was started in
   a) 1980 b) 1985
   c) 1970 d) 1975

146. Which of the following organization deals with the animal conservation
   a) ILRI b) FAO
   c) OIE d) WOAH
147. Operation Floof I was launched in 1970 by National Dairy Development Board with agreement with
   a) Indian Council of Agricultural Research
   b) World Food Programme
   c) United Nation Development Programme
   d) National Nutrition Mission
148. Good quality fibres are produced from Indian goats of
   a) Himalyan region b) Central region
   c) Eastern region d) Southern region
149. India's first cloned indigenous cattle 'Ganga' is of which breed
   a) Sahiwal b) Red Sindhi
   c) Rathi d) Gir
150. Which of these is correct regarding National Kamdhenu Breeding Centre
   a) Development and conservation of Indigenous breeds
   b) Nucleus Herd for all the Indigenous cattle and buffalo breeds
   c) Established at Itarsi and Nellore
   d) All of these
151. Double humped camels in India are found in
   a) Laddakh b) Jaiselmer
   c) Kutch d) Malwa

Answer Key

1	a	2	b	3	a	4	c	5	d	6	d	7	b
8	c	9	b	10	c	11	b	12	c	13	b	14	a
15	b	16	a	17	b	18	d	19	c	20	a	21	a
22	a	23	b	24	a	25	d	26	d	27	d	28	d
29	d	30	c	31	d	32	a	33	d	34	d	35	d
36	d	37	b	38	a	39	b	40	c	41	c	42	d
43	a	44	b	45	d	46	b	47	b	48	a	49	b
50	b	51	d	52	d	53	a	54	c	55	d	56	d
57	d	58	a	59	b	60	c	61	c	62	b	63	a
64	b	65	b	66	b	67	c	68	c	69	c	70	b
71	b	72	c	73	d	74	b	75	c	76	c	77	d
78	b	79	a	80	a	81	c	82	a	83	a	84	b
85	c	86	c	87	b	88	b	89	c	90	a	91	a
92	d	93	a	94	a	95	a	96	b	97	b	98	b

99	c	100	c	101	b	102	b	103	c	104	a	105	b
106	b	107	a	108	a	109	b	110	c	111	b	112	a
113	c	114	c	115	a	116	a	117	c	118	b	119	a
120	c	121	a	122	c	123	b	124	b	125	d	126	b
127	b	128	b	129	a	130	c	131	b	132	c	133	c
134	a	135	d	136	b	137	b	138	c	139	b	140	b
141	a	142	b	143	c	144	b	145	c	146	b	147	b
148	a	149	d	150	d	151	a						

2

Breeds of Livestock and Poultry

Pratistha Shrivastava

Department of Veterinary Parasitology, Institute of Veterinary Science & Animal Husbandry, Siksha O Anusandhan, Bhubaneswar, Odisha

Introduction

CATTLE BREEDS

The genus *Bos* is classified into *Bos indicus* and *Bos taurus*. *Bos indicus* belongs to tropical region and have hump whereas *Bos taurus* belongs to temperate region and is humpless.

Milch breeds are Red Sindhi, Gir, Sahiwal, Tharparkar.

Dual purpose or general utility breeds are Nimari, Kankrej, Nellore, Dangi, Rathi, Deoni, Hariana, Krishna Valley, Ongole.

Draught breeds are Amritmahal, Nagori, Khillari, Vechur, Bachaur, Siri, Ponwar, Kangayam, Bargur, Malvi, Hallikar.

Cross-breeds

Jersind = Jersey x Red Sindhi.

Frieswal = HF x Sahiwal.

Jerthar = Jersey x Tharparkar.

Karan Swiss = Brown Swiss x Sahiwal.

Karan Fries = HF x Tharparkar.

Sunandini = Brown Swiss x Non descript.

Jamaica Hope = 80% Jersey, 15% Sahiwal, 5% HF.

Taylor = Short horn bull x Native cow.

BUFFALO BREEDS (*Bubalus bubalis*)

Buffalo breeds are classified as Riverine type (Water buffalo) and Swamp buffalo.

Murrah group includes Murrah, Nili-Ravi, Kundi, Godavari.

Gujarat group includes Surti, Jaffarabadi, Mehsana.

UP group includes Bhadawari and Tarai.

South India group includes Toda and South Kanara.

Central India group includes Nagpuri, Jerangi, Kalahandi, Sambalpur, Pandharpuri, Manda.

Cross-breeds :

Mehsana = Murrah x Surti.

SHEEP BREEDS (*Ovis aries*)

Cross-breeds of sheep:

Hissardale = Bikaneri ewe x Australian Merino ram.

Avikalin = Rambouillet ram x Malpura ewe.

Avivastra = Rambouillet ram x Chokla ewe.

Avimans = Malpura & Sonadi x Dorset & Suffolk.

Bharat Merino = Chokla & Nali x Merino & Rambouillet.

Kashmir Merino = Gaddi, Bhakarwal, Poonchi x Merino & Rambouillet.

Indian Karakul = Marwari, Malpura, Sonadi x Karakul.

Nilgiri synthetic = Nilgiri x Merino & Rambouillet.

Patanwadi Synthetic = Patanwadi x Merino & Rambouillet.

Exotic breeds of sheep :

Fine wool breeds : Merino and Rambouillet.

Fur breeds : Karakul.

Mutton breeds : Dorset, Suffolk and Southdown.

Long coarse wool breeds : Lincoln and Leicester.

North temperate region breeds : Gaddi, Bhakarwal, Poonchi, Gurez, Rampur Bushai, Karnah, Changthangi.

North-western arid and semi-arid region breeds : Nali, Marwari, Jaisalmeri, Pugal, Magra, Malpura, Patanwadi.

Southern peninsular region breeds : Nellore, Mandya, Deccani, Hassan, Bellary, Madras Red.

Eastern region breeds : Garole, Ganjam, Chottanagpuri.

GOAT BREEDS (*Capra hircus*)

Exotic goat breeds : Saanen, Alpine, Angora, Anglo-Nubian, Toggenburg, Boer, Orenberg.

North temperate region breeds : Chegu, Changthangi, Gaddi.

North-western arid and semi-arid region breeds : Jamunapari, Barbari, Jhakrana, Beetle, Sirohi, Kutchi, Marwari.

Southern peninsular region breeds : Malabari, Osmanabadi, Sangamneri.

Eastern region breeds : Black Bengal, Ganjam.

PIG BREEDS (*Sus domesticus*)

Indian breeds : Ghoongroo, Niang Megha, Agonda goan, Tenyi Vo, Nicobari, Doom.

Exotic breeds :

English breeds : Large White Yorkshire, Middle White Yorkshire, Berkshire, Tamworth.

Denmark breeds : Landrace.

U.S.A) breed : Duroc, Chester-White, Poland-China.

HORSE BREEDS (*Equus caballus*)

Indian breeds : Kathiawari, Manipuri, Marwari, Spiti, Zanskari, Bhutia.

CAMEL BREEDS (*Camelus dromedaries*)

Indian breeds : Bikaneri, Jaisalmeri, Mewari, Kutchi, Kharai.

POULTRY BREEDS (*Gallus gallus domesticus*)

Classifiaction of Poultry breeds.

Asiatic breeds : Brahma, Cochin, Langshan.

American breeds : Plymouth rock, Wyandotte, Rhode Island Red, Rhode Island White, Jersey Black Giant, New Hampshire.

English breeds : Australorp, Cornish, Dorking, Orpington, Sussex.

Mediterranean breeds : White Leghorn, Minorca, Ancona, Andalusian.

Mediterranean breeds have white color ear lobe.

Asiatic breeds, American breeds and English breeds have red color ear lobe.

In most of the breeds the colour of skin is yellow except in Australorp, Dorking, Orpington, Sussex, Minorca and Andalusian.

Shank is feathered in Asiatic breeds only.

All the breeds lays brown shelled eggs except Mediterranean breeds.

Mediterranean breeds lays white shelled eggs.

Aseel is a gaming bird.

Kadaknath breed is known as 'Kalamasi'. The comb, wattle and tongue are purple in color. This is the breed having maximum disease resistance. It's meat has aphrodisiac property (stimulate sexual desire).

White Leghorn is the best layer breed in the world.

Questions

1. Which among the following is the highest milk producing breed of buffalo ?
   a) Nili-Ravi b) Murrah
   c) Surti d) Mehsana
2. Which breed of buffalo is having sickle shaped horns ?
   a) Surti b) Bhadawari
   c) Murrah d) Mehsana
3. Which among the following buffalo breed have highest milk fat percentage ?
   a) Surti b) Bhadawari
   c) Murrah d) Jaffarabadi
4. Which of the following is the heaviest breed of buffalo ?
   a) Murrah b) Mehsana
   c) Surti d) Jaffarabadi
5. Which among the following is known as the dwarf breed of buffalo ?
   a) Nagpuri b) Murrah
   c) Jerangi d) Surti

6. The home track of Murrah buffalo is ?
   a) Madhya Pradesh b) Gujarat
   c) Punjab d) Telangana
7. The home track of Nili-Ravi is ?
   a) Ferozpur, Punjab b) Delhi
   c) Maharashtra d) Kerala
8. The home track of Jaffarabadi breed is ?
   a) Maharashtra b) Madhya Pradesh
   c) Uttar Pradesh d) Gujarat
9. The home track of Surti breed is ?
   a) Gujarat b) Assam
   c) Odisha d) Kerala
10. The home track of Mehsana breed is ?
   a) Odisha b) Andhra Pradesh
   c) Gujarat d) Punjab
11. The home track of Bhadawari breed is ?
   a) Agra, Uttar Pradesh b) Odisha
   c) West Bengal d) Tamil Nadu
12. Which of the following buffalo breed have copper colour body coat ?
   a) Murrah b) Mehsana
   c) Surti d) Bhadawari
13. Mehsana breed of buffalo is a cross of which of the following ?
   a) Murrah x Surti b) Surti x bhadawari
   c) Bhadawari x Murrah d) None of the above
14. The home track of Jerangi breed of buffalo is ?
   a) Tamil Nadu b) West Bengal
   c) Odisha d) Madhya Pradesh
15. Which among the following is the most violent breed of buffalo ?
   a) Toda b) Jerangi
   c) Nagpuri d) Murrah
16. Which of the following cattle breed is having longest lactation period ?
   a) Ayrshire b) Brown Swiss
   c) Jersey d) Holstein Friesian
17. Which of the following cattle breed is the highest milk producer in the world ?
   a) Holstein Friesian b) Jersey
   c) Brown Swiss d) Ayrshire
18. Which of the following cattle breed have the highest milk lactose %?
   a) Brown Swiss b) Jersey
   c) Ayrshire d) Hereford

19. Which of the following is the first crossbred cattle developed in India ?
  a) Taylor b) Jamaica Hope
  c) Frieswal d) Jersind
20. Which among the following is not a milch purpose breed of cattle ?
  a) Gir b) Kankrej
  c) Sahiwal d) Red Sindhi
21. Which among the following cattle breed have longest lactation period among desi breeds ?
  a) Sahiwal b) Tharparkar
  c) Red Sindhi d) Gir
22. Which of the following cattle breed have highest disease resistant property ?
  a) Red Sindhi b) Gir
  c) Tharparkar d) Rathi
23. Which among the following is the best dual purpose breed of cattle ?
  a) Kankrej b) Nimari
  c) Hariana d) Rathi
24. Heaviest Indian cattle breed having famous gait 'Sawai-Chal' is ?
  a) Kankrej b) Dangi
  c) Ongole d) Hariana
25. Which of the following cattle breed is pure white in colour ?
  a) Nimari b) Mewati
  c) Rathi d) Ongole
26. Which of the following is the best draught-purpose breed of India ?
  a) Vechur b) Amritmahal
  c) Siri d) Khillari
27. Which of the following is the smallest cattle breed in the world ?
  a) Siri b) Ponwar
  c) Vechur d) Hallikar
28. Which of the following cattle breed is known as the Pride of Tamil Nadu ?
  a) Malvi b) Hallikar
  c) Kankrej d) Kangayam
29. Which among the following is not a hilly breed of cow ?
  a) Badri b) Siri
  c) Ponwar d) Kankrej
30. Nimari breed of cattle is a cross of which of the following ?
  a) Gir, Rathi and Nagori b) Gir and Khillari
  c) Red Sindhi, Sahiwal and Tharparkar d) None of the above
31. The home track of Kankrej is?
  a) Madhya Pradesh b) Hisar
  c) Rann of Kutch (Guajarat) d) Andhra Pradesh

32. Mewati breed of cattle is a cross of which of the following ?
 a) Gir and Khillari b) Gir and Dangi
 c) Gir, Rathi and Nagori d) None of the above
33. Rathi breed of cattle is a cross of which of the following ?
 a) Gir, Rathi and Nagori b) Gir and Khillari
 c) Red Sindhi, Sahiwal and Tharparkar d) Gir and Dangi
34. The home track of Vechur is ?
 a) Kottayam (Kerala) b) Bihar
 c) Uttar Pradesh d) Rajasthan
35. The home track of Amritmahal is ?
 a) Uttar Pradesh b) Rajasthan
 c) Gujarat d) Karnataka
36. The home track of Malvi is ?
 a) Karnataka b) Madhya Pradesh
 c) Gujarat d) Assam
37. Hissardale is a cross of which of the following ?
 a) Rambouillet ram x Chokla ewe b) Rambouillet ram x Malpura ewe
 c) Bikaneri ewe x Australian Merino ram d) None of the above
38. Avikalin is a cross of which of the following ?
 a) Rambouillet ram x Malpura ewe b) Rambouillet ram x Chokla ewe
 c) Bikaneri ewe x Australian Merino ram d) Rambouillet ram x Dorset
39. Avivastra is a cross of which of the following ?
 a) Rambouillet ram x Malpura ewe b) Rambouillet ram x Chokla ewe
 c) Bikaneri ewe x Australian Merino ram d) Rambouillet ram x Dorset
40. Exotic fine wool breed of sheep is ?
 a) Lincoln b) Karakul
 c) Leicester d) Merino
41. Exotic fur breed of sheep is ?
 a) Dorset b) Lincoln
 c) Karakul d) Merino
42. Exotic mutton breed of sheep is?
 a) Dorset b) Karakul
 c) Merino d) Rambouillet
43. Exotic long coarse wool breed of sheep is ?
 a) Lincoln b) Leicester
 c) Both d) None
44. Which of the following breed is best fine wool breed in the world ?
 a) Merino b) Rambouillet
 c) Karakul d) Dorset

45. Which of the following is the largest and heaviest breed of sheep in the world ?
 a) Leicester b) Lincoln
 c) Southdown d) Suffolk

46. Which of the following breed of sheep has mousey grey face ?
 a) Leicester b) Lincoln
 c) Southdown d) Suffolk

47. Which of the following is the best mutton breed of sheep ?
 a) Dorset b) Southdown
 c) Suffolk d) None of the above

48. Which of the following sheep breed is known as the "Indian Merino" ?
 a) Nali b) Marwari
 c) Nellore d) Chokla

49. Which of the following sheep breed has canary coloration of wool ?
 a) Mandya b) Ganjam
 c) Marwari d) Nail

50. Which of the following sheep breed has highest disease resistance ?
 a) Marwari b) Pugal
 c) Mandya d) Ganjam

51. Which among the following is a triple purpose sheep breed ?
 a) Pugal b) Ganjam
 c) Marwari d) Chokla

52. Which of the following sheep breed has yellow streak above eyebrow ?
 a) Nellore b) Pugal
 c) Chokla d) Gaddi

53. Which among the following is the tallest breed of sheep in India ?
 a) Nellore b) Pugal
 c) Chokla d) Gaddi

54. Which breed of sheep is also known as "Goat like Sheep" ?
 a) Chokla b) Gaddi
 c) Ganjam d) Nellore

55. Which of the following is the best mutton breed of India ?
 a) Mandya b) Garole
 c) Nellore d) Bhakarwal

56. Which among the following is the smallest sheep breed ?
 a) Bhakarwal b) Gaddi
 c) Chokla d) Mandya

57. Which of the following is the most prolific sheep breed of India ?
 a) Garole b) Gaddi
 c) Ganjam d) Bhakarwal

58. Best kullu shawls are made by the wool of which breed of sheep ?
   a) Gurez b) Gaddi
   c) Garole d) Mandya
59. Which among the following breed is biggest among Kashmir breeds ?
   a) Gurez b) Bhakarwal
   c) Chokla d) Gaddi
60. Which among the following goat breed is known as the 'milk queen' ?
   a) Alpine b) Saanen
   c) Angora d) Toggenburg
61. The home track of Saanen is which of the following ?
   a) Switzerland b) Africa
   c) Turkey d) India
62. Which of the following breed of goat is famous for 'Mohair' ?
   a) Alpine b) Angora
   c) Saanen d) Toggenburg
63. Which of the following breed of goat is known as '**sheep like goat**' ?
   a) Saanen b) Angora
   c) Anglo-nubian d) Boer
64. Which of the following breed is known as the **Jersey of goat ?**
   a) Toggenburg b) Anglo-Nubian
   c) Saanen d) Orenburg
65. Which of the following is the most outstanding dual-purpose breed of goat ?
   a) Anglo-Nubian b) Saanen
   c) Toggenburg d) Alpine
66. In which of the following goat breed horns are absent ?
   a) Anglo-Nubian b) Saanen
   c) Toggenburg d) Alpine
67. Which of the following exotic goat breed have maximum adaptability ?
   a) Saanen b) Boer
   c) Alpine d) Toggenburg
68. Which of the following is the best meat type breed used for cross-breeding for meat ?
   a) Boer b) Alpine
   c) Saanen d) Anglo-Nubian
69. The home tract of Toggenburg is ?
   a) South Africa b) England
   c) Kazakhstan d) Switzerland
70. The home track of Anglo-Nubian is ?
   a) India b) England
   c) Switzerland d) Africa

71. The home track of Alpine breed is ?
   a) Turkey   b) Switzerland
   c) Africa   d) India
72. The home track of Angora breed is ?
   a) Turkey   b) Switzerland
   c) Africa   d) India
73. Which of the following breed does not belong to North temperate region ?
   a) Chegu   b) Chanthangi
   c) Gaddi   d) Barbari
74. Which of the following goat breed does not belong to Southern peninsular region ?
   a) Malabari   b) Ganjam
   c) Osmanabadi   d) Sangamneri
75. Which of the following goat breed does not belong to Eastern region ?
   a) Black bengal   b) Ganjam
   c) Both   d) None
76. Which of the following breed does not belong to North-western arid and semi-arid region ?
   a) Jhakrana   b) Kutchi
   c) Barbari   d) Chegu
77. The home track of Jamunapari breed is ?
   a) Etawah   b) Punjab
   c) Haryana   d) Telangana
78. The home track of Barbari breed is ?
   a) Punjab   b) Haryana
   c) Etawah   d) Ladakh
79. The home track of Beetle breed is ?
   a) Kutchi   b) Kerala
   c) Alwar   d) Punjab
80. The home track of Kutchi breed is ?
   a) Ladakh   b) Osmanabad
   c) Haryana   d) Gujarat
81. The home track of Chanthangi is ?
   a) Ladakh   b) Agra
   c) Kerala   d) Haryana
82. The home track of malabari is ?
   a) Kerala   b) Rajasthan
   c) Assam   d) Odisha
83. Which of the following breed is the biggest and most majestic breed of Indian goat ?
   a) Baarbari   b) Chegu
   c) Jamunapari   d) Jhakrana

84. Which of the following goat breed is having Roman nose appearance ?
 a) Jhakrana b) Jamunapari
 c) Kutchi d) Black Bengal
85. Which of the following goat breed is known as the city breed ?
 a) Barbari b) Osmanabadi
 c) Malabari d) Kutchi
86. Which of the following goat breed is the dwarf breed and highly suitable for stall feeding ?
 a) Jhakrana b) Chegu
 c) Malabari d) Barbari
87. Which of the following Indian goat breed have maximum milk fat % ?
 a) Barbari b) Malabari
 c) Jamunapari d) Kutchi
88. Which of the following goat breed is famous for tanning purpose ?
 a) Jamunapari b) Malabari
 c) Jhakrana d) Osmanabadi
89. Which of the following goat breed have corkscrew shaped horns ?
 a) Kutchi b) Osmanabadi
 c) Jhakrana d) Jamunapari
90. Which of the following is the best chevon breed of India ?
 a) Chegu b) Changthangi
 c) Jamunapari d) Black Bengal
91. Which among the following is the highly prolific goat breed of India ?
 a) Black Bengal b) Jamunapari
 c) Chegu d) Beetle
92. Which among the following is Pashmina producing breed of goat ?
 a) Jamunapar b) Chegu
 c) Beetle d) Black Bengal
93. Which among the following breed is used to obtain best quality Kashmiri rug or shawl ?
 a) Changthangi b) Malabari
 c) Jamunapari d) None of the above
94. The home track of Sangamneri breed is ?
 a) Pune b) Punjab
 c) Assam d) Hyderabad
95. The home track of Large White Yorkshire is which of the following ?
 a) Denmark b) England
 c) Switzerland d) None of the above
96. The home track of Tamworth is which of the following ?
 a) Denmark b) England
 c) Switzerland d) None of the above

97. The home track of Berkshire is which of the following ?
   a) Denmark b) England
   c) Switzerland d) None of the above
98. The home track of Landrace is which of the following ?
   a) Denmark b) England
   c) Switzerland d) None of the above
99. Which among the following is the heaviest breed of pig ?
   a) Tamworth b) Landrace
   c) Berkshiret d) Large White Yorkshire
100. Which among the following is an excellent pork breed ?
   a) Landrace b) Tamworth
   c) Berkshire d) Middle White Yorkshire
101. Which of the following breed is black in color with 6 white marks on body ?
   a) Landrace b) Berkshire
   c) Tamworth d) Large White Yorkshire
102. Which among the following breed is golden red in colour ?
   a) Middle White Yorkshire b) Berkshire
   c) Tamworth d) Middle White Yorkshire
103. Which among the following breed is known for lean meat ?
   a) Middle White Yorkshire b) Tamworth
   c) Middle White Yorkshire d) Large White Yorkshire
104. Which among the following breed is known to have highest quality bacon in the world ?
   a) Landmark b) Berkshire
   c) Middle White Yorkshire d) Large White Yorkshire
105. Which among the following breed have white body colour with some black skin spots (Freckles) ?
   a) Berkshire b) Tamworth
   c) Middle White Yorkshire d) Landrace
106. The home track of Ghoongroo breed of pig is ?
   a) Meghalaya b) Assam
   c) West Bengal d) Nagaland
107. The home track of Tenyi Vo breed of pig is ?
   a) Nagaland b) Assam
   c) Andaman & Nicobar d) None of the above
108. Which among the following is the best Indian breed of horse ?
   a) Manipuri b) Spiti
   c) Zanskari d) Kathiawari

109. Which among the following breed of Indian horse is known for their intelligence so used for polo, military and racing ?
   a) Manipuri   b) Spiti
   c) Zanskari   d) Kathiawari
110. The home track of Zanskari breed is ?
   a) Leh & Ladakh   b) Himachal Pradesh
   c) Marwar   d) Manipur
111. Which among the following breed of camel is also known as swimming camel ?
   a) Kutchi   b) Bikaneri
   c) Mewari   d) Kharai
112. Which of the following breed of camel is tolerant to high saline water ?
   a) Jaisalmeri   b) Bikaneri
   c) Kharai   d) Mewari
113. Which of the following type of camel is riding type ?
   a) Hill camel   b) Riverine camel
   c) Desert type   d) None of the above
114. Which of the following type of camel is/are baggage type ?
   a) Hill camel   b) Riverine camel
   c) Both   d) None
115. Which of the following breed of poultry produces white-shelled eggs ?
   a) English breeds   b) Mediterranean breeds
   c) American breeds   d) Asiatic breeds
116. Which of the following breed have pea-comb ?
   a) Brahma   b) Cochin
   c) Leghorn   d) Australorp
117. Which of the following breed have rose-comb ?
   a) Minorca   b) Rhode Island White
   c) Both   d) None
118. The colour of ear lobe is white in which breed ?
   a) Brahma   b) Ancona
   c) Orpington   d) Jersey Black Giant
119. The colour of ear lobe is red in which breed ?
   a) Australorp   b) Minorca
   c) Ancona   d) Leghorn
120. Which of the following breed have white skin colour ?
   a) Rhode Island Red   b) Jersey Black Giant
   c) Australorp   d) Minorca
121. tWhich of the following breed have yellow skin colour ?
   a) Rhode Island Red   b) Australorp
   c) Orpington   d) Andalusian

122. Which of the following breed is having bluish-black color of shank ?
a) Cornish b) Minorca
c) Langshan d) New Hampshire

123. Which of the following breed is having yellow shank colour ?
a) Sussex b) Orpington
c) Dorking d) Plymouth rock

124. Which of the following breed is having dark slate shank colour ?
a) Cornish b) Australorp
c) New Hampshire d) Orpington

125. Which of the following breed is having white shank colour ?
a) Cornish b) Sussex
c) Plymouth rock d) Cochin

126. Feathered shank is a character of which of the following breed ?
a) Mediterranean breed b) English breed
c) Asiatic breed d) American breed

127. Which among the following is the best layer breed in the world ?
a) White Leghorn b) Cornish
c) Orpington d) Plymouth rock

128. Which among the following is the best broiler breed in the world ?
a) Rhode Island Red b) Jersey Black Giant
c) Cornish d) White Leghorn

129. Which of the following is the heaviest breed of poultry ?
a) Andalusian b) Jersey Black Giant
c) Kadaknath d) Aseel

130. Which of the following is the lightest breed of poultry ?
a) Aseel b) Chittagong
c) Brahma d) Kadaknath

131. Which of the following breed of poultry lays blue shelled eggs ?
a) Busra b) Cochin
c) Andalusian d) Cornish

132. Which among the following is/are referred to as table bird ?
a) English breed b) Asiatic breed
c) Mediterranean breed d) American breed

133. Which among the following is best dual purpose breed of poultry ?
a) English breed b) Asiatic breed
c) Mediterranean breed d) American breed

134. Which among the following Indian breed is known for excellent fighting quality ?
a) Cochin b) Aseel
c) Kadaknath d) Chittagong

135. Which among the following Indian breed is known for its majestic gait ?
a) Aseel b) Kadaknath
c) Chittagong d) Busra

136. Which among the following Indian breed is known as **Kalamasi** ?
a) Busra b) Chittagong
c) Brahma d) Kadaknath

137. Which among the following is maximum disease resistant poultry breed ?
a) Kadaknath b) Brahma
c) Cochin d) Aseel

138. Which of the following Indian poultry breed is known as **Malay** ?
a) Kadaknath b) Aseel
c) Chittagong d) Busra

139. Which of the following is known as **Shanghai fowl** ?
a) White Leghorn b) Cochin
c) Aseel d) None of the above

140. The origin of Aseel breed is which of the following ?
a) Odisha b) Gujarat
c) Maharashtra d) Andhra Pradesh

141. The origin of kadaknath breed is ?
a) Odisha b) Gujarat
c) Jhabua, Madhya Pradesh d) Haryana

142. The home track of Chittagong breed is ?
a) Odisha b) Madhya Pradesh
c) Haryana d) Assam

143. The home track of Busra breed is ?
a) Odisha b) Gujarat
c) Madhya Pradesh d) Assam

144. The home track of White Leghorn is ?
a) China b) Switzerland
c) Italy d) India

145. The home track of Cochin is ?
a) India b) Italy
c) Germany d) China

146. Which among the following is the best camel breed in India ?
a) Kharai b) Mewari
c) Jaisalmeri d) Bikaneri

147. The home track of Badri breed of cattle is ?
a) Andaman & Nicobar b) Odisha
c) Uttarakhand d) Nagaland

148. The home track of Kodi Adu breed of goat is ?
a) Telangana b) Tamil Nadu
c) Andhra pradesh d) Kerala

149. The home track of Chevaadu breed of sheep is ?
a) Tamil Nadu b) Telangana
c) Andhra Pradesh d) Kerala

150. The home track of Kendrapada breed of sheep is ?

a) West Bengal | b) Madhya Pradesh
c) Uttar Pradesh | d) Odisha

Answer Key

1	b	2	a	3	b	4	d	5	c	6	c	7	a
8	d	9	a	10	c	11	a	12	d	13	a	14	c
15	a	16	c	17	a	18	a	19	a	20	b	21	d
22	c	23	c	24	a	25	d	26	b	27	c	28	d
29	d	30	b	31	c	32	c	33	c	34	a	35	d
36	b	37	c	38	a	39	b	40	d	41	c	42	a
43	c	44	a	45	b	46	c	47	c	48	d	49	d
50	a	51	c	52	b	53	a	54	d	55	c	56	d
57	a	58	b	59	a	60	b	61	a	62	b	63	b
64	b	65	a	66	c	67	d	68	a	69	d	70	b
71	c	72	a	73	d	74	b	75	d	76	d	77	a
78	c	79	d	80	d	81	a	82	a	83	c	84	b
85	a	86	d	87	a	88	c	89	a	90	d	91	a
92	b	93	a	94	a	95	b	96	b	97	b	98	a
99	d	100	d	101	b	102	c	103	b	104	a	105	d
106	c	107	a	108	d	109	a	110	a	111	d	112	c
113	c	114	c	115	b	116	a	117	c	118	b	119	a
120	c	121	a	122	c	123	d	124	b	125	b	126	c
127	a	128	c	129	b	130	d	131	c	132	a	133	d
134	b	135	a	136	d	137	a	138	c	139	b	140	d
141	c	142	a	143	b	144	c	145	d	146	d	147	c
148	b	149	a	150	d								

3

General Identification and Tagging for Selection and Rearing of Livestock

A.K. Srivastava, and K.J. Ankuya

Department of Livestock Production Management, College of Veterinary Science and Animal Husbandry, Kamdhenu University, Sardarkrushinagar, Gujarat 385506

Introduction

Identification of animals is must as a requirement in the daily management to spot and identify a particular animal in a herd/group/flock.

Objectives of Identification

- Identification is done to carry out routine work efficiently.
- For registration and recording of the parentage in breeding programme / birth
- Identification required at time of transportation and Insurance and loan from Bank.
- For individual feeding of animals.
- During milking
- During sale, for participation of animals in the rally, show and exhibition.
- For treating the animal, heat detection etc.
- It is necessary for in case of theft and loss of animal for complain and search of animal.

Selection of Identification Method

- Depends very much on Need and personal preference and limitations of the livestock.
- Hot branding not useful for thin skin animals
- Very useful to combine several methods.
- Branding for livestock once/twice a year
- So after birth Ear tattooing is done and branding in next season.

Factors considered for selection of Identification Method

- The cost
- The ease of application
- The ease of reading
- Susceptibility to alteration
- Performance

SYSTEMS OF IDENTIFICATION

A. NATURAL SYSTEM

B. ARTIFICIAL SYSTEM

A. NATURAL SYSTEM: Various markings on the body parts are used to identify the particular animal

- White Marks on fore head
- White muzzle and switch
- White Marks on legs
- White Marks on ear and tail
- Acquired marks: like wound, scars, surgical scars, collar marks are also used by different owners

B. ARTIFICIAL SYSTEM

1. Name and Photographs
2. Tattooing
3. Branding
4. Tagging
5. Ear notching / Flesh marks
6. Number plates
7. Wing / Leg bands
8. Toe punching
9. Colour marking Temporary methods: Chalk/grease marker/ Potassium permanganate /Black/light coloured paints
10. Electronic Chip / Transponders
11. Muzzle printing
12. Retinal Image

Numbering System

- Whatever method used – some sort of Numbering system should be used
- Each number should give maximum information and should be unique
- For Example Students registration No. (04-0496- 2023) and Vehicle No.(GJ-08BB 1234)
- First two digits --- year of birth and Rest digits --- sequence no. of birth
- Sixteenth calf born in year 2012 --- 12 16
- For a herd only less than 100 calving in a year
- If more than 100 calving ------ 12 016
- Male and female separate number

  Female odd number --- 501, 503, 505 ....

  Male Even number --- 502, 504, 506 ....
- Swine the piglets it is better to use litter no. in one year and individual no. within litter is given in another ear

BASIC RULES FOR NUMBERING

- Never repeat the same number on different animal
- Convey as much as information possible with minimum figures
- Keep it simple so it can be easily understood by the Stockman
- Be sure that tags, tattoos, brands and other equipment are readily and consistently available

Questions

1. Which of the following is not an objective of identification in animals?
   a) To carry out routine work efficiently.
   b) For registration and recording of the parentage in breeding programme / birth
   c) Required at time of transportation and Insurance and loan from Bank.
   d) For increasing milk production of individual animals.
2. Broadly identification systems have been classified in
   a) Two groups b) Three groups
   c) Four groups d) Five groups
3. Various markings on the body parts are used to identify the particular animal, this system is
   a) Artificial system b) Natural system
   c) Temporary system d) Permanent system
4. Generally animal is given any name such as their origin, place of purchase, owner's name, physical appearance, name of river, the system of identification is
   a) Artificial system b) Natural system
   c) Temporary system d) Permanent system
5. Tattooing is one of the _____________ of identification
   a) Natural system and temporary method
   b) Natural system and permanent method
   c) Artificial system and Temporary method
   d) Artificial system and Permanent method
6. Which of the following is most popular method of identification for animals?
   a) Tattooing b) Branding
   c) Ear tagging d) Wing band
7. What is the principle of tattooing?
   a) When piercing hole (wound) heals, the dye is retained under the skin and it leaves a permanent mark.
   b) The tattooing ink deposited on the skin and it is permanent.
   c) Presence of corrosive substance in the tattooing ink, acts as burning agent and causes a permanent mark.
   d) Tattooing ink destroys hair follicles located under several layers of the skin and leaved a permanent scar on the skin of the animal.

8. Which of the following part of the body, tattooing is not done?
   a) In the external ear,
   b) Internal side of lips.
   c) In the Jugular groove.
   d) Below the base of tail.

9. Identify the principle of hot branding?
   a) The skin is pierced with needle and branding liquid is deposited in the skin and the liquid is retained under the skin which, leaves a permanent mark.
   b) The numbers marks are created with knife on the skin of animal.
   c) Presence of corrosive substance in the branding ink, acts as burning agent and causes a permanent mark.
   d) Branding destroys hair follicles located under several layers of the skin and leaved a permanent scar on the skin of the animal.

10. Identify the principle of cold branding?
   a) The skin is pierced with needle and branding liquid is deposited in the skin and the liquid is retained under the skin which, leaves a permanent mark.
   b) The branding solution is deposited on the skin and it is temporary in nature.
   c) Presence of corrosive substance in the branding ink, acts as burning agent and causes a permanent mark.
   d) Branding destroys hair follicles located under several layers of the skin and leaved a permanent scar on the skin of the animal.

11. The best method of identification for the calves within 24 hrs of birth
   a) Hot branding
   b) Ear tattooing
   c) Ear tagging
   d) Cold branding

12. Dermatoglyphics is also known as
   a) Hot branding
   b) Muzzle printing
   c) Iris imaging
   d) RFID

13. Branding is done at thigh region of the animal
   a) To save the skin from damage
   b) It is easy to perform branding action at thigh
   c) It is easy to observe the numbers at thigh region
   d) None of the above

14. Branding deteriorates the quality of
   a) Bone
   b) Horn
   c) Hide
   d) Meat

15. Branding is recommended at which of the following body part
   a) Tail which is situated at the side of the hide
   b) Head which comes at the centre of the hide
   c) Limbs which comes at the lower part of the hide
   d) Thigh which is situated at the marginal end of the hide.

16. Ear notching is most preferable method of identification in
    a) Goat b) Buffaloes
    c) Birds d) Swine
17. Cold branding destroys
    a) Hair only
    b) Pigment producing cells / melanocytes
    c) Hair follicle
    d) None of the above
18. In hot branding, time of application of hot iron number rod at the site which is devoid of hair
    a) 3-5 seconds b) 5-10 seconds
    c) 30-35 seconds d) 90-100 seconds
19. The major advantage of plastic tags
    a) They are available in various colours
    b) They are available with pre-printed number
    c) They are self-piercing
    d) They are readable from a distance
20. In branding the numbers should be separated by at least ___ cm from each other
    a) 1.0 cm b) 2.0 cm
    c) 2.5 cm d) 5.0 cm
21. Which of the following will be observed if the ear notches are too small?
    a) It will deform the shape of ear b) It will be close soon
    c) It will cause drooping of ear d) All of the above
22. In hot branding, time of application of hot iron number rod at the site with hair
    a) 3-5 seconds b) 5-10 seconds
    c) 30-35 seconds d) 90-100 seconds
23. Which of the following will be observed if the ear notches are too large?
    a) It will deform the shape of ear
    b) It will be close soon
    c) It will cause erection of the ear
    d) It will be easily hidden by the hairs
24. In cold branding, time of application of number rod at the site is about
    a) 5 seconds b) 10 seconds
    c) 30 seconds d) 90 seconds
25. In cold branding method of identification, time of application of number rod at the site for white calf is about
    a) 15 seconds b) 30 seconds
    c) 90 seconds d) 150 seconds

26. Animals are photographed to get which of the following view of the animal?
    a) Side view or profile b) Rear view
    c) Hind view d) All of the above
27. In white cattle, the cold branding destroys which of the following
    a) Hair only
    b) Pigment producing cells / melanocytes
    c) Hair follicle
    d) All the above
28. Appropriate site to apply the ear tags
    a) One third of the way out from base of ear
    b) Tip of the ear
    c) Base of the ear
    d) At any place in the ear
29. Biometric method of identification includes:
    a) Retinal imaging b) Iris imaging
    c) Muzzle printing d) All of the above
30. Abbreviation of RFID
    a) Rare frequency internal device
    b) Retinal frequency identification device
    c) Radio frequency identification device
    d) Rosset frequency internal device
31. Tag punches are used with which of the following type of ear tags?
    a) Non-piercing tags b) Self -piercing tags
    c) Both the option (a) and (b) d) None of the above
32. Components of RFID includes
    a) Reader and Antenna b) Transponder
    c) Computer system d) All of the above
33. For taking three dimensional photo-graphsof animals, the angle should be,
    a) 30 degree b) 45 degree
    c) 60 degree d) 90 degree
34. For taking photographs of the animals, distance between animal and camera should be
    a) 3 time length of animal b) Twice the length of animal
    c) Length of animal d) Half length of animal
35. The most appropriate method of identification for the young calf is
    a) Hot branding b) Ear tattooing
    c) Ear tagging d) Ear notching

36. The most common method of identification for the swine and beef cattle is
   a) Branding b) Ear tattooing
   c) Ear tagging d) Ear notching
37. Branding is mostly used in which of the animal
   a) Sheep b) Goat
   c) Pigs d) Horse
38. The part to be heated of branding rods for hot branding preferably should be made up of
   a) Iron b) Copper
   c) Brass d) Zinc
39. If the part to be heated of branding rods for hot branding is made of copper, advantage (s) is (are)
   a) Copper retains heat better than iron
   b) Hair does not stick to copper number as it stick to iron
   c) More contact surface can be obtained with copper than iron
   d) Both the option (a) and (b)
40. The branding rods for cold / freezing branding preferably should be
   a) Branding rods should be flat on the contact surface of the letter or figure
   b) Branding rods should have a shallow groove on the contact surface of the letter or figure
   c) Branding rods same as hot branding rods
   d) None of the above
41. In hot branding the iron branders should be heated to
   a) White hot b) Bright red hot
   c) Bluish red hot d) No colour change
42. The best suitable method of identification for birds
   a) Branding b) Tattooing
   c) Wing bands d) Wing notching
43. Toe punching is suitable method of identification for
   a) Ducks b) Guinea pig
   c) Chicken d) Rat and Mice
44. The best suitable method for group identification of animals
   a) Tattooing b) Colour / paint markings
   c) Tagging d) Ear notching
45. What is (are) the objective (s) for the identification in livestock?
   a) Accurate recording thereby avoiding the mistakes which are otherwise likely} to occur by likely the farmer, manager and attendants.
   b) Prevention of disputes over lost, stolen or strayed stock
   c) Managing herd health, AI performance, testing as well as routine operation and processing.
   d) All of the above

46. Which of the following is required for the freeze branding in the animals?
    a) Liquid Nitrogen
    b) Corrosive liquid
    c) Gentian Blue
    d) Malachite Green
47. Identify the correct statement
    a) In chemical branding melanin producing cells gets destroyed, hence colourless hairs appear on the branded area.
    b) In hot branding melanin producing cells gets destroyed, hence colourless hairs appear on the branded area.
    c) In freeze branding melanin producing cells gets destroyed, hence colourless hairs appear on the branded area.
    d) All statements are correct.
48. Which of the following is required for the cold branding in the animals?
    a) Liquid Nitrogen
    b) Corrosive liquid
    c) Gentian Blue
    d) Malachite Green
49. Identify the correct statement
    a) Tagging is a temporary method of identification
    b) Tagging is permanent method of identification
    c) In self piercing type of tags a hole is first made with a tag punch in the upper edge of the ear then tag is placed.
    d) In non piercing type of tags, ithas sharp ends and be directly fixed to the ear with the forceps.
50. Which of the following is required for the Freeze branding in the animals?
    a) Corrosive liquid
    b) Gentian Blue
    c) Malachite Green
    d) Solid Carbon di oxide
51. Which is the most suitable time for the putting identification marks in the animals?
    a) Soon after its birth
    b) Soon after weaning
    c) Soon after puberty
    d) Soon after parturition
52. Which is the most prevailing method of identification used by the farmers having few numbers of animals?
    a) Tattooing
    b) Ear tagging
    c) Name
    d) Branding
53. Appropriate method to apply the ear tags
    a) On the lower edge of the ear with number on the top
    b) Tip of the ear with number on the bottom
    c) On the upper edge of the ear with number on the top
    d) At any place in the ear with number on the top

54. Major disadvantage of the tattooing is
    a) It is permanent method of identification
    b) Animal must be caught and the inside of the ear cleaned to be able to read the identification number
    c) It can be done immediately after birth
    d) It decreases the look of the animal
55. Major objection of the ear tagging method of identification
    a) It is permanent method of identification
    b) The tags may be lost
    c) It cannot be done immediately after birth
    d) It decreases the value of the animal
56. Which is the most suitable method for identification in the avian species?
    a) Tattooing
    b) Wing notching
    c) Wing bands
    d) Branding
57. In birds the most appropriate time to apply the wing band is
    a) First day ofhatching
    b) First day of grower stage
    c) At pullet stage
    d) Soon after initiation of laying
58. In birds the most appropriate time to apply the leg band is
    a) First day of hatching
    b) During chick stage
    c) duringgrower stage
    d) At adult stage
59. Small farmers generally don't practice a specific marking system for their animals because
    a) They don't have enough resources to do the identification of their animals
    b) They don't understand the importance of identification system of animals
    c) They know their animals and can identify them individually
    d) They think that it is harmful for the animals
60. Which of the following is not an objective of the identification?
    a) Maintenance of proper records on dairy farms.
    b) Popper feeding of animals
    c) Better management practices whenever required
    d) For increased milk production
61. Which of the following is not an objective of the identification?
    a) For increased growth rate of animals
    b) Identification number is required for registration of purebred animal
    c) Popper breeding of animals
    d) Identification is required for animals in animal shows and fairs
62. Which of the following identification method is used in the calf on the day of its birth
    a) Tattooing
    b) Ear notching
    c) Ear tags
    d) Branding

63. Which of the following identification method is not appropriate for the sheep

a) Tattooing b) Ear notching

c) Ear tags d) Branding

64. The most suitable method of identification for precision dairy farming is

a) RFID b) Muzzle printing

c) Ear tags d) Branding

65. The temperature of liquid nitrogen used for freeze branding method of identification is

a) - 60 ^{0}C b) - 96 ^{0}C

c) -196 ^{0}C d) - 296 ^{0}C

66. The temperature of dry ice used for freeze branding method of identification is

a) - 60 ^{0}C b) - 78^{0}C

c) - 90 ^{0}C d) - 196 ^{0}C

67. The temperature of dry ice used for freeze branding method of identification is

a) - 78^{0}F b) - 109^{0}F

c) - 119^{0}F d) - 196 ^{0}F

68. The dry ice used for freeze branding method of identification is

a) Solid Carbon di oxide –at 78.5^{0}C b) Solid Nitrogen oxide –at 78.5^{0}C

c) Solid Carbon di oxide –at 88.5^{0}C d) Solid Nitrogen oxide –at 88.5^{0}C

69. In freeze branding method of identification, time of application of number rod at the site is

a) Less than 20 seconds b) 30 seconds to 60 seconds

c) 90 seconds to 120 seconds d) More than 150 seconds

70. Painting numbers on the horns and rumps

a) A permanent method of identification

b) A temporary method of identification

c) It used for identification of pure bred animals

d) Popular method of identification in breeding programmes

71. Which of the following identification method is temporary in nature

a) Tattooing b) Ear notching

c) Ear tags d) Branding

72. Which of the following identification method is permanent in nature

a) Colour marking b) Number plate

c) Ear tags d) Ear Tattooing

73. Which of the following identification method is highly painful and not permitted by Animal Welfare Board

a) Tattooing b) Ear notching

c) Ear tags d) Colour marking

74. Which of the following identification method is used generally for short duration.
   a) Tattooing
   b) Ear notching
   c) Ear tags
   d) Number plates
75. Which of the following identific ation method is used generally at the time of transportation?
   a) Branding
   b) Ear tags
   c) Number plates
   d) Ear notching
76. Which of the following identification method is used generally at the time of show and exhibition of animals?
   a) Branding
   b) Number plates
   c) Ear tags
   d) Ear notching
77. Which of the following identification method is used generally during animal fairs and Competitions ?
   a) Number plates
   b) Branding
   c) Ear tags
   d) Ear notching
78. Which of the following statement is incorrect regarding number plates identification method?
   a) It can be easily applied
   b) It is permanent method of identification
   c) It can be placed around the neck strap or neck chain.
   d) It can be used at the time of transportation, show, exhibition animal fair and Competitions.
79. Number Plates of various shapes and sizes bearing name and address placed on which body parts
   a) Around the neck strap
   b) Tied in the neck chain
   c) Around horns
   d) All the above
80. Wing bands and leg bands are generally made up of
   a) Aluminium
   b) Copper
   c) Iron
   d) PVC
81. The first official identification systems were documented in
   a) 16th century
   b) 17th century
   c) 18th century
   d) 19th century
82. In which country the first official identification systems were used Uruguay for instance maintained at that time a register of hot brands
   a) Belgium
   b) Uruguay
   c) England
   d) Switzerland
83. Which type of identification systems was officially used for the animals for the first time
   a) Register of ear tags
   b) Register of Tattooing
   c) Register of cold brands
   d) Register of hot brands

84. Livestock ear tags were developed in which year
   a) 1750 b) 1799
   c) 1847 d) 1903
85. First time ear tags were used for identification of which species
   a) Sheep b) Cattle
   c) Horse d) Pig
86. First time ear tags were used for identification of which breed of sheep
   a) Merino b) Corriedale
   c) Rambouillet d) Dorset
87. First time ear tags were developed in under the direction of Sir Joseph Banks, who was
   a) President of Uruguay b) President of the Royal Society
   c) President of Belgium d) President of USFDA
88. First time ear tags were used for identification of sheep flock which was established for
   a) King George III b) President of USA
   c) President of Uruguay d) President of Belgium
89. The purpose of "Private" or "Management" identification is
   a) A proof of ownership and protection of stock theft.
   b) A basis for improved herd management trough differentiation of individual performance
   c) A way of automating the operation of technical equipment's (dairy parlours, automated feeding systems, weighing and drafting systems etc.
   d) All the above
90. The purpose of "Official" or "National" identification is
   a) Animal disease control and eradication (Tuberculosis, Brucellosis etc.) programme
   b) Herd Improvement programme through collection of precise data
   c) High level pedigree herds monitoring in all best breeds
   d) All the above
91. The purpose of "Official" or "National" identification is
   a) Production and movement control of livestock
   b) Control of sanitary crises (BSE, Foot & Mouth Disease, Plague etc.), and contention through knowledge of herd locations and movements
   c) Ensuring the certification of herd based warranties for farmers' loans
   d) All the above
92. The purpose of "Official" or "National" identification is
   a) Production and movement control of livestock
   b) Consumer confidence in Food safety through traceability
   c) Market access for meat and dairy exporters
   d) All the above

93. Which of the following factors should be considered while selecting an appropriate identification system?
    a) Size of the operation
    b) Visibility from a distance
    c) Application methods
    d) All the above

94. Which of the following factors should be considered while selecting an appropriate identification system?
    a) Equipment's required for identification
    b) Cost of the identification system
    c) Duration of identification
    d) All the above

95. Which of the following factors should be considered while selecting an appropriate identification system?
    a) Nature of identification (temporary or permanent)
    b) Visibility from a distance
    c) Type of records kept
    d) All the above

96. Branding is not an appropriate identification system for
    a) Cattle
    b) Pigs
    c) Camels
    d) Horses

97. Dyes and paints mark the on animals usually lasts for
    a) Less than a week
    b) Less than a fortnight
    c) Less than a month
    d) Less than 3 months

98. Identify the incorrect statement from the following
    a) Caustic chemicals (Caustic soda paste, caustic potash) were proposed as an alternative to hot iron for branding in cattle
    b) Caustic branding is difficult to apply with accuracy and gives irregular results
    c) It is a less painful method than the hot branding method hence recommended identification method
    d) Caustic branding method has an advantage that it does not use fire

99. When the swelling appears at branded site, in cold branding identification system?
    a) 5 seconds
    b) 5 minutes
    c) 5 hours
    d) 5 days

100. When the swelling disappears at branded site, in cold branding identification system?
    a) 5 hours after branding
    b) 24 hours after branding
    c) 5 days after branding
    d) 10 days after branding

101. When the top layer of skin sheds at branded site, in cold branding identification system?
    a) 1 day after branding
    b) 5 days after branding
    c) 15 days after branding
    d) 30 days after branding

102. At what time the white hairs start to grow at branded site, in cold branding identification system?
  a) 15 day after branding b) 30 days after branding
  c) 60 days after branding d) 90 days after branding

103. When the white hairs grow completely at branded site, in cold branding identification system?
  a) 1 month after branding b) 2 months after branding
  c) 3 months after branding d) 6 months after branding

104. In cold branding identification system, what is the application time of branded stamp on black hair weaned animal?
  a) 45 Seconds b) 1 Minute
  c) 1 Minute 15 seconds d) 2 Minutes 15 Seconds

105. In cold branding identification system, what is the application time of branded stamp on dark red hair weaned animal?
  a) 45 Seconds b) 1 Minute
  c) 1 Minute 15 seconds d) 2 Minutes 15 Seconds

106. In cold branding identification system, what is the application time of branded stamp on yellow hair weaned animal?
  a) 45 Seconds b) 1 Minute
  c) 1 Minute 15 seconds d) 2 Minutes 15 Seconds

107. In cold branding identification system, what is the application time of branded stamp on white hair weaned animal?
  a) 45 Seconds b) 1 Minute
  c) 1 Minute 15 seconds d) 2 Minutes 15 Seconds

108. In cold branding identification system, what is the application time of branded stamp on weaned animal?
  a) 45 Seconds b) 1 Minute
  c) 1 Minute 15 seconds d) 2 Minutes 15 Seconds

109. In cold branding identification system, what is the application time of branded stamp on yearling animal?
  a) 45 Seconds b) 1 Minute
  c) 1 Minute 15 seconds d) 2 Minutes 15 Seconds

110. In cold branding identification system, the application time of branded stamp on yearling animal and weaned animals is
  a) 45 Seconds
  b) Yearling animal 60 Seconds and weaned animals 45 Seconds
  c) Yearling animal 45 Seconds and weaned animals 60 Seconds
  d) 1 Minute

111. In cold branding identification system, the application time of branded stamp depends on
   a) Age of the animal
   b) Colour of the hair
   c) Both Age and colour of the hair
   d) None of the above

112. In cold branding identification system, the application time of branded stamp is
   a) More on white hair animal than the black hair animal
   b) More on black hair animal than the white hair animal
   c) Colour of the hair has no effect on application time
   d) None of the above

113. Pigs must be notched
   a) Within 7 days of birth
   b) Within 15 days of birth
   c) Just before weaning
   d) Any time

114. Ear tags should be installed
   a) Before the first cartilage rib of the ears
   b) Between the first and second cartilage rib of the ear
   c) Between the second and third cartilage rib of the ear
   d) Between the third and fourth cartilage rib of the ear

115. Incidence of tag loss due to tag tearing through ear in lambs is about
   a) 1%
   b) 2 %
   c) 5%
   d) 10%

116. Median duration for ear tag retention is about
   a) 112 days
   b) 272 days
   c) 322 days
   d) 382 days

117. Which of the following is a part of an electronic animal identification system?
   a) Transponder
   b) Transceiver/Reader
   c) Software/Data
   d) All the above

118. Which of the following is a not a part of an electronic animal identification system?
   a) Transponder
   b) Transceiver/Reader
   c) Pulsator
   d) Software/Data

119. First farm in India to use RFID microchips that can be injected into the animal's body is
   a) Cattle yard, NDRI, Karnal
   b) The Kopordem farm at Valpoi in Sattari Taluk in North Goa
   c) LRS, Katupakkam, TANUVAS, Chennai
   d) Sahiwal Farm CIRC, Meerut

120. The Kopordem farm at Valpoi in Sattari Taluk in North Goa has become the first farm in India
   a) To use RFID microchips that can be injected into the animal's body
   b) To use muzzle printing in the dairy animals
   c) To use electronic ear tags on the animals
   d) To use Electronic collars that can be tied to the animal's body

121. The average expected life span of the electronic ear tags is
    a) 1 year b) 3 years
    c) 5 years d) 10 years

122. The advantages of an electronic animal ID system is (are)
    a) Qualification for specific marketing programs
    b) Reduction in data entry errors
    c) Increased efficiency in the capture of data
    d) All the above

123. The advantages of an electronic animal ID system is (are)
    a) Reduced data errors reading tags
    b) Unique ID for each animal
    c) Instant ability to generate management reports
    d) All the above

124. The disadvantages of an electronic animal ID system is (are)
    a) Increased expense for animal ID supplies
    b) No guarantee of additional market value
    c) Increased complexity
    d) All the above

125. The disadvantages of an electronic animal ID system is (are)
    a) Not all equipment and tags are ISO compliant
    b) Challenges with technical issues (collision, interference)
    c) Short read ranges between scanner and tags
    d) All the above

126. The main principle behind the muzzle printing method of identification is
    a) The lines and dotted pattern from a muzzle print are specific for each animal
    b) It is easy method of identification
    c) It does not interfere the animals body
    d) It is very accurate method of identification

127. When two prints of the same animal are compared, there must be ______ identifiable matching lines or dots common to both prints.
    a) Three b) Six
    c) Nine d) Twelve

128. What is (are) the problem (s) associated with muzzle printing method of identification?
    a) Use of too much ink
    b) A build-up of moisture on the animal's nose
    c) Improper holding the animalstill, which can result in a smeared, unreadable print
    d) All the above

129. Retinal imaging usesthe patterns of
   a) Rods in the Retina
   b) Cones in the Retina
   c) Retinal blood vessels to produce a unique image of each eye
   d) Pupil in the eyes
130. Which of the following identification system is considered having low value for animal welfare?
   a) Hot branding
   b) Tattooing
   c) Ear tagging
   d) Electronic ear tags
131. Which of the following identification system is considered having low value for animal welfare?
   a) Ear tattooing
   b) Ear notching
   c) Ear tagging
   d) Electronic chip
132. Which of the following identification system is considered having good value for animal welfare?
   a) Ear tattooing
   b) Metal ear tags
   c) Retinal imaging
   d) Plastic ear tags
133. Select appropriate statement

   Statement 1: Identification is required for registration and recording of the parentage in breeding programme / birth.

   Statement 2: Identification is required at time of transportation, Insurance and loan from Bank.
   a) Statement 1 is correct while Statement 2 is wrong
   b) Statement 2 is correct while Statement 1 is wrong
   c) Both Statement 1 and statement 2 are correct
   d) Both Statement 1 and statement 2 are wrong
134. Select appropriate statement

   Statement 1: Identification is required during sale, for participation of animals in the rally, show and exhibition.

   Statement 2: Identification required to increase the milk production potential in dairyanimals.
   a) Statement 1 is correct while Statement 2 is wrong
   b) Statement 2 is correct while Statement 1 is wrong
   c) Both Statement 1 and statement 2 are correct
   d) Both Statement 1 and statement 2 are wrong
135. Select appropriate statement

   Statement 1: In a examination of the ears of over 700 sheep, approximately 28% of the animals suffered slight to moderate ear damage associated with plastic ear tags,

   Statement 2: Poor application of ear tags can result in infections and ear damage, and this is more marked in young calves.

a) Statement 1 is correct while Statement 2 is wrong
b) Statement 2 is correct while Statement 1 is wrong
c) Both Statement 1 and statement 2 are correct
d) Both Statement 1 and statement 2 are wrong

136. Select appropriate statement

Statement 1: In Natural system of identification various markings on the body parts are used to identify the particular animal,

Statement 2: In Artificial System of identification, acquired markslike wound, scars, surgical scars, collar marks are used for identification.

a) Statement 1 is correct while Statement 2 is wrong
b) Statement 2 is correct while Statement 1 is wrong
c) Both Statement 1 and statement 2 are correct
d) Both Statement 1 and statement 2 are wrong

137. Select appropriate statement

Statement 1: Name and photographs of the animals are classified as Natural system of identification.

Statement 2: Tattooing and ear tagging are classified as Artificial System of identification.

a) Statement 1 is correct while Statement 2 is wrong
b) Statement 2 is correct while Statement 1 is wrong
c) Both Statement 1 and statement 2 are correct
d) Both Statement 1 and statement 2 are wrong

138. Select appropriate statement

Statement 1: Tattooing is the artificial and temporary method of identification system.

Statement 2: Tattooing is the most popular method of identification for animals.

a) Statement 1 is correct while Statement 2 is wrong
b) Statement 2 is correct while Statement 1 is wrong
c) Both Statement 1 and statement 2 are correct
d) Both Statement 1 and statement 2 are wrong

139. Select appropriate statement

Statement 1: Ear tagging is the artificial and temporary method of identification system.

Statement 2: Ear tagging is the most popular method of identification for animals.

a) Statement 1 is correct while Statement 2 is wrong
b) Statement 2 is correct while Statement 1 is wrong
c) Both Statement 1 and statement 2 are correct
d) Both Statement 1 and statement 2 are wrong

140. Select appropriate statement

Statement 1: Freeze branding destroys hair follicles located under several layers of the skin and leaved a permanent scar on the skin of the animal.

Statement 2: In cold branding, presence of corrosive substance in the branding ink, acts as burning agent and causes a permanent mark.

a) Statement 1 is correct while Statement 2 is wrong
b) Statement 2 is correct while Statement 1 is wrong
c) Both Statement 1 and statement 2 are correct
d) Both Statement 1 and statement 2 are wrong

141. Select appropriate statement

Statement 1: Principle of tattooing describes that when piercing hole (wound) heals, the dye is retained under the skin and it leaves a permanent mark.

Statement 2: Principle of tattooing describes that presence of corrosive substancein the tattooing ink, acts as burning agent and causes a permanent mark.

a) Statement 1 is correct while Statement 2 is wrong
b) Statement 2 is correct while Statement 1 is wrong
c) Both Statement 1 and statement 2 are correct
d) Both Statement 1 and statement 2 are wrong

142. Select appropriate statement

Statement 1: In Hot branding numbers marks are created with hot knife on the skin of animal.

Statement 2: Hot branding destroys hair follicles located under several layers of the skin and leaved a permanent scar on the skin of the animal.

a) Statement 1 is correct while Statement 2 is wrong
b) Statement 2 is correct while Statement 1 is wrong
c) Both Statement 1 and statement 2 are correct
d) Both Statement 1 and statement 2 are wrong

143. Select appropriate statement

Statement 1: In hot branding, hot iron number rod should be placed at the site which is devoid of hair for 30 seconds.

Statement 2: In hot branding the numbers should be separated by at least 10 cm from each other.

a) Statement 1 is correct while Statement 2 is wrong
b) Statement 2 is correct while Statement 1 is wrong
c) Both Statement 1 and statement 2 are correct
d) Both Statement 1 and statement 2 are wrong

144. Select appropriate statement

Statement 1: The most appropriate method of identification for the young calf is ear tattooing.

Statement 2: The most common method of identification for the swine and beef cattle is ear notching

a) Statement 1 is correct while Statement 2 is wrong

b) Statement 2 is correct while Statement 1 is wrong

c) Both Statement 1 and statement 2 are correct

d) Both Statement 1 and statement 2 are wrong

145. Select appropriate statement

Statement 1: The temperature of dry ice used for freeze branding method of identification is- 78^{0}C.

Statement 2: The temperature of dry ice used for freeze branding method of identification is - 109^{0}F

a) Statement 1 is correct while Statement 2 is wrong

b) Statement 2 is correct while Statement 1 is wrong

c) Both Statement 1 and statement 2 are correct

d) Both Statement 1 and statement 2 are wrong

146. Select appropriate statement

Statement 1: The dry ice used for freeze branding method of identification isSolid Carbon di oxide –at 78.5^{0}C

Statement 2: In freeze branding method of identification, time of application of number rod at the site is 3-5 seconds

a) Statement 1 is correct while Statement 2 is wrong

b) Statement 2 is correct while Statement 1 is wrong

c) Both Statement 1 and statement 2 are correct

d) Both Statement 1 and statement 2 are wrong

147. Select appropriate statement

Statement 1: The best suitable method of identification for chicken is wing bands.

Statement 2: Toe punching is suitable method of identification for ducks.

a) Statement 1 is correct while Statement 2 is wrong

b) Statement 2 is correct while Statement 1 is wrong

c) Both Statement 1 and statement 2 are correct

d) Both Statement 1 and statement 2 are wrong

148. Select appropriate statement

Statement 1: Major disadvantage of the tattooing is that animal must be caught and the inside of the ear cleaned to be able to read the identification number.

Statement 2: Major objection of the ear tagging method of identification that it cannot be done immediately after birth.

a) Statement 1 is correct while Statement 2 is wrong
b) Statement 2 is correct while Statement 1 is wrong
c) Both Statement 1 and statement 2 are correct
d) Both Statement 1 and statement 2 are wrong

149. Select appropriate statement

Statement 1: In birds the most appropriate time to apply the wing band is at adult stage.

Statement 2: In birds the most appropriate time to apply the leg band is at first day of hatching.

a) Statement 1 is correct while Statement 2 is wrong
b) Statement 2 is correct while Statement 1 is wrong
c) Both Statement 1 and statement 2 are correct
d) Both Statement 1 and statement 2 are wrong

150. Select appropriate statement

Statement 1: Branding system of identification is most appropriate for the sheep.

Statement 2: The most suitable method of identification for precision dairy farming is muzzle printing.

a) Statement 1 is correct while Statement 2 is wrong
b) Statement 2 is correct while Statement 1 is wrong
c) Both Statement 1 and statement 2 are correct
d) Both Statement 1 and statement 2 are wrong

Answer Key

1	d	2	a	3	b	4	a	5	d	6	c	7	a
8	c	9	d	10	c	11	b	12	b	13	a	14	c
15	d	16	d	17	b	18	a	19	d	20	c	21	b
22	b	23	a	24	c	25	d	26	d	27	c	28	a
29	d	30	c	31	a	32	d	33	b	34	a	35	b
36	d	37	d	38	b	39	d	40	b	41	b	42	c
43	a	44	b	45	d	46	a	47	c	48	b	49	a
50	d	51	a	52	c	53	c	54	b	55	b	56	c
57	a	58	d	59	c	60	d	61	a	62	a	63	d
64	b	65	c	66	b	67	b	68	a	69	b	70	b
71	c	72	d	73	b	74	d	75	c	76	b	77	a
78	b	79	d	80	a	81	c	82	b	83	d	84	b

85	a	86	a	87	b	88	a	89	d	90	d	91	d
92	d	93	d	94	d	95	d	96	b	97	c	98	c
99	b	100	c	101	d	102	c	103	c	104	a	105	b
106	c	107	d	108	a	109	b	110	b	111	c	112	a
113	a	114	c	115	c	116	b	117	d	118	c	119	b
120	a	121	d	122	d	123	d	124	d	125	d	126	a
127	b	128	d	129	c	130	a	131	b	132	c	133	c
134	a	135	c	136	a	137	b	138	d	139	c	140	b
141	a	142	b	143	d	144	c	145	c	146	a	147	c
148	a	149	d	150	b								

4

Animal Handling and Restraining

Jessy Bagh[1], Rajarshree Rath[1], Annada Das[2], and Kaushik Satyaprakash[3]

[1]*Department of Livestock Production and Management, CVSc & AH, OUAT Bhubaneswar, Odisha*

[2]*Department of Livestock Products Technology, Faculty of Veterinary and Animal Sciences, WBUAFS, Kolkata, West Bengal*

[3]*Department of Veterinary Public Health and Epidemiology, Faculty of Veterinary and Animal Sciences, RGSC, BHU, Mirzapur, Uttar Pradesh*

Introduction

Handling and restraining is done to perform different management technique like drenching, dressing, vaccination etc safely, correctly, quickly and painlessly.

Procedure

- Handling should be done gently
- Animal should not be shouted or beaten, always try to call/speak before touching.
- Approach animal from behind and from their left side
- Head and neck portion should be handled first
- Always have the owner or attendant along with you while handling strange animals

Common appliances used in controlling animals

1. **Rope**: essential tool most often used for restraining animals. Cotton rope is preferred for strength, safety and easy to make knots
2. **Halter**: It is used as a least harsh of all restrain methods for animals. Halter are used to teach the animal to lead, to routinely handle them for day to day activities. Halter for horses are made of leather
3. **Anti cow kicker**: it is used for some heifers or cows who react violently while milking or examining the udder. It is also used for animal which are in habit of kicking or jumping up and down during the examination of udder or milking process.

   Anti-cow kicker consists of two metal spring clips connected by a chain. The clips are fitted on the tendo- Achilles region of the hind leg in such a way that in front of the hock chain hangs. Left clip has another smaller clip to which the tail can be fixed.
4. **Bull nose ring**: Nose ring is fitted to the nasal septum of bulls which help a lot for securing and leading the bull as because it causes pain while escaping.

5. **Bull holder**: It helps leading bull for any purpose. It has got a short, central rod, one end of the rod to which two semicircular "bent finger like structure" is affixed and the free smooth ends can be separated and brought close to each other by means of a keeper attached to the centralrod. The other end of the rod is attached with a ring which is used as a handle.
6. **Bull Leader or bull pole**: It is used to lead bulls when attached to the nose ring, which is a pole of 1.5 m length made up of either bamboo or wood. One end of the pole is fixed to a hook and spring lever device. By pulling the rope tied to the spring lever, the hook can be slipped in to the bull nose ring and locked. The hook can be released by reverse action
7. **Drink water gag**: used for examination of mouth by keeping them in between two jaws
8. **Muzzle**: It is made up of rope, string bamboo splits, wire netting, leather/straps which are used to envelope mouth of animals, to prevent them from bitting, self-sucking milk, eating, bedding materials, licking medicine etc applied on the body.
9. **Neck cradle**: It is used to immobilized the neck of animals to prevent the loop from licking of wounds or bandages on their body. This cradle is applied to the neck and tied along the crest to immobilize the neck
10. **Trevis**: this can be used as a best restrain method for many of the management techniques like ear tagging, dehorning and artificial insemination and also for treating animals

Handling of cows: A cow is restrained by grasping both the horns and the nostrils.

Handling Bulls: Bulls are handle with help of nose ring, bull leader. Older bulls should always wear halter. Aggressive bulls may be blind folded by blinkers before handling.

Handling sheep and Goats: To examine a particular animal in a flock, all of them may be brought to a corner and packed tightly to an enclosure. Sheep and goats can be hold by two ways :1) Jaw or chin hold 2) Leg or flank hand

Handling Young Lambs and Kids: For castration and docking, the young lambs and kids are held in a vertical position with the lamb's or kid 's back against the holder. The rear and fore cannon of left and right side are held by left and right hand respectively and then raised on a fixed object in an upright position

Casting: When animals are done for certain examination like shoeing, nail clipping, management of dystocia or prolapse is not feasible in standing position, casting of animal is vital. Commonly used casting method is Reuff's method.

Mutiple Choice Question

1. Throwing animal to the ground is known as:

   a) Casting b) Restraining

   c) Grooming d) Floating

2. Which of the following tools is not used for handling?

   a) Rope b) Bull nose ring

   c) Muzzle d) Ear notcher

3. What is process of controlling the animal?
   a) Restraining b) Castration
   c) Casting d) Ringing
4. How handling should be done?
   a) Gently b) Rudely
   c) Cruelly d) Loudly
5. From which side cow should be approached?
   a) Back b) Front
   c) Top d) None
6. Which part of cattle should be handle first?
   a) Head and neck b) Hind leg
   c) Tail d) Back
7. Anti – cow kicker is fitted to which part of the leg
   a) Archilles tendon of hind leg b) Elbow region of fromt leg
   c) Rump area d) Interdigital space
8. An instrument which has got a short, central rod, one end of the rod to which two semicircular "bent finger like structure" is affixed is known as:
   a) Bull nose ring b) Bull leader
   c) Anti cow kicker d) Muzzle
9. What are the methods of handling Sheep?
   a) Jaw or chin hold b) Leg or flank hand
   c) Both d) None
10. A portion of rope not being worked with except to wrap the running end is known as:
   a) Working part of rope b) Standing part of rope
   c) Blight d) Hitch
11. A turn of rope used for restraining that doesn't cross itself is:
   a) Bight b) Loop
   c) Hitch d) Working end
12. Tension knot of the rope is known as:
   a) Hitch b) Bight
   c) Loop d) Halter
13. Which among the following is a leat harsh method among all restraining method
   a) Halter b) Bull nose ring
   c) Bull leader d) Muzzle
14. Which of the following is not proper attitude for handling of animal
   a) Patient b) Organized approach
   c) Determination d) Rush

15. Which among the following is not a anti- anxiety drugs to facilitate small animal handling?
    a) Diphenhydramine b) Chlorphrniramine
    c) Acepromazine d) Diclofenac
16. What are the risks of animal handling?
    a) Physical injury b) Chemical
    c) Hazadrous manual tasks d) All of the above
17. What are the principle of animal handling?
    a) To avoid excitement of animal
    b) Reducing of stress while handling
    c) Performance and productivity improvement
    d) All of these
18. Muzzle is located in which region? :
    a) Head b) Nose
    c) Mouth d) Tail
19. Why do a good handler gathers knowleged regarding the basic behavior of the farm animal?
    a) Better handling facilitation
    b) Reducing stress
    c) Improve animal welfare and handlersafe
    d) All of the above
20. Studying of animal behavior while handling is known as:
    a) Ethology b) Cosmology
    c) Ichnology d) Ecology
21. Which of the following is not a fundamental animal instincts?
    a) Hunger b) Thirst
    c) Fear d) Colour blind
22. What are the essential element of animal behavior and handling?
    a) Flight zone b) Blind spot
    c) Point of balance d) All of above
23. Which is the personal space where the animal feels comfortable (minimum distance distance between animal and threat)?
    a) Blind spot b) Point of balance
    c) Flight zone d) None
24. Area immediately behind the tail where animal cannot perceive a handler is known as:
    a) Blind spot b) Point of balance
    c) Flight zone d) None

25. "Point of balance" is located in which portion of the animal?
    a) Shoulder b) Rump
    c) Head d) Leg
26. Minimum time duration required for a excited cow to get into normal for handling is:
    a) 30 mint b) 60 mint
    c) 15 mint d) 5 mint
27. A cow first kicks to which direction in stress while handling?
    a) Forward b) Kick Out
    c) Backward d) Kept quite
28. Which among the following are the signs of distress in animal handling
    a) Snoring b) Pawing
    c) Raised ears d) All of the above
29. When does the flight zone of animal dimishes?
    a) Rough handling b) Frequent gentle handling
    c) Both (a) and (b) d) None of the above
30. Anti - cow kicker is used in cows during which activities
    a) Milking b) Examination of Udder
    c) Examination of teats d) All of the above
31. Which of the following is used for handling the animals for longer duration?
    a) Trevis b) Rope
    c) Bull leader d) Muzzle
32. How is common method of handling mice ?
    a) By tail b) By body
    c) By leg d) By neck
33. How is the common method of handling rat ?
    a) By tail b) By body
    c) By leg d) By neck
34. What are the 3R in consideration for animal welfare?
    a) Replacing b) Refining
    c) Reducing d) All of the above
35. How is rabbit handle?
    a) By grabing scruff of the neck in one hand and while other hand placing in rump portion
    b) By tail
    c) By leg
    d) None

36. How is cats handle?
    a) By grasping and holding the back of the head between thumb and fingers
    b) By shoulder
    c) By leg
    d) By tail
37. In which species do E- collar tools is used?
    a) Dog b) Cattle
    c) Sheep d) Horse
38. The mouth examination in cattle is which of the following is used?
    a) Drinkwater's gag b) Linton's gag
    c) Travis d) Drenching gun
39. For mouth examination in sheep which of the following is used?
    a) Drinkwater's gag b) Linton's gag
    c) Travis d) Drenching gun
40. Which of the following is commonest and efficient method of casting cattle/buffalo?
    a) Reuff's Method b) Alternative method
    c) Criss-cross method d) None
41. Pigs are mostly identified by
    a) Tattooing b) Alternative method
    c) Criss-cross method d) None
42. Which of the following is used to prevent kicking in cows
    a) Milkman's rope b) Anti-cow-kicker
    c) Under-Kinch d) All the above
43. At what age nose ring should be applied on bulls
    a) 2 years b) 1.5 years
    c) 2.5 years d) 3 years
44. Device used to immobilize neck of large animals
    a) Cradles b) Nose ring
    c) Mouth gags d) Bull holder
45. Common devises used for restraining sheep are
    a) Linton's mouth gag b) Portable sheep stock
    c) Both a & b d) None of the above
46. Shape of wood in portable sheep stock
    a) X shaped b) V shaped
    c) Y shaped d) A shaped
47. Animals are approached generally from which side?
    a) From right side b) From left side
    c) From centre d) All of the above

48. Which body part of a horse should you avoid when approaching from the rear to prevent startling it?
    a) Tail
    b) Hooves
    c) Ears
    d) Mane
49. What is the primary purpose of proper livestock handling and restraining techniques?
    a) Entertainment
    b) Animal welfare and safety
    c) Crop production
    d) Pest control
50. Understanding the flight zone of livestock is crucial
    a) To calculate their weight
    b) To determine their age
    c) To predict their behaviour and maintain a safe distance
    d) To identify their gender
51. Restraining of animals are generally done for which of the following reasons?
    a) Hoof Trimming
    b) Dressing of affected hoofs and shoeing
    c) Extricating nails, thorns or glass pieces
    d) All of the above
52. Which type of rope is most preferred for restraining cattle
    a) Cotton ropes which is strong, safe and easy to make knots
    b) Strong nylon or polypropylene ropes with smooth surfaces
    c) Wire cables that can cause cuts and injuries
    d) Leather ropes that offer good grip
53. Extremely vicious animals are controlled by
    a) Casting
    b) Narcotic drugs
    c) Halter
    d) Nose ring
54. The most effective way to restrain a sheep for veterinary care is
    a) Trevis or crush
    b) Lassos and rope halters
    c) Casting rope
    d) Round it up into a corner of the field or pen and pack tightly
55. The purpose goal of proper cattle restraint is to:
    a) Perform procedures like vaccination and hoof care
    b) Assert dominance over the animal
    c) Punish the animal for unwanted behaviour
    d) Restrict its movement for entertainment purposes
56. Which of the following should NOT be done while approaching an animal
    a) Approach the animal from behind and on their left side
    b) Call the animal and speak to it before touching it
    c) Carry a stick and signal the animal that you are fearful of it
    d) First handle the head and neck regions of the animal

57. Chutes with headgates are beneficial because:
   a) They completely immobilize the animal, making procedures easier
   b) They provide safe access to specific body parts while minimizing stress
   c) They allow handlers to dominate the animal through physical force
   d) They are inexpensive and easy to build on any farm
58. The most common way to restrain a pig for examination of head and neck regions is
   a) Pig Catcher   b) Twitch on the upper jaw
   c) Casting of pigs   d) Pig net
59. The best way to approach a herd of unfamiliar animals is to
   a) Walk directly towards them in a confident manner
   b) Remain calm, move slowly, and avoid sudden movements
   c) Make loud noises to announce your presence
   d) Approach from behind to avoid startling them
60. Which of the following is incorrect about casting the animals
   a) Casting means throwing the animal on the ground
   b) Pregnant animals should not be casted
   c) Animals are thrown on hard surfaces with stones, bricks, wooden pieces on ground
   d) Animals can be casted on either side
61. Which of the following is NOT a primary reason for casting cattle?
   a) Conducting hoof training and shoeing
   b) Performing surgical operations
   c) Performing dehorning and branding
   d) Training calves for obedience
62. Which of the following is true about using a muzzle
   a) Prevent animals from biting, self-sucking of mil, licking medicines
   b) Should not be fitted tightly
   c) Removed at the time of feeding
   d) All of the above
63. When handling poultry, it is crucial to
   a) Grab them by the wings to lift them off the ground
   b) Pick them up gently by their feet, supporting their body
   c) Toss them in the air and catch them to demonstrate control
   d) Chase them around the coop until they tire out and can be captured
64. The most common narcotic drug used for controlling cattle and buffalo is
   a) Choral hydrate   b) Largactil
   c) Chlorpromazine compounds   d) Barbiturates

65. Which of the following is important while handling cattle
    a) Use force and harsh commands to maintain control
    b) Understand their natural flight response and respect their space
    c) Rely solely on equipment like ropes and halters
    d) Treat them roughly to demonstrate your authority
66. How should a horse be treated in the stable?
    a) All movements must be loud and firm to desensitize the horse
    b) All movements must be quick
    c) All movements must be carried out slowly, calmly and considerately
    d) All movements must be performed terribly.
67. How do you encourage a horse to turn around when it is facing the back of the stable?
    a) Call their name. If that doesn't work, use a treat or food bucket
    b) Come back later when they are at the door
    c) Hit them on the butt with the halter
    d) Come to their front lines and hunt them down
68. Which natural instinct is restricted in the horse's stable?
    a) Flight b) Fighting
    c) Both options are correct d) None
69. What type of halter does not tear or break easily under pressure and is extremely durable?
    a) Leather halter b) Control halter
    c) Nylon halter d) Cotton head collar
70. What type of halter works by putting extra pressure on the horse?
    a) Nose and head that give the handler additional control when leading or handling?
    b) Leather head collar
    c) Control head collar
    d) Nylon head collar
    e) Cotton head collar
71. How does a halter fit correctly on the horse's head?
    a) 4 fingers placed below the protruding cheekbone - 4 fingers wide between them noseband and front of nose.
    b) 2 fingers placed below the prominent cheekbone - 2 fingers wide between them noseband and front of nose.
    c) 3 fingers placed below the prominent cheekbone - 3 fingers wide between them noseband and front of nose.
    d) 1 finger placed below the prominent cheekbone - 3 fingers wide between them noseband and front of nose

72. At what height should the horse be tied?
    a) In a relaxed state, lower than the head, attached to a solid object
    b) When relaxed, higher than your head, attached to a snappable object
    c) At the same level as your head when relaxed, attached to a snap-on object
    d) None
73. What length should the rope be when tying a horse?
    a) It should be long enough to allow the horse to move freely and turn its body around
    b) It should restrict their head and neck movements
    c) Sufficiently long to allow movement of the head and neck without allowing this they should turn around
    d) all of the above
74. What type of knot should be used to tie a horse?
    a) A reef knot
    b) A quick release knot
    c) A Boa knot
    d) A small loosening knot
75. Where should you stand if you consider the horse to be a veterinarian or farrier?
    a) On the opposite side of the worker
    b) On the same side of the horse as the worker
    c) Directly in front of or slightly to the side of the worker
    d) Directly behind the worker or slightly to the side
76. Where should the handler stand when restraining the horse for a show or inspection?
    a) On the opposite side of the observer
    b) On the same side of the horse as the observer
    c) Directly in front or slightly to the side without blocking the view Observer
    d) Directly behind the observer or slightly to the side
77. Why should the horse be trained to stand upright?
    a) It prevents the horse from bucking or rearing up when riding
    b) The horse only needs to be taught to stand straight when competing
    c) It promotes good manners and also makes it easier to get promoted
    d) It promotes bad manners
78. How do you lead a horse correctly?
    a) Hold the horse's head and turn toward the horse to try to pull it forward
    b) Hold the lead rope in your right hand, approximately 5 cm below the horse's Chin, hold the loose part of the lead rope in your left hand
    c) Attach the rope to yourself, wrap it around your hand, or place it around your fingers through the metal loop on the halter or the bit ring.
    d) None

79. When should the correct PPE be worn when handling or leading a horse?
   a) Every time you handle or lead a horse
   b) When handling an excited or unfamiliar horse
   c) When handling a familiar, calm horse
   d) all of the above
80. How should the gate be positioned when a horse is released into the pasture?
   a) Slightly open
   b) Closed
   c) Left wide open
   d) Wide open on the right
81. When should you avoid entering the field to catch a horse?
   a) You should never take horses to pasture
   b) When the horses are impetuous or fight
   c) If there are more than four horses on the field
   d) None
82. How should you behave if a horse is difficult to catch?
   a) Stay calm and patient
   b) Get angry
   c) Be loud and chase the horse around
   d) Do nothing
83. How many horses should you lead at the same time when leaving or bringing in the field time to maintain security?
   a) 1 horse
   b) 2 horses
   c) 3 horses
   d) 4 horses
84. How should a horse be positioned before being put out to pasture?
   a) Facing the gate
   b) Looking at the playing field
   c) The horse's head above the gate and the handler on the other side of the gate
   d) Directed upwards
85. Which answer is NOT a reason to check the field regularly?
   a) To provide them with suitable pastures and to ensure their safety
   b) To prevent the field from being flooded
   c) To keep the horse and the field in good condition
   d) None
86. In which direction should the goal ideally open towards the playing field?
   a) Only inwards
   b) Both internally and externally
   c) Only to the outside
   d) None
87. What restraint methods might be used when leading or handling an unruly horse?
   a) A control halter or bridle
   b) A nylon or leather halter
   c) A lunge whip or school whip
   d) Neck support

88. Why is it important to understand animal behavior during handling?
   a) To maximize speed
   b) To ensure safety, reduce stress and improve efficiency
   c) Ignore signs of distress
   d) To restrict access to feeds
89. What conditions should be observed when handling newborns or young animals?
   a) Ignoring special care needs
   b) Provide proper nutrition, warmth and care
   c) Restricting access to feed
   d) Use of crowded spaces
90. Why is the use of calm handling techniques recommended?
   a) To increase production costs
   b) To ensure safety, reduce stress and improve animal welfare
   c) To restrict access to the feed
   d) Ignoring animal behavior
91. Why is it important to pay attention to hygiene and hygiene when handling poultry?
   a) To increase production costs
   b) To prevent the spread of disease and ensure product safety
   c) To restrict access to the feed
   d) Ignore signs of distress
92. Which of the following injuries is commonly associated with mishandling large livestock farm animals such as cattle and can lead to bone damage?
   a) Avulsion   b) Sprain
   c) Fracture   d) Bruise

e) Farm workers who improperly restrain or handle poultry may risk what kind of poultry there are injuries, often caused by fluttering or violent movements?
   a) Torn ligaments   b) Dislocation
   c) Avulsion   d) Lacerations

93. Farm workers who forcibly restrain animals may expose themselves to bites or kicks that increase the risk of which of the following injuries?
   a) Tendinitis   b) Herniated discs
   c) Avulsion   d) Bruise
94. What procedure is important to ensure the welfare of livestock and poultry during handling and transport?
   a) Rough handling and quick movements
   b) Provide adequate space and ventilation and reduce stress
   c) Restricting access to food and water
   d) Mixing different species without supervision

95. What is a prerequisite for ensuring animal welfare during handling and transport?
   a) Rough handling, rapid movements and overcrowding
   b) Provide adequate space and ventilation and reduce stress
   c) Restricting access to food and water
   d) Ignoring signs of stress and illness

96. Why is it important to provide appropriate training and guidance to staff for handling livestock and poultry?
   a) To increase production costs
   b) To improve skills, knowledge, safety and animal care
   c) Restrict access to veterinary care
   d) To reduce equipment consumption

97. What is the main goal of proper animal handling techniques?
   a) Profit maximization
   b) Ensuring animal welfare and reducing stress
   c) Acceleration of growth rates
   d) Reduction in feed costs

98. What training is essential for staff involved in animal husbandry?
   a) Advanced mathematics
   b) Proper animal behaviour and handling techniques
   c) History and geography
   d) Basic computer skills

99. Why is the use of excessive force when handling livestock not recommended?
   a) Increases production efficiency
   b) Ensures the safety of animals
   c) Causes stress, injuries and reduces productivity
   d) Reduces feed consumption

100. What are the essential requirements for personnel involved in poultry processing?
   a) Wear appropriate protective clothing and footwear
   b) Ignoring bird behavior and signs of distress
   c) Restricting access to clean water
   d) Haste and excessive use of force

101. Why is the use of appropriate handling equipment essential to the safety of farm animals?
   a) To increase production costs
   b) To ensure appropriate restraint and movement and minimize injury
   c) Restrict access to veterinary care
   d) To minimize feed consumption

102. What conditions should be observed when handling poultry?
   a) Ignore signs of illness
   b) Providing adequate housing and avoiding overcrowding
   c) Reduction of ventilation
   d) Use of excessive force

103. Why is understanding certain livestock species and their needs so important?
   a) Ignore special requirements
   b) To adapt handling techniques and ensure welfare
   c) Restrict access to veterinary care
   d) Reducing feed consumption

104. Why is continuous observation and monitoring essential when handling animals?
   a) Ignoring the behavior and needs of animals
   b) To identify problems, ensure safety and adapt handling techniques
   c) Restrict access to veterinary care
   d) To reduce access to food and water

105. Improper lifting or handling techniques can result in the following injuries especially when transporting heavy livestock?
   a) Tendinitis   b) Sprain
   c) avulsion   d) Dislocation

106. Which of the following represents a restriction on the improper handling of livestock and poultry?
   a) Increased production rates
   b) Increased risk of disease and reduced productivity
   c) Improved animal welfare
   d) Reduced feed consumption

107. What is a limitation of inadequate training of personnel handling livestock and Poultry?
   a) Improved animal handling skills and safety
   b) Increased productivity and efficiency
   c) Increased risk of injury to animals and staff
   d) Reduced equipment consumption

108. Why is regular monitoring and maintenance of equipment essential in animal husbandry poultry management?
   a) To increase production costs
   b) To ensure safety, efficiency and functionality
   c) Restrict access to food and water
   d) To reduce labor costs

109. Which answer does NOT mean the horse is happy or relaxed?

a) Ears directed forward or to the side, relaxed muscle tension.

b) Ears pointed back, head lowered, eyes half closed.

c) Ears flat back on the neck, tense body language.

d) None

Answer Key

1	a	2	d	3	a	4	a	5	a	6	a	7	a
8	d	9	c	10	b	11	a	12	b	13	a	14	d
15	d	16	d	17	d	18		19	d	20		21	d
22	d	23	c	24	a	25	a	26	a	27	a	28	d
29	b	30	d	31	a	32	a	33	b	34	d	35	a
36	a	37	a	38	a	39	b	40	a	41	a	42	d
43	b	44	a	45	c	46	c	47	b	48	c	49	b
50	c	51	d	52	a	53	b	54	d	55	a	56	c
57	b	58	a	59	b	60	c	61	d	62	d	63	b
64	a	65	b	66	c	67	a	68	a	69	c	70	
71		72	c	73	c	74	b	75	b	76	c	77	c
78	b	79	a	80	b	81	b	82	a	83	a	84	a
85	b	86	b	87	a	88	b	89	b	90	b	91	b
92	d	93	c	94	b	95	b	96	b	97	b	98	b
99	c	100	a	101	b	102	b	103	b	104	b	105	b
106	b	107	c	108	b	109	c						

5

Climate Change Impact on Livestock Production

R.R.K. Sinha, Alok Bharti, Ravikant Nirala and Abhay Kumar

Bihar Veterinary College, Bihar Animal Sciences University, Patna, Bihar

Introduction

Globally, the climate change is clearly evident in the form of changing weather pattern, and this has direct and indirect bearing on livestock production. Scientific evidence from multiple resources indicates that, without a doubt, climate is changing. It is also possible to suggest with increased confidence that climate is changing because of increased human activities which have serious repercussions on social and economic development. Greenhouse gases absorb heat from the sun in the atmosphere and reduce the amount of heat escaping into space. This extra heat has been found to be the primary cause of observed changes in the climate system over the 20th century. Livestock make a necessary and important contribution to global calorie, protein supplies and important micro nutrients such as B12, iron, calcium. They produce 17% of calories consumed globally and 33% of protein. Livestock can increase the world's edible protein balance by transforming inedible protein found in forage into forms that people can digest. Climate change poses serious threats to livestock production. Various climate model projections suggest that by the year 2100, mean global temperature may be 1.1–6.4 °C warmer than in 2010. Increased temperatures, shifts in rainfall distribution, increased frequency of extreme weather events and consequent increased heat stress and reduced water availability are expected to adversely affect livestock production and productivity around the world both directly and indirectly.

Climate change affects livestock directly through heat stress, altered availability of water and feed resources, and increased prevalence of diseases, as well as indirectly through its impact on grazing lands, feed crop yields, and the socio-economic environment. Here's a closer look at these impacts:

1. Heat Stress

One of the most immediate effects of climate change on livestock is heat stress. High temperatures can lead to a range of physiological problems in animals, including reduced feed intake, lower fertility rates, and in severe cases, heat stroke. Dairy cows, for instance, produce less milk and have lower reproductive performance during heat stress periods. Similarly, meat-producing animals like pigs and poultry show reduced growth rates under high temperatures, which can affect the overall productivity of farms.

2. Water and Feed Availability

Climate change can lead to more frequent and severe droughts, impacting the availability of water and feed for livestock. Water scarcity not only affects animal hydration but also the production of feed crops, leading to higher feed costs and potential nutritional deficiencies. Additionally, changes in rainfall patterns and increased evaporation rates can reduce the productivity of pastures and rangelands, further challenging the sustainability of grazing systems.

3. Disease Prevalence

The distribution and prevalence of livestock diseases are influenced by climate conditions. Warmer temperatures and increased humidity can promote the growth and survival of pathogens and parasites. Climate change can also expand the habitats of various vectors, such as ticks and mosquitoes, leading to the spread of vector-borne diseases to new areas. This not only affects animal health and welfare but also requires greater efforts and resources for disease management and control.

4. Impact on Grazing Lands

The quality and quantity of forage available on grazing lands are directly affected by climate change. Altered precipitation patterns, increased temperatures, and the occurrence of extreme weather events such as floods and droughts can degrade pastures and reduce their carrying capacity. These forces livestock producers to invest in supplementary feed, alter stocking rates, or even relocate their operations, which can have significant economic implications.

5. Socio-economic Impact

The socio-economic impact of climate change on livestock production is profound. Small-scale farmers and pastoralists, particularly in developing countries, are especially vulnerable to climate-induced changes. These communities often depend heavily on livestock for their livelihoods, and their limited capacity to adapt to changing conditions can exacerbate poverty and food insecurity. Moreover, the global nature of agricultural markets means that climate impacts in one region can have ripple effects on food prices and availability worldwide.

Climate adaptation in livestock

Climate change will have far-reaching consequences for dairy and meat production, especially in vulnerable parts of the world where it is vital for nutrition and livelihoods. The impact of climate change can heighten the vulnerability of livestock systems and exacerbate existing stresses upon them, such as drought. Ensuring good animal welfare will be paramount to addressing these challenges; breeds suited to the local environment are often more robust and resilient than industrially farmed breeds.

Conclusion

Adapting to the impacts of climate change on livestock production requires a multi-faceted approach. Strategies include improving the genetic resilience of livestock to heat stress, developing sustainable water management practices, enhancing pasture and feed crop resilience, implementing integrated disease management programs, and investing in research and development. Additionally, policies and practices that reduce greenhouse gas emissions from livestock production can contribute to mitigating the overall impact of climate change. Building resilience in livestock systems is crucial for ensuring food security, supporting rural economies, and protecting the welfare of billions of animals globally in the face of a changing climate.

MCQ on Impact of Climate Change on Livestock Production

1. What is a direct impact of climate change on livestock?
   a) Improved feed quality b) Increased growth rates
   c) Heat stress d) Lower veterinary costs
2. How does heat stress affect dairy cows?
   a) Increases milk production b) Decreases feed intake
   c) Improves fertility d) Reduces water consumption
3. What is a consequence of reduced water availability due to climate change?
   a) Increased pasture growth b) Higher feed costs
   c) Decreased animal diseases d) Improved animal welfare
4. Climate change can lead to an increased prevalence of which of the following?
   a) Frostbite in livestock b) Vector-borne diseases
   c) Genetic mutations d) Cold stress incidents
5. How might climate change indirectly affect livestock production?
   a) By increasing global meat demand
   b) Through altering grazing land productivity
   c) By reducing the cost of farm inputs
   d) Through decreasing atmospheric CO2 levels
6. Which livestock is particularly vulnerable to heat stress?
   a) Fish b) Pigs
   c) Bees d) Sheep
7. What adaptation strategy can help livestock cope with heat stress?
   a) Decreasing water availability
   b) Providing shade and cooling systems
   c) Reducing feed intake
   d) Increasing the herd size
8. Drought conditions can lead to:
   a) Improved forage quality
   b) Increased water resources
   c) Nutritional deficiencies in livestock
   d) Lower electricity consumption on farms
9. What role does climate change play in the spread of livestock diseases?
   a) It has no significant impact
   b) It reduces disease incidence
   c) It can change disease dynamics and spread
   d) It solely affects aquatic species

10. Climate change impacts on livestock can exacerbate:
    a) Technological advancements
    b) Food security
    c) Genetic diversity
    d) Urbanization trends
11. Which strategy is NOT effective in adapting to climate change in livestock production?
    a) Intensive breeding for heat tolerance
    b) Overgrazing to maximize short-term gains
    c) Improved water harvesting techniques
    d) Changing livestock species or breeds to more resilient ones
12. What is a potential socio-economic impact of climate change on livestock farming?
    a) Decreased dependence on livestock for livelihoods
    b) Increased resilience to market fluctuations
    c) Greater vulnerability for smallholder and subsistence farmers
    d) More stable global meat prices
13. How does climate change affect the nutritional value of pasture and forage crops?
    a) Increases protein content uniformly
    b) No significant impact
    c) Can reduce nutritional quality
    d) Leads to higher carbohydrate content in all plant species
14. Which of the following is an indirect effect of climate change on livestock through feed crops?
    a) Enhanced taste of feed
    b) Increased crop yields across all regions
    c) Fluctuations in feed prices
    d) Uniform feed availability globally
15. Increased CO_2 levels can affect plant growth. How does this relate to livestock production?
    a) Leads to decreased feed costs due to higher crop yields
    b) No effect, as CO_2 levels do not affect plants
    c) Can change the nutritional profile of crops, and so animal feed quality
    d) Increases meat quality directly
16. What is an effective disease management strategy in the context of climate change?
    a) Reducing genetic diversity
    b) Using antibiotics indiscriminately
    c) Integrated disease surveillance and control
    d) Ignoring vector control practices
17. Climate change may require livestock producers to:
    a) Focus solely on increasing herd size
    b) Shift to monoculture farming practices
    c) Consider alternative and more resilient livestock species
    d) Avoid investing in technology and infrastructure

18. What impact does extreme weather events have on livestock?
    a) They have a calming effect on animals
    b) Increase in feed efficiency
    c) Lead to loss of livestock and infrastructure
    d) Enhance animal breeding cycles
19. Reducing greenhouse gas emissions from livestock can:
    a) Worsen climate change impacts
    b) Have no effect on climate change
    c) Mitigate the overall impact of climate change
    d) Increase the vulnerability of livestock to diseases
20. The increase in ambient temperatures affects livestock reproduction by:
    a) Enhancing fertility rates uniformly
    b) Causing heat stress that can lower fertility
    c) Increasing gestation periods
    d) Having no impact on reproduction
21. Adaptation measures in livestock production to combat climate change include all EXCEPT:
    a) Ignoring early warning systems for extreme weather
    b) Genetic selection for traits conferring resilience to climate stressors
    c) Enhancing water use efficiency
    d) Diversifying livestock and crop systems
22. What is the role of technology in adapting livestock production to climate change?
    a) It is largely irrelevant
    b) To increase dependency on chemical inputs
    c) To enhance resilience through better management and efficiency
    d) To reduce the need for human labor only
23. How can climate change affect the availability of grazing land?
    a) It can increase availability uniformly worldwide
    b) It does not affect grazing land
    c) Can lead to degradation and reduced carrying capacity
    d) Ensures more consistent quality of pasture
24. The shift in geographical distribution of certain diseases due to climate change means that livestock producers must:
    a) Focus only on traditional diseases
    b) Prepare for emerging and re-emerging diseases
    c) Ignore changes in disease patterns
    d) Rely solely on natural immunity

25. Climate change has the potential to disrupt which of the following in livestock production?
    a) Only the internal temperature regulation of animals
    b) Feed and water supply, disease patterns, and production efficiency
    c) The global positioning of farms only
    d) None of the above
26. Which of the following best describes the impact of climate change on feed crop production for livestock?
    a) Guaranteed increase in yields globally
    b) Unaffected by changing climate conditions
    c) Potential for reduced yields and altered nutritional content
    d) Increased yields due to higher CO_2 levels only
27. In the face of climate change, water conservation practices in livestock production are important because:
    a) Water is infinite and needs to be conserved for future use only
    b) They help mitigate the effects of drought and ensure sustainability
    c) Livestock do not actually need much water
    d) Climate change does not affect water resources
28. The relationship between livestock production and climate change is:
    a) One-way, with climate change affecting livestock only
    b) Bidirectional, as livestock production also contributes to climate change
    c) Non-existent, as they do not influence each other
    d) Only relevant in tropical regions
29. Adaptation to climate change in livestock production may require changes in:
    a) Only livestock genetics
    b) Management practices, genetics, and infrastructure
    c) The price of meat and dairy products only
    d) Public perception only
30. The ultimate goal of adapting livestock production to climate change is to:
    a) Maximize short-term profits
    b) Ensure long-term sustainability and resilience
    c) Reduce the global livestock population
    d) Eliminate the need for veterinary services
31. How does climate change primarily affect livestock?
    a) By improving pasture quality
    b) By reducing the incidence of pests
    c) By increasing heat stress
    d) By decreasing feed and water availability

32. Which greenhouse gas is predominantly produced by ruminant digestion and contributes to climate change?
    a) Carbon dioxide (CO_2)
    b) Nitrous oxide (N_2O)
    c) Methane (CH_4)
    d) Chlorofluorocarbons (CFCs)
33. What adaptation strategy can help livestock cope with increased heat stress due to climate change?
    a) Decreasing water availability
    b) Reducing shade and shelter
    c) Implementing heat-tolerant animal breeds
    d) Increasing the use of antibiotics
34. Climate change can lead to a higher incidence of certain diseases in livestock due to:
    a) Improved veterinary medicines
    b) The expansion of disease vectors into new areas
    c) Less interaction between wild and domestic animals
    d) Decreased humidity and rainfall
35. Which of the following is a direct impact of climate change on livestock water resources?
    a) Increased water quality
    b) Increased water availability in all regions
    c) Reduced water availability due to drought
    d) Unchanged water consumption by animals
36. How does climate change affect the nutritional quality of forage that livestock depend on?
    a) Increases protein content uniformly
    b) No significant impact
    c) Decreases diversity of available forage
    d) Can reduce nutritional quality due to plant stress
37. Mitigation strategies to reduce the carbon footprint of livestock production include:
    a) Increasing the number of livestock
    b) Improving feed efficiency and management
    c) Reducing efforts to capture methane emissions
    d) Encouraging deforestation for pasture expansion
38. The concept of 'climate-smart agriculture' includes the following practices except:
    a) Increasing the use of fossil fuels in production
    b) Promoting sustainable land management
    c) Enhancing resilience to climate impacts
    d) Improving productivity in a sustainable manner

39. Increased carbon dioxide levels can affect plant growth and forage quality. This is known as:
    a) The albedo effect
    b) Carbon fertilization effect
    c) Methane feedback loop
    d) Nitrous oxide paradox
40. What role does livestock play in contributing to climate change?
    a) They have no impact on greenhouse gas emissions
    b) They primarily emit nitrous oxide through waste
    c) They are a major source of methane emissions
    d) They absorb carbon dioxide through respiration
41. What is a primary socio-economic impact of increased heat stress on livestock due to climate change?
    a) Increased livestock productivity
    b) Decreased need for water
    c) Reduced livestock productivity
    d) Increased availability of forage
42. How does climae change affect the livelihoods of pastoral communities?
    a) By increasing the predictability of weather patterns
    b) By decreasing the incidence of livestock diseases
    c) By reducing grazing land and water resources
    d) By increasing the global market price for meat
43. Climate change can lead to conflicts among livestock farming communities due to:
    a) Increased cooperation over water resources
    b) Reduced competition for grazing lands
    c) Enhanced community resilience
    d) Scarcity of water and grazing land
44. What adaptation strategy can help livestock farming communities cope with the economic impacts of climate change?
    a) Decreasing the size of their herds
    b) Diversifying income sources
    c) Relocating to urban areas
    d) Focusing solely on livestock farming
45. Which of the following is a potential impact of climate change on dairy farming?
    a) Increased milk production year-round
    b) Decreased vulnerability to heat stress
    c) Increased costs for cooling and water
    d) Decreased feed costs
46. The increased incidence of livestock diseases due to climate change affects farming communities by:
    a) Reducing the need for veterinary services
    b) Decreasing the cost of livestock management
    c) Increasing livestock mortality rates
    d) Enhancing genetic diversity of livestock

47. Climate-induced migration among livestock farming communities is often a result of:
    a) Improved pasture management techniques
    b) Increased availability of agricultural land
    c) Loss of grazing land and water
    d) Decreased livestock diseases
48. Insurance schemes for livestock farmers affected by climate change can:
    a) Increase vulnerability to climate risks
    b) Discourage adaptation measures
    c) Provide a safety net against climate-related losses
    d) Lead to overgrazing and land degradation
49. How does climate change impact the nutritional security of communities dependent on livestock?
    a) By increasing the diversity of available food
    b) By improving the nutritional content of livestock products
    c) By reducing the availability and quality of livestock products
    d) By decreasing food prices
50. The role of women in livestock farming communities can be particularly affected by climate change due to:
    a) Increased leisure time
    b) Reduced workload in livestock management
    c) Enhanced access to resources and decision-making
    d) Limited access to resources and increased workload
51. Investing in what area is considered crucial for enhancing the resilience of livestock farming communities to climate change?
    a) Reducing livestock numbers universally
    b) Focusing solely on crop agriculture
    c) Research and development for climate-resilient livestock breeds
    d) Eliminating traditional knowledge systems
52. What is an indirect socio-economic effect of climate change on livestock farming communities?
    a) Direct loss of livestock due to heat stress
    b) Immediate reduction in feed costs
    c) Shifts in agricultural labor markets
    d) Instant increase in water availability
53. How does climate change exacerbate gender inequalities in livestock farming communities?
    a) By equally distributing resources between genders
    b) By providing more education opportunities for women
    c) By increasing women's access to land and capital
    d) By increasing women's burdens and reducing their access to resources

54. Community-based adaptation strategies for climate change in livestock farming include:
    a) Ignoring traditional knowledge and practices
    b) Sole reliance on government support
    c) Collective action and sharing of best practices
    d) Focusing on individual efforts only
55. The introduction of climate-resilient livestock breeds can impact farming communities by:
    a) Decreasing genetic diversity
    b) Increasing dependence on technological solutions
    c) Improving productivity and livelihoods
    d) Reducing the need for adaptation strategies
56. What is a primary effect of drought on livestock production?
    a) Increased feed availability
    b) Improved water quality
    c) Reduced feed availability
    d) Decreased livestock diseases
57. Floods can directly impact livestock by causing:
    a) Enhanced growth rates
    b) Increased feed efficiency
    c) Loss of habitat
    d) Decreased water needs
58. Which of the following is a common indirect effect of drought on livestock?
    a) Increased forage quality
    b) Reduced water scarcity
    c) Increased vulnerability to diseases
    d) Decreased production costs
59. How can livestock producers mitigate the impact of drought on their herds?
    a) By reducing the size of their herds
    b) Increasing the size of their herds
    c) Decreasing water supplies
    d) Ignoring weather forecasts
60. During floods, what is a crucial action for livestock safety?
    a) Moving livestock to higher ground
    b) Keeping livestock in low-lying areas
    c) Reducing feed intake
    d) Increasing water consumption
61. Drought conditions can lead to a shortage of which essential resource for livestock?
    a) Sunlight
    b) Oxygen
    c) Water
    d) Shelter
62. What long-term strategy can help livestock production systems become more resilient to floods and droughts?
    a) Decreasing genetic diversity in herds
    b) Increasing reliance on a single water source
    c) Developing drought- and flood-tolerant forage varieties
    d) Reducing the number of water storage facilities

63. Floods can lead to an increased risk of which condition in livestock?
    a) Dehydration
    b) Foot rot and other hoof diseases
    c) Heat stress
    d) Weight gain
64. How does drought affect the nutritional value of forage for livestock?
    a) Increases protein content
    b) No significant effect
    c) Decreases overall nutritional value
    d) Makes forage more palatable
65. Which management practice is effective in protecting livestock during extreme weather events such as floods?
    a) Maintaining a single, large water source
    b) Constructing elevated housing and shelters
    c) Decreasing herd mobility
    d) Ignoring weather warnings
66. What is a potential effect of prolonged drought on livestock breeding?
    a) Increased fertility rates
    b) No impact on breeding cycles
    c) Decreased birth rates
    d) Shorter gestation periods
67. Floods can contaminate water sources, leading to an increased risk of:
    a) Drought
    b) Waterborne diseases
    c) Sunburn
    d) Frostbite
68. Which adaptation measure can help livestock cope with the scarcity of water during droughts?
    a) Providing salt licks
    b) Reducing shade areas
    c) Implementing water-saving technologies
    d) Increasing grain feed
69. The immediate aftermath of a flood can disrupt livestock production by causing:
    a) An oversupply of feed
    b) Improved access to markets
    c) Transportation challenges
    d) Lower humidity levels
70. Drought resilience in livestock can be improved through:
    a) Selective breeding for traits such as drought tolerance
    b) Increasing the concentration of livestock in small areas
    c) Delaying the provision of water to increase tolerance
    d) Sole reliance on natural water sources
71. How does climate change primarily affect the quality of grazing land for livestock?
    a) By uniformly increasing land fertility
    b) Through increased variability in rainfall
    c) By decreasing daytime temperatures
    d) Through decreased carbon dioxide levels

72. What is a direct impact of prolonged drought conditions on grazing lands?
    a) Enhanced plant growth
    b) Increased water availability
    c) Reduced forage quality and quantity
    d) Lowered soil acidity
73. Climate change can lead to an increase in which of the following on grazing lands?
    a) Soil moisture
    b) Invasive plant species
    c) Perennial grasses
    d) Ice cover
74. Increased CO_2 levels associated with climate change may initially benefit grazing lands by:
    a) Reducing plant growth
    b) Increasing plant growth
    c) Decreasing soil fertility
    d) Increasing soil salinity
75. How does the alteration of precipitation patterns affect livestock grazing lands?
    a) By making them consistently wetter
    b) Through the promotion of desertification
    c) By reducing erosion
    d) Through decreased evaporation rates
76. What effect does climate change have on the water supply for grazing lands?
    a) Stabilizes seasonal water supplies
    b) Increases water supply reliability
    c) Leads to more frequent and severe droughts
    d) Decreases evapo-transpiration rates
77. Climate change is expected to increase the frequency of which phenomenon, impacting grazing lands negatively?
    a) Snowfall
    b) Wildfires
    c) Frosts
    d) Heavy rainfall events
78. The encroachment of shrubs onto grazing lands, a consequence of climate change, results in:
    a) Improved soil quality
    b) More stable water supplies
    c) Decreased forage availability for livestock
    d) Reduced erosion
79. What strategy can help mitigate the effects of climate change on grazing lands?
    a) Reducing livestock numbers
    b) Increasing the use of fertilizers
    c) Planting non-native grass species
    d) Rotational grazing practices
80. How does climate change affect the nutritional content of forage on grazing lands?
    a) Increases protein content across all plant species
    b) Leads to a uniform increase in nutritional quality
    c) Can decrease the nutritional value of forage
    d) Does not affect nutritional content

81. What impact does the increased frequency of extreme weather events have on grazing lands?
   a) Makes them more resilient
   b) Reduces the incidence of invasive species
   c) Causes soil compaction and erosion
   d) Increases biodiversity
82. Climate change-induced alterations in grazing land ecosystems can lead to:
   a) A decrease in predator species
   b) Increased carbon sequestration
   c) Shifts in plant and animal species composition
   d) Lower atmospheric CO2 levels
83. The melting of permafrost due to global warming affects grazing lands in Arctic regions by:
   a) Decreasing available land for grazing
   b) Increasing the land available for grazing
   c) Reducing methane emissions
   d) Enhancing permafrost stability
84. Sustainable management practices on grazing lands, important in the context of climate change, include:
   a) Increasing stock density
   b) Monoculture planting
   c) Integrated pest management
   d) Removal of all woody plants
85. Which of the following is a predicted outcome of climate change for grazing lands in semi-arid regions?
   a) Reduced evapo-transpiration
   b) Increased rainfall and flooding
   c) More frequent and intense droughts
   d) Decrease in daytime temperatures
86. The phenomenon of 'green-up' in grazing lands refers to:
   a) The conversion of forests into grazing land
   b) The early onset of spring vegetation growth due to warmer temperatures
   c) The implementation of sustainable grazing practices
   d) The restoration of degraded grazing lands
87. In the context of climate change, adaptive grazing management might include:
   a) Strictly maintaining historical stocking rates
   b) Flexibility in stocking rates based on forage availability
   c) Elimination of all grazing to protect soil
   d) Year-round grazing without rotation
88. Climate change impacts on grazing land hydrology can lead to:
   a) More predictable water cycles
   b) Decreased incidence of flash floods
   c) Changes in stream flows and water availability
   d) Increased water storage capacity in soils

89. Increased atmospheric CO2 levels can affect plant species composition on grazing lands by:
   a) Favoring C4 over C3 plants
   b) Favoring C3 over C4 plants
   c) Uniformly benefiting all plant types
   d) Reducing the growth of all plants

90. What role does biodiversity play in the resilience of grazing lands to climate change?
   a) High biodiversity generally reduces resilience
   b) Biodiversity has no impact on resilience
   c) High biodiversity can increase resilience to climate impacts
   d) Only specific species contribute to resilience, not biodiversity

91. Warmer climates can increase the population of which type of livestock pests?
   a) Ice-adapted species
   b) Desert-adapted species
   c) Tropical and subtropical vectors
   d) Arctic vectors

92. The melting of permafrost due to global warming can potentially release:
   a) Previously unknown beneficial bacteria
   b) Ancient viruses with no current immunity in livestock
   c) Heat-resistant pathogens
   d) Cold-loving bacteria beneficial to livestock

93. How does climate change affect the vaccination strategies for livestock diseases?
   a) Makes them more effective year-round
   b) Requires adjustments due to shifting disease patterns
   c) Eliminates the need for vaccinations
   d) None of the above

94. Increased carbon dioxide levels can lead to more lush vegetation, which can affect livestock diseases by:
   a) Reducing food availability and increasing disease
   b) Increasing the habitat for disease-carrying insects
   c) Directly killing off disease vectors
   d) None of the above

95. Climate change-induced stress in livestock can lead to:
   a) Improved disease resistance
   b) A weakened immune system, making them more susceptible to diseases
   c) No change in disease susceptibility
   d) Increased lifespan

96. Drought conditions associated with climate change can lead to an increased prevalence of which disease due to concentrated animal populations around dwindling water sources?
   a) Aquatic diseases
   b) Airborne diseases
   c) Contagious ecthyma (Orf)
   d) Anthrax

97. Which climate change effect can exacerbate the spread of avian influenza among poultry?
    a) Decreased rainfall
    b) Increased interaction with wild birds migrating over longer distances
    c) Colder summer temperatures
    d) Higher CO_2 levels in the atmosphere
98. Rising temperatures can change the epidemiology of livestock diseases by:
    a) Making all diseases less common
    b) Creating a uniform disease profile worldwide
    c) Affecting the seasonal and geographic distribution of diseases
    d) Only affecting tropical regions
99. How does climate variability affect parasitic diseases in livestock?
    a) By making parasites less virulent
    b) By disrupting the life cycles of parasites, potentially reducing their numbers
    c) By creating more favorable conditions for parasite survival and reproduction
    d) Climate has no effect on parasitic diseases
100. What is the impact of heavy and unpredictable rainfall patterns on livestock disease management?
    a) Makes disease management easier due to predictable patterns
    b) Leads to more consistent and effective use of preventative measures
    c) Can wash away preventive treatments and increase disease spread through water
    d) Has no real impact on disease management
101. The reduction in biodiversity due to climate change can affect livestock diseases by:
    a) Decreasing the number of diseases
    b) Increasing disease resistance in livestock
    c) Leading to the emergence of new diseases and pests
    d) Making existing diseases less virulent
102. Which approach is recommended for managing livestock diseases in a changing climate?
    a) Reducing dependence on chemical treatments
    b) Increasing the use of antibiotics as a preventive measure
    c) Integrated disease management combining vaccination, biosecurity, and environmental management
    d) Focusing solely on genetic resistance
103. Climate change can influence the nutritional content of forage crops, affecting livestock health by:
    a) Increasing their resistance to diseases
    b) Making them more susceptible to nutritional deficiencies and related diseases
    c) No impact as livestock can adapt quickly to changes in nutritional content
    d) Improving the taste of forage crops without affecting nutritional content

104. What is the role of remote sensing technology in managing climate change impacts on livestock diseases?
   a) It has no role in managing livestock diseases
   b) It can predict climate change but not its impact on diseases
   c) It helps in early detection of disease outbreaks by monitoring environmental changes
   d) It is only used for weather prediction

105. How does the alteration in sea levels influence saltwater intrusion into freshwater resources, affecting livestock?
   a) It has no significant impact on livestock
   b) Leads to improved water quality for livestock
   c) Can cause water scarcity and increase the risk of salinity-related diseases
   d) Only affects coastal livestock farms

106. Increased atmospheric CO_2 levels contribute to plant growth. How does this affect livestock diseases?
   a) Enhances plant defenses against diseases, indirectly benefiting livestock
   b) May lead to overgrazing, stressing the livestock and increasing disease susceptibility
   c) Directly reduces livestock diseases by improving air quality
   d) No effect; plant growth and livestock diseases are unrelated

107. What impact does climate change have on the practice of mixed farming and its relation to livestock disease dynamics?
   a) Encourages monoculture practices, reducing disease spread
   b) Increases biodiversity, thereby reducing disease prevalence
   c) Can lead to closer interaction between livestock and crops, potentially increasing disease vectors
   d) Has no impact on farming practices or disease dynamics

108. The increased use of air conditioning in barns to combat heat stress in livestock can lead to:
   a) Lower disease rates due to controlled environments
   b) Increased respiratory diseases due to poor air quality
   c) No change in disease prevalence
   d) Enhanced growth rates overshadowing any disease increases

109. Climate change's impact on migratory patterns of birds can affect livestock by:
   a) Decreasing the chance of disease transmission
   b) Increasing biodiversity and ecological balance
   c) Introducing new pathogens to which livestock have no immunity
   d) Having no effect as birds and livestock do not share diseases

110. The relationship between climate change and antimicrobial resistance in livestock diseases is characterized by:
   a) No correlation; antimicrobial resistance is solely a result of drug misuse
   b) An indirect effect, where climate stressors can increase the use of antibiotics, potentially leading to higher resistance rates
   c) A direct increase in resistance due to higher temperatures alone
   d) A decrease in antimicrobial resistance due to climate-induced changes in disease vectors

111. Climate change can influence the distribution of vector-borne diseases in livestock by:
   a) Decreasing the range of vectors
   b) Limiting vector lifespan
   c) Expanding the habitats suitable for vectors
   d) Eradicating disease vectors

112. Which factor related to climate change is known to increase the prevalence of respiratory diseases in livestock?
   a) Increased CO_2 levels   b) Higher temperatures
   c) Increased humidity   d) Decreased rainfall

113. How does climate change potentially affect the lifecycle of parasites affecting livestock?
   a) By shortening their lifecycle, reducing disease spread
   b) By extending their active and reproductive periods
   c) By limiting their mobility and spread
   d) By making them less resilient to environmental conditions

114. Increased temperatures associated with climate change can lead to a higher incidence of which type of diseases in livestock?
   a) Frostbite   b) Heat stress-related conditions
   c) Cold-related respiratory diseases   d) None of the above

115. What impact does climate change have on the availability of clean water sources for livestock, potentially affecting disease prevalence?
   a) Improves water quality and availability
   b) Has no significant impact
   c) Reduces water quality and availability, increasing disease risk
   d) Increases water availability but reduces quality

116. Floods, becoming more common due to climate change, can lead to an increase in:
   a) Drought-resistant diseases   b) Waterborne diseases
   c) Heat stress conditions   d) Vector inactivity

117. Climate change can alter the geographic range of livestock diseases by:
    a) Restricting diseases to their current locations
    b) Causing diseases to move into previously unaffected areas
    c) Eliminating diseases in warmer areas
    d) Decreasing overall disease prevalence
118. Which of the following is a direct effect of warmer winters on livestock disease prevalence?
    a) Reduced survival of disease vectors
    b) Increased survival and activity of disease vectors
    c) Decreased livestock immunity
    d) None of the above
119. Climate change is expected to increase the risk of which disease in areas with increased rainfall and humidity?
    a) Dehydration-related conditions
    b) Skin diseases, such as fungal infections
    c) Respiratory diseases caused by dry air
    d) Diseases related to extreme cold
120. The alteration of migration patterns in wild animals due to climate change can affect livestock diseases by:
    a) Decreasing the genetic diversity of livestock
    b) Reducing the incidence of diseases
    c) Introducing new diseases to livestock populations
    d) Improving livestock resilience to diseases
121. How does the increase in CO_2 levels associated with climate change potentially affect plant-based diseases affecting livestock?
    a) By decreasing the nutritional value of plants, weakening livestock
    b) By increasing the growth rate of pathogenic fungi
    c) By eradicating plant diseases
    d) No significant effect
122. What role does climate change play in the development of antibiotic resistance in livestock diseases?
    a) No significant role
    b) Directly reduces antibiotic resistance
    c) May accelerate the spread of antibiotic resistance due to increased disease pressure
    d) Completely eliminates antibiotic-resistant diseases
123. Rising sea levels, a result of climate change, can affect livestock disease by:
    a) Improving coastal farmland salinity
    b) Reducing the habitat for disease vectors
    c) Increasing the salinity of freshwater sources, affecting livestock health
    d) Decreasing overall humidity levels

124. Extreme weather events, more frequent due to climate change, can lead to livestock diseases by:
   a) Forcing livestock into closer quarters, increasing transmission rates
   b) Decreasing the livestock population directly
   c) Improving livestock health and resilience
   d) Reducing the prevalence of chronic diseases

125. Drought conditions can exacerbate which type of diseases in livestock?
   a) Diseases related to excessive moisture, such as foot rot
   b) Respiratory diseases due to improved air quality
   c) Parasitic infestations due to concentrated animal populations around water sources
   d) Cold-related diseases due to decreased temperatures

126. Climate change impacts the nutrient cycle in grazing lands, which can affect livestock diseases by:
   a) Enhancing the immunity of livestock through improved nutrition
   b) Reducing the occurrence of diseases due to better plant health
   c) Leading to nutritional deficiencies that weaken livestock
   d) Increasing the protein content in forage, reducing disease susceptibility

127. How does increased atmospheric humidity, a result of climate change, affect ectoparasite populations on livestock?
   a) Decreases their survival rate
   b) Has no significant impact
   c) Increases their survival and reproduction rates
   d) Reduces their reproductive cycle duration

128. The shift in plant species composition due to climate change can influence livestock diseases by:
   a) Reducing the variety of diseases
   b) Eliminating all plant-based diseases
   c) Changing the types of diseases due to new plant-host vectors
   d) Directly increasing livestock immunity to diseases

129. Which climate change effect can lead to an increased risk of bluetongue virus in livestock?
   a) Cooler temperatures reducing vector populations
   b) Increased carbon sequestration
   c) Warmer and wetter conditions favoring vector proliferation
   d) Reduced rainfall and drier conditions

130. How does the alteration of seasonal patterns by climate change affect disease outbreaks in livestock?
   a) Makes outbreaks more predictable
   b) Has no effect on the timing or severity of outbreaks
   c) Can lead to more unpredictable and severe outbreaks
   d) Limits outbreaks to winter months
131. The expansion of arid areas due to climate change is likely to increase the prevalence of:
   a) Waterborne diseases
   b) Diseases associated with high moisture levels
   c) Tick-borne diseases due to decreased host availability
   d) Heat stress and related conditions
132. Climate change affects the biological control agents of livestock pests by:
   a) Making them more effective across all regions
   b) Reducing their effectiveness due to mismatched life cycles with pests
   c) Increasing their population indiscriminately
   d) No effect, as biological agents adapt quickly
133. An increase in extreme weather events can disrupt veterinary supply chains, leading to:
   a) More consistent disease management
   b) Improved access to veterinary medicines
   c) Delays in disease treatment and prevention
   d) Decreased costs for livestock healthcare
134. The effect of climate change on feed crop production can indirectly influence livestock disease by:
   a) Ensuring a stable supply of nutritious feed
   b) Causing nutritional deficiencies that may predispose livestock to disease
   c) Eliminating the need for supplemental feed
   d) Decreasing the reliance on feed crops
135. Altered wind patterns due to climate change can affect livestock diseases by:
   a) Decreasing the dispersal of airborne pathogens
   b) Increasing the dispersal and range of airborne pathogens
   c) Having no impact on the spread of diseases
   d) Reducing overall wind speeds globally
136. Climate-induced changes in agricultural practices can lead to livestock diseases by:
   a) Reducing the diversity of crops, limiting disease vectors
   b) Forcing shifts to crops that may host new diseases
   c) Eliminating the use of pesticides and herbicides
   d) Increasing the genetic diversity of livestock

137. Increased CO_2 levels can contribute to the growth of which type of pathogens affecting livestock?
   a) Pathogens that are less virulent
   b) Pathogens that thrive in lower temperatures
   c) Fungal pathogens due to changes in plant physiology
   d) Viruses due to increased UV radiation

138. How do warmer ocean temperatures affect marine-based diseases that can impact coastal livestock?
   a) By decreasing the survival rate of marine pathogens
   b) Increasing the range and virulence of marine pathogens
   c) Eliminating all marine-based diseases
   d) Cooling the ocean, reducing pathogen spread

139. The interaction between climate change and wildlife can affect livestock diseases by:
   a) Isolating wildlife from livestock, reducing disease transmission
   b) Decreasing the biodiversity necessary for disease spread
   c) Facilitating the cross-species transmission of pathogens
   d) Completely separating disease ecosystems

140. Mitigation strategies against climate change-induced livestock diseases include:
   a) Reducing genetic diversity among livestock
   b) Increasing the use of broad-spectrum antibiotics
   c) Enhancing surveillance and early detection systems
   d) Ignoring climate predictions in agricultural planning

141. How does climate change primarily affect water availability for livestock?
   a) By uniformly increasing rainfall worldwide
   b) Through more frequent and severe droughts
   c) By creating new freshwater sources
   d) None of the above

142. Which of the following feed crops is most susceptible to yield fluctuation due to extreme weather conditions caused by climate change?
   a) Genetically modified crops designed for drought resistance
   b) Traditional cereal grains like wheat and corn
   c) Deep-rooted crops like alfalfa
   d) Cactus and other drought-resistant forages

143. Climate change can alter the nutritional quality of pastures by:
   a) Increasing their protein content consistently
   b) Decreasing the diversity of plant species available
   c) Increasing the fiber content, making them less digestible
   d) None of the above

144. Increased CO_2 levels can affect plant growth. How does this impact livestock feed availability?
   a) Leads to increased yields of all crop types
   b) Primarily boosts the growth of C3 plants over C4 plants, affecting feed variety
   c) Reduces overall feed crop yields due to accelerated weed competition
   d) Has no significant effect on feed availability

145. Adaptation strategies for ensuring water availability for livestock in a changing climate include:
   a) Expanding desert grazing areas
   b) Relying on natural water sources without human intervention
   c) Implementing water harvesting and storage systems
   d) Decreasing livestock numbers to reduce water demand

146. The impact of climate change on feed crop pests and diseases is expected to:
   a) Decrease significantly due to higher temperatures
   b) Increase, affecting both yield and quality of livestock feed
   c) Remain unchanged as pests and diseases adapt at the same rate as crops
   d) Only affect crops in cooler, temperate regions

147. Which livestock adaptation strategy can help cope with reduced feed quality due to climate change?
   a) Increasing reliance on synthetic feeds
   b) Supplementing diets with vitamins and minerals
   c) Focusing solely on grazing without supplements
   d) Reducing livestock numbers to match available feed quality

148. How does climate change-induced heat stress affect livestock's water needs?
   a) Decreases water needs as animals eat less
   b) Increases water needs due to higher respiration rates
   c) Has no effect on water needs but changes feeding behavior
   d) Reduces overall metabolic rates, decreasing water needs

149. What role does agroforestry play in mitigating the effects of climate change on livestock feed and water availability?
   a) Provides shade and reduces evaporation from soil and water sources
   b) Agroforestry has no impact on livestock resources
   c) Increases competition for water between trees and feed crops
   d) Reduces land available for feed crops

Answer Key

1	c	2	b	3	b	4	b	5	b	6	b	7	b
8	c	9	c	10	b	11	b	12	c	13	c	14	c
15	c	16	c	17	c	18	c	19	c	20	b	21	a
22	c	23	c	24	b	25	b	26	c	27	b	28	b
29	b	30	b	31	c	32	c	33	c	34	b	35	d
36	d	37	b	38	a	39	b	40	c	41	c	42	c
43	d	44	b	45	c	46	c	47	c	48	c	49	c
50	d	51	c	52	c	53	d	54	c	55	c	56	c
57	c	58	c	59	a	60	a	61	c	62	c	63	b
64	c	65	b	66	c	67	b	68	c	69	c	70	a
71	b	72	c	73	b	74	b	75	b	76	c	77	b
78	c	79	d	80	c	81	c	82	c	83	a	84	c
85	c	86	b	87	b	88	c	89	b	90	c	91	c
92	b	93	b	94	b	95	b	96	d	97	b	98	c
99	c	100	c	101	c	102	c	103	b	104	c	105	c
106	b	107	c	108	b	109	c	110	b	111	c	112	c
113	b	114	b	115	c	116	b	117	b	118	b	119	b
120	c	121	b	122	c	123	c	124	a	125	c	126	c
127	c	128	c	129	c	130	c	131	d	132	b	133	c
134	b	135	b	136	b	137	c	138	b	139	c	140	c
141	b	142	b	143	b	144	b	145	c	146	b	147	b
148	b	149	a	150	b								

6

Impact of Stress on Livestock Production

R.R.K. Sinha, Abhay Kumar, Kaushalendra Kumar and Alok Bharti

Bihar Veterinary College, Bihar Animal Sciences University, Patna, Bihar

Introduction

Livestock production plays a critical role in global food security and economic sustainability. However, various stressors can significantly impact the well-being and productivity of livestock animals. Stress in livestock can arise from various sources such as environmental conditions, management practices, transportation, social interactions, and disease. Understanding the impact of stress on livestock production is essential for ensuring animal welfare and optimizing productivity. Although many factors can be involved, climatic factors are among the first and crucial limiting factors of the development of animal production in warm regions. In addition, global warming will further accentuate heat stress related problems in livestock. The first and foremost stress the livestock are exposed as a result of climate change is the heat stress. Among the environmental variables affecting animals, heat stress seems to be one of the intriguing factors making animal production challenging in many geographical locations in the world. Although animals can adapt to the hot climate, nevertheless the response mechanisms that ensures survival are also detrimental to performance. The vulnerability of livestock to heat stress varies according to species, genetic potential, life stage and nutritional status. By far heat stress seems to be the most important factors affecting drastically ruminant livestock production under changing climatic condition. Heat stress has severe consequences both on production and reproduction in livestock.

Impact of heat stress on livestock growth, production and reproduction

High ambient temperatures, solar radiation, and humidity are environmental stressing factors that affect animals. Heat stress is one of the most important stressors especially in hot regions of the world. In humid tropics along with extended periods of high ambient temperature and humidity, the primary non-evaporative means of cooling (viz., conduction, convection and radiation) becomes less effective with rising ambient temperature, and hence under such conditions, an animal becomes increasingly reliant upon evaporative cooling in the form of sweating and panting to alleviate heat stress (Kimothi and Ghosh, 2005). Increased summer temperature leads to depressed and low feed intake, reduction in body weight of animals, and lower milk production. In addition the cellular and molecular stress responses have an effect on mammary gland metabolism, energy partitioning and immune status. Under extreme conditions there may also be an increase on mortality rates. Heat stress reduces libido, fertility and embryonic survival in animals. Enhanced heat dissipation during heat stress may also lead to electrolyte losses (Coppock et al., 1982). Reproductive processes in the male and female animal are very sensitive to disruption by hyperthermia, with the most pronounced consequences being reduced quantity and quality of sperm production in males and decreased fertility in females. The poor reproductive performance in buffaloes especially during summer months is due to inefficiency in maintaining the thermo-regulation under high environmental temperature and relative humidity (RH) as those have dark skin and sparse coat of body hair which absorb more heat along with poor heat dissipation mechanism due to less number of sweat glands (Marai and Haeeb, 2010). Similarly, heat stress in lactating dairy cows causes significant loss of serum Na+and K+ (West, 1999) and also reduces birth weights of Holstein calves (Collier et al., 1982). High ambient temperature can adversely affect the structure and physiology of cells as well as functional and metabolic alterations in cells and tissues including cells of immune system (Iwagami, 1996). Heat stress in lactating animals results in dramatic reduction in roughage intake, gut motility and rumination which alters dietary protein utilization and body protein metabolism (Ames *et al.*, 1980). Temperature extremes can influence disease resistance in dairy calves (Stott *et al.*, 1976). In poultry, heat stress interferes with the broilers comfort and suppresses productive efficiency, growth rate, feed conversion and live weight gain (Etches *et al.*, 1995; Yalcin et al., 1997) due to changes in behavioural, physiological and immunological responses. With rise in ambient temperature, the poultry bird has to maintain a balance between heat production and heat loss. This forces the bird to reduce its feed consumption by 5% to reduce heat from metabolism to a tune for every 1°C rise in temperature between 32-38°C (Sohail *et al.*, 2012). Heat stress limits the productivity of laying hens, as reflected by egg production and egg quality, as the bird diverts feed metabolic energy to maintain its body temperature and also lower egg production and egg quality (Hsu *et al.*, 1998). The resulting hyperventilation decreases CO2 blood levels, which may decrease egg shell thickness (Campos, 2000). Plasma triiodothyronine and thyroxine, which are important growth promoters in animals, adversely affect heat-stressed broiler chickens (Sahin *et al.*, 2001). There are direct effects on organ and muscle metabolism during heat exposure which can persist after slaughter (Gregory, 2010); however, chronic heat exposure negatively affects fat deposition and meat quality in broilers (Imik *et al.*, 2012). In addition, heat stress is associated with depression of meat chemical composition and quality in broilers (Dai *et al.*, 2012). High temperature and humidity results in increased meat pH, less expressed juice, cooking loss and drip loss. Chronic heat stress decreased the proportion of breast muscle, while increasing the proportion of thigh muscle in broilers (Lara and Rostagno, 2013) and protein content lower and fat deposition higher in birds subjected to hot climate (Zhang *et al.*, 2012). Heat stress causes decrease in production performance, as well as reduced eggshell thickness and increased egg breakage (Lin *et al.*, 2004). Additionally, heat stress has been shown to cause a significant reduction of egg weight, egg shell weight, eggshell per cent (Lara and Rostagno, 2013) and all phases of semen production in breeder cocks (Banks *et al.*, 2005). In hotter climate, immune suppressing effect of heat stress is more on broilers and laying hens (Ghazi *et al.*, 2012) and will alter global disease distribution (Guis *et al.*, 2012) through changes in climate.

Management Strategies to Mitigate Stress

Improving Environmental Conditions: Providing adequate shelter, ventilation, and temperature control can help mitigate environmental stressors such as heat, cold, and humidity. Access to clean water and nutritious feed is essential for maintaining optimal health and reducing stress in livestock.

- **Optimizing Management Practices:** Implementing low-stress handling techniques, reducing stocking densities, and minimizing transportation stress can help mitigate stress in livestock. Proper handling during routine procedures such as vaccination, handling, and transportation can reduce fear and anxiety in animals.
- **Nutritional strategies:** Heat stressed animals are more likely to have lower reproductive and productive performance. Feeding high quality forages and balanced rations will decrease some of the effects of heat stress and will boost performance of the animals. During hot dry summer there is decrease in dietary feed intake which is responsible for the reduced productivity. In this situation the approaches like frequent feeding, improved forage quality, use of palatable feeds, good nutrition balance and greater nutrient density are required.
- **Enhancing Welfare Standards:** Adopting welfare-friendly housing systems, providing enrichment activities, and promoting social interactions among animals can improve welfare and reduce stress in livestock. Ensuring adequate space, comfortable resting areas, and opportunities for natural behaviors can enhance the overall well-being of animals.
- **Monitoring and Health Management:** Regular monitoring of animal health, early detection of stress-related issues, and prompt intervention can prevent disease outbreaks and mitigate the impact of stress on livestock production. Implementing vaccination programs, parasite control measures, and biosecurity protocols are essential for maintaining herd or flock health.

Multiple choices questions on Impact of Stress on Livestock Production:

1. What is stress in livestock production?
   a) Positive influence on productivity
   b) Negative influence on productivity
   c) Irrelevant to productivity
   d) Seasonal variation
2. Which of the following is a physical manifestation of stress in livestock?
   a) Increased appetite b) Decreased heart rate
   c) Weight gain d) Decreased feed intake
3. How does stress affect reproduction in livestock?
   a) Improves fertility b) No effect on fertility
   c) Reduces fertility d) Increases gestation period
4. Which hormone is often elevated in stressed livestock?
   a) Serotonin b) Dopamine
   c) Cortisol d) Insulin

5. What impact does stress have on the immune system of livestock?
   a) Boosts immunity b) No effect on immunity
   c) Suppresses immunity d) Shortens lifespan
6. How does stress influence animal behavior?
   a) Calming effect b) No effect on behavior
   c) Aggressive or abnormal behavior d) Decreased alertness
7. Which of the following is NOT a source of stress in livestock production?
   a) Transportation b) Social isolation
   c) Consistent routine d) Disease outbreaks
8. What role does nutrition play in mitigating stress in livestock?
   a) Exacerbates stress b) No effect on stress
   c) Helps reduce stress d) Increases susceptibility to stress
9. What effect can environmental factors have on stress levels in livestock?
   a) None b) Minor fluctuations
   c) Significant impact d) Only affects certain breeds
10. How does stress affect meat quality in livestock?
   a) Enhances meat quality b) No effect on meat quality
   c) Reduces meat quality d) Lengthens aging process
11. Which of the following is a behavioral sign of stress in livestock?
   a) Increased grooming b) Decreased vocalization
   c) Increased aggression d) Increased social interaction
12. What effect does stress have on milk production in dairy cows?
   a) Increases milk production b) No effect on milk production
   c) Reduces milk production d) Increases milk fat content
13. Which management practice can help reduce stress during handling and transportation?
   a) Rough handling
   b) Mixing unfamiliar animals
   c) Providing adequate space
   d) Transportation during extreme temperatures
14. What is the primary impact of stress on poultry production?
   a) Increased egg production b) Improved growth rate
   c) Decreased feed efficiency d) Decreased mortality rate
15. How does stress affect the incidence of diseases in livestock?
   a) Decreases disease susceptibility b) No effect on disease susceptibility
   c) Increases disease susceptibility d) Increases vaccine effectiveness
16. What impact does stress have on the overall productivity of a livestock operation?
   a) Increases productivity b) No effect on productivity
   c) Decreases productivity d) Reduces labor requirements

17. Which of the following factors contributes to heat stress in livestock?
    a) Cool ambient temperature
    b) Adequate ventilation
    c) High humidity
    d) Low stocking density
18. What effect does stress have on the metabolic rate of livestock?
    a) Decreases metabolic rate
    b) No effect on metabolic rate
    c) Increases metabolic rate
    d) Reduces appetite
19. Which of the following is NOT a potential consequence of chronic stress in livestock?
    a) Reduced fertility
    b) Increased disease resistance
    c) Poor growth
    d) Decreased meat quality
20. How does stress during early development affect livestock?
    a) No long-term effects
    b) Improves resilience
    c) Increases susceptibility to stress later in life
    d) Decreases appetite
21. Which of the following is an example of a nutritional strategy to reduce stress in livestock?
    a) Providing high-energy diets
    b) Limiting access to clean water
    c) Reducing dietary fiber
    d) Decreasing protein intake
22. What impact does stress have on the sleep patterns of livestock?
    a) Increases sleep duration
    b) No effect on sleep patterns
    c) Decreases sleep duration
    d) Alters sleep quality
23. How does stress affect the social hierarchy within a livestock group?
    a) Strengthens hierarchy
    b) No effect on hierarchy
    c) Disrupts hierarchy
    d) Increases aggression
24. Which of the following is a psychological sign of stress in livestock?
    a) Increased activity level
    b) Decreased anxiety
    c) Depression-like behavior
    d) Enhanced learning ability
25. What impact does stress have on the water intake of livestock?
    a) Increases water intake
    b) No effect on water intake
    c) Decreases water intake
    d) Reduces need for water
26. How does stress affect the composition of milk in dairy cows?
    a) Increases milk fat content
    b) No effect on milk composition
    c) Reduces milk protein content
    d) Improves milk flavor
27. Which of the following factors exacerbates stress during transportation of livestock?
    a) Short travel duration
    b) Smooth road conditions
    c) High stocking density
    d) Ample bedding material
28. What impact does stress have on the reproductive hormones of livestock?
    a) Increases hormone levels
    b) No effect on hormone levels
    c) Decreases hormone levels
    d) Alters hormone receptors

29. How does stress affect the susceptibility of livestock to respiratory diseases?
    a) Decreases susceptibility
    b) No effect on susceptibility
    c) Increases susceptibility
    d) Enhances vaccine effectiveness
30. What is the primary effect of stress on the gastrointestinal tract of livestock?
    a) Improves nutrient absorption
    b) Decreases gut motility
    c) Increases appetite
    d) Reduces gastric acid secretion
31. Which of the following is a symptom of heat stress in poultry?
    a) Increased egg production
    b) Panting
    c) Decreased water consumption
    d) Increased feed intake
32. How does stress affect the behavior of grazing animals?
    a) Decreases grazing activity
    b) No effect on grazing behavior
    c) Increases grazing activity
    d) Reduces social interactions
33. Which of the following measures can help alleviate heat stress in livestock?
    a) Providing access to shade
    b) Increasing stocking density
    c) Limiting access to water
    d) Restricting ventilation
34. What impact does stress have on the respiration rate of livestock?
    a) Decreases respiration rate
    b) No effect on respiration rate
    c) Increases respiration rate
    d) Alters lung capacity
35. How does stress during gestation affect the offspring of livestock?
    a) No effect on offspring
    b) Increases birth weight
    c) Impairs growth and development
    d) Reduces mortality rate
36. Which of the following is a symptom of stress-related diseases in livestock?
    a) Decreased heart rate
    b) Increased feed intake
    c) Diarrhea
    d) Reduced body temperature
37. How does stress affect the susceptibility of livestock to metabolic disorders?
    a) Decreases susceptibility
    b) No effect on susceptibility
    c) Increases susceptibility
    d) Enhances metabolic efficiency
38. Which of the following management practices can help reduce stress during weaning?
    a) Abrupt separation from the dam
    b) Grouping unfamiliar calves
    c) Delaying weaning age
    d) Providing access to forage
39. What impact does stress have on the blood glucose levels of livestock?
    a) Increases blood glucose levels
    b) No effect on blood glucose levels
    c) Decreases blood glucose levels
    d) Reduces insulin sensitivity
40. How does stress affect the growth rate of young livestock?
    a) Enhances growth rate
    b) No effect on growth rate
    c) Reduces growth rate
    d) Accelerates puberty onset
41. Which of the following is a consequence of stress-induced aggression in livestock?
    a) Enhanced social cohesion
    b) Decreased risk of injury
    c) Increased morbidity
    d) Improved reproductive success

42. How does stress affect the milk let-down reflex in dairy cows?
    a) Strengthens the reflex b) No effect on the reflex
    c) Impairs the reflex d) Shortens lactation period
43. What impact does stress have on the heart rate of livestock?
    a) Decreases heart rate b) No effect on heart rate
    c) Increases heart rate d) Alters blood pressure
44. Which of the following is a symptom of stress-related respiratory disorders in poultry?
    a) Wheezing b) Decreased respiratory rate
    c) Increased lung capacity d) Improved oxygenation
45. How does stress affect the susceptibility of livestock to metabolic disorders?
    a) Decreases susceptibility b) No effect on susceptibility
    c) Increases susceptibility d) Enhances metabolic efficiency
46. Which of the following management practices can help reduce stress during weaning?
    a) Abrupt separation from the dam b) Grouping unfamiliar calves
    c) Delaying weaning age d) Providing access to forage
47. What impact does stress have on the blood glucose levels of livestock?
    a) Increases blood glucose levels b) No effect on blood glucose levels
    c) Decreases blood glucose levels d) Reduces insulin sensitivity
48. How does stress affect the growth rate of young livestock?
    a) Enhances growth rate b) No effect on growth rate
    c) Reduces growth rate d) Accelerates puberty onset
49. Which of the following is a consequence of stress-induced aggression in livestock?
    a) Enhanced social cohesion b) Decreased risk of injury
    c) Increased morbidity d) Improved reproductive success
50. How does stress affect the milk let-down reflex in dairy cows?
    a) Strengthens the reflex b) No effect on the reflex
    c) Impairs the reflex d) Shortens lactation period
51. What impact does stress have on the heart rate of livestock?
    a) Decreases heart rate b) No effect on heart rate
    c) Increases heart rate d) Alters blood pressure
52. Which of the following is a symptom of stress-related respiratory disorders in poultry?
    a) Wheezing b) Decreased respiratory rate
    c) Increased lung capacity d) Improved oxygenation
53. How does stress affect the susceptibility of livestock to metabolic disorders?
    a) Decreases susceptibility b) No effect on susceptibility
    c) Increases susceptibility d) Enhances metabolic efficiency

54. Which of the following management practices can help reduce stress during weaning?
    a) Abrupt separation from the dam
    b) Grouping unfamiliar calves
    c) Delaying weaning age
    d) Providing access to forage
55. What impact does stress have on the blood glucose levels of livestock?
    a) Increases blood glucose levels
    b) No effect on blood glucose levels
    c) Decreases blood glucose levels
    d) Reduces insulin sensitivity
56. How does stress affect the growth rate of young livestock?
    a) Enhances growth rate
    b) No effect on growth rate
    c) Reduces growth rate
    d) Accelerates puberty onset
57. Which of the following is a consequence of stress-induced aggression in livestock?
    a) Enhanced social cohesion
    b) Decreased risk of injury
    c) Increased morbidity
    d) Improved reproductive success
58. How does stress affect the milk let-down reflex in dairy cows?
    a) Strengthens the reflex
    b) No effect on the reflex
    c) Impairs the reflex
    d) Shortens lactation period
59. What impact does stress have on the heart rate of livestock?
    a) Decreases heart rate
    b) No effect on heart rate
    c) Increases heart rate
    d) Alters blood pressure
60. Which of the following is a symptom of stress-related respiratory disorders in poultry?
    a) Wheezing
    b) Decreased respiratory rate
    c) Increased lung capacity
    d) Improved oxygenation
61. How does stress affect the susceptibility of livestock to metabolic disorders?
    a) Decreases susceptibility
    b) No effect on susceptibility
    c) Increases susceptibility
    d) Enhances metabolic efficiency
62. Which of the following management practices can help reduce stress during weaning?
    a) Abrupt separation from the dam
    b) Grouping unfamiliar calves
    c) Delaying weaning age
    d) Providing access to forage
63. What impact does stress have on the blood glucose levels of livestock?
    a) Increases blood glucose levels
    b) No effect on blood glucose levels
    c) Decreases blood glucose levels
    d) Reduces insulin sensitivity
64. How does stress affect the growth rate of young livestock?
    a) Enhances growth rate
    b) No effect on growth rate
    c) Reduces growth rate
    d) Accelerates puberty onset
65. Which of the following is a consequence of stress-induced aggression in livestock?
    a) Enhanced social cohesion
    b) Decreased risk of injury
    c) Increased morbidity
    d) Improved reproductive success

66. How does stress affect the milk let-down reflex in dairy cows?
   a) Strengthens the reflex
   b) No effect on the reflex
   c) Impairs the reflex
   d) Shortens lactation period

67. What impact does stress have on the heart rate of livestock?
   a) Decreases heart rate
   b) No effect on heart rate
   c) Increases heart rate
   d) Alters blood pressure

68. Which of the following is a symptom of stress-related respiratory disorders in poultry?
   a) Wheezing
   b) Decreased respiratory rate
   c) Increased lung capacity
   d) Improved oxygenation

69. How does stress affect the susceptibility of livestock to metabolic disorders?
   a) Decreases susceptibility
   b) No effect on susceptibility
   c) Increases susceptibility
   d) Enhances metabolic efficiency

70. Which of the following management practices can help reduce stress during weaning?
   a) Abrupt separation from the dam
   b) Grouping unfamiliar calves
   c) Delaying weaning age
   d) Providing access to forage

71. What impact does stress have on the blood glucose levels of livestock?
   a) Increases blood glucose levels
   b) No effect on blood glucose levels
   c) Decreases blood glucose levels
   d) Reduces insulin sensitivity

72. How does stress affect the growth rate of young livestock?
   a) Enhances growth rate
   b) No effect on growth rate
   c) Reduces growth rate
   d) Accelerates puberty onset

73. Which of the following is a consequence of stress-induced aggression in livestock?
   a) Enhanced social cohesion
   b) Decreased risk of injury
   c) Increased morbidity
   d) Improved reproductive success

74. How does stress affect the milk let-down reflex in dairy cows?
   a) Strengthens the reflex
   b) No effect on the reflex
   c) Impairs the reflex
   d) Shortens lactation period

75. What impact does stress have on the heart rate of livestock?
   a) Decreases heart rate
   b) No effect on heart rate
   c) Increases heart rate
   d) Alters blood pressure

76. Which of the following is a symptom of stress-related respiratory disorders in poultry?
   a) Wheezing
   b) Decreased respiratory rate
   c) Increased lung capacity
   d) Improved oxygenation

77. How does stress affect the susceptibility of livestock to metabolic disorders?
   a) Decreases susceptibility
   b) No effect on susceptibility
   c) Increases susceptibility
   d) Enhances metabolic efficiency

78. Which of the following management practices can help reduce stress during weaning?

a) Abrupt separation from the dam
b) Grouping unfamiliar calves
c) Delaying weaning age
d) Providing access to forage

79. What impact does stress have on the blood glucose levels of livestock?

a) Increases blood glucose levels
b) No effect on blood glucose levels
c) Decreases blood glucose levels
d) Reduces insulin sensitivity

80. How does stress affect the growth rate of young livestock?

a) Enhances growth rate
b) No effect on growth rate
c) Reduces growth rate
d) Accelerates puberty onset

81. Which of the following is a consequence of stress-induced aggression in livestock?

a) Enhanced social cohesion
b) Decreased risk of injury
c) Increased morbidity
d) Improved reproductive success

82. How does stress affect the milk let-down reflex in dairy cows?

a) Strengthens the reflex
b) No effect on the reflex
c) Impairs the reflex
d) Shortens lactation period

83. What impact does stress have on the heart rate of livestock?

a) Decreases heart rate
b) No effect on heart rate
c) Increases heart rate
d) Alters blood pressure

84. Which of the following is a symptom of stress-related respiratory disorders in poultry?

a) Wheezing
b) Decreased respiratory rate
c) Increased lung capacity
d) Improved oxygenation

85. How does stress affect the susceptibility of livestock to metabolic disorders?

a) Decreases susceptibility
b) No effect on susceptibility
c) Increases susceptibility
d) Enhances metabolic efficiency

86. Which of the following management practices can help reduce stress during weaning?

a) Abrupt separation from the dam
b) Grouping unfamiliar calves
c) Delaying weaning age
d) Providing access to forage

87. What impact does stress have on the blood glucose levels of livestock?

a) Increases blood glucose levels
b) No effect on blood glucose levels
c) Decreases blood glucose levels
d) Reduces insulin sensitivity

88. How does stress affect the growth rate of young livestock?

a) Enhances growth rate
b) No effect on growth rate
c) Reduces growth rate
d) Accelerates puberty onset

89. Which of the following is a consequence of stress-induced aggression in livestock?

a) Enhanced social cohesion
b) Decreased risk of injury
c) Increased morbidity
d) Improved reproductive success

90. How does stress affect the milk let-down reflex in dairy cows?
   a) Strengthens the reflex
   b) No effect on the reflex
   c) Impairs the reflex
   d) Shortens lactation period
91. What impact does stress have on the heart rate of livestock?
   a) Decreases heart rate
   b) No effect on heart rate
   c) Increases heart rate
   d) Alters blood pressure
92. Which of the following is a symptom of stress-related respiratory disorders in poultry?
   a) Wheezing
   b) Decreased respiratory rate
   c) Increased lung capacity
   d) Improved oxygenation
93. How does stress affect the susceptibility of livestock to metabolic disorders?
   a) Decreases susceptibility
   b) No effect on susceptibility
   c) Increases susceptibility
   d) Enhances metabolic efficiency
94. Which of the following management practices can help reduce stress during weaning?
   a) Abrupt separation from the dam
   b) Grouping unfamiliar calves
   c) Delaying weaning age
   d) Providing access to forage
95. What impact does stress have on the blood glucose levels of livestock?
   a) Increases blood glucose levels
   b) No effect on blood glucose levels
   c) Decreases blood glucose levels
   d) Reduces insulin sensitivity
96. How does stress affect the growth rate of young livestock?
   a) Enhances growth rate
   b) No effect on growth rate
   c) Reduces growth rate
   d) Accelerates puberty onset
97. Which of the following is a consequence of stress-induced aggression in livestock?
   a) Enhanced social cohesion
   b) Decreased risk of injury
   c) Increased morbidity
   d) Improved reproductive success
98. How does stress affect the milk let-down reflex in dairy cows?
   a) Strengthens the reflex
   b) No effect on the reflex
   c) Impairs the reflex
   d) Shortens lactation period
99. What impact does stress have on the heart rate of livestock?
   a) Decreases heart rate
   b) No effect on heart rate
   c) Increases heart rate
   d) Alters blood pressure
100. Which of the following is a symptom of stress-related respiratory disorders in poultry?
   a) Wheezing
   b) Decreased respiratory rate
   c) Increased lung capacity
   d) Improved oxygenation
101. How does stress affect the susceptibility of livestock to metabolic disorders?
   a) Decreases susceptibility
   b) No effect on susceptibility
   c) Increases susceptibility
   d) Enhances metabolic efficiency

102. Which of the following management practices can help reduce stress during weaning?

a) Abrupt separation from the dam b) Grouping unfamiliar calves
c) Delaying weaning age d) Providing access to forage

103. What impact does stress have on the blood glucose levels of livestock?

a) Increases blood glucose levels b) No effect on blood glucose levels
c) Decreases blood glucose levels d) Reduces insulin sensitivity

104. How does stress affect the growth rate of young livestock?

a) Enhances growth rate b) No effect on growth rate
c) Reduces growth rate d) Accelerates puberty onset

105. Which of the following is a consequence of stress-induced aggression in livestock?

a) Enhanced social cohesion b) Decreased risk of injury
c) Increased morbidity d) Improved reproductive success

106. How does stress affect the milk let-down reflex in dairy cows?

a) Strengthens the reflex b) No effect on the reflex
c) Impairs the reflex d) Shortens lactation period

107. What impact does stress have on the heart rate of livestock?

a) Decreases heart rate b) No effect on heart rate
c) Increases heart rate d) Alters blood pressure

108. Which of the following is a symptom of stress-related respiratory disorders in poultry?

a) Wheezing b) Decreased respiratory rate
c) Increased lung capacity d) Improved oxygenation

109. How does stress affect the susceptibility of livestock to metabolic disorders?

a) Decreases susceptibility b) No effect on susceptibility
c) Increases susceptibility d) Enhances metabolic efficiency

110. Which of the following management practices can help reduce stress during weaning?

a) Abrupt separation from the dam b) Grouping unfamiliar calves
c) Delaying weaning age d) Providing access to forage

111. What impact does stress have on the blood glucose levels of livestock?

a) Increases blood glucose levels b) No effect on blood glucose levels
c) Decreases blood glucose levels d) Reduces insulin sensitivity

112. How does stress affect the growth rate of young livestock?

a) Enhances growth rate b) No effect on growth rate
c) Reduces growth rate d) Accelerates puberty onset

113. Which of the following is a consequence of stress-induced aggression in livestock?

a) Enhanced social cohesion b) Decreased risk of injury
c) Increased morbidity d) Improved reproductive success

114. How does stress affect the milk let-down reflex in dairy cows?
    a) Strengthens the reflex
    b) No effect on the reflex
    c) Impairs the reflex
    d) Shortens lactation period
115. What impact does stress have on the heart rate of livestock?
    a) Decreases heart rate
    b) No effect on heart rate
    c) Increases heart rate
    d) Alters blood pressure
116. Which of the following is a symptom of stress-related respiratory disorders in poultry?
    a) Wheezing
    b) Decreased respiratory rate
    c) Increased lung capacity
    d) Improved oxygenation
117. How does stress affect the susceptibility of livestock to metabolic disorders?
    a) Decreases susceptibility
    b) No effect on susceptibility
    c) Increases susceptibility
    d) Enhances metabolic efficiency
118. Which of the following management practices can help reduce stress during weaning?
    a) Abrupt separation from the dam
    b) Grouping unfamiliar calves
    c) Delaying weaning age
    d) Providing access to forage
119. What impact does stress have on the blood glucose levels of livestock?
    a) Increases blood glucose levels
    b) No effect on blood glucose levels
    c) Decreases blood glucose levels
    d) Reduces insulin sensitivity
120. How does stress affect the growth rate of young livestock?
    a) Enhances growth rate
    b) No effect on growth rate
    c) Reduces growth rate
    d) Accelerates puberty onset
121. Which of the following is a consequence of stress-induced aggression in livestock?
    a) Enhanced social cohesion
    b) Decreased risk of injury
    c) Increased morbidity
    d) Improved reproductive success
122. How does stress affect the milk let-down reflex in dairy cows?
    a) Strengthens the reflex
    b) No effect on the reflex
    c) Impairs the reflex
    d) Shortens lactation period
123. What impact does stress have on the heart rate of livestock?
    a) Decreases heart rate
    b) No effect on heart rate
    c) Increases heart rate
    d) Alters blood pressure
124. Which of the following is a symptom of stress-related respiratory disorders in poultry?
    a) Wheezing
    b) Decreased respiratory rate
    c) Increased lung capacity
    d) Improved oxygenation
125. How does stress affect the susceptibility of livestock to metabolic disorders?
    a) Decreases susceptibility
    b) No effect on susceptibility
    c) Increases susceptibility
    d) Enhances metabolic efficiency

126. Which of the following management practices can help reduce stress during weaning?
   a) Abrupt separation from the dam
   b) Grouping unfamiliar calves
   c) Delaying weaning age
   d) Providing access to forage
127. What impact does stress have on the blood glucose levels of livestock?
   a) Increases blood glucose levels
   b) No effect on blood glucose levels
   c) Decreases blood glucose levels
   d) Reduces insulin sensitivity
128. How does stress affect the growth rate of young livestock?
   a) Enhances growth rate
   b) No effect on growth rate
   c) Reduces growth rate
   d) Accelerates puberty onset
129. Which of the following is a consequence of stress-induced aggression in livestock?
   a) Enhanced social cohesion
   b) Decreased risk of injury
   c) Increased morbidity
   d) Improved reproductive success
130. How does stress affect the milk let-down reflex in dairy cows?
   a) Strengthens the reflex
   b) No effect on the reflex
   c) Impairs the reflex
   d) Shortens lactation period
131. What impact does stress have on the heart rate of livestock?
   a) Decreases heart rate
   b) No effect on heart rate
   c) Increases heart rate
   d) Alters blood pressure
132. Which of the following is a symptom of stress-related respiratory disorders in poultry?
   a) Wheezing
   b) Decreased respiratory rate
   c) Increased lung capacity
   d) Improved oxygenation
133. How does stress affect the susceptibility of livestock to metabolic disorders?
   a) Decreases susceptibility
   b) No effect on susceptibility
   c) Increases susceptibility
   d) Enhances metabolic efficiency
134. Which of the following management practices can help reduce stress during weaning?
   a) Abrupt separation from the dam
   b) Grouping unfamiliar calves
   c) Delaying weaning age
   d) Providing access to forage
135. What impact does stress have on the blood glucose levels of livestock?
   a) Increases blood glucose levels
   b) No effect on blood glucose levels
   c) Decreases blood glucose levels
   d) Reduces insulin sensitivity
136. How does stress affect the growth rate of young livestock?
   a) Enhances growth rate
   b) No effect on growth rate
   c) Reduces growth rate
   d) Accelerates puberty onset
137. Which of the following is a consequence of stress-induced aggression in livestock?
   a) Enhanced social cohesion
   b) Decreased risk of injury
   c) Increased morbidity
   d) Improved reproductive success

138. How does stress affect the milk let-down reflex in dairy cows?
   a) Strengthens the reflex b) No effect on the reflex
   c) Impairs the reflex d) Shortens lactation period
139. What impact does stress have on the heart rate of livestock?
   a) Decreases heart rate b) No effect on heart rate
   c) Increases heart rate d) Alters blood pressure
140. Which of the following is a symptom of stress-related respiratory disorders in poultry?
   a) Wheezing b) Decreased respiratory rate
   c) Increased lung capacity d) Improved oxygenation
141. How does stress affect the susceptibility of livestock to metabolic disorders?
   a) Decreases susceptibility b) No effect on susceptibility
   c) Increases susceptibility d) Enhances metabolic efficiency
142. Which of the following management practices can help reduce stress during weaning?
   a) Abrupt separation from the dam b) Grouping unfamiliar calves
   c) Delaying weaning age d) Providing access to forage
143. What impact does stress have on the blood glucose levels of livestock?
   a) Increases blood glucose levels b) No effect on blood glucose levels
   c) Decreases blood glucose levels d) Reduces insulin sensitivity
144. How does stress affect the growth rate of young livestock?
   a) Enhances growth rate b) No effect on growth rate
   c) Reduces growth rate d) Accelerates puberty onset
145. Which of the following is a consequence of stress-induced aggression in livestock?
   a) Enhanced social cohesion b) Decreased risk of injury
   c) Increased morbidity d) Improved reproductive success
146. How does stress affect the milk let-down reflex in dairy cows?
   a) Strengthens the reflex b) No effect on the reflex
   c) Impairs the reflex d) Shortens lactation period
147. What impact does stress have on the heart rate of livestock?
   a) Decreases heart rate b) No effect on heart rate
   c) Increases heart rate d) Alters blood pressure
148. Which of the following is a symptom of stress-related respiratory disorders in poultry?
   a) Wheezing b) Decreased respiratory rate
   c) Increased lung capacity d) Improved oxygenation
149. How does stress affect the susceptibility of livestock to metabolic disorders?
   a) Decreases susceptibility b) No effect on susceptibility
   c) Increases susceptibility d) Enhances metabolic efficiency

150. Which of the following management practices can help reduce stress during weaning?

a) Abrupt separation from the dam
b) Grouping unfamiliar calves
c) Delaying weaning age
d) Providing access to forage

Answer Key

1	b	2	d	3	c	4	c	5	c	6	c	7	c
8	c	9	c	10	c	11	c	12	c	13	c	14	c
15	c	16	c	17	c	18	c	19	b	20	c	21	
22	c	23	c	24	c	25	a	26	c	27	c	28	c
29	c	30	b	31	b	32	a	33	a	34	c	35	c
36	c	37	c	38	d	39	a	40	c	41	c	42	c
43	c	44	a	45	c	46	d	47	a	48	c	49	c
50	c	51	c	52	a	53	c	54	d	55	a	56	c
57	c	58	c	59	c	60	a	61	c	62	d	63	a
64	c	65	c	66	c	67	c	68	a	69	c	70	d
71	a	72	c	73	c	74	c	75	c	76	a	77	c
78	d	79	a	80	c	81	c	82	c	83	c	84	a
85	c	86	d	87	a	88	c	89	c	90	c	91	c
92	a	93	c	94	d	95	a	96	c	97	c	98	c
99	c	100	a	101	c	102	d	103	a	104	c	105	c
106	c	107	c	108	a	109	c	110	d	111	a	112	c
113	c	114	c	115	c	116	a	117	c	118	d	119	a
120	c	121	c	122	c	123	c	124	a	125	c	126	d
127	a	128	c	129	c	130	c	131	c	132	a	133	c
134	d	135	a	136	c	137	c	138	c	139	c	140	a
141	c	142	d	143	a	144	c	145	c	146	c	147	c
148	a	149	c	150	d								

7

Body Condition Scoring

R R K Sinha, Alok Bharti, Ravikant Nirala and Amita

Bihar Veterinary College, Bihar Animal Sciences University, Patna, Bihar

Introduction

The body condition scoring (BCS) is a subjective estimate of the energy reserves in adipose tissues of an animal. It is an acceptive, non-invasive, quick and inexpensive method to estimate degree of fatness. It is a means of accurately determining body condition of dairy cows, independent of body weight and frame size. It is evinced that the profile of lactating cows in milch barn is different e.g. some may be in early lactation and the others may either be in mid or late lactation. The observations on body condition status of animal will help the manager to adopt corrective management measures, thus enabling to improve the production profile of an animal. Hence, body condition scoring may be used as an efficient tool in this regard. Although many may consider this as a nutritional management practice, but changing BCS have implications on milk yield, health, reproduction, longevity and overall profitability of an animal. Body Condition Scoring (BCS) is a system used to evaluate the overall health and nutritional status of animals by assessing their body fat and muscle mass. Body condition influences productivity, reproduction, health, and longevity of animals. Thinness or fatness can be a clue to underlying nutritional deficiencies, health problems, or improper herd management. If done on a regular basis, body condition scoring can be used to troubleshoot problems and improve the health, longevity, and productivity of the herd. Presence of fat deposits in certain body areas like the tail base, around the loin, behind the shoulders, or on the neck indicates the conditioning of animals. This method is commonly applied to various domestic animals, including dogs, cats, horses, and livestock such as cattle and sheep.

The score helps owners, veterinarians, and animal caretakers make informed decisions about the animal's feeding regime and overall care to optimize their health and productivity. The BCS is generally given on a numerical scale, with the scale's range differing between species. The scoring system typically ranges from 1 to 9 or 1 to 5, depending on the species being evaluated:

Cattle

For **beef cattle**, the BCS scale typically ranges from 1 to 9; 1: Extremely emaciated with no fat cover. 5: Moderate condition. Backbone, ribs, and hip bones are not visibly protruding and have a good balance of muscle and fat. 9: Extremely obese with excessive fat cover. **Dairy cattle** may use a slightly different scale, often from 1 to 5 with 0.25-point increments, where; 1: Very thin, with bones easily visible. 3: Ideal condition with a good balance of fat and muscle. The backbone is slightly visible. 5: Overly conditioned with excess fat. Body condition scores (BCS) are an indirect estimate of energy balance.

Sheep and Goats

The BCS for sheep and goats usually ranges from 1 to 5; 1: Very thin with no fat around the tail base or over the ribs. 3: Good condition. The spine is palpable but with a good cover of fat, and fat around the tail base is beginning to be more pronounced. 5: Obese with a thick layer of fat over the loin and ribs, and possibly fat deposits in the brisket and flanks.

Horses

Horses are typically scored on a scale from 1 to 9; 1: Poor condition, with the animal being extremely emaciated. 5: Moderate condition. The backbone is not prominently visible, ribs cannot be seen but can be easily felt, and the neck and shoulders blend smoothly into the body. 9: Extremely fat or obese, with a crease down the back due to fat along the spine, and fat deposits over the ribs, tailhead, shoulders, and neck. The ideal score for most horses is between 5 and 6, indicating a well-balanced amount of fat coverage over the body without being overweight.

Dogs and Cats

For dogs and cats, the body condition scoring systems often range from 1 to 5 or 1 to 9. A score of 1 indicates the animal is severely underweight, showing signs of emaciation, while a score at the highest end of the scale indicates obesity. An ideal score would be in the middle of the scale, indicating a well-proportioned body where you can feel the ribs but not see them, and the animal has a visible waist when viewed from above.

Advantage of assessing Body condition scoring

Regular body condition scoring helps in adjusting feed rations to ensure animals maintain an optimal condition that supports their health, productivity, and reproductive performance. BCS is an important tool to prevent health issues related to poor nutrition such as infertility, lameness, and increased susceptibility to diseases. Regular body condition scoring is recommended as part of a comprehensive health management practice. It's important to note that BCS should be considered alongside other factors like weight, age, and breed characteristics for a comprehensive assessment of an animal's health and well-being.

MCQ. On Body Condition Scoring

1. What does BCS stand for in livestock management?
   - a) Body Composition Score
   - b) Body Condition Score
   - c) Body Count Score
   - d) Body Category Score
2. What is the ideal BCS range for most dairy cattle for optimal productivity?
   - a) 1-3
   - b) 4-6
   - c) 7-9
   - d) 2-4
3. Which livestock species is commonly assessed using Body Condition Scoring?
   - a) Poultry
   - b) Swine
   - c) Cattle
   - d) All of the above

4. Why is Body Condition Scoring important in livestock management?
   a) Helps in determining the sale value of the animal
   b) Aids in making nutritional and management decisions
   c) It's only used for breeding purposes
   d) None of the above
5. Which BCS would indicate that a cow is extremely emaciated?
   a) 1 b) 5
   c) 9 d) 6
6. How often should livestock producers perform Body Condition Scoring?
   a) Once a year b) Only before breeding season
   c) Regularly throughout the year d) Never, it's not necessary
7. What aspect of livestock productivity can be directly affected by BCS?
   a) Milk production b) Reproductive efficiency
   c) Growth rates d) All of the above
8. In beef cattle, a BCS lower than what number is considered too thin for breeding?
   a) 3 b) 4
   c) 5 d) 6
9. Which tool is essential for accurately assessing BCS in livestock?
   a) Ultrasound b) Weight scale
   c) Visual observation and palpation d) DNA analysis
10. What is the primary goal of managing livestock with appropriate BCS?
   a) To ensure the animals look visually appealing
   b) To maximize productivity and health
   c) To reduce the cost of feed
   d) To increase the sale price per animal
11. What does BCS stand for in the context of livestock?
   a) Body Composition Scale b) Body Condition Scoring
   c) Balanced Carbohydrate Supply d) Body Caloric System
12. In the typical BCS scale, what is the range for an animal considered to have an ideal body condition?
   a) 1-3 b) 3-5
   c) 4-6 d) 6-9
13. Which of the following animals would be classified as "Moderate" on the BCS scale?
   a) Extremely emaciated b) Slightly fleshy
   c) Moderately thin d) Obese
14. Why is Body Condition Scoring important in livestock management?
   a) It helps to determine the breed of the animal.
   b) It is a subjective measure with no practical applications.
   c) It provides insight into the nutritional status of an individual animal.
   d) It only applies to dairy cattle.

15. Which production goal is influenced by Body Condition Scoring in livestock?
    a) Wool quality
    b) Milk production
    c) Egg size
    d) All of the above
16. What does a BCS of 1 indicate in livestock?
    a) Ideal body condition
    b) Obese
    c) Extremely emaciated
    d) Moderately fleshy
17. How often should farmers ideally conduct Body Condition Scoring in their livestock?
    a) Once a year
    b) Every 5 years
    c) Regularly throughout the production cycle
    d) Only during winter months
18. Which of the following factors should be considered alongside BCS for a comprehensive health assessment?
    a) Breed characteristics
    b) Age
    c) Weight
    d) All of the above
19. What adjustments can be made based on BCS in livestock management?
    a) Reproductive management decisions
    b) Dietary adjustments
    c) Health interventions
    d) All of the above
20. In a BCS of 8, what is the likely characteristic of the animal?
    a) Moderately fleshy
    b) Fat
    c) Moderately thin
    d) Very fat (obese)
21. What is the primary purpose of Body Condition Scoring (BCS) in livestock?
    a) To determine the age of the animal
    b) To assess the nutritional and health status of the animal
    c) To measure the weight of the animal
    d) To evaluate the breeding potential of the animal
22. In a BCS scale of 1 to 9 for cattle, what does a score of 1 indicate?
    a) Optimal condition
    b) Overweight
    c) Extremely emaciated
    d) Slightly underweight
23. Which livestock species commonly uses a BCS range from 1 to 5?
    a) Poultry
    b) Sheep
    c) Swine
    d) Cattle
24. How can BCS directly impact the reproductive efficiency of livestock?
    a) By influencing the animal's growth rate
    b) By affecting the animal's ability to conceive and carry a pregnancy to term
    c) By changing the color of the animal's coat
    d) By affecting the animal's milk production only

25. Which of the following best describes a BCS of 5 in cattle on a 1-9 scale?
    a) Emaciated b) Moderate
    c) Overweight d) Obese
26. Why is regular monitoring of BCS important in livestock management?
    a) It helps in planning the music playlist for barns
    b) It assists in determining the right time for marketing or slaughter
    c) It is only necessary for exotic animals
    d) It is required for compliance with animal welfare laws only
27. In which scenario might a higher BCS be desirable?
    a) Before breeding season to ensure optimal reproductive performance
    b) Before entering a weight loss competition
    c) When preparing animals for a long transport
    d) During a drought when feed is scarce
28. What management action is advised for livestock with a BCS significantly below the ideal range?
    a) Increase exercise to reduce weight
    b) Decrease water intake to limit weight gain
    c) Adjust diet to increase nutritional intake
    d) No action needed if the animal is still active
29. Which of the following is NOT a direct benefit of maintaining an ideal BCS in dairy cows?
    a) Increased milk production b) Improved hoof health
    c) Enhanced meat flavor d) Better reproductive performance
30. How often should BCS be assessed in a well-managed livestock operation?
    a) Once a year b) Only before breeding
    c) At regular intervals throughout the year d) Only at weaning
31. Which livestock species is NOT commonly assessed using a Body Condition Score?
    a) Cattle b) Sheep
    c) Pigs d) Chickens
32. A BCS of 1 in cattle indicates what condition?
    a) Obese b) Ideal condition
    c) Emaciated d) Moderately fleshy
33. For dairy cows, an ideal BCS at calving is usually:
    a) 2-3 b) 3-4
    c) 5-6 d) 7-8
34. Which of the following is a potential consequence of a high BCS in livestock?
    a) Increased fertility b) Decreased risk of diseases
    c) Increased risk of metabolic disorders d) Decreased feed costs

35. Body Condition Scoring in sheep is typically done by assessing fat cover in which area?
    a) Over the loin
    b) Along the back
    c) Behind the shoulder
    d) Tail head area
36. In beef cattle, a BCS of 7 indicates what condition?
    a) Thin
    b) Moderate
    c) Fleshy
    d) Emaciated
37. Why is BCS particularly important in breeding livestock?
    a) It determines the quality of the meat
    b) It affects the animal's growth rate
    c) It influences reproductive efficiency
    d) It changes the animal's coat color
38. Which of the following best describes the method of assessing BCS?
    a) Only visual inspection
    b) Only weighing the animal
    c) Both visual and physical examination
    d) Blood tests
39. A low BCS in livestock can indicate which of the following?
    a) Overfeeding
    b) Adequate nutrition
    c) Undernutrition
    d) Optimal health
40. In sheep, a BCS of less than 2 can lead to what issue in ewes?
    a) Increased wool production
    b) Decreased fertility
    c) Improved milk quality
    d) Enhanced growth rate in lambs
41. Which factor is NOT a direct outcome of optimal BCS in livestock?
    a) Improved disease resistance
    b) Increased lifespan
    c) Higher meat quality
    d) Enhanced feed efficiency
42. How can Body Condition Scoring directly impact livestock productivity?
    a) By influencing the animal's genetic makeup
    b) By determining the physical space the animal occupies
    c) By affecting reproduction and milk production
    d) By changing the animal's species
43. When should Body Condition Scoring be performed in cattle to make decisions about winter feeding strategies?
    a) At the beginning of the breeding season
    b) Just before calving
    c) At weaning
    d) During mid-summer
44. Which body part is NOT typically evaluated in cattle when performing Body Condition Scoring?
    a) Ribs
    b) Tailhead
    c) Loin area
    d) Hooves

45. What management practice can be directly influenced by BCS in dairy cows?
    a) Choosing the type of milk to produce
    b) Deciding when to initiate the breeding period
    c) Selecting the breed of cow for purchase
    d) Determining the color of the cow's coat

46. In the BCS system, what score is typically considered ideal for most breeding cattle?
    a) 1-2 b) 4-6
    c) 7-9 d) 3-4

47. What does a BCS of 1 indicate?
    a) The animal is extremely emaciated
    b) The animal has an ideal amount of fat
    c) The animal is slightly overweight
    d) The animal is extremely obese

48. Which livestock species is NOT commonly assessed using Body Condition Scoring?
    a) Cattle b) Sheep
    c) Goats d) Chickens

49. What is Body Condition Scoring (BCS) primarily used to assess in livestock?
    a) Genetic potential b) Feed efficiency
    c) Nutritional status d) Age

50. Which species is NOT commonly assessed using a 1-9 BCS scale?
    a) Cattle b) Sheep
    c) Pigs d) Goats

51. A BCS of 1 in cattle indicates what condition?
    a) Optimal condition b) Overweight
    c) Obese d) Extremely emaciated

52. Adjusting feed based on BCS can help improve:
    a) Wool quality in sheep b) Milk yield in dairy cows
    c) Running speed in horses d) Egg production in chickens

53. In cows, a BCS significantly lower than the ideal range can result in:
    a) Increased twin births b) Reduced fertility
    c) Enhanced milk flavor d) Longer lifespan

54. For beef cattle, a BCS of 6-7 at weaning is indicative of:
    a) Underfeeding b) Ideal feeding
    c) Slight overfeeding d) Severe overfeeding

55. Low BCS scores in livestock can lead to increased susceptibility to:
    a) Parasitic infections b) Broken limbs
    c) Sunburn d) None of the above

56. The ideal BCS for dairy cows at calving is:
 a) 2-3 b) 3-4
 c) 5-6 d) 7-8
57. Which of the following is a primary factor affecting the accuracy of BCS in dairy cattle, especially in high-yielding breeds?
 a) Color of the cow's coat
 b) Ambient temperature and housing conditions
 c) Phase of lactation
 d) Breed of the cow
58. In the context of sheep BCS, what condition could a consistent score of 1 indicate, considering adequate feed availability?
 a) Superior wool quality
 b) Genetic predisposition to leanness
 c) Underlying health issues such as dental problems
 d) Optimal condition for breeding
59. How does BCS at calving correlate with postpartum anestrus duration in beef cows?
 a) No correlation exists
 b) Higher BCS results in longer anestrus
 c) Lower BCS is associated with shorter anestrus
 d) Higher BCS is associated with shorter anestrus
60. Considering dairy cows, which BCS range at dry-off has been associated with optimal outcomes in terms of health, reproduction, and milk production in the next lactation?
 a) 2.5 to 3.0 b) 3.25 to 3.75
 c) 3.5 to 4.0 d) 4.5 to 5.0
61. In terms of feed adjustment based on BCS, which strategy is recommended for a beef cattle herd with an average BCS of 6 entering the winter feeding period?
 a) Increase energy intake to improve condition
 b) Maintain current feeding regimen
 c) Reduce energy intake to prevent over-conditioning
 d) Focus solely on protein supplementation
62. What is a potential consequence of maintaining a high BCS (e.g., 7 or above) in breeding ewes outside of the breeding season?
 a) Improved lambing rates
 b) Increased incidence of dystocia
 c) Decreased wool production
 d) Enhanced milk production for lambs
63. When assessing BCS in goats, which anatomical region is NOT typically considered due to its lack of reliability in reflecting body fat reserves?
 a) The loin b) The brisket
 c) The ribs d) The tailhead

64. In equine BCS assessment, which of the following is considered a critical area for determining fat deposition related to metabolic health risks?

a) Neck b) Hooves

c) Flank d) Shoulders

65. What specific physiological changes occur at the cellular level in livestock with a BCS of 1, impacting their metabolic processes?

a) Decreased lipolysis b) Upregulation of insulin receptors

c) Increased gluconeogenesis d) Enhanced mitochondrial activity

66. In highly productive dairy cows with a BCS of 8, what hormonal imbalance might be expected, and how does it affect milk production?

a) Elevated cortisol leading to increased lactose synthesis

b) Reduced growth hormone causing increased milk yield

c) Increased insulin sensitivity resulting in higher milk fat content

d) Elevated glucocorticoids suppressing milk production

67. What is the impact of a BCS of 3 on the fatty acid composition of adipose tissue in beef cattle, and how does this influence meat quality?

a) Increased saturated fats leading to improved marbling

b) Higher omega-3 fatty acids enhancing tenderness

c) Decreased monounsaturated fats improving flavor

d) Elevated trans fats negatively affecting meat texture

68. How can the body condition of pregnant ewes (BCS 2) influence epigenetic modifications in fetal development, specifically related to metabolic programming?

a) Upregulation of genes associated with lean muscle mass

b) Methylation changes in genes linked to increased feed efficiency

c) Activation of genes promoting early puberty in offspring

d) Downregulation of genes responsible for nutrient absorption

69. Considering seasonal variations, how does a harsh winter with limited forage availability impact the BCS of free-ranging bison herds, and what adaptive physiological changes might occur?

a) Increased BCS due to enhanced cold tolerance

b) Decreased BCS due to metabolic suppression

c) Maintenance of BCS through hibernation-like metabolic adjustments

d) Fluctuations in BCS unrelated to seasonal changes

70. In ruminants with a BCS of 9, how does the altered gut microbiota composition affect nutrient absorption and utilization?

a) Increased fiber digestion leading to improved energy efficiency

b) Enhanced nitrogen retention resulting in higher protein synthesis

c) Imbalanced microbial community reducing volatile fatty acid production

d) Suppressed methane production causing improved feed conversion

71. In camelids with a consistently low BCS (2-3) due to arid conditions, what long-term physiological adaptations might be observed to ensure survival?
    a) Enhanced water conservation through reduced urine production
    b) Increased susceptibility to parasitic infections for better nutrient extraction
    c) Development of thicker fur to conserve body heat
    d) Altered sleep patterns to optimize metabolic rate
72. How does a chronically high BCS (7-8) impact the immune function of poultry, specifically in terms of antibody response to vaccinations?
    a) Suppressed antibody production leading to decreased vaccine efficacy
    b) Enhanced humoral response resulting in prolonged immunity
    c) Upregulated cellular immunity causing autoimmunity
    d) Unaffected immune response due to the independent nature of BCS and vaccination
73. In beef cattle with a BCS of 5, how does their enteric methane production differ from cattle with a BCS of 3, and what physiological factors contribute to this difference?
    a) Increased methane emissions due to higher fiber intake
    b) Reduced methane production due to enhanced microbial diversity
    c) Similar methane emissions as BCS is not directly linked to rumen fermentation
    d) Fluctuating methane levels due to inconsistent forage quality
74. What role does a high BCS (8-9) play in altering the antioxidant capacity of grazing sheep, and how does this influence their susceptibility to oxidative stress-related diseases?
    a) Increased antioxidant activity leading to improved disease resistance
    b) Reduced antioxidant capacity causing susceptibility to infectious diseases
    c) Enhanced reactive oxygen species production with no impact on health
    d) Unaltered antioxidant status as BCS does not affect cellular redox balance
75. What physiological changes are primarily responsible for a decrease in BCS in lactating dairy cows?
    a) Decreased feed intake and increased milk production
    b) Increased feed intake and decreased milk production
    c) Decreased water consumption
    d) Increased water consumption and decreased feed intake
76. In dairy cows, a BCS loss greater than how many units postpartum is associated with delayed ovarian activity?
    a) 0.5 units
    b) 1 unit
    c) 1.5 units
    d) 2 units
77. For ewes, an optimal BCS for enhancing lambing rates and minimizing pregnancy toxemia is:
    a) 2-3
    b) 3-4
    c) 4-5
    d) 5-6

78. Which BCS range in beef cattle is most closely associated with an optimal immune response?

a) 4-5
b) 5-6
c) 6-7
d) 7-8

79. Adjusting the diet of a high-producing dairy cow with a BCS of 2.5 should prioritize:

a) Increasing fiber to promote rumen health
b) Maximizing energy density to recover body condition
c) Decreasing protein to avoid excessive body condition loss
d) Balancing micronutrients to enhance feed efficiency

80. In cattle, how does a pre-parturition BCS of less than 5 affect calving outcomes?

a) Increases the risk of dystocia
b) Decreases the time to first estrus
c) Increases calf vigor at birth
d) Has no significant effect on calving outcomes

81. The ideal BCS for dairy heifers at first breeding to ensure optimal reproductive and lactation performance is:

a) 2.5-3.0
b) 3.0-3.5
c) 3.5-4.0
d) 4.0-4.5

82. Adjusting the BCS of grazing beef cows before winter requires consideration of what key factor?

a) Increasing BCS by 1 unit to compensate for cold stress
b) Maintaining a constant BCS throughout the year
c) Decreasing BCS to improve mobility in snow
d) Focusing solely on micronutrient supplementation

83. What is the primary goal of adjusting nutrition based on BCS in dairy cows?

a) Increase milk production
b) Maintain stable body weight
c) Ensure optimal reproductive performance
d) Maximize feed cost savings

84. A beef cow with a BCS of 4 requires dietary adjustments to:

a) Increase energy intake before breeding
b) Decrease protein intake during lactation
c) Maintain current feed regimen
d) Reduce overall feed intake

85. For a dairy cow at a BCS of 3.5 post-calving, the nutritional focus should be on:

a) High-energy diets to regain body condition
b) High-fiber diets to stimulate rumination
c) Reduced feed intake to prevent obesity
d) Increased protein for milk production

86. In sheep with a BCS below the ideal range for breeding, the diet should be enriched with:
   a) Fibers to reduce weight loss
   b) Carbohydrates to increase energy
   c) Fats for slow energy release
   d) Proteins to enhance muscle growth
87. When managing the diet of a horse with a BCS of 6, what is a primary concern?
   a) Preventing weight gain
   b) Encouraging rapid weight loss
   c) Increasing muscle mass
   d) Enhancing coat shine
88. The dietary management for a dairy cow with a high BCS (above 3.5) during dry off period should focus on:
   a) Increasing energy density
   b) Limiting energy intake
   c) Supplementing with high levels of proteins
   d) Enhancing micronutrient supplementation
89. For lactating dairy cows with a low BCS (below 2.5), it is crucial to:
   a) Restrict water intake to concentrate nutrients
   b) Provide high-quality forage to improve condition
   c) Focus on weight maintenance rather than gain
   d) Decrease dietary energy sources
90. To improve the BCS of underconditioned beef cattle, the most effective dietary change is to:
   a) Increase the proportion of forage in the diet
   b) Supplement with grain-based concentrates
   c) Reduce overall feed intake for better digestion
   d) Add more roughage to slow down feed consumption
91. A ewe with a BCS of 3 aiming for optimal lambing outcomes should have a diet adjusted to:
   a) Decrease energy intake pre-lambing
   b) Increase protein levels pre-lambing
   c) Maintain a stable energy intake throughout pregnancy
   d) Gradually increase energy intake as lambing approaches
92. In managing goats with varying BCS, a common strategy is to:
   a) Provide uniform diets to all goats to simplify management
   b) Group goats by BCS and adjust diets accordingly
   c) Focus on high-energy diets regardless of BCS
   d) Limit protein intake to manage weight

93. The adjustment of nutritional management based on BCS is least likely to directly influence:
    a) Feed efficiency b) Coat color
    c) Reproductive performance d) Growth rates

94. For broodmares with a BCS of 5, the nutritional management leading up to foaling should:
    a) Emphasize calorie restriction to prevent excessive weight gain
    b) Increase caloric intake to support fetal growth
    c) Maintain a consistent diet as in non-pregnant states
    d) Focus solely on mineral supplementation

95. In managing a dairy cow's transition diet based on BCS, a cow with a BCS of 4 should:
    a) Be provided with a high-energy ration immediately post-calving
    b) Have restricted feed intake pre-calving to prevent fat mobilization
    c) Receive a balanced energy and protein diet to avoid metabolic disorders
    d) Focus on fiber-rich diets to prevent ketosis

96. Adjusting the diet of pigs based on BCS is crucial for:
    a) Enhancing meat quality in finishing pigs
    b) Decreasing gestation length in sows
    c) Increasing litter size
    d) Reducing feed costs across all stages

97. When a beef steer exhibits a BCS lower than desired for market, the most effective nutritional strategy is to:
    a) Increase dietary protein to enhance muscle development
    b) Focus on high-energy feeds to rapidly increase weight
    c) Implement a grass-fed regimen to improve meat quality
    d) Reduce feed intake to concentrate muscle growth

98. A low BCS in dairy cows (below 2.5) is associated with which reproductive issue?
    a) Increased milk production b) Decreased incidence of mastitis
    c) Extended postpartum anestrus d) Shortened gestation period

99. Optimal BCS for breeding in beef cows is generally considered to be:
    a) 2-3 b) 3-4
    c) 4-5 d) 5-6

100. In ewes, a BCS lower than ideal (below 2.5) can lead to:
    a) Increased twin births b) Reduced lambing rates
    c) Higher milk production d) Shorter lambing intervals

101. The BCS in sows that typically results in the highest fertility rates is:
    a) 2 b) 3
    c) 4 d) 5

102. How does a high BCS at calving (above 3.5) affect dairy cow fertility?
   a) Increases early pregnancy loss
   b) Shortens time to first estrus
   c) Enhances oocyte quality
   d) Reduces the incidence of dystocia

103. In beef cattle, a pre-breeding BCS of less than 5 is associated with:
   a) Higher pregnancy rates
   b) Decreased calving interval
   c) Increased embryonic loss
   d) Improved semen quality in bulls

104. For optimal reproductive performance in goats, the BCS should be maintained at:
   a) 1.5-2.0
   b) 2.0-2.5
   c) 2.5-3.0
   d) 3.0-3.5

105. An ideal BCS for horses to maintain fertility and successful pregnancy outcomes is:
   a) 4-5 on a 9-point scale
   b) 5-6 on a 9-point scale
   c) 6-7 on a 9-point scale
   d) 7-8 on a 9-point scale

106. Which of the following is a potential effect of over-conditioning (high BCS) in breeding sows?
   a) Increased litter size
   b) Reduced farrowing rates
   c) Enhanced milk production
   d) Shortened weaning to estrus interval

107. The effect of a low BCS in dairy cows on estrus behavior is:
   a) More pronounced estrus signs
   b) Shortened estrus duration
   c) Reduced visibility of estrus signs
   d) No impact on estrus behavior

108. Which BCS range is considered optimal for breeding in dairy heifers?
   a) 2.0-2.5
   b) 2.5-3.0
   c) 3.0-3.5
   d) 3.5-4.0

109. In broodmares, a BCS below 5 (on a 9-point scale) can result in:
   a) Increased incidence of twins
   b) Higher rates of early embryonic death
   c) Shortened gestation lengths
   d) Increased foaling rates

110. What is the impact of a BCS of 4 or above in beef cows at the time of calving on reproductive performance?
   a) Improved conception rates at first service
   b) Reduced time to first estrus postpartum
   c) Increased risk of postpartum anestrus
   d) No significant impact

111. How does maintaining an optimal BCS in ewes affect lamb survival rates?
   a) Increases lamb mortality
   b) Has no effect on lamb survival
   c) Decreases lamb mortality
   d) Only affects twins' survival rates

112. The relationship between BCS and reproductive efficiency in dairy cows is mediated primarily through:
   a) Milk yield b) Energy balance
   c) Protein intake d) Feed conversion ratio

113. A low BCS in dairy cows (below 2.5) is most likely associated with increased susceptibility to:
   a) Laminitis b) Ketosis
   c) Mastitis d) All of the above

114. In beef cattle, optimal BCS for minimizing the risk of infectious diseases is:
   a) 2-3 b) 3-4
   c) 4-5 d) 5-6

115. Over-conditioned (high BCS) sheep are at a higher risk of developing:
   a) Foot rot b) Pregnancy toxemia
   c) Internal parasitism d) Pneumonia

116. Which disease is associated with low BCS in lactating dairy cows?
   a) Displaced abomasum b) Bloat
   c) Hardware disease d) None of the above

117. An optimal BCS in dairy cows has been shown to reduce the incidence of:
   a) Metritis b) Milk fever
   c) Both A and B d) Neither A nor B

118. High BCS in sows is often related to increased risk of:
   a) Mastitis b) Lameness
   c) Metritis d) All of the above

119. Maintaining a BCS of 3-3.5 in dairy cows can help reduce the occurrence of:
   a) Ketosis b) Liver abscesses
   c) Ruminal acidosis d) All of the above

120. In horses, a high BCS (above 7 on a 9-point scale) is a risk factor for:
   a) Colic b) Laminitis
   c) Both A and B d) Neither A nor B

121. Which condition is NOT typically associated with a low BCS in goats?
   a) Caprine arthritis encephalitis b) Enterotoxemia
   c) Caseous lymphadenitis d) Parasitic infections

122. For beef cattle, an optimal BCS is crucial in preventing:
   a) Respiratory diseases b) Reproductive diseases
   c) Both A and B d) Neither A nor B

123. A dairy cow with a high BCS is more susceptible to:
   a) Subclinical ketosis b) Clinical mastitis
   c) Both A and B d) Neither A nor B

124. In sheep, a BCS lower than 2 can increase the risk of:
   a) Hypocalcemia b) Copper toxicity
   c) Pneumonia d) Foot abscesses

125. The most common disease associated with both high and low BCS in dairy cows is:
   a) Lameness b) Mastitis
   c) Metabolic disorders d) Respiratory diseases

126. Optimal BCS in broodmares is associated with decreased risk of:
   a) Uterine infections b) Retained placenta
   c) Both A and B d) Neither A nor B

127. A low BCS in beef cows (below 4) can contribute to increased susceptibility to:
   a) Bovine respiratory disease complex (BRDC)
   b) Bovine viral diarrhea (BVD)
   c) Both A and B
   d) Neither A nor B

128. How does BCS affect the immune response in livestock?
   a) High BCS always enhances the immune response
   b) Low BCS always enhances the immune response
   c) Optimal BCS supports a more effective immune response
   d) BCS has no impact on the immune response

129. In dairy cattle, managing BCS to avoid extremes is important to reduce the risk of:
   a) Rumen disorders b) Transition cow disorders
   c) Infectious diseases d) All of the above

130. What role does BCS play in the management of parasitic infections in sheep?
   a) No role
   b) Indirect role through influencing grazing behavior
   c) Direct role by affecting skin thickness and barrier functions
   d) Both B and C

131. A high BCS in lactating sows can lead to increased incidence of:
   a) Prolapse b) Agalactia
   c) Both A and B d) Neither A nor B

132. An ideal BCS in horses to minimize the risk of infectious diseases is:
   a) 4-5 on a 9-point scale b) 5-6 on a 9-point scale
   c) 6-7 on a 9-point scale d) 7-8 on a 9-point scale

133. Which of the following best describes the relationship between BCS and disease resistance in goats?
   a) A direct correlation; higher BCS always means higher disease resistance
   b) An inverse correlation; lower BCS means higher disease resistance
   c) A bell-shaped relationship; both high and low BCS can compromise disease resistance
   d) No correlation; BCS does not affect disease resistance

134. Improving BCS from low to optimal in dairy cows can have the greatest impact on reducing the risk of:
   a) External parasites b) Metabolic diseases
   c) Contagious mastitis d) Genetic disorders

135. The relationship between BCS and the incidence of lameness in dairy cattle is:
   a) Positive; higher BCS increases the risk
   b) Negative; higher BCS decreases the risk
   c) U-shaped; both high and low BCS increase the risk
   d) Insignificant; BCS has no impact on lameness

136. In broiler breeders, an optimal BCS is important to prevent:
   a) Ascites b) Fatty liver syndrome
   c) Osteoporosis d) All of the above

137. A primary reason to maintain an optimal BCS in breeding bulls is to reduce the risk of:
   a) Scrotal hernia b) Foot and leg problems
   c) Seminal vesiculitis d) All of the above

138. For dairy goats, an optimal BCS is critical to minimize the occurrence of:
   a) Ketosis b) Udder edema
   c) Caprine arthritis encephalitis d) A and B

139. Which is NOT a common effect of low BCS on disease resistance in livestock?
   a) Increased vulnerability to metabolic diseases
   b) Higher resistance to bacterial infections
   c) Compromised immune function
   d) Increased stress response

140. In the context of BCS and disease resistance, nutritional management should aim to:
   a) Maximize energy density in the diet at all times
   b) Ensure rapid weight gain before breeding season
   c) Avoid extremes of BCS to support optimal health and productivity
   d) Focus solely on protein intake

141. A low BCS in livestock can lead to a higher incidence of which condition due to impaired immune function?
   a) Genetic mutations b) Nutritional myodegeneration
   c) Infectious diseases d) None of the above

142. The impact of BCS on disease resistance in livestock is primarily mediated through:
   a) Genetic predisposition b) Immune system function
   c) Behavioral changes d) Environmental factors

143. A higher Body Condition Score (BCS) in livestock is generally associated with:
   a) Increased disease resistance b) Decreased disease resistance
   c) No impact on disease resistance d) Only affects respiratory diseases

144. How does a low BCS contribute to disease susceptibility in cattle?
    a) Weakens the immune system
    b) Increases vaccination effectiveness
    c) Enhances antibiotic resistance
    d) Improves overall health
145. In poultry, a low BCS can lead to increased susceptibility to:
    a) Avian influenza
    b) Feather color mutations
    c) Improved egg production
    d) Decreased coccidiosis risk
146. A BCS below the optimum range in sheep may increase the risk of:
    a) Foot rot
    b) Wool shedding
    c) Increased lambing rates
    d) Improved overall flock health
147. How does a low BCS impact the gastrointestinal health of ruminants?
    a) Reduces the risk of acidosis
    b) Increases the risk of bloat
    c) Enhances nutrient absorption
    d) Has no impact on gastrointestinal health
148. The relationship between BCS and disease resistance is primarily mediated through:
    a) Endocrine system
    b) Immune system
    c) Respiratory system
    d) Musculoskeletal system
149. In swine, a BCS below 3 may result in increased susceptibility to:
    a) Porcine reproductive and respiratory syndrome (PRRS)
    b) Improved growth rates
    c) Reduced litter size
    d) Enhanced resistance to common pig diseases
150. How does a low BCS in dairy cows affect mastitis risk?
    a) Increases mastitis risk
    b) Decreases mastitis risk
    c) Has no impact on mastitis risk
    d) Improves milk quality

Answer Key

1	b	2	b	3	d	4	b	5	b	6	c	7	d
8	b	9	c	10	b	11	b	12	c	13	c	14	c
15	d	16	c	17	c	18	d	19	d	20	b	21	b
22	c	23	b	24	b	25	b	26	b	27	a	28	c
29	c	30	c	31	d	32	c	33	b	34	c	35	c
36	c	37	c	38	c	39	c	40	b	41	a	42	c
43	c	44	d	45	b	46	b	47	a	48	d	49	c
50	c	51	d	52	b	53	b	54	c	55	a	56	b
57	c	58	c	59	d	60	b	61	c	62	b	63	b
64	a	65	c	66	d	67	a	68	b	69	c	70	c

71	a	72	a	73	b	74	b	75	a	76	c	77	b
78	b	79	b	80	a	81	b	82	a	83	c	84	a
85	a	86	b	87	a	88	b	89	b	90	b	91	d
92	b	93	b	94	b	95	c	96	a	97	b	98	c
99	c	100	b	101	b	102	a	103	c	104	c	105	b
106	b	107	c	108	c	109	b	110	c	111	c	112	b
113	d	114	c	115	b	116	a	117	c	118	d	119	a
120	c	121	b	122	c	123	c	124	d	125	b	126	c
127	a	128	c	129	d	130	d	131	c	132	b	133	c
134	b	135	c	136	d	137	b	138	d	139	b	140	c
141	c	142	b	143	a	144	a	145	a	146	a	147	b
148	b	149	a	150	a								

8

Fly Control and Management

***Ganesh K. Sawale*[1], *and G.P. Bharkad*[2]**

[1]*Department of Veterinary Pathology, Mumbai Veterinary College, Parel, Mumbai Maharashtra*

[2]*Department of Veterinary Parasitology, College of Veterinary & Animal Sciences Udgir, Maharashtra*

Introduction

Poultry manure provides an ideal habitat for fly breeding due to high manure moisture leading to increased fly populationand fly menace in poultry farm. The moisture, temperature and humid condition play important role in fly breeding. The flies on poultry farms are unacceptable as they act as a reservoir of many diseases and spread diseases to birds and human beings. In addition to spread of diseases, fly are nuisance to birds as they distract the birds as well as poultry farm employees, nearby farms and residence (Berry, 2003). High fly population contribute tapeworm infestation in flock and disseminate bacterial (like salmonella, fowl cholera, etc.) and viral diseases (Bird flu, New Castle disease, etc. in flocks. Fly population also causes public health issue leading to pressure on poultry farmers to control fly population on poultry farms to acceptable level. The flies on poultry farm includes House fly (*Muscadomestica*), little house fly (*Fanniacanicularis*), Black Garbage fly (*Hydrotaeaaenescens*), Dump flies (*H. aenescens, H. ignava, H. capensis*), Drosophila flies (*Drosophila repleta*), Soldier fly (*Hermetiaillucens*), Stable flies (*Stomoxyscalcitrans*), Drosophila flies (*Drosophila repleta*) and Blow flies (*Lucilia, Phormia*, and *Calliphora*) and black flies. The *Lucilia* species include *L. cuprina* and *L. sericata*(Axtell, 1999). Among these, the most common flies on farms are House fly and the little house fly. Both these fly are capable of movement up to 5 miles. Flies reproduce at very fast rate and each female can lay up to 1000 eggs over 30 day life cycle (Day, 2010). All flies go through four life cycle stages viz. egg, larva, pupa and adult. The eggs are laid in freshly voided faeces (manure) which is high in moisture (around 60 -80%). The larva hatch in moist manure (12 hours to 48 hours). The larva spin cocoon and pupate. The pupa in turn becomes adult. The complete lifecycle takes weeks to two months (Hess, *et al.*, 2019). The fly can be controlled by good management and sanitation programme, mechanical and chemical measures and biological control. The mechanical control of fly includes installation of doors that mechanically open and close, adjustment of exhaust fans, electrocuting light traps, odor-baited traps, etc. The chemical control of fly includes use of carbamates, pyrethroids and organoposphate insecticide. The biological fly control measure includes utilization of enemy of flies viz. entomic pathogenic fungi, nematode, beetle, parasitic wasp, etc.

1. The scientific name for House fly is ..
   a) *H. aenescens* b) *Muscadomestica*
   c) *Stomoxyscalcitrans* d) *L. cuprina*
2. The *Muscadomestica* is commonly called as ..
   a) The little House fly b) Common House fly
   c) Black garbage fly d) Dump fly
3. The adult *Muscadomestica*fly size (length) ranges from
   a) < 3 mm b) 3-5 mm
   c) 6-7 mm d) 8-10 mm
4. The house fly *Muscadomestica*under normal condition usually complete life cycle in
   a) <5 days b) 7-10 days
   c) 2-3 Months d) None of these
5. The egg of house fly *Muscadomestica* usually hatch in
   a) < 24 hours b) 1-2 week
   c) 1-2 Months d) None of these
6. The following statement are true for egg of *Muscadomestica*except.
   a) Eggs are white in colour
   b) Eggs are laid singly or piled in small group
   c) Eggs are 1.2 mm in length
   d) Egg are round in shape
7. The following statement are true for larva of *Muscadomestica*except.
   a) Larvae are white in colour
   b) Larvae are cylindrical in shape
   c) Head of larvae contain four pair of dark hooks
   d) Larvae are 3-9 mm in length
8. The following statement are true for larva of *Muscadomestica*except.
   a) Larvaego through three instars and full grown maggot
   b) Maggots are greasy and cream coloured
   c) Full grown maggot size ranges from 7-12 mm
   d) Low moisture required for survivalof larva
9. The optimal temperature for larval development of House fly is
   a) $4\text{-}12^{0}$ b) $35\text{-}38^{0}$
   c) $42\text{-}47^{0}$ d) All of these
10. The following statement are true for Pupa of *Muscadomestica*except.
   a) Pupa are 8 mm long
   b) Pupa varies in colour*viz*. red, yellow, brown or black
   c) Pupa are 15-20 mm long with tapering ends
   d) Pupa complete development in 2-6 days under optimal condition

11. The following statement are true for adult House flyexcept.
    a) House fly is 6-7 mm long
    b) Males are usually larger than female
    c) Female had relatively wide space between two eyes
    d) The thorax of house fly bears four narrow black stripes
12. The following statement are true for adult male House flyexcept.
    a) Eyes are closely placed (almost touches with each other)
    b) Males are usually smaller than female
    c) Underside of male is yellow in colour
    d) Males are usually larger than female
13. The adult house fly usually can survive for
    a) < a week
    b) 3-4 week
    c) > 2 months
    d) All of these
14. The following are the diseases transmitted by adult house fly as a transport vector except
    a) Salmonella infection in birds
    b) Fowl typhoid
    c) New Castle disease
    d) Avian malaria
15. The following statement are true for adult house fly for development stages except
    a) 10 days at 85 ^{0}F
    b) 21 days at 70 ^{0}F
    c) 45 days at 60 ^{0}F
    d) 9 days at 50 ^{0}F
16. The scientific name of little house fly is..
    a) *Muscadomesti*
    b) *Stomoxyscalcitrans*
    c) *L. cuprin*
    d) *Fanniacannicularis*
17. The *Fanniacannicularis* is commonly called as is
    a) House fly
    b) Littlehouse fly
    c) Stable fly
    d) Black garbage fly
18. The following statements are true for little house fly except…
    a) Its one half the size of common house fly
    b) Species often flies in circle
    c) Development from egg to adult requires 2-4 week under optimal condition
    d) Development from egg to adult requires less than week
19. The following statements are true for little house fly except..
    a) Its larger than common house fly
    b) Possess three brown stripes on thorax
    c) Its smaller than common house fly
    d) Adult complete life cycle in 15-28 days
20. The following statements are true for larvae of little house fly except..
    a) The larvae are flat or slender in shape
    b) Larvae are smaller (3.5 to 6 mm) than common house fly
    c) Larvae are brown in colour
    d) Larvae have smooth body surface

21. The life expectancy (survival) for little house fly is..
   a) 1-2 week
   b) 2-5 weeks
   c) 5-10 weeks
   d) 10-20 weeks
22. The scientific name for Black garbage fly is
   a) *Muscadomesti*
   b) *Fanniacannicularis*
   c) *Hydrotaeaaenescens*
   d) *Hydrotaeaaenescens*
23. The *Hydrotaeaaenescens(*fly) is commonly called as
   a) Common house fly
   b) Dump fly
   c) Black garbage fly
   d) Both b & c
24. The following statements are true for Black garbage fly except..
   a) The fly is shiny bronz-black in colour
   b) The fly is shiny green in colour
   c) Life cycle completes in 14-45 days
   d) Adult tend to stay on food source
25. The following statements are true for dump fly except..
   a) The adult fly is one half size of house fly
   b) The fly is slender in shape
   c) It's often called black garbage flies
   d) Adult tend to stay on poultry manure
26. The following statements are true for dump fly larvae except..
   a) The larvae are similar to house fly larvae but more slender and active
   b) The fly larvae prey on arthropod in the manure
   c) The black garbage fly is used as a biological control agent against the house fly
   d) The larvae are round in shape
27. The dump fly lays around …eggs over 7-10 days period.
   a) <50 eggs
   b) up to 170 eggs
   c) >500 eggs
   d) None of these
28. The scientific name of soldier fly is..
   a) *Muscadomesti*
   b) *Stomoxyscalcitrans*
   c) Hermetiaillucens
   d) *Fanniacannicularis*
29. The *Hermetiaillucens* is commonly called as is
   a) House fly
   b) Soldier fly
   c) Stable fly
   d) Black garbage fly
30. The following statements are true for soldier fly except..
   a) The solder fly oviposits egg masses on the drier portions of the manure
   b) A complete life cycle from egg to adult in poultry houses requires 40–60 days
   c) Adult fly have two wings
   d) Adults range from 40 to 50 mm in length

31. The following statements are true for soldier fly except..
    a) Adults range from 15 to 20 mm in length
    b) The adult's antennae are elongated with onesegments
    c) Adults have white coloration near the end of each leg
    d) The adult's antennae are elongated with three segments
32. The soldier fly lays around …eggs.
    a) <200 eggs b) 500 eggs
    c) 1000 eggs d) None of these
33. The following statements are true for soldier fly egg except.
    a) Eggs are oval in shape and 1mm in length
    b) The eggs hatch into larvae in about four days
    c) Eggs are pale yellow or creamy white in colour
    d) Eggs are laid in moist poultry manure
34. The following statements are true for soldier fly larvae except.
    a) Larvae are 27 mm in length and 6 mm in width
    b) The larvae are dull whitish in colour with small projecting head
    c) Larvae require around 14 days completing development
    d) Black soldier fly larvae are satiable feeders
35. The larvae of one the fly has been shown to be effective manure recyclers
    a) House fly b) Black soldier fly
    c) Stable fly d) Black garbage fly
36. The following statements are true for Drosophila flies except
    a) Adults are dull brown and prefer cooler area of poultry house for resting
    b) The flies are commonly called as Soldier fly
    c) Adults flies are 2 mm to 4 mm in size
    d) These are small, non-biting flies
37. The *Drosophila repleta*is commonly called as
    a) Dark eyed fruit fly b) Dark eyed vinegar fly
    c) Both a and b are true d) Only a is true
38. The Flies [Diptera] in the family Calliphoridae are commonly called as
    a) Blow flies b) Dark eyed vinegar fly
    c) Stable fly d) Soldier fly
39. The following statements are true for Blow flies except
    a) Adult lay their eggs on media rich in proteins (animal carcasses, broken egg)
    b) The adults are green, bronz or black in colour
    c) Larva to adult development occurs within a week perio
    d) Larva to adult development requires 3-4 week period

40. The following are the Blow flies except

a) *Lucili* b) *Phormia*

c) *Drosophila* d) *Calliphora*

41. The scientific name of green bottle fly is..

a) *Lucili* b) *Phormia*

c) *Drosophila* d) *Calliphora*

42. *Lucilia* is commonly called as is

a) Blue bottle fly b) Green bottle fly

c) Cluster fly d) Soldier fly

43. The scientific name of blue bottle fly is..

a) *Lucili* b) *Phormia*

c) *Drosophila* d) *Calliphora*

44. *Calliphora* is commonly called as is

a) Green bottle fly b) Blue bottle fly

c) Cluster fly d) Soldier fly

45. The following statements are true for Black flies except

a) Adult flies can bite to adult birds

b) Black flies are non-biting flies

c) Black flies are small and usually of 1.2 to 3 mm in size

d) Black flies are commonly called as buffalo gnats

46. The following statements are true for Black flies except

a) Black fly eggs are 0.18 to 0.46 mm long and somewhat irregular in shape

b) Black fly larvae are slender, 5 to 15 mm long

c) Adult lays eggs in stagnated water

d) Black fly pupae are 2 to 3 mm long with a respiratory organ on the thorax

47. The following statements are true for Black flies except

a) Adult lays eggs in running water

b) Female lays the egg after blood meal

c) Adults flies can transmit bacterial poultry diseases

d) Adults flies can transmit haemoprotozoan (*Leucocytozoon spp.*) poultry diseases

48. The important poultry disease transmitted by Black flies is/ are…

a) *Leucocytozooncauleryi* b) *Leucocytozoonsimondi*

c) *Plasmodium spp* d) Both a & b

49. The basic approaches for biological control of flies include(s)…

a) Encouragement of the populations of natural enemies already present

b) Use of chemical to kill larval and adult stages of fly

c) Use of mechanical control like traps, etc.

d) All of these

50. The mechanical control of flies include(s) all the following except...
   a) Encouragement of the populations of natural enemies already present
   b) Adjustment of exhaust fans
   c) Electrocuting light traps
   d) Use of odor-baited traps
51. The chemical control of flies include(s) all the following except...
   a) Use of carbamates
   b) Use of pyrethroids
   c) Use of Electrocuting light traps
   d) Use of organoposphate insecticide
52. The biological control of house fly is achieved by use of ...
   a) *Muscidifurax raptor* b) *Muscidifuraxzaraptor*
   c) *Spalangiacameroni.* d) Only a and b
53. The biological control of house fly is achieved by use of ...
   a) *Spalangianigroaenea* *b)* *Spalangianigra*
   c) *Spalangiacameroni.* *d)* *Spalangiaendius*
54. The chemical commonly used in fly bait is...
   a) Carbaryl b) Cyfluthrin
   c) Methomyl d) None of these
55. The chemical commonly used as feed additive for control of fly larvae is ...
   a) Carbaryl *b)* Cyromazine
   c) Methomyl *d)* *None of these*
56. The chemical commonly used for autosterlization of house fly is ...
   a) Triflumuron b) Cyromazine
   c) Methomyl d) None of these
57. The space spray or mist in poultry farm are commonly used for control of ...
   a) Large fly population b) Small fly population
   c) Large larval population d) None of these
58. The Bait stations can also help cont rol the fly population on poultry farms and contain...
   a) An insecticide b) Fly attractant like sugars
   C) BOTHA AND d) None of these
59. The vapour stripe is one of the method of fly control ...
   a) Mechanical control b) Biological control
   c) Chemical control d) None of these
60. The larvicideare used for fly control by ...
   a) Spraying larvicide on manure to kill larvae
   b) Feeding larvicide through feed to kill larvae developed in voided manure
   c) Both a and
   d) None of these

61. The larvadex is a larvicideused for fly control by ...
   a) Spraying on manure to kill larvae
   b) Feeding through feed to kill larvae developed in voided manure
   c) Larvadex is continuously given through oral route throughout life of birds
   d) None of these

References

Axtell RC. Poultry integrated pest management: status and future. Integrated pest management reviews. 1999 Mar;4:53-73.

Berry JG. Fly control in the poultry house. Oklahoma Cooperative Extension Service; 2003.

Day, ER. Poultry Area Fly Control. Livestock: Poultry Area Fly Control 2-5 In: Field Crops 2010.

Hess J, Macklin K, and Strother GR. Poultry Pest Management - Alabama Cooperative Extension System (aces.edu), 2019.

Answer Key

1	b	2	b	3	c	4	b	5	a	6	d	7	c
8	d	9	b	10	c	11	b	12	d	13	b	14	d
15	d	16	d	17	b	18	d	19	a	20	d	21	b
22	d	23	d	24	b	25	d	26	d	27	b	28	c
29	b	30	d	31	b	32	b	33	d	34	d	35	b
36	b	37	c	38	a	39	d	40	c	41	a	42	b
43	d	44	b	45	b	46	c	47	c	48	d	49	a
50	a	51	c	52	d	53	a	54	c	55	b	56	a
57	a	58	c	59	c	60	c	61	b				

9

Livestock Production and Livelihood Security

Jessy Bagh[1], Annada Das[2], and Kaushik Satyaprakash[3]

[1]Department of Livestock Production and Management, CVSc & AH, OUAT Bhubaneswar, Odisha

[2]Department of Livestock Products technology, Faculty of Veterinary and Animal Sciences, WBUAFS, Kolkata, West Bengal

[3]Department of Veterinary Public Health and Epidemiology, Faculty of Veterinary and Animal Sciences, RGSC, BHU, Mirzapur, Uttar Pradesh

Introduction

Livestock is a global resource with significant benefits to society in the form of food, income, nutrients, employment, insurance, traction, clothing and others.

Livestock sector of India holds among one of the largest globally. Around 20.5 million people depend on it on livestock for their livelihood. Livestock farming contributed 16% of small farm income households compared to an average of 14% for all rural households. provides livestock

Livelihood for two thirds of the rural population. Furthermore, it provides employment to around 8.8% of the workforce population in India. India has huge livestock populations. The livestock sector contributes 4.11% GDP and 25.6% of total agricultural GDP.

Livestock count

Livestock farming plays an important role in the farmers' economy. The farmers in India Maintaining a mixed farming system, i.e. H. a combination of agriculture and livestock farming in which production takes place. One company becomes the input of another company and thus realizes the resource efficiency.

Livestock farming serves as insurance against crop failures.

A production system consists of interconnected and interacting components (or subsystems). within the boundaries of which material and immaterial elements are located (subsystem, components) with goals and purposes that require inputs to produce outputs and whose balance is influenced by supporting, catalytic and opposing other systems and subsystems".

Livestock as a livelihood for the rural poor

The following describes the different roles of farm animals in the lives of small farmers and poor villagers

1. It cushions the risks of crop failure, unemployment and underemployment.

2. Improves the nutritional status of the family and enables domestic consumption of essential nutrients
3. Provides regular cash income
4. Providing draft, manure and fuel services
5. Contributes to improving socioeconomic status

Some of the limitations small farmers face:

1. Have meager resources
2. Limited access to resources, services, technology and market due to their low social economic status
3. Subsistence farming/livelihood
4. Poorly organized
5. Spread over a large area with poor transportation and communication facilities

Role of livestock in the rural economy

- Livestock serve farmers in different ways.
- Income: Livestock farming is a source of additional income, especially resource, for many families in India
- Arms that only hold a few animal heads. Cows and buffaloes provide a regular income with milk to livestock farmers through the sale of milk. Goat and sheep fullfill emergencies income , to meet requirements such as marriage, treatment of sick people, raising children, repairing houses, etc. The animals also serve as movable banks and assets that provide economic purposes security for the owners.
- Employment: A large number of people in India depend on less educated and unskilled people farming for their livelihood. But seasonal farming could create jobs for a maximum of 180 days per year. The country is becoming less and less dependent on livestock.
- They utilize their labor during the lean farming season.
- Food: Animal products such as milk, meat and eggs are an important source of animal protein
- to the members of the animal owners. The per capita availability of milk is about 355 g/day;
- eggs is 69/year;
- Social security: The animals provide social security to the owners in terms of their status in society.
- The families, especially the landless, who own animals are better off than those who do not.
- Gifting animals during marriage is a common phenomenon in different parts of the country.
- Animal husbandry is a part of Indian culture. Animals are used for various socio-religious purposes
- Features. cows for housewarming ceremonies; Rams, goats and chickens are sacrificed during the holiday seasons; bulls and cows are worshiped on various religious occasions. Many owners are developing bonding with their animals.

- Gender equality: Animal husbandry promotes gender equality. More than three quarters of the work
- The demand in animal production is met by women. The share of female employment in livestock farming

Multiple Choice Questions

1. Total livestock population in India:
   a) 535.78 million b) 302.79 Million
   c) 192.49 Million d) 145.12 million
2. Total Bovine population in India:
   a) 535.78 million b) 302.79 Million
   c) 192.49 Million d) 145.12 million
3. Total sheep population in India:
   a) 74.26 million b) 148.88 million
   c) 302.79 Million d) 192.49 Million
4. Total Goat population in India:
   a) 74.26 million b) 148.88 million
   c) 302.79 Million d) 192.49 Million
5. Total pig population in India:
   a) 74.26 million b) 148.88 million
   c) 9.06 Million d) 192.49 Million
6. Total horse population in India:
   a) 3.9 lakhs b) 3.4 lakhs
   c) 302.79 Million d) 192.49 Million
7. Total poultry in India is:
   a) 851.81million b) 302.79 Million
   c) 192.49 Million d) 145.12 million
8. Per capita milk availability in India ():
   a) 459 b) 322
   c) 392 d) 500
9. Per capitability of egg is:
   a) 101eggs/annum b) 62 eggs/annum
   c) 50 eggs/annum d) 200eggs/annum
10. Which of the following products is NOT a primary product that comes from farm animals?
    a) Meat b) Wool
    c) Grains d) Milk
11. Livestock plays a crucial role in many rural households.
    a) Social activities b) Economic **activities**
    c) Educational aspects d) Political aspects

12. Integrated livestock farming
    a) Reduce the dependence on animal products
    b) Promote monoculture
    c) Increase crop yields
    d) Enhance sustainability and productivity
13. What disease affects the lungs of cattle and can be transmitted to humans?
    a) Foot and mouth disease
    b) Brucellosis
    c) Tuberculosis
    d) Bovine spongiform encephalopathy
14. Goat farming is commonly referred to as goat farming
    a) Caprine farming
    b) Porcine farming
    c) Bovine farming
    d) Ovine farming
15. Which of the following is a major challenge for ranchers due to climate?
    a) Increase in feed availability
    b) Decreased water requirements
    c) Spread of diseases
    d) Enhanced breeding
16. What animal product is essential for the production of many vaccines?
    a) Meat
    b) Milk
    c) Blood
    d) Wool
17. The term "livestock insurance" primarily includes:
    a) Loss of crops due to livestock grazing
    b) Damage to livestock due to weather events
    c) Health insurance for
    d) Legal liabilities related to livestock
18. Silage is:
    a) A type of livestock breed
    b) Fermented fodder
    c) A disease in cattle
    d) A method of livestock breeding
19. What type of farm animal is primarily bred for its fur?
    a) Sheep
    b) Cattle
    c) Mink
    d) Goat
20. What factor significantly affects quality of meat products
    a) Age of the animal
    b) Color of the animal
    c) Weight of the animal
    d) Breed of the animal
21. The term "Rangeland" refers to:
    a) Land used for crop cultivation
    b) Land for housing livestock
    c) Pasture and grasslands for grazing livestock
    d) Wetlands used for fish farming

22. Which of the following diseases can be prevented by vaccination in poultry?
    a) Mad cow disease b) Newcastle disease
    c) Scrapie d) Foot and mouth disease
23. What type of farm animal is known as a "ship"?
    a) Camel b) Horse
    c) Cow d) Sheep
24. The main purpose of a feedlot is:
    a) Breeding livestock
    b) Grazing livestock
    c) Raising livestock to reach market weight
    d) Providing veterinary services to livestock
25. Which of the following is a primary source of income?
    a) Crop farming b) Fishing
    c) Livestock rearing d) Forestry
26. The technique of crossing is aimed at:
    a) Reduce genetic variability
    b) Improve desirable traits in livestock
    c) Decrease livestock productivity
    d) Increase susceptibility to diseases
27. Which among the following is not beneficial sustainable livestock production?
    a) Preservation of natural resources b) Reduced greenhouse gas emissions
    c) Increased land degradation d) Enhanced food security
28. The FAO defines "livestock" as:
    a) Only animals used for meat production
    b) Only
    c) Domesticated animals raised in an agricultural setting for various purposes
    d) Only wild animals
29. Which type of livestock mainly produces wool?
    a) Sheep b) Cattle
    c) Goat d) Poultry
30. What agricultural practice involves raising both animals?
    a) Monoculture farming b) Aquaculture
    c) Integrated farming d) Silviculture
31. Mastitis affects:
    a) The reproductive system of livestock
    b) The respiratory system of livestock
    c) The mammary glands of livestock
    d) The digestive system of lives

32. Which organization plays an important role in setting global standards and guidelines?
    a) WHO (World Health Organization)
    b) UNICEF (United Nations Children's Fund)
    c) FAO (Food and Agriculture Organization)
    d) UNESCO (United Nations
33. Livestock play a crucial role in the _______ supply of nutrients and organic matter in agriculture
    a) Reduction b) Preservation
    c) Decomposition d) Amplification
34. What percentage of India's agricultural GDP is contributed by livestock?
    a) 10% b) 20%
    c) 25% d) 30%
35. Globally, which continent has the highest livestock population?
    a) Europe b) Africa
    c) Asia d) North America
36. In India, which state has the highest cattle
    a) Uttar Pradesh b) Rajasthan
    c) Bihar d) Madhya Pradesh
37. The global meat production in 2022-2023 approximately was:
    a) 250 million tons b) 300 million tons
    c) 347 million tons d) 45 million tons
38. What percentage of the global workforce is engaged in the livestock sector
    a) 10% b) 25%
    c) 40% d) 50%
39. Which country is the largest exporter of beef in the world?
    a) Brazil b) India
    c) USA d) Australia
40. Globally, among livestock sector which animal species has highest population ?
    a) Cattle b) Sheep
    c) Goats d) Poultry
41. What percentage of India's livestock production is accounted for by smallholder farmers?
    a) 30% b) 50%
    c) 70% d) 90%
42. The global livestock sector accounts for what percentage of total global agricultural GDP
    a) 20% b) 30%
    c) 40% d) 50%

43. In India, what is the approximate annual growth rate of the poultry sector?
    a) 5% b) 10%
    c) 15% d) 20%
44. Which livestock sector contributes the most to greenhouse gas emissions globally?
    a) Poultry b) Cattle
    c) Sheep d) Goats
45. How many number of breeds has been registered by national Bureau of Animal Genetic resource in India
    a) 10 b) 20
    c) 30 d) 40
46. Globally, which region has the highest milk production?
    a) Europe b) Asia
    c) Africa d) North America
47. In India, which state leads in the production of goat meat?
    a) Uttar Pradesh b) Rajasthan
    c) Maharashtra d) Andhra Pradesh
48. What percentage of the global livestock sector's output is utilized for direct human
    a) 40% b) 50%
    c) 60% d) 70%
49. Which organization provides global statistics and data related to livestock production?
    a) WHO b) FAO
    c) UNESCO d) UNICEF
50. 19. In India, which breed of cattle is primarily reared for draft purposes?
    a) Jersey b) Holstein
    c) Ongole d) Sahiwal
51. Globally, which country has the largest sheep population?
    a) Australia b) China
    c) India d) New Zealand
52. The global trade value of dairy products in 2020 was approximately:
    a) $100 billion b) $150 billion
    c) $200 billion d) $250 billion
53. In India, what percentage of agricultural households are engaged in livestock rearing?
    a) 20% b) 40%
    c) 60% d) 80%
54. Which country is the largest importer of livestock products?
    a) China b) USA
    c) Russia d) Japan

55. The FAOSTAT database provides comprehensive data on:
   a) Livestock production only
   b) Crop production only
   c) Both livestock and crop production
   d) Agricultural machinery only
56. What percentage of the global arable land is used for livestock feed production?
   a) 10%
   b) 20%
   c) 30%
   d) 40%
57. Which livestock product contributes most to India's agricultural exports?
   a) Meat
   b) Milk
   c) Eggs
   d) Wool
58. Globally, which livestock sector is the fastest- growing?
   a) Poultry
   b) Cattle
   c) Sheep
   d) Goats
59. In India, the 'National Livestock Mission' aims to achieve an annual growth rate of:
   a) 5%
   b) 10%
   c) 15%
   d) 20%
60. What percentage of the global livestock sector's water footprint is ascribed to cattle?
   a) 50%
   b) 60%
   c) 70%
   d) 80%
61. Which organization publishes the 'State of the World's Animal Genetic Resources' report?
   a) WHO
   b) FAO
   c) UNESCO
   d) UNICEF
62. Globally, which livestock product has the highest trade volume?
   a) Beef
   b) Poultry
   c) Milk
   d) Sheep meat
63. Which region of India has highest poultry production?
   a) North India
   b) South India
   c) West India
   d) East India
64. What percentage of global agricultural GDP comes from livestock –related activities?
   a) 10%
   b) 20%
   c) 30%
   d) 40%
65. The 'Livestock Census' in India is conducted every:
   a) 2 years
   b) 5 years
   c) 10 years
   d) 15 years
66. Globally, which livestock sector consumes the most antibiotics?
   a) Cattle
   b) Poultry
   c) Sheep
   d) Goats

67. Which state has the highest buffalo population in India ?
    a) Punjab b) Uttar Pradesh
    c) Haryana d) Rajasthan
68. The Global Livestock Environmental assessment Model (GLEAM) is associated with:
    a) Measuring livestock biodiversity
    b) Assessing the environmental impact of livestock
    c) Monitoring livestock diseases
    d) Evaluating livestock genetics
69. In India, the 'National Dairy Plan' aims to:
    a) Increase meat production
    b) Improve milk production and distribution
    c) Boost poultry farming
    d) Enhance wool production
70. What percentage of India's livestock feed is imported?
    a) 5% b) 10%
    c) 15% d) 20%
71. Globally, which livestock product has seen the most significant increase in consumption over the past decade?
    a) Beef b) Poultry
    c) Milk d) Sheep meat
72. In India, which livestock species has the highest export potential?
    a) Cattle b) Sheep
    c) Goats d) Poultry
73. The 'Livestock Wealth Index' is a tool used to:
    a) Measure livestock productivity b) Assess the wealth of livestock
    c) Evaluate livestock diseases d) Rank livestock breeds
74. Globally, which organization focuses on sustainable livestock development?
    a) WHO b) FAO
    c) UNESCO d) UNICEF
75. In India, which state is known for its Murrah buffalo breed?
    a) Punjab b) Haryana
    c) Uttar Pradesh d) Rajasthan
76. What percentage of the global livestock sector's methane emissions come from enteric fermentation?
    a) 30% b) 40%
    c) 50% d) 60%
77. In India, which livestock product has the highest domestic consumption?
    a) Meat b) Milk
    c) Eggs d) Wool

78. Globally, which region has the highest egg production?
    a) Europe b) Asia
    c) Africa d) North America
79. The 'Livestock Emergency Guidelines and Standards (LEGS)' is associated with:
    a) Livestock breeding techniques
    b) Livestock health and disease control
    c) Livestock in emergencies and disasters
    d) Livestock market systems
80. In India, which livestock product has the highest per capita consumption?
    a) Meat b) Milk
    c) Eggs d) Wool
81. What percentage of the global livestock sector's land use is for grazing?
    a) 40% b) 50%
    c) 60% d) 70%
82. Livestock contribute significantly to livelihood security by providing income through:
    a) Wool production b) Egg production
    c) Milk production d) Leather production
83. In rural economies, livestock often serve as a form of:
    a) Entertainment b) Savings
    c) Currency d) Decoration
84. The primary role of livestock in livelihood security is:
    a) Enhancing social status
    b) Diversifying income sources
    c) Providing companionship
    d) Supporting environmental conservation
85. Livestock play a crucial role in livelih
    a) Seasonal income b) Irregular income
    c) Stable and regular income d) One
86. Which of the following is a key aspect of the role of livestock in livelihood security?
    a) Contributing to air quality b) Enhancing gender equality
    c) Reducing water consumption d) Decreasing soil fertility
87. Livestock rearing is often considered a reliable source of income because it:
    a) Depends on unpredictable factors
    b) Is immune to market fluctuations
    c) Is not influenced by climate conditions
    d) Provides a steady income steady income stream

88. The sale of livestock products such as milk, meat, and wool contributes to the _______ of rural households.
    a) Financial stability
    b) Emotional well
    c) Educational development
    d) Social networking

89. In many developing countries, small- scale livestock farming is a primary means of livelihood for:
    a) Urban populations
    b) Youth populations
    c) Tribal communities
    d) Government employees

90. Livestock contribute to livelihood security by providing employment opportunities in areas such as:
    a) Information technology
    b) Tourism
    c) Veterinary services
    d) Banking

91. The practice of agro –pastoralism involves:
    a) Solely focusing on crop cultivation
    b) Integrating livestock and crop farming
    c) Shifting cultivation
    d) Urban farming

92. Livestock ownership is often linked to:
    a) Higher rates of malnutrition
    b) Lower household income
    c) Improved food security
    d) Reduced access to education

93. In pastoral societies, livelihood security is closely tied to the well- being of:
    a) Agricultural crops
    b) Wildlife
    c) Forests
    d) Livestock herds

94. Which of the following is a challenge to the role of livestock in livelihood security?
    a) Decreased dependence on livestock products
    b) Improved veterinary healthcare
    c) Climate change affecting forage availability
    d) Increased market demand for livestock products

95. Livestock contribute to biodiversity conservation by:
    a) Reducing the population of wild animals
    b) Enhancing soil fertility
    c) Promoting monoculture
    d) Preserving indigenous livestock breeds

96. Livestock – based livelihoods are often vulnerable to :
    a) Government policies
    b) Technological advancements
    c) International trade agreements
    d) Urbanization

97. The concept of 'Fodder Banks' is associated with:
    a) Livestock vaccination
    b) Conservation of forage resources
    c) Livestock insurance
    d) Livestock breeding

98. Livestock contribute to climate change resilience by:
    a) Emitting greenhouse gases
    b) Enhancing carbon sequestration
    c) Promoting deforestation
    d) Depleting water resources
99. The 'Livestock Emergency Guidelines and Standards (LEGS)' focus on:
    a) Livestock marketing strategies
    b) Livestock in emergencies and disasters
    c) Livestock breeding techniques
    d) Livestock insurance policies
100. Which factor is NOT a benefit of livestock ownership for vulnerable communities?
    a) Social cohesion
    b) Income diversification
    c) Increased vulnerability to climate change
    d) Nutritional security
101. The 'Goat Banks' initiative is aimed at:
    a) Providing loans to farmers
    b) Conserving endangered goat species
    c) Promoting goat farming among women
    d) Facilitating goat milk production
102. The role of livestock in livelihood security is particularly significant for:
    a) Urban professionals
    b) Coastal communities
    c) Pastoral nomads
    d) Industrial workers
103. Which livestock species is often referred to as the "poor man's
    a) Goat
    b) Poultry
    c) Sheep
    d) Pigs
104. Livestock contribute to sustainable livelihoods by fostering:
    a) Dependency on external aid
    b) Over – reliance on crop farming
    c) Diversification of income source
    d) Environmental degradation
105. In agroecosystems, the presence of livestock is associated with:
    a) Increased soil erosion
    b) Improved soil fertility
    c) Reduced water quality
    d) Loss of biodiversity
106. The 'One Health'
    a) Spreading infectious diseases
    b) Providing ecosystem services
    c) Decreasing agricultural productivity
    d) Promoting deforestation
107. Livelihood security through livestock and poultry production is closely tied to:
    a) Industrial development
    b) Urbanization
    c) Agricultural diversity
    d) Information technology
108. The 'Blue Revolution' primarily focuses on the enhancement of livelihood security
    a) Poultry production
    b) Fish farming
    c) Dairy farming
    d) Beekeeping

109. Livestock and poultry are considered a source of sustainable income due to their ability to
   a) Produce high levels of greenhouse gases
   b) Adapt to climate change
   c) Contribute to deforestation
   d) Depend on external inputs

110. The concept of 'Zero Grazing' in livestock management refers to:
   a) Letting animals graze freely in open fields
   b) Keeping animals indoors and providing feed
   c) Focusing on organic farming practices
   d) Promoting extensive grazing systems

111. The 'Duck- Rice farming system' is an example of
   a) Monoculture
   b) Aquaculture
   c) Integrated farming
   d) Nomadic pastoralism

112. Livelihood security is enhanced through poultry farming by:
   a) Reducing household income
   b) Providing diverse products like eggs and meat
   c) Increasing reliance on crop farming
   d) Contributing to soil erosion

113. In the context of livelihood security, what is the significance of small ruminants like goat and sheep?
   a) They require extensive grazing lands
   b) They are resistance to diseases
   c) They contribute to income diversification
   d) They are primarily kept for aesthetic purposes

114. The 'Rural Poultry Development' initiative aims to:
   a) Increase urbanization
   b) Promote backyard poultry farming
   c) Discourage poultry production
   d) Eliminate

115. In livestock and poultry production, the term 'Flock Health Management' refers to:
   a) Managing the health of individual animals
   b) Managing the health of a group of animals
   c) Managing the health of crops
   d) Managing the health of aquati

116. Which of the following is a key factor affecting the success of backyard poultry farming for livelihood security?
   a) Use of intensive farming practices
   b) Dependence on external inputs
   c) Access to veterinary services
   d) Exclusively relying on wild species

117. Livelihood security through livestock and poultry production is negativel affected by:
   a) Crop diversification
   b) Adoption of sustainable farming practices
   c) Climate –resilient livestock breeds
   d) Disease outbreaks
118. 'Contract Farming' in the context of poultry production involves:
   a) Independent farming without external
   b) Farmers producing poultry products for a specific buyer
   c) Government – controlled farming practices
   d) Livestock production without market involvement
119. Which livestock species is commonly associated with the practice of transhumance, contributing to livelihood security in certain regions?
   a) Cattle b) Poultry
   c) Goats d) Pigs
120. 'Stall- feeding' in livestock management refers to
   a) Keeping animals in stalls and providing them with feed
   b) Allowing animals to graze freely in open fields
   c) Moving animals to different locations
   d) Utilizing natural resources for feeding livestock
121. The 'Livestock Extension Services' primarily focus on:
   a) Reducing livestock populations
   b) Promoting sustainable farming practices
   c) Discouraging backyard poultry farming
   d) Limiting access to veterinary care
122. In the context of livelihood security, the 'Tricho – Card' is associated with
   a) Livestock breeding b) Poultry nutrition
   c) Disease management in livestock d) Financial services for farmers
123. The practice of 'Silvopastoralism' involves integrating
   a) Livestock with crop farming b) Livestock with agroforestry
   c) Poultry with aquaculture d) Livestock with urbanization
124. Livestock and poultry contribute to food security by providing a source of:
   a) Carbohydrates b) Proteins
   c) Fats d) All of the above
125. The 'Rinder –pest eradication Program' eliminate a highly contagious disease affecting:
   a) Cattle b) Poultry
   c) Sheep d) Pigs

126. In the context of poultry farming, the term 'Free – Range' refers to:
   a) Rearing poultry in cages
   b) Providing unlimited access to grazing
   c) Rearing poultry
   d) Conducting poultry farming without any regulations

127. The 'Poultry Value Chain' includes activities such as:
   a) Crop farming
   b) Livestock breeding
   c) Poultry processing and marketing
   d) Urban development

128. 'Integrated Livestock –Fish Farming involes:
   a) Poultry and livestock farming
   b) Livestock farming and crop cultivation
   c) Poultry farming and aquaculture
   d) Livestock farming and forestry

129. In the context of livelihood security, the 'Vaccination Camps' aim to:
   a) Promote organic farming
   b) Control diseases in livestock and poultry
   c) Discourage vaccination for livestock
   d) Promote monoculture

130. Livestock and poultry production contribute to environmental sustainability by:
   a) Depleting natural resources
   b) Enhancing soil fertility
   c) Reducing biodiversity
   d) Contributing to deforestation

131. 'Agroforestry' in the context of livestock and poultry production involves:
   a) Rearing animals in forests
   b) Combining trees with livestock and poultry farming
   c) Clearing forests for farming
   d) Rearing only wild animals

132. 'Livestock Development Boards' in various countries focus on:
   a) Reducing livestock populations
   b) Promoting sustainable livestock farming
   c) Eliminating small –scale farmers
   d) Ignoring market dynamics

133. In the context of livelihood security, the 'Poultry Cooperative Societies' aim to:
   a) Promote individual farming practices
   b) Enhance market access for small –scale poultry farmers
   c) Discourage poultry farming
   d) Eliminate competition among poultry farmers

134. The 'Feed Conversion Ratio' in poultry farming refers to:
   a) The rate of conversion of poultry waste to energy
   b) The efficiency of converting feed into body mass
   c) The ratio of male to female poultry
   d) The rate of poultry egg production

135. Livestock and poultry production contribute to nutrition security by:
   a) Decreasing the availability of protein
   b) Increasing reliance on processed foods
   c) Providing essential nutrients like proteins and vitamins
   d) Promoting unhealthy dietary practices
136. 'Grassroots Innovations' in livestock and poultry production refer to:
   a) Traditional farming practices
   b) Modern farming techniques
   c) Innovations developed by local communities
   d) Government- led initiatives
137. Livestock and poultry farming contribute to cultural heritage by preserving
   a) Urban development
   b) Traditional knowledge and practices
   c) Industrial practices
   d) Modern technologies
138. The 'Livestock Credit Schemes' aim to:
   a) Promote overgrazing
   b) Encourage unsustainable farming practices
   c) Facilitate access to financial resources for livestock farmers
   d) Discourage livestock farming
139. Livestock and poultry production contribute to livelihood security by promoting:
   a) Monocultural farming
   b) Diversification of income sources
   c) Dependence on external market
   d) Fragmentation of land
140. 'Biosecurity Measures' in poultry farming are designed to:
   a) Promote disease transmission
   b) Enhance disease prevention and control
   c) Encourage open farming systems
   d) Neglect animal welfare
141. The 'Poultry Hatcheries' play a crucial role in:
   a) Promoting extensive grazing
   b) Producing day
   c) Discouraging poultry farming
   d) Ignoring market demands
142. Livestock and poultry production contribute to livelihood security by fostering:
   a) Environmental degradation
   b) Climate resilience
   c) Soil erosion
   d) Water scarcity
143. 'Mobile Veterinary Clinics' are essential for:
   a) Promoting disease outbreaks
   b) Providing timely healthcare services to livestock
   c) Ignoring animal welfare
   d) Disrupting agricultural markets

144. 'Livestock Insurance Schemes' aim to:
   a) Discourage livestock farming
   b) Promote risky farming practices
   c) Provide financial protection to livestock farmers
   d) Ignore the needs of small –scale farmers
145. In the context of livelihood security, 'Value Addition' in livestock and poultry production prefers to:
   a) Reducing the nutritional value of products
   b) Enhancing product quality and market value
   c) Neglecting product standards
   d) Ignoring consumer preferences
146. 'Livestock Markets' play a crucial role in:
   a) Promoting sustainable farming practices
   b) Facilitating trade and marketing of livestock products
   c) Ignoring consumer demands
   d) Discouraging small-scale farmers
147. The 'National Livestock Mission' in various countries aims to:
   a) Reduce livestock populations
   b) Promote sustainable livestock development
   c) Eliminate small- scale farmers
   d) Ignore market dynamics
148. The 'Livestock Extension Programs' aim to:
   a) Discourage livestock farming
   b) Provide training and support to livestock farmers
   c) Promote unsustainable farming practices
   d) Ignore technologic
149. Livestock and poultry production contribute to livelihood security by:
   a) Encouraging soil conservation
   b) Promoting responsible land use
   c) Enhancing agricultural biodiversity
   d) Reducing crop yields
150. 'Integrated Livestock Development Projects' aim
   a) Promote fragmented farming systems
   b) Integrate various components of livestock production
   c) Discourage community participation
   d) Ignore sustainable practices

Answer Key

1	a	2	b	3	a	4	b	5	c	6	b	7	a
8	a	9	a	10	c	11	b	12	d	13	c	14	a
15	c	16	c	17	b	18	b	19	c	20	d	21	c
22	b	23	a	24	c	25	c	26	c	27	c	28	c
29	c	30	c	31	c	32	c	33	d	34	c	35	c
36	a	37	c	38	c	39	a	40	d	41	d	42	c
43	c	44	b	45	c	46	a	47	b	48	b	49	b
50	c	51	b	52	b	53	d	54	a	55	c	56	c
57	b	58	a	59	b	60	c	61	b	62	c	63	a
64	d	65	b	66	b	67	b	68	b	69	b	70	a
71	b	72	c	73	b	74	b	75	b	76	d	77	b
78	b	79	c	80	b	81	c	82	c	83	b	84	b
85	c	86	b	87	d	88	a	89	c	90	c	91	b
92	c	93	d	94	c	95	d	96	a	97	b	98	b
99	b	100	c	101	c	102	c	103	a	104	c	105	b
106	b	107	c	108	b	109	b	110	b	111	c	112	b
113	c	114	b	115	b	116	c	117	d	118	b	119	a
120	a	121	b	122	c	123	b	124	d	125	a	126	b
127	c	128	c	129	b	130	b	131	b	132	b	133	b
134	b	135	c	136	c	137	b	138	c	139	b	140	b
141	b	142	b	143	b	144	c	145	b	146	b	147	b
148	b	149	c	150	b								

10

Animal Exhibition Rules and its Monitoring

Mamta[1], Rajneesh Sirohi[1], Ajay Kumar[1], Rashmi[2], and *Manish Kr. Singh*[3]

[1]*Department of Livestock Production and Management, DUVASU, Mathura Uttar Pradesh*

[2]*Department of Veterinary VAHE, DUVASU, Mathura, Uttar Pradesh*

[3]*Department of Poultry Science, DUVASU, Mathura, Uttar Pradesh*

Introduction

Animals are exhibited in various ways and events like in fairs, judging shows, in circuses, in zoos and as performing animals. Some famous animal fairs in northern part of the country are Sonepur cattle fair of Bihar. It is the largest cattle fair of Asia, held on the confluence of holy river Ganges and Gandak annually on KartikPoornima in the month of November for the trade of animals such as Cattle, horses,goats,donkeys,camels,birds and elephants. Haathi Bazaar is the major attraction of SonepurMela. Nagaur cattle fair held during the months of January and February. It is the second biggest cattle fair in India. Pushkar Cattle Fair,popularly known as camel fair held for five-days between the months of October and November.

Cattle shows are organized time to time where animals are judged for their different characteristics, selecting for their best type, possessing true breed characteristics, dairy conformation, good temperament, proper growth and development according to its age, with optimum condition of fleshing and free from defects. To take part in such shows animals are transported to different places. So, apart from knowledge of restraining methods, concept related to ageing, animal handling (flight zone, point of balance) animal behavioural consideration and welfare indicators are of much importance for transporting and presenting animals in any show. Some of the important rules and regulation related with animal exhibition are as follows-

Prevention of Cruelty to Animals Act, 1960, according to section 22 of which, it is prohibited to exhibit or train animals. In case a person is doing so, such a person shall possess legal documentation from the government. In addition, the Central Government has the authority to declare that a particular animal cannot be displayed for entertainment purposes by notifying it in its official gazette.

The Prevention of Cruelty to Draught and Pack Animals Rules, 1965, this rule has the provisions for the prevention and protection of animals from unnecessary pain, cruelty, torture when used to draw carriages and loaded with packs and people. Section 6 of this rule discuss the general condition for using different categories of working animals to carry vehicles. It also provides the rules for the use of draught and pack animals and the maximum load permitted on these animals while using them.

The Performing Animals Rules, 1973, as per this rule a performing animal means an animal that is used for entertainment through which the public are admitted through sales of tickets. No animal can be used for entertainment purposes until registration is done under the Act.

The Transport of Animals Rules, 1978, this rule provide the general conditions for the transport of animals, that is, they should be in good condition, fit for transportation. During transportation, pregnant, diseased, or young animals must be separated from other animals. Overloading of animals amounts to treating an animal cruelly under the provision of the Prevention of Cruelty to Animals Act, 1960.

The Animal Protection (Dogs) Rules, 2001, provide the rules relating to pets and street dogs.

Prevention of Cruelty to Animals (Regulation of Livestock Markets) Rules, 2017. according to this, animal market means a market place or sale-yard or any other premises or place to which animals are brought from other places and exposed for sale or auction and includes any lairage adjoining a market or a slaughterhouse and used in connection with it and any place adjoining a market used as a parking area by visitors to the market for parking vehicles and includes animal fair and cattle pound where animals are offered or displayed for sale or auction.

It has provision for a Committee for regulation of animal markets asThe District Animal Market Monitoring Committee which has many functions. It shall ensure that the traders and purchasers abide by the rules relating to transport of animals and also ensure that the animal market has adequate housing, shade, feeding troughs, water tanks with multiple taps and buckets, lighting, ramps at the appropriate height of vehicles, separate enclosures for sick and infirm animals, separate enclosures for young and pregnant animals, veterinary facility, feed storage area and feed supply, water supply, toilets, non-slippery flooring, provisions for proper disposal of dead animals from the animal market site, provisions to ensure hygiene, proper disposal of manure and bio-waste from animal market site, sand pits for rolling of equines, separate enclosures for different species of animals.

Different Animal welfare organizations and breeders societies also play important role in exhibition and marketing of animals having their contribution in animal health, advocacy, marketing and trades and research etc.

1. An official veterinarian of an exhibition shall
   1. Approve the cleaning and disinfection of exhibition premises
   2. Inspect all livestock admitted to the exhibition
   3. Maintaining tagging record
   4. Providing feed and water

   a) Only 1 is correct b) 1,2 and 3 are correct
   c) All are correct d) 1 and 2 are correct
2. Sheep and goat ....days before and after should not be exhibited

   a) 30 b) 15
   c) 60 d) 4

3. As per regulation of livestock market rules, 2017, animal market means

1.	Animal fare	2.	Cattle pound
3.	Lairage near slaughter house	4.	Any place for animal sale
a)	All are correct	b)	1 and 3 are correct
c)	2 and 4 are correct	d)	Only 1 is correct

4. Unfit animal for exhibition
   a) Non pregnant   b) Advance pregnant
   c) Young   d) Weak
5. Chairman of district animal market monitoring committee
   a) District collector   b) Chief veterinary officer
   c) Forest officer   d) Superintendent of police
6. Quorum for the meeting of district animal market monitoring committee
   a) 2 members   b) 4 members
   c) 6 members   d) 5 members
7. Chairman of animal market committee
   a) Chairman of local authority   b) District collector
   c) Forest range officer   d) Police inspector
8. Quorum for the meeting of district animal market monitoring committee
   a) 2 members   b) 4 members
   c) 6 members   d) 5 members
9. No animal market could be organized in a place which is situated
   a) Beyond 25 km from any state border
   b) Within 25 km from any state border
   c) Beyond 10km from any state border
   d) Within 10 km from any state border
10. Prevention of Cruelty to Animals (Regulation of Livestock Markets) Rules came into force in
   a) 2017   b) 2014
   c) 2015   d) 2018
11. Fractious animal means an animal
   a) That is likely to cause injury to other animal
   b) That has tendency to flee away
   c) That likely become feral
   d) That cannot be sold
12. Young animals are those which are
   a) Below six month of age   b) Below one year
   c) Below 3 months   d) Below two years

13. Which is not a prohibited practice in animal exhibition
    a) Hot branding and cold branding b) Casting
    c) Bishoping d) Sealing teats
14. No person shall handle an animal in an animal market by
    1. Lifting it off the ground 2. Dragging it along the ground
    3. Suspending it clear of the ground 4. Lifting by head, neck feet, tail
    a) Only 1 is correct b) 1,2 and 3 are correct
    c) All are correct d) 1 and 2 are correct
15. Providing feed and water to the animal in animal market is the duty of
    a) Animal owner b) Member secretory
    c) veterinarian d) SPCA member
16. Ensuring the adequate lighting in the animal market is the duty of
    a) Animal owner b) Member secretory
    c) veterinarian d) SPCA member
17. Declaration furnished to the Animal Market Committee shall be retained by it for a period of
    a) One year b) Six months
    c) 3 months d) 5 years
18. Declaration should be taken by the person bring animal to the animal exhibition regarding
    1. Identification of person
    2. Identification of animal
    3. Cattle has not been brought to the market for sale
    4. Cattle has not been brought to the market for slaughter
    a) Only 1 is correct b) 1,2 and 3 are correct
    c) All are correct d) 1 and 2 are correct
19. Theexpenses incurred by veterinary inspector in treating detained unfit animal in animal market is to be borne by
    a) Animal owner b) Member secretory
    c) veterinarian d) SPCA member
20. For loading and unloading of animals in animal market there should have
    a) Ramps with side railing b) Ramps without side railing
    c) Species wise designed ramps d) Permanent ramps
21. General conditions for registration of performing animals
    1. Animal not be transported more than 8 hours
    2. For ten or more such animals vet as regular employee
    3. Avoid training of performing animals
    4. Avoid breeding of performing animals
    a) Only 1 is correct b) 1,2 and 3 are correct
    c) All are correct d) 1 and 2 are correct

22. Grooming of exhibiting animal is important because
    1. It clean skin
    2. Make the coat glossy
    3. Make animal more docile
    4. Stimulate blood circulation
    a) All are correct
    b) Only 2 and 4 are correct
    c) Only 1 and 3 are correct
    d) 1,2 and 3 are correct
23. Grooming for the exhibiting animal is more effective if done
    a) One hour before milking
    b) At the time of milking
    c) Just after milking
    d) No impact of grooming
24. For implying body weight formula for cattle, which is incorrect
    a) Animal must stand on levelled ground
    b) Animal stand quietly
    c) Measure length from elbow joint to pin bone
    d) Measure length from shoulder point to pin bone
25. A young cattle calf have ....number of temporary teeth
    a) 20
    b) 32
    c) 24
    d) 34
26. Adult cattle have ....pair of incisors
    a) 1
    b) 2
    c) 3
    d) 4
27. A cattle having pair of permanent middle incisor erupted would have approximate age about
    a) 1 year
    b) 2 year
    c) 3 year
    d) 6 months
28. A cow is full mouth at age about
    a) 3 year
    b) 4 year
    c) 5 year
    d) 6 year
29. Permanent incisors which are last to erupt are
    a) Central
    b) Middle
    c) Lateral
    d) Corener
30. Proper concentration of chlorine sanitizer for washing udder
    a) 50-200 ppm
    b) 10-20 ppm
    c) 200-400 ppm
    d) 30-50 ppm
31. Solutions used for teat dip
    a) Chlorhexidine (0.5%)
    b) Iodine (0.5%)
    c) Hypochlorite (4%)
    d) All of these
32. Quality test for clean milk
    a) Strip cup test
    b) CMT
    c) MBRT
    d) All of these

33. Diseases spread through cows
    - a) Tuberculosis
    - b) Undulant fever
    - c) Anthrax
    - d) All of these
34. Disease spread through milkers
    - a) Thphoid
    - b) Paratyphoid
    - c) Scarlet fever
    - d) All of these
35. Animals which are used at or for the purpose of any entertainment to public through sale of tickets
    - a) Working animals
    - b) Performing animals
    - c) Domestic animals
    - d) Exhibit animals
36. Buffalo race sport in Karnataka
    - a) Kambala
    - b) Jallikattu
    - c) Sallikattu
    - d) Manjuvirattu
37. A sport having buffalo race in slushy paddy fields
    - a) Kambala
    - b) Jallikattu
    - c) Sallikattu
    - d) Manjuvirattu
38. Bringing of infected animals into market and other places is prohibited as per
    - a) PCID act 2009
    - b) PCA, 1960
    - c) Performing animals rules 1973
    - d) Draught and pack animal rule 1965
39. Organizing market, fair or exhibition of animal in controlled area is prohibited under
    - a) PCID act 2009
    - b) PCA, 1960
    - c) Performing animals rules 1973
    - d) Draught and pack animal rule 1965
40. Occurrence of disease cases in an area in excess of normal expectancy
    - a) Eradication
    - b) Endemic
    - c) Outbreak
    - d) Pandemic
41. As per dog breeding and marketing rules 2017 certificate of registration issued by state board shall be valid for a period of
    - a) 2 year
    - b) 4 year
    - c) 1 year
    - d) 5 year
42. As per dog breeding and marketing rules dogs cannot be sold as
    - a) Pups less than 8 weeks of age
    - b) Dogs over 6 month of age
    - c) Dogs without sterilization
    - d) Microchipped dogs

43. Which is true about sale of dogs as per dog breeding and marketing rules
    1. Pups can be displayed in public places for immediate sale
    2. Pup not sold within 6 month should be rehabilitated by the breeder
    3. Not sold to a pet shop operator without licence
    4. Pups cannot be displayed in public places for immediate sale
    a) 2,3 and 4 are correct
    b) 3 and 4 are correct
    c) 2 and 4 are correct
    d) 1 and 3 are correct
44. The establishment of a breeder who died before expiry of the period of registration
    a) Is granted to its legal heir forever
    b) Renewed to legal heir
    c) Licence is cancelled
    d) Granted to its legal heir until expiry
45. During its life span a female dog should not be exploited to give birth to more than
    1) 5 litters
    2) 7 litters
    3) 3 litters
    4) 8 litters
46. For mating purpose a male dog should be certified as healthy by a vet practitioner
    a) At least 10 days before mating
    b) At least 5 days before mating
    c) At least 20 days before mating
    d) At least 1 month before mating
47. A female dog should not be mated after the age of
    a) 8 years
    b) 5 years
    c) 6 years
    d) 10 years
48. As per performing animal rules, 1973, in a horse race whip can be used by licenced jockey
    a) Not more than 3 times in a race
    b) Not more than 2 times in a race
    c) Not more than 5 times in a race
    d) Not more than 8 times in a race
49. According to the law applicable to performing animals, which of the following is legal
    a) Snake charmer
    b) Dog show
    c) Bull fights
    d) Fortune telling parakeets
50. Infirmary is a place where
    a) Injured animals receive care and treatment
    b) Animals are registered
    c) Animals get rest
    d) Animals get feed and water
51. As per licencing of farrier rules, concerned person should have minimum of …. Implements and tools related to farriery
    a) 14
    b) 10
    c) 8
    d) 16

52. Registration of cattle premises rules, 1978 are applicable only to cities or towns which have a population of at least

a) 1 lakh b) 10,000

c) 1000 d) 10 lakh

53. An application for registration of cattle premises must contain information regarding

a) Number and type of animal kept

b) Purpose for which they are kept

c) Provision of housing and sanitation facilities

d) All of these

54. Establishment of society, SPCA established at

a) District level b) Tehsil level

c) Block level d) State level

55. As per draught and pack animal rules 1965, no person shall use any animal for more than

a) 9 hrs in a day in aggregate b) 9 hrs in a day in aggregate

c) 6 hrs continuously without rest d) 8 hrs continuously without rest

56. Statement true regarding general condition for use of draught and pack animal

a) Disintegrated after work

b) Use of spike is allowed

c) Harness rest directly on wither

d) Use animal >10 hrs in a day in aggregate

57. Preparation of show animals include

1. Hoof trimming
2. Feeding extra quantity of concentrate mixture
3. Attending to horns
4. Training of animals

a) 1,2,3 and 4 are correct b) 3 and 4 are correct

c) 2 and 4 are correct d) 1 and 3 are correct

58. For presenting a cow in a show, plan its breeding such that the cow may calve

a) About 3 months before show b) About 6 months before show

c) About 1 months before show d) About 10 days before show

59. Which statement is odd, if an animal calved long in advance of the date of show

1. They would look unduly thin 2. Show poor capacity

3. Chances of winning increases 4. Chances of winning decreases

60. for selecting a cow to be presented in heifer category which should be the best choice for an owner

a) 6 months b) 8 months

c) 10 months d) 12 months

61. For show preparations, clipping of hairs should not be done in
   a) Head b) Neck
   c) Tail d) Belly
62. Finalpreparations on the day of show by the cattle owner include
   1. Milking several hours before judging 2. Apply oil on horns and hooves
   3. Combing of switch of tail 4. Clean the halters and ropes
   a) 1,2,3 and 4 are correct b) 3 and 4 are correct
   c) 2 and 4 are correct d) 1 and 3 are correct
63. Ifnecessary, the fair officer can do the following except
   a) To prohibit the entry of any cattle
   b) To get the cattle in fair area immunized
   c) To isolated diseased cattle
   d) To left the dead animal to owner
64. The most widely accepted unit of sale for animal is
   a) Per animal b) Per pair
   c) Per group d) Per head
65. Largest cattle fair is
   a) Sonepur cattle fair b) Nagaur cattle fair
   c) Pushkar cattle fair d) Bateshwar cattle fair
66. Fair popularly known as camel fair is
   a) Sonepur cattle fair b) Nagaur cattle fair
   c) Pushkar cattle fair d) Bateshwar cattle fair
67. Pushkar cattle fair is held during month of
   a) October-November b) September- October
   c) November- December d) December- January
68. Sonepur cattle fair is held in
   a) U.P. b) Bihar
   c) M.P. d) Rajasthan
69. true about Sonepur cattle fair
   1. Held annualy on kartikpoornima
   2. Popular for haathi bazar
   3. It trades only cattle
   4. It trades domestic animals and birds
   a) 1,2, and 4 are correct b) 3 and 4 are correct
   c) 2 and 4 are correct d) 1 and 3 are correct
70. Cattle fair held along river Ganges
   a) Jhalawar cattle fair b) Nagaur cattle fair
   c) Sonepur cattle fair d) Bateshwar cattle fair

71. A feminine cow will have

a) Lean neck b) Thick neck

c) Short neck d) Irregular muscling

72. Characters evaluated for judging of dairy cow

1. Feminity 2. Balance

3. Size 4. Weight

a) 1,2, and 3 are correct b) 3 and 4 are correct

c) 2 and 4 are correct d) 1 and 3 are correct

73. Features for desirable frame and capacity of dairy cow

1. Broad muzzle
2. Wide chest floor
3. Large and deep heart girth
4. Depth of rib increase towards rear

a) 1,2, 3 and 4 are correct b) 3 and 4 are correct

c) 2 and 4 are correct d) 1 and 3 are correct

74. Desirable characteristics of rump

1. Wide hook bones
2. Prominent hook bones
3. Pin bones set slightly higher than hook bones
4. Pin bones set slightly lower than hook bones

a) 1, 4 are correct b) 3 and 4 are correct

c) 2 and 4 are correct d) 1 and 3 are correct

75. Desirable characteristics for feet and legs

1. Squarely placed feet 2. Deep heel

3. Proper angle 4. Slightly spaced toes

a) 1,2, 3 and 4 are correct b) 3 and 4 are correct

c) 2 and 4 are correct d) 1 and 3 are correct

76. Undesirable characteristics of legs

a) Sickle hocked b) Post legged

c) Cow hocked d) All of these

77. Evaluation of mammary system includes following parts

1. Udder 2. Median suspensory ligament

3. Teats 4. Mammary veins

a) 1,2, 3 and 4 are correct b) 3 and 4 are correct

c) 2 and 4 are correct d) 1 and 3 are correct

78. Factors affecting dairy character or appearance

a) Stage of lactation b) Feeding

c) Estrus d) Vaccination

79. Desirable BCS prior to calving is
   a) 3.5-4   b) 2.5-3.5
   c) 1.5-2.5   d) 4.5-5.5
80. The faults in dairy cattle which needs serious discrimination apart from score card are:
   1. Blind quarter   2. Udder oedema
   3. Webbed feet   4. Injured teats
   a) 1,2, and 3 are correct   b) 3 and 4 are correct
   c) 2 and 4 are correct   d) 1 and 3 are correct
81. The sequence of relative emphasis given to judging a heifer
   a) Feet and legs>frame>mammary system
   b) Mammary system>frame>feet and legs
   c) Frame> mammary system>feet and legs
   d) Feet and legs>mammary system> frame
82. The sequence of relative emphasis given to judging a cow
   a) Feet and legs>frame>mammary system
   b) Mammary system>frame>feet and legs
   c) Frame> mammary system>feet and legs
   d) Feet and legs>mammary system> frame
83. AWBI, the statutory advisory body on animal welfare laws was established in
   a) 1962   b) 1952
   c) 1972   d) 1942
84. The AWBI board have ….. Members
   a) 22   b) 24
   c) 20   d) 28
85. The provision of constitution of AWBI is given in …….chapter of PCA act 1960
   a) Chapter I   b) Chapter II
   c) Chapter III   d) Chapter IV
86. Act of cruelty as per PCA, 1960
   a) Overloading   b) Overriding
   c) Kicking   d) All of these
87. Cruelty does not apply if done in prescribed manner
   a) Dehorning   b) Dewclawing
   c) Devocalization   d) Phooka
88. Cruelty does not apply if done in prescribed manner
   a) Dehorning   b) Castration
   c) Branding   d) All of these

89. AWBI provides financial assistance to AWO as
    a) Regular grant b) Cattle rescue grant
    c) Natural calamity grant d) All of these
90. Thechairperson of SPCA is
    a) District magistrate b) Chief veterinary officer
    c) MLA d) AWO representative
91. Organization not involved in stray animal protection
    a) PFA b) HIS
    c) CZA d) PeTA
92. For ideal confirmation of a horse, the top of neck should be.......long as underside of horse's neck
    a) Twice b) Same
    c) Half d) Thrice
93. Thehighest point of horse body consider for taking its height
    a) Wither b) Poll
    c) Pin d) Back
94. For ideal confirmation of a horse, the top of back should be.......long as underside of horses back
    a) Twice b) Same
    c) Shorter d) longer
95. Undesirable back in horse's confirmation
    a) Roached back b) Swayback
    c) Ling backed d) All of these
96. Jallikattu is related with the festival of
    a) Pongal b) Bihu
    c) Onam d) brajutsav
97. Breed used in jallikattu
    a) Pullikulam b) Amritmahal
    c) Hallikar d) Kankrej
98. Jallikattu is observed in state of Tamil Nadu in the month of
    a) April b) December
    c) January d) March
99. The supreme court of India banned jallikattu in the year
    a) 2014 b) 2012
    c) 2000 d) 2004
100. handling of animals by behavioural methods include
    1. Offering water 2. Offering relished feed
    3. Blind folding 4. Grooming
    a) 1,2, 3 and 4 are correct b) 3 and 4 are correct
    c) 2 and 4 are correct d) 1 and 3 are correct

101. Physical restraint may only be used
    1. To administer sedatives
    2. To administer anaesthetics
    3. For short procedures causing limited pain
    4. Where sedatives are contraindicated
    a) 1,2, and 3 are correct b) 3 and 4 are correct
    c) 2 and 4 are correct d) 1 and 3 are correct

102. Negative mental state of animal
    1. Fear 2. Anxiety
    3. Stress 4. Injury
    a) 1,2, and 3 are correct b) 3 and 4 are correct
    c) 2 and 4 are correct d) 1 and 3 are correct

103. Foot trimming is required for bullock
    a) Which are used in agricultural purpose
    b) Which are to be shown in a show
    c) If hoof are not in proper shape and angle
    d) Which are used over concrete road

104. While using a pair of bullock in a cart
    1. Ensure bullock are of equal height and size
    2. There should be no cracks in yoke
    3. Bullock pull load by neck
    4. Do not use spiked sticks
    a) 1,2, 3 and 4 are correct b) 3 and 4 are correct
    c) 2 and 4 are correct d) 1 and 3 are correct

105. The authority to provide permission regarding use of animals for performance in films
    a) AWBI b) CZA
    c) Censor board d) PCA

106. In horses, the unshod feet need trimming
    a) Every 4 week b) Every 8 week
    c) Every 10 week d) Every 12 week

107. In horses, the shod feet need trimming
    a) Every 2- 4 week b) Every 6-8 week
    c) Every 8-10 week d) Every 10-12 week

108. Incorrect regarding pinjrapole
    a) Like a typical gaushala b) Presence of cow is incidental
    c) Founded in 1834 d) All of these

109. Which one is not the general objective of gaushala
    a) To house uneconomic cattle b) Production of pedigreed bull
    c) Conservation and upgrading d) Distribution of female calves

110. Which one is not a good handling practice?
a) Use positive interaction with animal b) Make excessive voice
c) Move animals in group d) Avoid staring animals

111. Physical indicator for welfare assessment of cattle
a) Milk yield b) Glucose
c) Cortisol d) Ectoparasite

112. Welfare input factors for welfare assessment of cattle are
a) Animal b) Environment
c) Stockman d) All of these

113. In normal ethogram, a dairy cow spent about ..... Hrs in resting
a) 8 hours b) 12 hours
c) 10 hours d) 18 hours

114. Common welfare issues with animals exhibited in circus
a) Poor caging b) Harsh training
c) Feed deprivation d) All of these

115. As per performing animal rules, an owner should have veterinarian as a regular employee if he has at least
a) 10 performing animals b) 20 performing animals
c) 30 performing animals d) 40 performing animals

116. Horse should not be transported
a) Within 24 hours of having race b) Within 36 hours of having race
c) Within 48 hours of having race d) Within 72 hours of having race

117. Registry of purebred dog in India is
a) KCI b) FEI
c) HIS d) CZA

118. Kennel club of India was established in
a) 1978 b) 1966
c) 1962 d) 1972

119. KCI registers litters of puppies
a) Whose sire and dam both been registered
b) Whose sire and dam are not already registered
c) Imported puppies
d) All of these

120. Main functions of animal welfare organizations
1. Promoting welfare education
2. Maintaining animal shelter
3. Cooperation with authorities
4. Propagation of non-vegetarianism
a) 1,2, 3 and 4 are correct b) 3 and 4 are correct
c) 2 and 4 are correct d) 1 and 3 are correct

121. National institute of animal welfare is located at
   a) Haryana b) Bihar
   c) Odisha d) Delhi
122. Standards for welfare in display of zoo animals is laid down by
   a) CZA b) NTCA
   c) NIAW d) AWBI
123. Head office for kennel club of India is situated at
   a) Chennai b) Chandigarh
   c) Bengaluru d) Delhi
124. Equestrian federation of India was constituted in
   a) 1967 b) 1957
   c) 1982 d) 1972
125. The governing body promoted equestrian sports in India is
   a) EFI b) FEI
   c) KCI d) RVC
126. The breed popular in the Mela of Kutch
   a) Banni b) Bhadawari
   c) Jaffrabadi d) Chilika
127. Poor transportation of animal to market area may cause
   a) Disease transmission b) Loss of body weight
   c) Bruising d) All of these
128. Common welfare issues while transporting animals
   a) Overstocking b) Poor ventilation
   c) Use of vehicle without modification d) All of these
129. Flight zone is
   a) The circle of safety around the animal b) entire range for grazing of animal
   c) Tendency of animal to flee d) Barn of the animal
130. Statement correct about flight zone
   a) Circle of safety
   b) Approaching animal head on will increase it
   c) Animal move when handler penetrate it
   d) All of these
131. Best place for a handle to work to handle animal
   a) At the edge of flight zone b) Deep in flight zone
   c) Far from flight zone d) Anywhere in flight zone
132. Prevention of Cruelty to Animals (Regulation of Livestock Markets) Rules came into action since
   a) 2017 b) 2014
   c) 2012 d) 1010

133. Unfit animal for exhibition as Prevention of Cruelty to Animals (Regulation of Livestock Markets) Rules,

a) Diseased b) Infirm

c) Fatigued d) All of these

134. Animal markets should be registered under

a) District animal market monitoring committee

b) District animal market exhibition committee

c) District animal sale committee

d) District animal show committee

135. Authority which can authorize an officer to inspect an animal market

1. State Board
2. local authority
3. District Animal Market Monitoring Committee
4. State Animal Husbandry Department

a) 1,2, 3 and 4 are correct b) 3 and 4 are correct

c) 2 and 4 are correct d) 1 and 3 are correct

136. for loading of ….. A written permission by DM is must apart from vet certificate

a) Cattle b) Bull

c) Camel d) Dog

137. In a market, a naturally died animal may not be

a) Incinerated b) Buried

c) Sold for leather d) All of these

138. An animal may not b permitted for sale if it is likely to give birth

a) During coming to the market b) Suring display in market

c) During return from market d) All of these

139. Prohibited practices during animal display

a) Using muzzle

b) Putting decorative material on animals

c) Forcing animal to dance

d) All of these

140. The size of cage for the birds to be displayed should have dimension

a) Twice the wing span b) Same as the wing span

c) Half of the wing span d) Nothing to do with wing span

141. Animal breeder'ssocieties works in the area of

a) Animal health b) Advocacy

c) Marketing and trade d) All of these

142. Tool used in training of elephants

a) Ankus b) Bull hook

c) Both are correct d) Trunk twitch

143. Animal that is not banned as performing animal is

1. Bear
2. Monkey
3. Tiger
4. Elephant

a) All are banned
b) Bear is not banned
c) monkey is not banned
d) none is banned

144. Behavioural indicators of pain in animal suffering mastitis

a) Milk yield and quality
b) Dry matter intake
c) Hock to hock distance while standing
d) Acute phase proteins

145. Indirect indicator of dairy animal welfare is

a) Milk yield
b) Rumination
c) Restlessness
d) Infertility

146. Major reason of culling dairy animal

a) Mastitis
b) Lameness
c) Infertility
d) All of these

147. Cutting of horn's pointed end in mature dairy cattle is

a) Dehorning
b) Horn tipping
c) Horn clipping
d) Horn shearing

148. Minimum space provided in vehicle per adult cattle during road transport

a) 0.8 m^2
b) 1.0m^2
c) 1.2 m^2
d) 1.4 m^2

149. Minimum space provided in vehicle for adult mare during road transport

a) 1.8 m^2
b) 1.0m^2
c) 1.2 m^2
d) 2.0 m^2

148. During road transport, the space required for goat in vehicle

a) Twice as for sheep
b) Half as for sheep
c) Same as for shorned sheep
d) Same as for unshorned sheep

Answer Key

1	b	2	a	3	a	4	b	5	a	6	b	7	a
8	d	9	a	10	a	11	a	12	a	13	b	14	c
15	a	16	b	17	b	18	c	19	a	20	a	21	d
22	a	23	a	24	c	25	a	26	d	27	c	28	c
29	d	30	a	31	d	32	d	33	d	34	d	35	b
36	a	37	a	38	a	39	a	40	c	41	a	42	a
43	a	44	d	45	a	46	a	47	a	48	a	49	b
50	a	51	a	52	a	53	d	54	a	55	a	56	a
57	a	58	d	59	c	60	d	61	d	62	a	63	d
64	a	65	a	66	c	67	a	68	b	69	a	70	c
71	a	72	a	73	a	74	a	75	a	76	d	77	a

78	a	79	a	80	a	81	a	82	b	83	b	84	a
85	b	86	d	87	a	88	d	89	d	90	a	91	c
92	a	93	a	94	c	95	d	96	a	97	a	98	c
99	a	100	a	101	a	102	a	103	c	104	a	105	a
106	a	107	b	108	a	109	a	110	b	111	d	112	d
113	b	114	d	115	a	116	a	117	a	118	a	119	d
120	a	121	a	122	a	123	a	124	a	125	a	126	a
127	d	128	d	129	a	130	d	131	a	132	a	133	d
134	a	135	a	136	c	137	c	138	d	139	d	140	a
141	d	142	c	143	a	144	c	145	d	146	d	147	b
148	d	149	d	150	d								

11

General Health Management and Productive Performance

Parag Acharya, and Abhijeet Fernandes

Scientist (LPM), RRTTS, Bhawanipatna, Odisha University Agriculture & Technology (OUAT), Bhubaneswar, Odisha

Assistant Professor (VGO), CoVS, Rampura Phul, GADVASU, Ludhiana, Punjab

Introduction

Livestock plays a pivotal role in sustaining the livelihood of millions of people worldwide, particularly in rural and semi-urban communities. Beyond providing food products such as milk, meat and eggs, livestock also contribute to income generation, draught power, manure for agriculture and socio-cultural functions in many regions. The health and productive performance of livestock animals are central to achieving the economic, nutritional and ecological goals of animal husbandry. Any compromise in animal health or productivity directly impacts farmers' income, food security, and national agricultural output.

Animal health is the foundation of productive and sustainable livestock farming. Good health ensures animals can grow, reproduce and perform at their genetic potential. Conversely, disease, poor nutrition and environmental stress can severely reduce productivity and increase mortality. Common health challenges in livestock include infectious diseases (bacterial, viral, and parasitic), metabolic disorders and management-related stress conditions. Moreover, zoonotic diseases—those transmissible to humans—are of growing concern in the context of public health and food safety.

Preventive health management, including timely vaccinations, deworming, hygienic practices and bio-security measures, can significantly reduce the incidence of disease. An effective health program also includes early disease detection, prompt veterinary intervention and stress reduction strategies. Preventing diseases is not only more economical than treatment but also crucial in reducing the misuse of antibiotics and combating antimicrobial resistance (AMR), which is a growing global threat.

Productive performance in livestock includes key traits such as growth rate, reproductive efficiency, milk yield, egg production, feed conversion efficiency and work output. These traits are primarily influenced by four major factors: genetic potential, nutrition, management practices and overall health status. The genetic makeup of an animal determines its inherent capacity for production, setting the baseline for performance. Building upon this, nutrition plays a vital role as a cornerstone of productivity—balanced feeding is essential for supporting growth, reproduction, lactation, immune function and general well-being. Reproductive efficiency, in particular, is a critical determinant of profitability in breeding animals; indicators such as regular estrous cycles, successful conception and healthy offspring reflect optimal reproductive performance. Beyond internal factors, the external environment also plays a crucial role. Proper housing and environmental management help reduce stress and the incidence of diseases, thereby enhancing productivity. Animals must be protected from extreme weather, given adequate ventilation and ensured constant access to clean water and sufficient space. Inadequate housing can result in heat stress, respiratory issues, and physical injuries. Complementing all these factors, sound husbandry practices—including regular cleaning, proper waste disposal, timely weaning and a well-planned vaccination schedule—further support animal health and welfare. Additionally, gentle handling and maintaining herd hierarchy minimize stress-related productivity losses, ensuring that animals can perform to their full potential.

There is a direct correlation between animal health and productive performance. For example, a dairy cow suffering from mastitis not only produces less milk but may also require costly treatment and longer recovery time, affecting overall farm profitability. Similarly, parasitic infections in goats or sheep can lead to weight loss, anaemia and poor reproductive outcomes. Health issues in poultry, such as coccidiosis or respiratory infections, can lead to reduced egg laying and feed inefficiency.

Chronic or subclinical diseases, although not immediately apparent, can also cause long-term productivity losses. Subclinical mastitis, mineral deficiencies and early-stage parasitic infestations often go unnoticed but gradually erode the animal's performance. Therefore, routine monitoring and health assessment are vital to ensure animals are not only disease-free but also performing at their full potential.

Extreme weather conditions, particularly during summer and monsoon seasons, can adversely affect livestock health and performance. Heat stress leads to reduced feed intake, lower fertility and increased susceptibility to disease, especially in high-yielding breeds. Seasonal changes also influence the incidence of vector-borne diseases and reproductive cycles in many species.

Mitigating the impact of climate involves providing adequate shade, clean drinking water, good ventilation and nutritional support including electrolytes and antioxidants during heat waves. Livestock farmers need to be trained on climate-resilient practices and early warning systems for disease outbreaks associated with seasonal shifts.

Recent advancements in livestock management technologies—such as wearable health monitors, automated milking machines, AI-based breeding tools and mobile apps for disease tracking—are transforming animal agriculture. These innovations help monitor health parameters in real-time, identify early signs of disease and ensure timely interventions.

Moreover, data-driven decision-making, supported by livestock health records, breeding logs and production data, helps in identifying trends, managing herd performance and improving profitability. Such tools are increasingly becoming accessible even to smallholder farmers, supported by government and private sector initiatives.

Sustainable livestock farming ensures that animals are healthy, the environment is protected and public health is not compromised. Reducing the use of antibiotics, improving waste management and preventing zoonoses are essential components of this holistic approach

1. .... is a method of oral administration of drug ?

   a) Balling guns b) Drenching

   c) Dose syringes d) All of the above

2. .... is a method of giving liquid medicine or suspension to cattle & buffalo ?
   a) Balling guns b) Drenching
   c) Dose syringes d) All of the above
3. .... is used to administer small amounts of liquids and suspension, especially to horses and pigs ?
   a) Balling guns b) Drenching
   c) Dose syringes d) All of the above
4. .... instrument is placed on top of the tongue of cattle & buffalo to give boluses, capsules and tablets.
   a) Balling guns b) Drenching
   c) Dose syringe d) All of the above
5. Which of the following is the advantage of parenteral route of drug administration?
   a) Danger of acute drug reaction is minimal
   b) Bioavailability is faster and more predictable
   c) Gastric irritation and vomiting are avoided
   d) Both b & c
6. Which of the following is the advantage of oral route of drug administration?
   a) Safe b) Sterility is not required
   c) Liver enzymes are by-passed d) Both a & b
7. Which of the following is correct?
   a) S/C route- Injection beneath the skin, on top of muscle layer
   b) I/M route- Injection directly in major muscle mass
   c) I/D route- Needle inserted between the layers of skin
   d) All are correct
8. Which of the following is correct regarding Intra Peritoneal route of drug administration?
   a) Drug absorption rapid than SC but slower than IV
   b) Route not recommended for horses
   c) Only a is correct
   d) Both a & b are correct
9. Epidural injection is given at the..............
   a) Jugular vein
   b) sacro-coccygeal vertebral junction
   c) Peritoneal cavity
   d) None of the above
10. Which of the following route of drug administration is preferred for faster bioavailability of drug
   a) Oral b) Topical
   c) Parentral d) All

11. Intravenous drug administration is generally done at..............vein
    a) Cephali
    b) Radial
    c) Jugular
    d) Coccygeal
12. Pessary is generally placed in...........
    a) Rectum
    b) Uterus
    c) Stomach
    d) Vagina
13. Major cause of calf mortality is
    a) FMD
    b) Calf scour & Pneumonia
    c) Naval ill
    d) None
14. Early weaned calves, if kept in group housing system are susceptible to
    a) Hair ball formation
    b) Anaemia
    c) Polyneuritis
    d) Rickets
15. Hair ball (Trichobezoar) formation in the stomach of calves can be due to
    a) Pica
    b) Biting
    c) High Fiber
    d) Inter-licking
16. Cross-sucking among calves is more common........
    a) Immediately before natural milk sucking
    b) Immediately after pail milk feeding
    c) During milk sucking
    d) Before weaning
17. Intersucking or self sucking in cows can be prevented by –
    a) Modified bull nose ring with spines on outer semicircular portion.
    b) Neck cradles
    c) Neem oil at teats
    d) All of the above
18. In a well managed dairy farm, what should be the maximum limit of mortality in case of calf and adult cattle?
    a) 10 % & 5 %
    b) 15 % & 10 %
    c) 15 % & 5 %
    d) 20 % & 10 %
19. Which of the following disinfectant is used for the treatment of naval cord in calf?
    a) $KMnO_4$
    b) Tincture Iodine
    c) Formalin
    d) Phenyle
20. Pica is mainly due to
    a) Boredom
    b) Imbalance of dietary Ca:P
    c) High protein diet
    d) High fiber diet
21. Buller-steer syndrome is seen mostly due to
    a) Late weaning
    b) Limited exercise
    c) High dietary fiber
    d) Early weaning

22. Ketosis in dairy cattle is due to deficiency of
    a) Mineral b) Energy
    c) Protein d) Fatty acid
23. Spontaneous ketosis is most commonly prevalence during
    a) 1-2 weeks of lactation b) 2-3 weeks of lactation
    c) 3-5 weeks of lactation d) 4-6 weeks of lactation
24. Predominate ketone body found in buffalo
    a) Acetoacetate b) B-hydroxybutyrate
    c) Acetone d) Isopropanol
25. Dietary deficiency of which nutrient may lead to a high incidence of ketosis
    a) Cobalt b) Manganese
    c) Phosphorus d) All
26. Nervous sign of ketosis is due to
    a) Acetoacetate b) B-hydroxybutyrate
    c) Acetone d) Isopropyl alcohol
27. Capricious appetite & hide bound condition are the common clinical finding in
    a) Ketosis b) Milk fever
    c) PPH d) Monday morning sickness
28. Test used to detect ketone bodies in milk
    a) Rothera test b) Sodium nitroprusside test
    c) Bromocresol purple test d) All
29. Crawling & frog leg attitude like behaviour commonly seen in
    a) Milk fever b) Downer cow syndrome
    c) Obturator paralysis d) All
30. For strategic transition cow management, metabolic parameters need to be accessed
    a) NEFA in the last week of prepartum & BHBA in the 1st week postpartum
    b) NEFA & BHBA in the 1st week of postpartum
    c) NEFA & BHBA in the last week of prepartum
    d) None
31. A total DCAD amount (range of) is effective in controlling milk fever
    a) -100 to -200 mEq/kg feed DM b) -50 to -100 mEq/kg feed DM
    c) -200 to -300 mEq/kg feed DM d) None
32. Sternal recumbency with lateral kinking of neck & lateral recumbency with generalized flaccidity seen in which stage of milk fever
    a) 1st & 2nd b) 2nd & 3rd
    c) 1st & 3rd d) 3rd & 2nd
33. Lactation tetany in dairy animal occur due to
    a) Mg deficiency b) Ca deficiency
    c) P deficiency d) All

34. Pregnancy toxemia in cattle is also known as
    a) Ketosis b) Fat cow syndrome
    c) Milk fever d) DCS
35. Which nutrient deficiency associated with hepatic lipidosis condition in cow ?
    a) Mg b) Choline
    c) Biotin d) Thiamine
36. Most important disease of dairy cows for bringing maximum loss to dairy industry throughout the world ?
    a) Mastitis b) Brucellosis
    c) Tuberculosis d) FMD
37. Which of the following is the most succeptible for bacterial contamination of milk ?
    a) Udder b) Milker
    c) Milk utensils d) None of the above
38. Which test is commonly done in lactating herd of cattle & buffalo for regular screening of mastitis?
    a) CMT b) Strip cup
    c) PCR d) Tuberculin
39. What is the minimum number of bacteria present in milk that is drawn aseptically from the udder of healthy cow?
    a) 500 bacteria / ml b) 100 bacteria / ml
    c) 1000 bacteria/ ml d) 50 bacteria / ml
40. The somatic cell count / ml of milk should be .... in 'good' grade milk.
    a) Less than 0.2 million b) Less than 0.4 million
    c) Between 0.2 – 0.4 million d) Less than 50,000
41. Which is a good disinfectant for dairy utensils, udders and milker's hand ?
    a) Bleaching Powder b) Phenol
    c) Boric Acid d) QAC
42. Which of the following is used for sterilization of water supply and disinfection of sheds after disease outbreak?
    a) Bleaching Powder b) Phenol
    c) Boric Acid d) QAC
43. The common antiseptic solution used as teat dip after milking is
    a) Povidone Iodine
    b) Pottasium permanganate
    c) Povidone Iodine or Pottasium permanganate
    d) None
44. Which of the following is used to disinfect dairy utensils, udders, milker's hand etc?
    a) Quick lime b) Bleaching powder
    c) Cetrimide d) Washing soda

45. Protecting the health status of animals in a herd by limiting the introduction of disease is known as:

a) Isolation   b) Quarantine
c) Disinfection   d) Biosecurity

46. Segregation of animals suffering from infectious disease form healthy herd is known as

a) Isolation   b) Quarantine
c) Disinfection   d) Vaccination

47. Segregation of apparently healthy animals, especially animals being brought into the herd for first time from the healthy herd is known as

a) Isolation   b) Quarantine
c) Disinfection   d) Vaccination

48. The process by which the number of bacteria and other microorganisms are reduced enough to prevent diseases to an acceptable public health standard?

a) Cleaning   b) Sanitization
c) Disinfection   d) Vaccination

49. What is the quarantine period for 'Rabies'?

a) 21 days   b) 2 months
c) 6 months   d) None

50. To make any surface free of pathogenic microorganism is known as

a) Isolation   b) Quarantine
c) Disinfection   d) Vaccination

51. Cannibalism is generally seen in

a) Cattle   b) Pig
c) Poultry   d) Horse

52. Method of pregnancy diagnosis in small ruminant is

a) Rectal palpation   b) Abdominal palpation
c) Cuboni test   d) Cocking of tail

53. Rapid plate /Agglutination test is done for screening of ....disease in farm condition.

a) Tuberculosis   b) Paratuberculois
c) Brucellosis   d) Mastitis

54. Most sanitary method of carcass disposal is

a) Burial   b) Burning
c) Both a & b   d) None

55. Which among the following statements is false

a) External parasites are major problem in humid regions
b) Internal parasites are more menacing in arid region
c) Sweating also aids in evaporative heat loss in horses
d) Both a and b are false

56. In which of the following disease carcass is not opened for PM examination.
   a) TB
   b) FMD
   c) Anthrax
   d) All of the above

57. Consequence of FMD is
   a) Decreased milk yield
   b) Permanent hoof damage
   c) Abortion in advance stage of pregnancy
   d) All of the above

58. Which of the following is correct regarding *Brucella abortus ?*
   a) Being present in udder and milk, they do not induce inflammatory reactions in the udder (mastitis)
   b) The *Brucella* organism induce placentitis and abortion when they are present in the uterus
   c) Only a is correct
   d) Both a & b are correct

59. Calf hood vaccination is done for
   a) FMD
   b) HS
   c) BQ
   d) Brucellosis

60. Which of the following is correct?
   a) Single time vaccination provides lifelong immunity in case of Theileriosis & Brucellosis
   b) Males are not vaccinated against Brucellosis
   c) Cattle are vaccinated against Mastitis
   d) Only a & b are correct

61. 'Tuberculin test' is done for screening of .... disease in farm condition.
   a) TB
   b) JD
   c) Brucellosis
   d) None of the above

62. 'Johnin test' is done for screening of .... disease in farm condition.
   a) TB
   b) JD
   c) Brucellosis
   d) None of the above

63. The group of animals depend on external environment for thermoregulation are called
   a) Ectotherms
   b) Endotherms
   c) Homeotherms
   d) None of the above

64. .... is responsible for metestrous bleeding in cattle & buffalo ?
   a) Increase in estrogen
   b) Decline in estrogen
   c) LH surge
   d) All of the above

65. The hormone melatonin is secreted by the gland
   a) Pineal
   b) Thymus
   c) Adrenal
   d) Mammary

66. Mulberry heart disease in pig is caused by
    a) Vitamin A
    b) Vitamin E
    c) Selenium
    d) Vitamin E & Selenium
67. Swine flu is caused by
    a) Influenza type virus A
    b) Influenza type virus B
    c) Influenza type virus C
    d) Influenza type virus D
68. Feeding of raw garbage in swine spreads ....disease.
    a) Vesicular exanthema
    b) Piglet anemia
    c) Swine fever
    d) Swine erysipelas
69. Goose stepping in pigs occurs due to deficiency of
    a) Folic acid
    b) Pantothenic acid
    c) Niacine
    d) Zinc
70. Pig is vaccinated against:
    a) FMD
    b) HS
    c) Swine Erysipelas
    d) All
71. Which of the following animals is a long day breeder?
    a) Sheep
    b) Horse
    c) Cow
    d) All of the above
72. .... route of injection is not preferred in horses ?
    a) Intra Peritoneal
    b) Intra Muscular
    c) Epidural
    d) Both a & c
73. The site of ovulation in Mare is
    a) Ovulation fossa
    b) Germinal disc
    c) Ovulation ridge
    d) Margo plicatus
74. Which of the species has longest duration of estrous ?
    a) Goat
    b) Sheep
    c) Sow
    d) Mare
75. Split esturs and prolonged estrus are common in
    a) Swine
    b) Bovine
    c) Canine
    d) Equine
76. Dogs are often vaccinated against following diseases except -
    a) Parvo
    b) Distemper
    c) Ringworm
    d) Hepatitis
77. Ventriculocordectomy is commonly known as -
    a) Docking
    b) Debarking
    c) Castration
    d) Spaying
78. Binge or rapid eating behaviour is seen more commonly in
    a) Dog
    b) Cat
    c) Calf
    d) None of the above

79. Potato soup like pus is a characteristic feature of
    a) Pseudomonas b) Trichomoniasis
    c) Campylobacteriasis d) Brucellosis
80. Cocking of the tail is a characteristic pregnancy behavior exhibited by
    a) Giraffe b) Camel
    c) Horse d) Donkey
81. .... is always associated with threatened abortion.
    a) Mummification b) Maceration
    c) Both d) None
82. Longest mating time is observed in
    a) Bull b) Stallion
    c) Dog d) Boar
83. Scrotal hernia is most common in
    a) Bull b) Boar
    c) Stallion d) Buck
84. Fertile life of ova in cattle genital tract is-
    a) 5-10 hr b) 10-12 hr
    c) 20-24 hr d) None of the above
85. Fertile life of sperm in cattle genital tract is –
    a) 5-10 hr b) 15-24 hr
    c) 30-48 hr d) None of the above
86. Milk ejection test used for pregnancy diagnosis is based on injection of
    a) Prolactin b) Prostaglandins
    c) Oxytocin d) Cabergoline
87. Which of the following is common in occurrence
    a) Male pseudohermaphrodite b) Female pseudohermaphrodite
    c) True hermaphrodite d) All
88. Heifer test is usually performed for the diagnosis of
    a) Freemartinism b) White heifer disease
    c) Trichomoniasis d) Campylobacteriosis
89. Gestation period is equal to length of estrous cycle in
    a) Rhinoceros b) Kangaroo
    c) Elephant d) Camel
90. Which of the following chemical test is performed in urine for PD in mare
    a) AZ test b) Mucin test
    c) Cuboni test d) All
91. A-Z test of pregnancy diagnosis is also known as
    a) Rabbit test b) Mare test
    c) Cat test d) Rat test

92. FSH and LH are secreted by
 a) Alpha cells of acidophils
 b) Beta cells of acidophils
 c) Delta cells of basophils
 d) Beta cells of basophils

93. Placentophagy is more common in
 a) Canine
 b) Swine
 c) Porcine
 d) Equine

94. Persistent hymen is seen in
 a) Freemartins
 b) Hermaphrodites
 c) White heifer's disease
 d) None of the above

95. Vaginal biopsy is a useful method of pregnancy diagnosis in
 a) Cow
 b) Ewe
 c) Sow
 d) Mare

96. Block to polyspermy in mammalian ova occurs at
 a) Vitelline membrane
 b) Zona pellucida (zona reaction)
 c) None
 d) All of the above

97. For evaluating the herd fertility of a dairy farm, the best parameter will be
 a) Calving to conception interval
 b) Days open
 c) Calving index
 d) Submission rate

98. As per the Minimum Standard Protocol for production of bovine semen in India, a bull should be free from which of the following diseases?
 a) Brucellosis, Vibrosis, Trichomoniasis, TB, JD, IBR
 b) Brucellosis, Vibrosis, BVD, TB, JD, Leptospirosis
 c) Brucellosis, Trichomoniasis, BVD, Leptospirosis, JD, IBR
 d) Brucellosis, IBR, BVD, TB, JD, FMD

99. Which of the following are the four cardinal signs of pregnancy diagnosis in cattle & buffalo
 1. Slipping of fetal membrane
 2. Palpation of amniotic vesicle
 3. Palpataion of placentome
 4. Palpataion of fetus
 5. Fremitus & fetal bump

 Choose the correct option
 a) 1, 2, 3 & 4
 b) 2, 3, 4 & 5
 c) 1, 2, 3 & 5
 d) 1, 2, 4 & 5

100. Which of the following is a preventive type of antioxidant used in as semen additives
 a) Catalase
 b) Vit. C
 c) Vit. E
 d) Xanthine

101. In breeding soundness examination of bull, if the angle of tarsal is greater, it will give rise to the condition of
 a) Post leg
 b) Sickle hock
 c) Toe-in
 d) Corkscrew

102. Hooded cervix is present in
   a) Ewe b) Cow
   c) Mare d) Bitch
103. Uterine torsion is most common in __________ breed of buffalo
   a) Surti b) Murrah
   c) Jaffrabadi d) All
104. Which of the following hormone could be given orally to manipulate reproduction?
   a) Progesterone b) Mifepristone
   c) Kisspeptin d) All
105. Testosterone con c) in castrated animal is
   a) <0.5 ng/ ml b) 1 ng/ ml
   c) 2 ng/ ml d) 0.5-1.5 ng/ ml
106. Frenzied galloping, staggering & straddling gait, convulsion with head retraction are some of the clinical signs of
   a) Milk fever b) Lactation tetany
   c) Nervous ketosis d) Rabies
107. Hook shaped glans penis is present in
   a) Camel b) Sow
   c) Rodent d) Ram
108. Poll gland secretions contain pheromone in
   a) Camel b) Kangaroo
   c) Giraffe d) All
109. Highest testicular growth occurs in
   a) 1-6 months b) 6-12 months
   c) 12-18 months d) After puberty
110. Capped cervix is a pregnancy sign in
   a) Mare b) Ewe
   c) Sow d) Camel
111. 1st ET calf is -
   a) Prima b) Holi
   c) Virgil d) Frosty II
112. 1st IVF buffalo calf is
   a) Saubhagya b) Samrupa
   c) Pratham d) Polly
113. 1st cloned buffalo is
   a) Saubhagya b) Samrupa
   c) Pratham d) Polly
14. 1st transgenic sheep is
   a) Saubhagya b) Samrupa
   c) Pratham d) Polly

115. AS per MSP for frozen semen production, scrotal circumference & body weight of bulls should be measured at
   a) 3 & 1 month resp. b) Every month
   c) Fortnightly d) 2 & 1 month resp.
116. In which species suckling is not related to oxytocin release?
   a) Mare b) Sheep
   c) Goat d) Sow
117. Example of induced ovulatory is
   a) Camel b) Cat
   c) Ewe d) Both a & b
118. Which hormone is termed as "Obstetrical & Surgical pituitrin"
   a) Oxytocin, ADH b) Vasoprerssin, ADH
   c) ADH, Oxytocin d) None
119. Sudden luteinizing hormone release (LH surge) is not observed in
   a) Mare b) Buffalo
   c) Bitch d) Cow
120. Hulet method of pregnancy diagnosis is practiced in which of the following species.
   a) Ewe b) Sow
   c) Buffalo d) Mare
121. A: Ewe is a short-day breeder.
   R: Ewes staying at equator region may breed at any time of the year.
   Choose the correct option
   a) Both A & R true b) Both A & R false
   c) A is true but R is false d) A is false but R is true
122. Breech presentation is more common in
   a) Bitch b) Queen
   c) Ewe d) Sow
123. Copious micturition indicates completion of parturition in
   a) Sow b) Cow
   c) Mare d) Ewe
124. Non-sexual erection of penis is known as
   a) Pederasty b) Priaprism
   c) Carnal intercourse d) Satyriasis
125. Anti-agglutinin in semen is secreted by
   a) Seminal Vesicle b) Bulbourethral Gland
   c) Prostate Gland d) Epididymis
126. Vermiform appendage is present in penis of
   a) Bull b) Boar
   c) Ram d) Stallion

127. The order of milking in a herd should be for prevention of mastitis -
   1. Healthy younger cows
   2. Older healthy cow
   3. Healthy cows with mastitis history
   4. Cows with quarter producing abnormal milks

   a) 1,2,3,4 b) 4,3,2,1
   c) 2,1,3,4 d) 3,4,2,1

128. In cattle, milk progesterone test is more reliable for diagnosing
   a) Non-Pregnancy b) Pregnancy
   c) Mucometra d) Hydrometra

129. Homologous organ of Bulbourethral gland in female is
   a) Gartner's duct b) Bartholin gland
   c) Vestibular gland d) None of the above

130. Male seeking behaviour with subsequent "harem" activity seen in
   a) Ewe b) Doe
   c) Sow d) Mare

131. Intersexuality are more common in which species
   a) Cattle & Sheep b) Sheep & Pig
   c) Pig & Goat d) Sheep & Goat

132. Elevated tail head in nymphomanic cows is also called as
   a) Sterility Hump b) Sterility Head
   c) Buller Syndrome d) None of the above

133. Repeat breeding due to delayed ovulation in cows can be treated with
   a) Lutalyse b) Folligon
   c) Chorulon d) All

134. Species most & least resistant for luteolytic effect of PGF2α
   a) Equine & Canine b) Feline & Canine
   c) Canine & Feline d) Swine & Canine

135. The ligament responsible for udder breakdown in cows?
   a) Median suspensory ligament b) Lateral suspensory ligament
   c) Both of the above d) None of the above

136. Gestation length is inversely related to litter size in all farm animals except
   a) Cow b) Bitch
   c) Ewe d) Sow

137. Cortisol is transferred from dam to foetus in many species except
   a) Cow b) Ewe
   c) Mare d) None of the above

138. Lateral & sternal recumbency parturition occurs in
   a) Mare & Cow b) Sow & mare
   c) Cow & bitch d) Cow & Sow

139. Male foetuses are heavier than female at birth in all species except

a) Bovine b) Equine

c) Canine d) Porcine

40. The hormone responsible for inhibition of let down of milk ?

a) Oxytocin b) Adrenalin

c) Thyroxine d) Cytokine

141. Effective disinfectant to prevent entry of FMD virus to herd/ farm are

a) Sodium hydroxide (2%) b) Sodium carbonate (4%)

c) Citric acid (0.2%) d) All

142. Piglet anemia is associated with deficiency of

a) Copper b) Cobalt

c) Manganese d) Iron

143.

	Animal		**Temperature** (°F)
A	Cattle	1	103.0-summer & 98.3 – winter
B	Buffalo	2	100.6
C	Goat	3	101.6
D	Horse	4	103

a) a-2, b-1, c-4, d-3 b) a-3, b-1, c-4, d-2

c) a-1, b-3, c-4, d-2 d) a-1, b-2, c-4, d-3

144.

	Animal		**Pulse rate**
A	Cattle	1	40
B	Buffalo	2	60
C	Sheep	3	32
D	Horse	4	70

a) a-2, b-1, c-4, d-3 b) a-3, b-1, c-4, d-2

c) a-1, b-3, c-4, d-2 d) a-1, b-2, c-4, d-3

144.

	Animal		**Respiration rate**
A	Cattle	1	5
B	Goat	2	8
C	Camel	3	25
D	Horse	4	10

a) a-2, b-1, c-4, d-3 b) a-3, b-1, c-4, d-2

c) a-1, b-3, c-4, d-2 d) a-4, b-3, c-1, d-2

145. Which of the following animal is normally considered as free from breeding problem ?

a) Cattle b) Buffalo

c) Pig d) Goat

146.

	Poison		Antidote
a	Bleaching powder	1	Epsom
b	Lead salt	2	Starch gruel
c	Iodine	3	Ferric peroxide
d	Arsenic	4	White of egg

a) a-2, b-1, c-4, d-3 c) a-1, b-3, c-4, d-2

b) a-3, b-1, c-4, d-2 d) a-4, b-1, c-2, d-3

147.

	Poison		Antidote
a	HCN	1	Atropine sulphate
b	Organophosphates	2	Strong tea
c	Strychnine	3	Amyl nitrite
d	Tobaco	4	Tannic acid

a) a-2, b-1, c-4, d- c) a-1, b-3, c-4, d-2

b) a-3, b-1, c-2, d-4 d) a-4, b-1, c-2, d-3

148. Which hormone is responsible for maternal behaviour in cattle?

a) Oxytocin b) Prolactin

c) Estrogen d) All of the above

149. Daily normal resting time in high producing dairy cows –

a) 6- 8 hr b) 8- 10 hr

c) 10-12 hr d) 12- 14 hr

150. Male sex drive in domestic animal is synonymous to –

a) Puberty b) Sexual maturity

c) Libido d) None of the above

151. Stimulation of reproductive activity by the presence and activity of other members of the species is known as –

a) Fraser Darling effect b) Group effect

c) Induced effect d) All of the above

152. Behavioural problem in farm animal is known as –

a) Anomolous behaviour b) Etho- anomalies

c) Atypical behaviour d) All of the above

153. Habit or action of animals which are detrimental to themselves and other-

a) Anomolous behaviour b) Etho- anomalies

c) Atypical behaviour d) Vices

154. Repeated activities of animals which have no obvious purpose or benefit –
   a) Anomolous behaviour b) Etho- anomalies
   c) Stereotypes d) Vices

155. If a cow is mounting on another cow from head side, then the condition is –
   a) Animal mounting is in early heat
   b) Animal not mounting is in early heat
   c) Both animals are in heat
   d) None of the above

Answer Key

1	d	2	b	3	c	4	a	5	d	6	d	7	d
8	d	9	b	10	c	11	c	12	d	13	b	14	a
15	d	16	b	17	d	18	a	19	b	20	b	21	d
22	b	23	b	24	b	25	a	26	d	27	a	28	b
29	b	30	a	31	a	32	b	33	a	34	b	35	b
36	a	37	a	38	a	39	a	40	a	41	d	42	a
43	c	44	c	45	d	46	a	47	b	48	b	49	c
50	c	51	c	52	b	53	c	54	b	55	d	56	c
57	d	58	d	59	d	60	d	61	a	62	b	63	a
64	b	65	a	66	d	67	a	68	a	69	b	70	d
71	b	72	d	73	a	74	d	75	d	76	c	77	b
78	a	79	b	80	b	81	b	82	d	83	b	84	c
85	c	86	b	87	a	88	a	89	b	90	c	91	d
92	c	93	a	94	c	95	c	96	b	97	d	98	a
99	a	100	a	101	a	102	a	103	a	104	a	105	a
106	b	107	a	108	a	109	a	110	a	111	a	112	c
113	b	114	d	115	a	116	c	117	d	118	a	119	a
120	a	121	a	122	b	123	a	124	b	125	c	126	c
127	a	128	a	129	b	130	a	131	c	132	a	133	c
134	a	135	b	136	d	137	b	138	a	139	b	140	b
141	d	142	d	143	b	144	a	145	d	146	d	147	d
148	b	149	b	150	d	151	c	152	a	153	d	154	d
155	c												

12

Livestock Housing and Ventilation Management

Ajay Kumar, Mamta, Rajneesh Sirohi, and Yajuvendra Singh

College of Veterinary Science and Animal Husbandry, DUVASU, Mathura Uttar Pradesh

Introduction

A system of housing is more are less synonymous to the system of management of livestock. Housing is essential to protect the animals from adverse climatic condition (rains, hot and chilly winds). Housing also help to maintain normal health of animals by proper feeding watering and reducing environmental stresses. Housing allows the animals for proper rest, moderate exercise, suitable micro-environment and proper ventilation which are essential for comfort of the animals. While selecting the site a site for establishment of a dairy farm some points should be considered regarding topography, soil, nearby market, availability of labour, electricity, water etc. The housing system can be divided in to two type viz. conventional housing and loose housing system. The conventional housing system may be single row or double row depending upon the number of animals. The dairy farm consists of various building for different classes of livestock like calf shed/ lamb/kid/piglet pens, milking barn, maternity pen, cow shed, heifer shed, shearing room, slaughter house of pig etc. The ancillary structure of a farm are stores for keeping feed materials, equipment, milk house, silo, generator room, pump houses, AI centers, workers retiring room, office etc. The floor should be impervious and non-slippery. The floor should have a gradient toward the drain of 1 in 40 in covered area and 1in 60 in the open area for easy drainage of urine and washing of animals. The roof should be light, strong, durable, bad conductor of heat. The slopping of roof is better as they make allowance for air space and light along with roof ventilation. The wall is generally made up to a height of 1.5 m with open space supported by pillar for ventilation and sun light. In conventional housing system the open space are covered with wire mesh to prevent entry of birds, which can spread diseases directly or indirectly by contaminated feed and water. Isolation box for keeping sick animals should be located well away from other animal shed. In construction they are more or less similar to maternity pen. The lactating cow should be provided with clean and hygienic housing to prevent from any mammary infections. The cow dung removed periodically from animal shed & disposed to manure pits. The manure pit should be located minimum 200 meters away from the milking barn. Care should be taken to prevent the advance pregnant cows from being injured by slipping on floors, crowding through doors, mounting cows, that in heat fighting etc. At 2-3 weeks before calving they are to be shifted to individual pens. The calving pen should be well ventilated, clean, well bedded and free from unnecessary disturbances. Fitness of the bull is essential for quality semen production. Regular exercise helps to get rid from excess fat deposition and prevent over growth of hooves. Bull may be exercise through providing open area in a pen. In case of bull confinement, bull exerciser can be used for exercising 1-2 hrs daily. Milking parlors is fully covered barn in which the milch animals are milked. t is located at central place with all other buildings around it. The milking animals can be secured by stanchions or neck chains either in tail to tail or head to head to head arrangement. The length and width of the standing place depends on size of animals and may varying from 1.5 to 1.7 meter length and 1.05 to 1.20 meter width with a slope of 1 in 40 towards drain or gutter. Dipping tank may be made of galvanized steel sheet or constructed of brick in cement mortar. It should be located at one side of the yard. Foot bath may be of galvanized steel sheets or brick in cement mortar at the entrance to the yard to protect from foot rot disease. It should be well embedded in the soil. Shearing room should consist of two compartments with a dividing wall. One room is for storing wool and shearing tools, and the other for storing feed and medicines. The door of it should be 1 m wide and 2 m high in front side. It may have two windows of 0.7 m wide and 1.2 m high each, on each of long sides of room. One holding pen for about 30 sheep in front and the other holding pen behind shearing shed should be provided to hold shorn sheep after shearing. The shepherd house meant for caretaker and it should be located at a convenient place in yard. It should have a door (1 x 2 m) on the long side of the shed facing the passage of yard.Ultimately, then, the housing system should be designed with animal production, behaviour, thermal comfort, and microclimate modification in mind.

1. How many extra animals can be can be accommodated to loose housing system
   a) 10-15 %   b) 15-20 %
   c) 20-25%   d) 25-30 %
2. How many numbers of maternity pens is required in a dairy farm
   a) 5 %   b) 10 %
   c) 15 %   d) 20%
3. What are the ancillary structure of a dairy farm
   a) Store for feeding materials   b) Milk house
   c) Silo pit & AI centre   d) All of the above
4. What is fall of the roof of animal house
   a) 0.45 m   b) 0.60 m
   c) 0.75 m   d) 0.95 m
5. The height 15 feet at ridge and 8 feet at right side is necessary to give
   a) Essential washing space   b) Essential feeding space
   c) Essential air space   d) None of the above
6. Floor space (covered area) required for heifer
   a) 2 m^2 b) 4 m^2
   c) 6 m^2
7. Floor space (open area) required for bullock
   a) 5 m^2 b) 7 m^2
   c) 9 m^2 d) 11 m^2

8. The dimension of calving box for covered area
   a) 3 X 4 m^2 b) 3 X 5 m^2
   c) 3 X 6 m^2 d) 3 X 7 m^2
9. Dairy farm shed the pitch for thatched roof should be
   a) 15^0 b) 25^0
   c) 35^0 d) 45^0
10. The floor of dairy farm should have on gradient of
    a) 1 in 10 towards the drains b) 1 in 20 towards the drains
    c) 1 in 30 towards the drains d) 1 in 40 towards the drains
11. What is the carrying capacity of one hectare land
    a) 2-3 cows b) 5-6 cows
    c) 8-10 cows d) 12-14 cows
12. Covered and open area(m^2) required for milking buffalo respectively are
    a) 3.5 & 7.5 b) 4.0 & 8.0
    c) 2.5 & 5.0 d) 4.5 & 9.5
13. Lying time of lactating buffalo depend upon
    a) Ventilation b) Type of feeding
    c) Type of housing d) Angle of pitch
14. Loose housing system is example of
    a) Extensive systemq b) Intensive system
    c) Semi- intensive system d) Backyard
15. A hectare land producing 600 quintal fodder per year can support
    a) 2 cows b) 4 cows
    c) 6 cows d) 8 cows
16. Distance between two pillar should be
    a) 1-2 meter b) 2-3 meter
    c) 3-4 meter d) 4-5 meter
17. Wire fencing height for cattle & buffaloes
    a) 100 cm b) 120 cm
    c) 150 cm d) 180 cm
18. Painting of roof should be done by
    a) Upper surface- white colour b) Inner surface- dark colour
    c) both d) None of the above
19. Single row system should be adopted when the number of animal
    a) <7 b) ~10
    c) >15 d) < 15
20. Conventional system of housing is least common for
    a) Swine b) Equine
    c) Bovine d) All of the above

21. Quarantine means
    a) Maintaining animal for transport separately
    b) Segregation of disease animal
    c) Maintaining advance pregnant animal separately
    d) Maintaining of newly purchase animals separate housing system
22. In livestock housing, the wall thickness should not be exceed
    a) 15 cm b) 25 cm
    c) 35 cm d) 45 cm
23. Which gate works best for a dairy farm
    a) Sliding gate b) Single gate
    c) Hinged gate d) None of these
24. The air space needed for a cow is
    a) 200 ft^3 b) 400 ft^3
    c) 600 ft^3 d) 800 ft^3
25. When cleaning of floor and utensils in dairy farm the washing soda should be used
    a) 1% solution b) 3% solution
    c) 6 % solution d) 9 % solution
26. Conventional housing system is also known as
    a) Tie barn b) Stanchion barn
    c) Bot d) Ranch
27. The highest point of roof is
    a) Span b) Overhang
    c) Eave d) Ridge
28. Feeding space for adult cattle as per BIS standard
    a) 35-50 cm b) 60-75 cm
    c) 85-100 cm d) 115-130 cm
29. Corrugated asbestos sheet are material of option for constructing
    a) Partition b) Floor
    c) Pillar d) Roof
30. Floor space requirement for a buffaloes under conventional housing system
    a) Covered area x 2 b) Open area x 2
    c) Paddock area x 2 d) None of these
31. Usually the number of advance pregnant buffaloes kept per pen is
    a) One b) Two
    c) Three d) Four
32. Covered area and open area requirement for heifer & dry cow respectively are
    a) 2.0-4.0 & 3.5- 7.0 m^2 b) 1.0- 1.5 & 4.0-8.0 m^2
    c) 1.5- 2.5 & 12.0-12.0 m^2 d) All of the above

33. Drainage system in a cattle farm should be
    a) Pipe system b) Open type
    c) Closed type d) None of these
34. Width of foundation of livestock house should be
    a) Half of wall b) Equal to wall
    c) Two to four times than wall d) All of the above
35. A particular area within the home range defended by animals against intruder is
    a) Core area b) Territory
    c) Home range d) Critical area
36. Which amongst the following roof materials are considered best for dairy animals in hot arid environment
    a) Thatch b) Plastic
    c) Asbestos d) None of the above
37. Floor space (covered) required for bullock is
    a) 3.5 m^2 b) 7.0 m^2
    c) 4.0 m^2 d) 8.0 m2
38. The climatic conditions directly surrounding the animal is called
    a) Micro-environment b) Macro- environment
    c) Both d) None of the above
39. Materials are considered best for bedding on pacca floor for dairy animals
    a) Dry leave b) Sow-dust
    c) Sand d) Wheat straw
40. Which of the following is the most limiting resource at a dairy farm enterprise
    a) Land b) Labor
    c) Livestock d) Capital
41. Slope of ramp for loading of cattle in truck should not exceed
    a) 5-10 degree b) 20-25 degree
    c) 30-35 degree d) 40-45 degree
42. A animals requires rest per day for optimal production
    a) 5-6 hrs b) 13-14 hrs
    c) 18-19 hrs d) None of the above
43. Best advantage of round barn is
    a) Even distribution of light b) Easy cleaning of gutter
    c) Centrally located silo d) Low cost
44. Manger space requirement for calf is
    a) 40-50 cm b) 60-75 cm
    c) 80-95 cm d) None of the above

45. Handling yard used for
   a) Vaccination b) Marking
   c) Weighing d) All of the above
46. Inlet and outlet area required for from house of cow is
   a) 81sq. cm b) 91 sq. cm
   c) 111 sq. cm d) 121 sq. cm
47. Manger best suited for dairy farm
   a) Continuous without partitioned b) Covered
   c) Single isolated manger d) Continuous with fixed partitioned
48. Materials are considered best for bedding on pacca floor for dairy animals
   a) Dry leave b) Sow-dust
   c) Sand d) Wheat straw
49. The instrument to measure humidity in animal housing is
   a) Psychrometer b) Hygrometer
   c) Wet bulb & dry bulb thermometer d) All of the above
50. Flexible & more affordable housing for dairy animal
   a) Conventional housing system b) Tie barn
   c) Loose housing system d) None of the above
51. Most of the dairy detergent are made of
   a) Water softener b) Alkali form
   c) Acidic form d) Wheat straw
52. Width of manger shed should be
   a) 75 cm b) 75 m
   c) 75 mm d) 7.5 m
53. Floor space requirement for dairy cows is
   a) 50-60 square feet b) 70-80 square feet
   c) 110-120 square feet d) > 150 square feet
54. The housing of cattle also known as
   a) Deep litter system b) Barn system
   c) Free range system d) Loose housing system
55. The roof system between two wall having a distance more than 6 meter is
   a) Collar beam truss b) Couple close roof
   c) Single slope roof d) King post truss
56. The distance of animal & camera should be placed at
   a) Half the length of animal b) Twice length of animal
   c) Three time of length of animal d) Four time of length of animal
57. Which is better when construction of dairy building
   a) Grow into b) Go into
   c) Jump into d) All of the above

58. Water drinking spacing of a dairy farm should be
    a) 1/10 of feeding space
    b) 1/20 of feeding space
    c) Equal to feeding space
    d) None of the above
59. The width of building from one wall to the other is known as
    a) Span
    b) Pitch
    c) Eave
    d) None of the above
60. Pregnant animals are transferred to the maternity pens
    a) 2-3weeks before expected date of calving
    b) 5-6 weeks before expected date of calving
    c) 8-9 weeks before expected date of calving
    d) None of the above
61. The degree of slop provided to the sides of the roof in a farm building
    a) Plinth
    b) Run
    c) Pitch
    d) Span
62. Newborn calf below one month of age should be house
    a) In group of 30 in shed
    b) Well ventilated individual cage
    c) In group of 50 in shed
    d) In group of 50 in calf pen
63. One can regulate the direction of the predominant airflow by
    a) Tree wind break
    b) Homestead windward side
    c) Both
    d) None of the above
64. Managers' offices and residences are frequently referred to as
    a) Complementary room
    b) Ancillary room
    c) Homestead
    d) None of the above
65. Isolation implies
    a) Segregation of animal
    b) New purchase animal introduced
    c) Mixing of new animal
    d) All of the above
66. The important things to think about when housing dairy animals are as follows:
    a) Nearby market
    b) Design of farm building
    c) Location of site
    d) All of the above
67. The parturition in milking parlor is highly
    a) Undesirable
    b) Desirable
    c) Both
    d) None of these
68. The resources which remain unchanged irrespective of the level of production are called as-
    a) Fixed cost
    b) Variable cost
    c) Both
    d) None of these
69. Resources which changed with level of production are known as
    a) Fixed cost
    b) Variable cost
    c) Both
    d) All of the above

70. Veterinary aid , maintenance, labour etc. makes which component cost
   a) Recurring cost b) Non-recurring cost
   c) Fixed cost d) Variable cost
71. Livestock, equipments, land, building etc. makes which component cost
   a) Fixed capital b) Fixed cost
   c) Recurring cost d) Non-recurring cost
72. Variable cost includes
   a) Feed b) Electricity
   c) Labour d) All of the above
73. When the business activity is zero, total cost equal to
   a) Marginal cost b) Variable cost
   c) Fixed cost d) None of these
74. The average amount of man hours/ cow/ annum under conventional housing system
   a) 25 min/cow/day b) 150 man hrs /cow/year
   c) Both d) Non of these
75. Depreciation is frequently viewed as
   a) Recurring cost b) Fixed capital
   c) Fixed cost d) Variable cost
76. What is understood depreciation rate for kaccha and pucca shed
   a) 5 % & 2% b) 2 % & 5 %
   c) 2 % & 1 % d) 1 % & 2 %
77. In a crossbred dairy farm, what should be the optimal ratio of Dry : Milch animals
   a) 35: 65 b) 25: 75
   c) 35: 65 d) None of these
78. In a buffalo dairy farm, what should be the optimal ratio of Dry : Milch animals
   a) 35: 65 b) 25: 75
   c) 30: 70 d) None of these
79. In a zebu dairy farm what should be the optimal ratio of Dry : Milch animals
   a) 35: 65 b) 25: 75
   c) 30: 70 d) None of these
80. In a dairy farm, 50–60% of the total man hours are utilized for
   a) Feeding b) Breeding
   c) Cleaning d) Milking
81. How many milkers required a dairy farm for 100 dairy cows
   a) 8-10 b) 15-20
   c) 20-25 d) None of these
82. The number of hours of labour needed each day per adult unit in conventional housing
   a) 5 minute b) 25 minute
   c) 45 minute d) 60 minute

83. The number of hours of labour needed each day per adult unit in loose housing
 a) 16 minute b) 20 minute
 c) 25 minute d) 30 minute

84. One acre of good pasture will carry about how many goat
 a) 9-10 b) 15-16
 c) 18-19 d) 24-25

85. Which of the following is the ideal material for roofing of cattle shed
 a) Corrugated plain sheet b) Stone
 c) Earth d) Tiles

86. Dipping tank should be located at
 a) Centre of yard b) Near to office
 c) One side of yard d) All of the above

87. Storage space required for 100 kg of loose hay
 a) 0.6 m^2 b) 0.8 m^2
 c) 1.2 m^2 d) 1.6 m^2

88. Standard degree of purity of air for animal houses should not be lower than
 a) 66.80 % b) 76.67 %
 c) 86.45 % d) 96.70 %

89. Straw per quintal require space
 a) 3 m^3 b) 6 m^3
 c) 9 m^3 d) 12 m^3

90. Grain per quintal require a space of
 a) 0.6 m^3 b) 0.12 m^3
 c) 0.8 m^3 d) 0.17 m^3

91. In loose housing is better than conventional housing
 a) Easy to heat detection b) Easy to expansion in future
 c) Low cost d) All of the above

92. What is the purpose of housing in dairy animal
 a) Provide micro-environment
 b) Protect from wild animal
 c) Protect from adverse climatic condition
 d) All of the above

93. Animals housed in loose housing are kept free except during
 a) Medication & milking b) Calving
 c) Heat detection & feeding d) All of the above

94. It is necessary to provide a wallowing tank for
 a) Sheep & Goat b) Cattle & Buffalo
 c) Equine & Swine d) Buffalo & Pig

95. The depth of foot bath for cattle should be
a) 0.1 m
b) 0.3 m
c) 0.6 m
d) 0.9 m

96. For dairy animals houses, the recommended amount of fresh air supply per hour
a) 45 m^3/h
b) 85 m^3/h
c) 105 m^3/h
d) 115 m^3/h

97. In order to maximize the sunlight's benefits, the barn's long axis should be oriented as
a) North-South direction
b) East-West direction
c) North- East direction
d) West- South direction

98. The pitch angle for thatch roof should be
a) 12-18°
b) 25-30°
c) 35°
d) 45°

99. The pitch angle for sheet roof should be
a) 12-18°
b) 25-30°
c) 35°
d) 45°

100. The conventional housing system is also known as
a) Enclosed barn
b) Tie barn
c) Stanchion
d) All of the above

101. The conventional housing system teaser bull used for
a) Heat detection
b) Pregnancy diagnosis
c) Bio-stimulation
d) None of the above

102. In which housing system spread of disease is more
a) Head to head system
b) Tail to tail system
c) Both
d) None of these

103. Covered space requirement for down-calver
a) 80-100 sq ft
b) 100-120 sq ft
c) 180-200 sq ft
d) >200 sq ft

104. The open area surrounded by wall or fences is known as
a) Shelter
b) Pen
c) Sty
d) Paddock

105. Which of the livestock housing system labour efficient
a) Head to Head system
b) Tail to Tail system
c) Both
d) All of the above

106. Which of the following is an example of inlet
a) Metal grating
b) Direct pipe
c) Window
d) All of the above

107. What is the objective of providing shelter to dairy animals
   a) Better control of disease b) Reduce the wastage of feed
   c) Micro-Environment d) All of the above
108. Corrugated asbestos sheet, king truss are associated to
   a) Floor b) Wall
   c) Roof d) None of the above
109. Solid manure is usually collected & removed from shed
   a) Twice daily b) Thrice daily
   c) Per day d) None of the above
110. Specialized ventilator are
   a) King system b) Findlay system
   c) Both d) None of the above
111. Wall may be constructed with following materials like
   a) Brick b) Stone
   c) Concrete d) All of the above
112. Which of the following soil are best suited for building construction
   a) Loam b) Sand
   c) Clay d) Chalk
113. Which of the following milking parlour suitable for large herd
   a) Abreast parlour b) Tandem parlour
   c) Rotary parlour d) Herringbone parlour
114. What is the purpose of water supply to dairy farms
   a) Washing animals b) Cleaning of housing
   c) Irrigation of fodder crop d) All of the above
115. Floor space requirement for farrowing sow (covered area)
   a) 4-6 m^2 b) 7-9 m^2
   c) 13- 15 m^2 d) 17-19 m^2
116. Height of fence for housing of goat should be
   a) 100 cm b) 125 cm
   c) 150 cm d) 200 cm
117. The fender (guard rails) are provided for the housing of
   a) Goat b) Sheep
   c) Pig d) Cattle& Buffaloes
118. Type of floor more suitable for housing of goat in tropical regions
   a) Sand b) Mud
   c) Concrete d) Brick
119. Which of the following is ancillary structure in sheep housing
   a) Store b) Shearing room
   c) Weighing room d) None of the above

120. Pig house is also known as
   a) Barn b) Kennel
   c) Sty d) Stable
121. Which of the following is ancillary structure in pig housing
   a) Weighing room b) Milking parlor
   c) Garbage room d) Shearing room
122. Houses of horse are usually known as
   a) Sty b) Stable
   c) Kennel d) Kettling
123. Which type floor more suitable for housing of pig
   a) Sand b) Brick
   c) Concrete d) Mud
124. Goat are browsing nature, feed racks are provided
   a) Under region b) Elevated region
   c) Corner of the floor d) None of the above
125. Each pen in dairy farm accommodate maximum how many cattle
   a) 1 b) 20
   c) 30 d) 50
126. Dipping tank is essential for sheep due to
   a) Removal of ecto-parasite b) Removal of endo-parasite
   c) Removal of dung from body d) Prevent infestation with maggot
127. Inlet and outlet area in house of goat and sheep for cross-ventilation
   a) 4-5 sq cm b) 7-8 sq cm
   c) 11-12 sq cm d) 18-19 sq cm
128. Space requirement for ram or buck is
   a) 1 m^2/ animal b) 2 m^2 / animal
   c) 3.4 m^2/ animal d) 5 m^2/ animal
129. Exercise paddock for 100-125 goats
   a) 12 m x 18 m b) 16 m x 22 m
   c) 22 m x 30 m d) 26 m x 36 m
130. The height of ceiling in sheep or goat in dry and heavy rain fall area
   a) 125 cm dry & 180 cm rain fall b) 300 cm dry & 220 cm rain fall
   c) 325 cm dry & 280 cm rain fall d) None of the above
131. Height of shed for goat should be
   a) 3-5 m b) 5-7 m
   c) > 10 m d) None of the above
132. Guard rail should be provided in farrowing pens
   a) 15 cm above floor level b) 25 cm above floor level
   c) 35 cm above floor level d) 45 cm above floor level

133. The dimension of farrowing pen should be
  a) 40-80 sq ft b) 80-100 sq ft
  c) 120-180 sq ft d) > 200 sq ft

134. Inlet and outlet area for air cross-ventilation required sty of pig should be
  a) 6-15 sq cm b) 8 18 sq cm
  c) 10-20 sq cm d) None of the above

135. Fresh air required by pig per hours is
  a) 14 m^3 b) 28 m^3
  c) 42 m^3 d) 56 m^3

136. Guard rails prevent sow from crushing their
  a) Piglet b) Back
  c) Feet d) None of the above

137. Pig house temperature should not be below
  a) 30°F b) 50°F
  c) 60°F d) 80°F

138. Housing of pregnant pig in farrowing crate is done for
  a) Last ten days of gestation period b) Throughout gestation period
  c) 28-30 days transition period d) None of the above

139. Space requirement for ewe or nanny is
  a) 1 m^2/ animal b) 2 m^2/ animal
  c) 3 m^2/ animal d) 4 m^2/ animal

140. Each pen in dairy farm accommodate maximum how many newborn calf
  a) 10 b) 20
  c) 30 d) 40

141. Each pen in goat farm accommodate maximum how many goat
  a) 10 b) 40
  c) 60 d) 75

142. Paved area required for a cow is
  a) 100 sq ft b) 200 sq ft
  c) 300 sq ft d) 400 sq ft

143. Total land percentage for proper layout of dairy farm (road, building & paddock)
  a) 4 % b) 8%
  c) 16 % d) 24 %

144. In which housing system feed distribution is easier
  a) Head to head system b) Tail to tail system
  c) Both d) All of the above

145. Calve kept individual stalls up to the
  a) 8 weeks of age b) 10 weeks of age
  c) 12 weeks of age d) 14 weeks of age

146. Which of the following system of pig housing
a) Open air system b) Indoor system
c) Combination system d) All of the above

147. Under semi-intensive system goat are grazed for
a) 1-2 hrs b) 3-4 hrs
c) 5-6 hrs d) 10-11hrs

148. The height hay racks of goat above the ground should be
a) 0.5 m b) 1.0 m
c) 2.0 m d) 3.0 m

149. The height of the outer wall of manger (feeding trough) should be
a) 50 cm b) 100 cm
c) 150 cm d) 200 cm

150. The site of establishment of a dairy farm should be selected
a) Nearby market b) Labour availability
c) Type of soil d) All of the above

Answer Key

1	a	2	a	3	d	4	c	5	c	6	a	7	b
8	a	9	c	10	d	11	c	12	b	13	c	14	c
15	b	16	b	17	c	18	c	19	b	20	a	21	d
22	c	23	c	24	d	25	b	26	c	27	d	28	b
29	d	30	a	31	a	32	a	33	b	34	c	35	b
36	a	37	a	38	a	39	c	40	d	41	b	42	b
43	d	44	a	45	d	46	b	47	a	48	c	49	d
50	c	51	b	52	a	53	a	54	b	55	d	56	c
57	a	58	a	59	a	60	a	61	c	62	b	63	a
64	c	65	a	66	d	67	a	68	a	69	b	70	d
71	a	72	d	73	c	74	c	75	c	76	a	77	b
78	a	79	c	80	d	81	a	82	b	83	a	84	a
85	a	86	c	87	d	88	d	89	a	90	d	91	d
92	d	93	d	94	d	95	b	96	d	97	a	98	c
99	a	100	a	101	a	102	a	103	b	104	d	105	b
106	d	107	d	108	c	109	a	110	c	111	d	112	a
113	c	114	d	115	b	116	c	117	c	118	a	119	b
120	c	121	c	122	b	123	c	124	b	125	d	126	a
127	a	128	c	129	a	130	b	131	a	132	b	133	b
134	a	135	b	136	a	137	c	138	c	139	a	140	c
141	c	142	a	143	b	144	a	145	a	146	d	147	c
148	a	149	b	150	d								

13

Animal and Poultry Feed and Fodder Production Management

Neeti Lakhani[1], Gurslamat Singh[1], and Preeti Lakhani[2]

[1]*Department of Animal Nutrition, College of Veterinary Science, Rampura Phu, GADVASU, Bathinda, Punjab*

[2]*Department of Veterinary Physiology, Lala Lajpat Rai University of Veterinary and Animal Sciences (LUVAS), Hisar, Haryana*

Introduction

Animal and poultry feed and fodder production management is a vital aspect of the agricultural industry, playing a pivotal role in sustaining livestock health and productivity. This intricate domain encompasses a myriad of practices, technologies, and strategies aimed at producing high-quality feed and fodder to meet the nutritional needs of various animal species, ensuring their optimal growth, development, and overall well-being. Feed and fodder production management involves the cultivation, processing, and formulation of feed ingredients tailored to the specific dietary requirements of different animals. From traditional practices to modern, technology-driven methodologies, this field has evolved significantly to address the growing demands of an expanding livestock industry.

The cornerstone of effective feed and fodder management lies in understanding the nutritional needs of animals. Different species exhibit varying dietary preferences and nutritional requirements, necessitating a diverse array of feed formulations. Whether it's ruminants like cattle and goats, monogastric animals such as pigs and poultry, or niche species like aquaculture, each category demands a unique blend of nutrients for optimal growth, reproduction, and disease resistance.

The production of animal feed and fodder involves a meticulous process that starts from sourcing raw materials. These materials can range from grains, legumes, and oilseeds to forages, by-products, and supplements rich in proteins, carbohydrates, fats, vitamins, and minerals. Careful selection and quality assessment of these ingredients are imperative to ensure the final feed meets nutritional standards and is free from contaminants or toxins that might compromise animal health.

Furthermore, feed formulation requires a precise balance of nutrients, often necessitating the expertise of nutritionists and animal scientists. They utilize scientific principles to design diets that maximize growth efficiency, support immune function, and minimize environmental impacts such as excess nutrient excretion. Modern feed production also incorporates technological advancements to enhance efficiency and quality. Mechanized processes for grinding, mixing, and pelleting ensure uniformity in feed texture and composition. Moreover, innovations in nutritional science, such as the utilization of enzymes and additives, aid in improving feed digestibility and nutrient absorption, thereby optimizing animal performance.

Fodder management, on the other hand, primarily revolves around the cultivation, preservation, and utilization of forage crops and grasses. These crops serve as a crucial source of nutrients for grazing animals and are also harvested and conserved as silage or hay for feeding during lean seasons. Efficient fodder management involves selecting appropriate forage species, employing sustainable cultivation practices, and employing preservation techniques like ensiling, haymaking, or silage baling to maintain nutrient quality and palatability. Additionally, advancements in hydroponic fodder systems enable year-round production of nutrient-rich sprouted grains, offering a viable alternative in regions with limited arable land or adverse climatic conditions.

The significance of feed and fodder management extends beyond mere nutrition; it directly influences animal health, productivity, and the overall economy. Well-managed diets contribute to reduced mortality rates, improved reproduction, enhanced product quality (such as milk, meat, and eggs), and ultimately, increased profitability for farmers and stakeholders across the supply chain. However, challenges persist within this domain, including fluctuating ingredient costs, sustainability concerns regarding resource utilization, and the need for continuous innovation to meet evolving nutritional demands. Moreover, ensuring feed safety and quality standards remain paramount, considering their direct impact on animal health and consumer safety. Sustainable practices are increasingly gaining traction in feed and fodder production management. Techniques like precision farming, utilization of alternative protein sources (such as insects or microbial-derived proteins), and adopting circular economy principles by repurposing by-products contribute to minimizing environmental footprints while ensuring a consistent supply of high-quality feed.

In conclusion, animal and poultry feed and fodder production management form the backbone of a thriving livestock industry. Its multifaceted nature demands a delicate balance between traditional wisdom and modern innovation to meet the growing global demand for safe, nutritious, and sustainable animal products. As the industry continues to evolve, advancements in technology, coupled with a deep understanding of animal nutrition, will play pivotal roles in shaping the future of feed and fodder production.

1. Maintenance type roughage contains....................DCP

   a) 3-5% b) less than 3%

   c) 8-10% d) 1%

2. For storage of grains moisture level should not be more than..................

   a) 14% b) 25%

   c) 30% d) 35%

3. DCP is a good source of

   a) Calcium b) Phosphorus

   c) both d) None

4. Molasses is a rich source of

   a) Protein b) Cellulose

   c) Complex Carbohydrates d) Soluble Sugars

5. Factors affecting deterioration of feed during storage
   a) Physical b) Mechanical
   c) Biological d) All
6. star gazing in poultry occur due to
   a) Biotin b) Vitamin B1
   c) Mn d) All
7. Curled toe paralysis in occur due to Deficiency of
   a) Riboflavin b) Folacin
   c) Zn d) None
8. Temperature of stored grains should be
   a) 25°C b) 15°C
   c) 35°C d) 45°C
9. Enlarged hock, dermatitis Enlarged hock, dermatitis occur due to Deficiency of
   a) Riboflavin b) Vit D3
   c) Zn d) None
10. Microcytic, hyperchromic anaemia in poultry occur due to Deficiency of
    a) Fe b) Cu
    c) Both d) None
11. Muscular dystrophy with white areas of degeneration in skeletal muscle in chick, ducks, poult
    a) Vit E b) Se
    c) Both d) None
12. Polyneuritis in chick occur due to Deficiency of
    a) Biotin b) Vitamin B1
    c) Mn d) All
13. Encephalomalacia in chick occur due to Deficiency of
    a) Vit E b) Vit B1
    c) Vit B12 d) None
14. Molasses cause problem of diarrhoea because of high level of
    a) Carbohydrates b) Potassium
    c) Sodium d) Protein
15. Prussic acid is anti-nutritional factor present in the
    a) Sal seed meal b) Jowar white
    c) Tapioca meal d) GNC
16. .... anti-nutritional factor present in the cotton seed meal
    a) Prussic acid b) Saponin
    c) Gossypol d) Ricin

17. According to BIS 1374: 2007 Crude Protein (%) requirements for meat type Pre-starter chicken

a) 20 b) 21
c) 22 d) 23

18. According to BIS 1374: 2007 Crude Protein (%) requirements for meat type starter chicken

a) 20 b) 21
c) 22 d) 23

19. According to BIS 1374: 2007 Crude Protein (%) requirements for meat type finisher chicken

a) 20 b) 21
c) 22 d) 23

20. According to BIS 1374: 2007 ME requirements for meat type Pre-starter chicken

a) 3000 b) 3200
c) 3100 d) 3300

21. According to BIS 1374: 2007 ME requirements for meat type starter chicken

a) 3000 b) 3200
c) 3100 d) 3300

22. According to BIS 1374: 2007 ME requirements for meat type finisher chicken

a) 3000 b) 3200
c) 3100 d) 3300

23. According to BIS 1374: 2007 Crude Protein (%) requirements for chick layer

a) 20 b) 18
c) 17 d) 16

24. According to BIS 1374: 2007 Crude Protein (%) requirements for grower layer

a) 20 b) 18
c) 17 d) 16

25. According to BIS 1374: 2007 Crude Protein (%) requirements for layer phase I

a) 20 b) 18
c) 17 d) 16

26. According to BIS 1374: 2007 ME requirements for chick layer

a) 2800 b) 2500
c) 2600 d) 2400

27. According to BIS 1374: 2007 ME requirements for grower layer

a) 2800 b) 2500
c) 2600 d) 2400

28. According to BIS 1374: 2007 ME requirements for layer phase I

a) 2800 b) 2500
c) 2600 d) 2400

29. According to BIS 1374: 2007 ME requirements for layer phase II
    a) 2800 b) 2500
    c) 2600 d) 2400
30. 11th essential amino acid in poultry is
    a) Lysine b) Glycine
    c) Methionine d) Tryptophane
31. Glycine can be synthesized from creatine and serine as long as ……… Is not deficient.
    a) Folic acid b) Vit B12
    c) Pyridoxine d) All
32. Ornithine and glycine are used in liver for
    a) Detoxification b) Precursor
    c) Enzyme metabolism d) None
33. First limiting amino acid on soya free diet in poultry
    a) Lysine b) Methionine
    c) Arginine d) Isoleucine
34. Most limiting amino acid on soya diet in poultry
    a) Lysine b) Methionine
    c) Arginine d) isoleucine
35. Threonine is limiting amino acid in
    a) Wheat b) Sorghum
    c) Both d) None
36. Blood meal is rich in
    a) Lysine b) Isoleucine
    c) Both d) None
37. Corn gluten is rich in
    a) Tryptophan b) Isoleucine
    c) Both d) None
38. Sesame seed is rich in
    a) Lysine b) Methionine
    c) Both d) None
39. Soyabean is rich in
    a) Lysine b) Methionine
    c) Both d) None
40. Lysine toxicity is overcome by
    a) Arginine b) Glycine
    c) Both d) None
41. Tryptophane toxicity is overcome by
    a) Arginine b) Glycine
    c) Threonine d) All

42. Isoleucine alleviated the toxic effect of
    a) Valine b) Leucine
    c) Both d) None
43. Excess level of valine and leucine in poultry leads to
    a) Isoleucine deficiency
    b) Induce enzyme that catabolize branched chain Amino acids
    c) Both
    d) None
44. Example of amino acid antagonism
    a) Lysine -methionine b) Lysine – arginine
    c) Arginine – methionine d) all
45. Metabolic body weight of 1.75 kg adult hen
    a) 1.2 kg b) 1 kg
    c) 1.52 kg d) 1.67 kg
46. NEm reuirement of 1.75 kg adult hen
    a) 114 Kcal/day b) 120 Kcal/day
    c) 126 Kcal/day d) 130 Kcal/day
47. Activity increment for broiler is ....% of ME
    a) 37% b) 50%
    c) 75% d) 82%
48. NEm = ... of MEm
    a) 37% b) 50%
    c) 75% d) 82%
49. Under stress condition supplementation of ...... vitamine is helpful
    a) A & D b) C & E
    c) B1 & B12 d) A & K
50. Protein requirement (P) for egg production is a sum of: maintenance requirements (M)daily egg output (E) requirement for live weight gain (G)requirement for feather growth (F)
    a) M+G b) M+E
    c) M+G+E d) M+G+E+F
51. Penguin like squat in hens is due to
    a) Niacin b) Zn
    c) Vit D3 d) Folacin
52. Exudative diathesis in poultry caused by
    a) Vit E b) Se
    c) Both d) None
53. Enlarged hearts in poults caused by
    a) Cobalt b) Copper
    c) Se d) Riboflavin

54. Encephalomalacia is caused by deficiency of
    a) Vit A b) Vit E
    c) Vit B6 d) Magnesium
55. Hyperirritability is caused by deficiency of
    a) Vit A b) Vit E
    c) Vit B6 d) Magnesium
56. Cervical paralysis is caused by
    a) Niacin b) Zn
    c) Vit D3 d) Folacin
57. Ataxia due to elevation in the cerebrospinal fluid pressure upon the brainstem
    a) Vit A b) Vit E
    c) Vit B6 d) Magnesium
58. Scaliness on the feet of chicks
    a) Niacin b) Zn
    c) Vit D3 d) All
    e) Both a & b
59. Frizzled and rough feather in poults
    a) Ca b) Zn
    c) Pantothenic acid d) all
60. Depigmentation in turkey
    a) Cobalt b) Copper
    c) Se d) Riboflavin
61. Feed restriction is recommended up to
    a) 21-22 weeks b) 18-20 weeks
    c) 39-30 weeks d) 72 weeks
62. Heat stress cause reduce electrolyte intake and leads to
    a) Acidosis b) Alkalosis
    c) Ascites d) Cannibalism
63. Recommended level of calcium in ration of layers
    a) 3-3.5% b) 3.5-4%
    c) 4-4.5% d) 4.5-5%
64. Layer phase I is upto
    a) 22 weeks b) 26 weeks
    c) 36 weeks d) 56 weeks
65. Layer phase II is up to
    a) 22-26 weeks b) 26-36 weeks
    c) 36-56 weeks d) 57 onwards
66. Layer phase II is
    a) 22-26 weeks b) 26-36 weeks
    c) 36-56 weeks d) 57 onwards

67. Early embryo death can cause by
    a) Vit A b) Vit B12
    c) Vit E d) All
68. Parrot beak (crooked beak) in embryo is seen because of
    a) Riboflavin deficiency b) Biotin deficiency
    c) Pantothenic deficiency d) Vit A
69. Clubbed down embryos occur deficiency to
    a) Riboflavin deficiency b) Biotin deficiency
    c) Pantothenic deficiency d) Vit A
70. Safer upper limit of salt in water for poultry
    a) 1500 ppm b) 2000 ppm
    c) 2500 ppm d) 3000 ppm
71. Most susceptible to aflatoxin
    a) Guinea fowls b) Duck
    c) Emu d) Turkey
72. Least susceptible to aflatoxin
    a) Guinea fowls b) Duck
    c) Emu d) Turkey
73. Tapioca meal contains
    a) Prussic acid b) Tannin
    c) Trypsin inhibitor d) All
74. Egg yolk colour
    a) Chlorophyll b) Carotene
    c) Xanthophylls d) None
75. First published work in India on scientific feeding
    a) Nutritive value of Indian cattle feeds and the feeding of animals
    b) Principal of animal nutrition and feed technology
    c) Available fuel values
    d) Manual of cattle feeding
76. Comparative type feeding standards are
    1. Thaer's hay equivalent 2. Fjord's Scandinavian feed unit
    3. Kellner's feeding standard 4. Armsby feeding standard
    5. Wolff's feeding standard
    6. Wolff-lehmann's feeding standard
    7. Haecker's feeding standard
    a) 1 & 2 b) 3 & 4
    c) 4 & 5 d) 6 & 7

77. Production type feeding standards are

1. Thaer's hay equivalent
2. Fjord's Scandinavian feed unit
3. Kellner's feeding standard
4. Armsby feeding standard
5. Wolff's feeding standard
6. Wolff-lehmann's feeding standard
7. Haecker's feeding standard

a) 1 & 2
b) 3 & 4
c) 4 & 5
d) 6 & 7

78. DCP required per unit metabolic body weight is

a) 2 gm
b) 2.23 gm
c) 2.84 gm
d) 3 gm

79. DCP requirement for cattle body weight of 400, 450 & 500kg respectively is

a) 200, 230, 250g
b) 250, 280, 300g
c) 230, 250 ,280g
d) 150, 170, 200g

80. TDN required per unit metabolic body weight is

a) 27.87 gm
b) 31.33gm
c) 33.74 gm
d) 35.45 gm

81. TDN requirement for cattle body weight 400, 450 & 500kg respectively is

a) 2.4, 2.7 ,3 kg
b) 3, 3.4, 3.7 kg
c) 3.4, 3.7, 4.2 kg
d) 1.7, 2, 3 kg

82. Additional amount of DCP and CP provided in last trimester of cattle is

a) 130g , 250g
b) 90 g, 216 g
c) 250g, 130g
d) 216g, 90 g

83. BIS recommended mineral mixture containing salt is

a) Type I
b) Type II
c) Both
d) None

84. Recommended level of crude protein in BIS type I cattle feed

a) 18
b) 20
c) 22
d) 23

85. Recommended level of crude protein in BIS type II cattle feed

a) 18
b) 20
c) 22
d) 23

86. Using legume, total portion of green roughage is reduced to

a) 1/4 of total roughage
b) 1/3 of total roughage
c) 2/3 of total roughage
d) 3/4 of total roughage

87. Energy rich concentrate feedstuffs contain

a) < 20 % protein
b) > 20 % protein
c) > 35 % protein G
d) > 30 % protein

88. Protein rich concentrate feedstuffs contain
a) < 20 % protein b) > 20 % protein
c) < 15 % protein d) < 10 % protein

89. 1/10th the plants are in bloom
a) Early bloom b) Mid bloom
c) Late bloom d) Full bloom

90. 1/10 to 2/3 plants are in bloom
a) Early bloom b) Mid bloom
c) Late bloom d) Full bloom

91. 2/3 or more plants are in bloom
a) Early bloom b) Mid bloom
c) Late bloom d) Full bloom

92. Dry matter requirement of buffalo
a) 2-2.5 % of B.W b) 2.5-3 % of B.W
c) Both d) none

93. Dry matter requirement of Cow
a) 2-2.5 % of B.W b) 2.5-3 % of B.W
c) Both d) none

94. RQ of fat is
a) 7 b) 0.07
c) 1 d) 0.7

95 Popping is done at temperature
a) 370° C - 425° C b) 148.9° C
c) 121°C -148.9° C d) 100° C

96. Roasting is done at temperature
a) 370°C - 425° C b) 148.9° C
c) 121°C -148.9°C d) 100° C

97. Steam rolling at atmospheric pressure is done at
a) 370° C - 425° C b) 148.9° C
c) 121°C -148.9° C d) 100° C

98. Steam rolling at 20-60 psi pressure is done at
a) 370° C - 425° C b) 148.9° C
c) 121°C -148.9° C d) 100° C

99. Aflatoxin containing fungus are
a) Aspergillus b) Fusarium
c) Phomosis d) Peniciliin

100. Zearalenone containing fungus are
a) Aspergillus b) Fusarium
c) Phomosis d) Peniciliin

101. Fumonisins are contained by ……..

a) *F. culmorum* b) *F. verticillioides*
c) *F. germearum* d) *F. sporotrichoid*

102. For silage making mixture of the grasses or cereal fodder and legumes should be

a) 3:1 b) 1:1
c) 5:1 d) None

103. Dry matter of the crop that has to ensiled should be

a) 20-25 % b) 25-28%
c) 45% d) 30-35%

104. A.I.V method of silage making is developed by

a) Harshey b) Wolff
c) Vitranen d) Vansoest

105. A.I.V method of silage making contain

a) 2N $H2SO_4$ b) 2N HCOOH
c) 2N NH_3 d) ALL

106. pH of good quality silage is

a) 4.8 b) 4.2-4.5
c) 3.5-4.2 d) All

107. pH of very good quality silage is

a) 4.8 b) 4.2-4.5
c) 3.5-4.2 d) All

108. Flieg index is calculated by the amount of

a) Lactic acid b) Butyric acid
c) Acetic acid d) all

109. Silo-filler's disease is related to

a) NO b) NH3
c) VFAs d) all

110. Sweet clover disease is caused by

a) Lipoxygenase b) Rachitogenic
c) Dicoumarol d) 1-amino-D-proline

111. Which of the following is Anti. Vit A & Anti. Vit E

a) Lipoxygenase b) Rachitogenic
c) Dicoumarol d) 1-amino-D-proline

112. Which of the following is Anti. Pyridoxine is

a) Lipoxygenase b) Rachitogenic
c) Dicoumarol d) 1-amino-D-proline

113. Raw soyabean contain which anti vitamin

a) Lipoxygenase b) Rachitogenic
c) Dicoumarol d) 1-amino-D-proline

114. Linseed contain which anti vitamin
   a) Lipoxygenase
   b) Rachitogenic
   c) Dicoumarol
   d) 1-amino-D-proline
115. Which of the following is Anti. Vit D
   a) Lipoxygenase
   b) Rachitogenic
   c) Dicoumarol
   d) 1-amino-D-proline
116. Cytochrome oxidase contain
   a) Copper
   b) Molybdenum
   c) Mn
   d) Zn
117. Pyruvate carboxylase containe
   a) Copper
   b) Molybdenum
   c) Mn
   d) Zn
118. Xanthine dehydrogenase contain
   a) Copper
   b) Molybdenum
   c) Mn
   d) Zn
119. Zn containing enzyme is
   a) Carbonic anhydrase
   b) Carboxypeptidase
   c) Alkaline phosphatase
   d) All of the above
120. Ceruloplasmin use .... for iron utilization
   a) Copper
   b) Molybdenum
   c) Mn
   d) Zn
121. Ca binding proteins is
   a) Cadmolin
   b) Osteopontin
   c) Both A & B
   d) None
122. Calcium absorption is hindered by
   a) Phosphorus
   b) Magnesium
   c) Oxalates
   d) Phytates
123. Big head disease is due to
   a) High level of fiber
   b) High level of phosphorus
   c) High level of ca
   d) None of the above
124. high molybdenum and zinc rich soil cause .... Mineral deficiency in animal
   a) Mo
   b) Zn
   c) Calcium
   d) Copper
125. Copper deficiency is caused by
   a) Cadmium & Zn
   b) Calcium phytate
   c) Ferrous sulphide
   d) All

126. Parakeratosis in pigs is caused by
a) Mo b) Zn
c) Calcium d) Copper

127. Father of nutrition
a) Anotnie Lavoisier b) Laplace
c) Lazaro spallanzani d) Armsby

128. Animal calorimeter is designed by
a) Anotnie Lavoisier b) Laplace
c) Lazaro spallanzani d) Armsby

129. Founder of modern experimental methods in animal feeding experiments
a) Anotnie Lavoisier b) Laplace
c) Lazaro spallanzani d) Francois Magendie

130. fermentation hypothesis to explain forage utilization by ruminants was given by
a) Nathan zuntz b) J.V.Liebig
c) Atwater d) Babcock

131. First human respiration calorimeter was designed by
a) Nathan zuntz b) J.V.Liebig
c) Atwater d) Babcock

132. Term probiotic is coined by
a) Atwater b) Fuller
c) Babcock d) Parker

133. Microbes used as probiotics
a) Lactobacillus acidophilus b) Saccharomyces cerevisiae
c) Bifidobacterium bifidum d) All of the above

134. Probiotics used in swine is
a) *L . acidophilus* b) *S. faecium*
c) Both d) None

135. .... have good effect on yeast in monogastric is
a) MOS b) FOS
c) Both d) None

136. .... encourage the growth of beneficial bacteria
a) MOS b) FOS
c) Both d) None

137. By-product of cereals left after harvesting
a) Stower b) Fodder
c) Hay d) Straw

138. Aerial parts with ears & husk is called
a) Stower b) Fodder
c) Hay d) Straw

139. Aerial parts without ears & husk is called
   a) Stower   b) Fodder
   c) Hay   d) Straw
140. Outer covering of beans & peas
   a) Hull   b) Stover
   c) Husk   d) Shells
141. Dry Outer covering of grains
   a) Hull   b) Stover
   c) Husk   d) Shells
142. Hard Outer covering of nuts
   a) Hull   b) Stover
   c) Husk   d) Shells
143. Bloat causing glycosides are
   a) Cyanogens   b) Saponin
   c) Glucosinolates   d) All of the above
144. Antinutritional factor contained by almonds
   a) Dhurrin   b) Linamarin
   c) Amygdalin   d) Phaseolunatin
145. Antinutritional factor contained by jowar
   a) Dhurrin   b) Linamarin
   c) Amygdalin   d) None
146. Antinutritional factor contained by cassava
   a) Dhurrin   b) Linamarin
   c) Amygdalin   d) None
147. Crop milk in pigeons' production stops at
   a) 1–2-week   b) 2-3 week
   c) 3-4weeks   d) 4-5 weeks
148. Crop milk for nourish young pigeons up to
   a) 2 days   b) 3 days
   c) 5 days   d) 1 week
149. Mammalian muscle contain glycogen
   a) 0.5-1%   b) 2.26%
   c) 5%   d) 10%
150. Ratio of urea and water for urea treatment of straw
   a) 1:1   b) 1:2
   c) 1:5   d) 1:10

Answer Key

1	a	2	a	3	c	4	d	5	d	6	b	7	a
8	b	9	c	10	c	11	c	12	b	13	a	14	b
15	c	16	c	17	d	18	c	19	a	20	a	21	c
22	b	23	a	24	d	25	b	26	a	27	b	28	c
29	d	30	b	31	d	32	a	33	a	34	b	35	c
36	a	37	b	38	b	39	a	40	c	41	c	42	c
43	c	44	b	45	c	46	c	47	b	48	d	49	b
50	d	51	c	52	c	53	b	54	b	55	d	56	d
57	a	58	e	59	d	60	c	61	a	62	b	63	a
64	c	65	c	66	d	67	d	68	b	69	a	70	d
71	b	72	a	73	a	74	c	75	a	76	a	77	b
78	c	79	b	80	c	81	b	82	a	83	b	84	c
85	b	86	a	87	a	88	b	89	a	90	b	91	d
92	b	93	a	94	d	95	a	96	b	97	d	98	c
99	a	100	b	101	b	102	a	103	d	104	c	105	a
106	b	107	c	108	d	109	a	110	c	111	a	112	d
113	a	114	d	115	b	116	a	117	c	118	b	119	d
120	a	121	c	122	e	123	b	124	d	125	d	126	b
127	a	128	b	129	d	130	a	131	c	132	d	133	d
134	c	135	A	136	b	137	d	138	b	139	c	140	a
141	c	142	d	143	b	144	c	145	a	146	b	147	c
148	b	149	a	150	d								

14

Animal Reproduction and Breeding Management

***Rajesh Kumar*[1], *and Manoj Kumar Verma*[2]**

[1]*Department of Veterinary Gynaecology & Obstetrics, College of Veterinary Science & Animal Husbandry, Acharya Narendra Deva University of Agriculture & Technology Ayodhya, Uttar Pradesh*

[2]*Department of Animal Genetics & Breeding, College of Veterinary Science & Animal Husbandry, Acharya Narendra Deva University of Agriculture & Technology Ayodhya, Uttar Pradesh*

Introduction

Animals worldwide provide meat, milk, eggs, draft power, skins, transportation, and a variety of other useful items. India has a vast livestock population with a diverse spectrum of species. Animal husbandry plays an important role in the life of rural farmers. Animal breeding is an area of science concerned with sound animal husbandry methods. Animal breeding is the use of genetics and reproductive physiology to improve the genetic makeup of animals. The goal of animal breeding is to improve not only individual animals, but the entire animal population. The breeder has two basic tools namely selection and breeding for genetic improvement of livestock. The kinds of selection are natural and artificial selection. In artificial selection, breeder has choice to choose superior animals over the average of population for desired traits and allow them to produce offspring for future generation. Animals are selected using four criteria (basis): individual selection, pedigree selection, family selection, and progeny testing selection. Individual selection selects animals based on their own performances. Individuals are chosen through pedigree selection using ancestral records. In Family selection, individuals are selected on the basis family member's records. In progeny testing, animal are selected on the basis of their progeny performances. There are 3 methods of selection to improve the genetic potential of livestock i.e. tendem, independent culling level and selection index/total score methods. Mating system refers to the general pattern by which male and female mate within a population. Basically Inbreeding and out breeding are two mating system practiced in livestock practices. Inbreeding is mating of related individual having a common ancestor within 4-6 previous generations, while out breeding is the mating between the unrelated individuals.

Multiple Choice Questions

1. Post partum uterine involution

    a) 15-20 days b) 25-30 days

    c) 30-35 days d) 35-40 days

2. Sperm reservoirs in cattle
   a) Uterotubal junction — b) Endometrial glands
   b) Cervical crypts — d) Both a & b
3. Sperm capacitation in cattle
   a) Uterus — b) Isthmus
   c) Posterior vagina — d) Both a & b
4. Fertilization site in cattle
   a) Ampula — b) Isthmus
   c) Junction between Both a & b — d) None of these
5. Axoneme is responsible for
   a) Sperm survivability — b) Sperm capacitation
   c) Sperm motility — d) None of these
6. PGE_2 exhibit
   a) Luteotrophic action — b) Luteolytic action
   c) Both — d) None of these
7. $PGF_2\alpha$ exhibit
   a) Luteotrophic action — b) Luteolytic action
   c) Both — d) None of these
8. Half life of FSH
   a) 1-2hr — b) 2-2.5hr
   c) 3-3.5hr — d) None of these
9. Half life of PMSG
   a) 6 days — b) 7 days
   c) 8 days — d) 10 days
10. Exogenous oxytocin has a luteolytic effect in
   a) Cattle — b) Goat
   c) Mare — d) Both a & b
11. pH of bull semen
   a) 5.4-6.8 — b) 6.4-6.8
   c) 6.4-7.8 — d) 7-7.4
12. Diagnostic method early conception factor (ECF) ____hrs of fertilization
   a) 24 hours — b) 48 hours
   c) 24-48 hours — d) 48-72 hours
13. Diagnostic method real time ultra sound done ___ days of gestation
   a) 9-10 days — b) 10-12 days
   c) 13-21 days — d) 30 days
14. Diagnostic method progesterone concentration in plasma or milk done ___ days of gestation
   a) 9-10 days — b) 10-12 days
   c) 13-21 days — d) 21-24 days

15. Diagnostic method pregnancy associate glycoprotein (bPAG) done ___ days of gestation
    a) 9-10 days
    b) 10-12 days
    c) 13-21 days
    d) 24 days
16. Diagnostic method pulpation of the allantochorindone ___ days of gestation
    a) 9-10 days
    b) 34 days
    c) 30 days
    d) 38 days
17. Diagnostic method palpation of placentomes done ___ days of gestation
    a) 70 days
    b) 80 days
    c) 90 days
    d) 100 days
18. Diagnostic method palpation of Fremitus done ___ days of gestation
    a) 85 days
    b) 90 days
    c) 95 days
    d) 100 days
19. Diagnostic method palpation of fetus is done ___ days of gestation
    a) 100 days
    b) 110 days
    c) 120 days
    d) 130 days
20. Diagnostic method oestrone sulphate in blood and milk ___ days of gestation
    a) 100 days
    b) 105 days
    c) 110 days
    d) 115 days
21. Genital fold develop into
    a) Penis
    b) Labia majora
    c) Labia minora
    d) All of these
22. Genital tubercle develop into
    a) Penis
    b) Labia majora
    c) Labia minora
    d) All of these
23. Genital swelling develop into
    a) Penis
    b) Labia majora
    c) Labia minora
    d) All of these
24. Round ligament of the uterus and proper ligament of the ovary develop from
    a) Mesentery
    b) Gubernaculum
    c) Mesonephric tubules
    d) Urogenital sinus
25. Duct part of epoophoron develop from
    a) Mesonephric duct
    b) Para mesonephric duct
    c) Urogenital sinus
    d) Genital swelling
26. Paraurethral Gland develop from
    a) Mesonephric duct
    b) Para mesonephric duct
    c) Urogenital sinus
    d) Genital swelling

27. Bartholin Gland develop from
    a) Mesonephric duct b) Para mesonephric duct
    c) Urogenital sinus d) Genital swelling
28. Initiation of formation of placenta in cow
    a) 18 days b) 19 days
    c) 21 days d) 22 days
29. Embryonic attachment to the uterus in cow
    a) 8 days b) 10 days
    c) 12 days d) 14 days
30. Amniotic fluid originate from
    a) Fetal urine b) Respiratory track secretion
    c) Meternal circulation d) All of the above
31. Who is known as father of animal breeding
    a) Robert Bakewell b) R A Fisher
    c) J L Lush d) S Wright
32. Which of the following is domesticated as first animal by human being ?
    a) Dog b) Cattle
    c) Sheep d) Goat
33. The latest animal domesticated by human being-
    a) Cattle b) Buffalo
    c) Sheep d) Horse
34. The chicken was first time in-
    a) America b) China
    c) India d) Russia
35. The first herd book for livestock is associated with?
    a) English thoroughbred horses b) Shorthorn Cattle
    c) Angus Cattle d) Dutch Friesian cattle
36. The genetic improvement by selection in a generation is the function of-
    a) Variability in the trait b) Heritability
    c) Selection intensity d) All of the above
37. Which of the following defines the average age of the parents when their offspring were born?
    a) Age at maturity b) Generation interval
    c) Calving interval d) None of the above
38. The correlated response to selection is equal to-
    a) $Cr_y = i.h_x.h_y.r_g.\sigma_{p(y)}$ b) $Cr_y = i.h^2_y.r_g.\sigma_{p(y)}$
    c) $Cr_y = i.h^2_x.r_g.\sigma_{p(y)}$ d) None of the above

39. In which of the following selection method, taking only one trait at a time for genetic improvement of livestock?

a) Tendem
b) Independent culling Level
c) Total score/Selection index
d) All of the above

40. In which of the following selection method, taking two or more traits at a time for genetic improvement of livestock?

a) Tendem
b) Independent culling Level
c) Total score/Selection index
d) Both 'b' and 'c'

41. Which of the following is the best method of selection?

a) Tendem
b) Independent culling Level
c) Total score/Selection index
d) None of the following

42. In which method, Each trait having a minimum standard for selection?

a) Tendom
b) Independent culling Level
c) Total score/Selection index
d) None of the following

43. The intensity of selection depends with number traits considered 'n' is-

a) n
b) 1/n
c) $1/\sqrt{n}$
d) $1/n^2$

44. The effect of out breeding is more prominent on what type of gene action

a) Additive
b) Non-additive
c) Both 'a' & 'b'
d) None of the above

45. Selection associated with

a) Introduction of new gene
b) Increase the frequency of favorable gene
c) Both 'a' and 'b'
d) None of the above

46. Selection is useful for those traits which are governed by-

a) Additive genes
b) Dominant genes
c) Epistatic genes
d) All of the above

47. In cattle improvement program, sib selection is suggested for –

a) Sex linked traits
b) Sex limited traits
c) Sex influenced traits
d) None of the above

48. Standardized selection differential is also known as-

a) Selection intensity
b) Response to selection
c) Accuracy of selection
d) Selection load

49. Which of the following institute develop the Vrandavani cattle

a) IVRI, Izatnagar
b) NDRI, Karnal
c) DUVASU, Mathura
d) CIRC, Meerut

50. Which crossbred cattle is developed by ICAR-NDRI Karnal?

a) Frieswal
b) Sunandini
c) Karan Fries
d) Jerthar

51. The first crossbred cattle developed in India is-
 a) Taylor b) Sunandini
 c) Jerthar d) Frieswal
52. Which of the following crossbred sheep is developed for mutton purpose?
 a) Avikaline b) Avivastra
 c) Avimanas d) Hisardale
53. Which of the following crossbred sheep is developed for carpet wool?
 a) Avikaline b) Avivastra
 c) Avimanas d) Hisardale
54. Which Indian cattle breed possesses the peculiar gait "Swai chal"?
 a) Sahiwal b) Hariana
 c) Kankrej d) Amrit mahal
55. Which of the following increases the generation interval in cattle breeding program
 a) Progeny testing b) MOET
 c) Both 'a' and 'b' d) None of the above
56. New breed can be developed by-
 a) Inbreeding b) Cross breeding
 c) Grading up d) None of the above
57. Based on the experience of cross breeding result of cattle in India, the level of exotic inheritance should be
 a) 50-62.5% b) 62.5-75%
 c) Below to 50% d) Above to 75%
58. In which of the following there is maximum chance of inbreeding
 a) Progeny testing b) ONBS
 c) CNBS d) Out-crossing
59. Which of the followings has shorter generation interval in genetic improvement programme
 a) Adult MOET b) Juveline MOET
 c) Hybrid/Mixed MOET d) None of the above
60. Inbreeding within ancestral line is known as-
 a) Line breeding b) Close breeding
 c) Top crossing d) None of the above
61. Out breeding enhances the-
 a) Fitness b) Growth
 c) Fitness as well as growth d) None of the above
62. Which type of gene interaction possessed dominance and overdominance?
 a) Allelic b) Non-allelic
 c) Both 'a' and 'b' d) None of the above

63. Greatest inbreeding coefficient is obtained in matting between-
   a) Full sibs
   b) Half sibs
   c) Uncle & niece
   d) Grandson & grandmother
64. What will be the inbreeding coefficient for half sib matting
   a) 6.25%
   b) 12.5%
   c) 25%
   d) 50%
65. In which of the following matting, the primary aim of breeder is to increase the homozygosity for outstanding ancestors?
   a) Close inbreeding
   b) Line inbreeding
   c) Out crossing
   d) Grading up
66. How many times required in grading up matting program to produce pure breed from non-descript population?
   a) 2-3 generation
   b) 4-5 generation
   c) 6-7 generation
   d) Above the 10 generation
67. The cause of the heterosis is
   a) Variation in gene frequency between two population
   b) Dominance
   c) Epistasis & Overdominance
   d) All of the above
68. Which one of the following is the milder form of inbreeding?
   a) Line inbreeding
   b) Close inbreeding
   c) Out-crossing
   d) None of the above
69. In order to practice inbreeding, matted individuals must share common ancestors within-
   a) 2-3 generation
   b) 4-6 generation
   c) 7-9 generation
   d) 10 or more generation
70. Which one of the following is required to construct the selection index?
   a) Heritability of the trait
   b) Economic valve of the trait
   c) Both a & b
   d) None of the above
71. The value of a pedigree depends upon the-
   a) Closeness of relationship between individual and ancestors
   b) Heritability of the trait
   c) Both a & b
   d) None of the above
72. Higher intensity of selection can be practiced in-
   a) Males in dairy cattle
   b) Females in dairy cattle
   c) Females in swine
   d) None of the above
73. For effective progeny testing requires-
   a) As many sires on set as possible
   b) Random matting of dams
   c) Both a & b
   d) None of the above

74. Who use the selection index in animal breeding?
    a) Hazel & Smith b) Comstock
    c) Fisher d) Lush
75. Generally the traits associated with fitness-
    a) Low heritable b) Medium heritable
    c) High Heritable d) None of the above
76. Generally the traits associated with fitness-
    a) Alike in descent b) Unlike in descent
    c) Alike in State d) None of the above
77. In phenomenon of heterosis , the crossbred progenies-
    a) Exceed the mid parent
    b) Exceed the average of superior parents
    c) Exceed the average of inferior parents
    d) All of the above
78. Which of the following is not a cause of heterosis?
    a) Dominance b) Overdominance
    c) Epistasis d) Additive gene action
79. How many breeds are involved in criss-crossing ?
    a) Two b) Three
    c) Four d) Five
80. The mildest form of outbreeding is-
    a) Out crossing b) Cross breeding
    c) Grading up d) Species hybridization
81. The widest form of out breeding is –
    a) Out crossing b) Cross breeding
    c) Grading up d) Species hybridization
82. Which of the following breed give black color poultry meat?
    a) Karaknath b) Aseel
    c) Bursa d) Naked neck
83. Which of the following poultry bird is known for pugnacity?
    a) Kadaknath b) Aseel
    c) Bursa d) Ghagus
84. Which of the following buffalo is reared for fat percentage
    a) Muraah b) Mehsana
    c) Bhadawari d) Nili Ravi
85. According to National cattle breeding policy of India, the improvement of well defined Indian breeds can be made through-
    a) Selective breeding b) Cross breeding
    c) Grading up d) Top crossing

86. Mehsana buffalo is the result of cross between-
   a) Murrah and Nili Ravi b) Murrah and Surti
   c) Jaffarabadi and Surti d) Bhadawari and Nagpuri
87. Pien-niu is a species hybrid developed by crossing of-
   a) Cattle and buffalo b) Cattle and Mithun
   c) Cattle and Yak d) Cattle and Zebra
88. Which of the following exotic cattle has excellent heat tolerance power?
   a) Holstein Friesian b) Brown Swiss
   c) Jersey d) Ayrshire
89. Which of the following buffalo having highest population share with respect to total indigenous buffalo population?
   a) Murrah b) Mehsana
   c) Nili Ravi d) Surti
90. Which of the following buffalo having conservation status as risk?
   a) Murrah b) Bhadawari
   c) Nagpuri d) Toda
91. The least variable trait of the farm animal is-
   a) Age at first calving b) Service period
   c) Gestation period d) Lactation length
92. Reciprocal recurrent selection is generally used for genetic improvement of the-
   a) Cattle b) Sheep
   c) Buffalo d) Poultry
93. Which of the following breeding program can reduce the generation interval?
   a) Progeny testing b) MOET
   c) Both of the above d) None of the above
94. The superiority of the selected parents over the population mean from which are selected is known as
   a) Selection differential b) Response to selection
   c) Selection index d) None of the above
95. The mean superiority of the progeny of selected parents over the population mean is called as-
   a) Selection differential b) Response to selection
   c) Selection index d) None of the above
96. Annual genetic gain of a herd depends upon-
   a) Heritability b) Selection intensity
   c) Generation interval d) All of the above
97. The most efficient method of sire evaluation is –
   a) Sire daughter average b) Contemporary comparison
   c) Best linear unbiased prediction d) Best linear unbiased estimation

98. Matting between unrelated individuals within the same breed is called-
    a) Out crossing b) Cross breeding
    c) Grading up d) Species hybridization
99. Matting between individuals different breed is called-
    a) Out crossing b) Cross breeding
    c) Grading up d) Species hybridization
100. Matting between individuals different species is called-
    a) Out crossing b) Cross breeding
    c) Grading up d) Species hybridization
101. Mating among the progenies of the same generation having same level of inheritance is called as-
    a) Test cross mating b) Back cross mating
    c) Inter se mating d) None of the above
102. Genetic assortative mating is associated with-
    a) Inbreeding b) Outbreeding
    c) Both 'a' and 'b' d) None of the above
103. when two inbred lines of the same breed cross, it is-
    a) Incrossing b) Incross breeding
    c) Top incrossing d) Top incross breeding
104. Progeny of mating of animals from inbred lines of two different breeds-
    a) Incrossing b) Incross breeding
    c) Top incrossing d) Top crossing
105. Ancestral records of an individual are compiled in-
    a) History sheet b) Performance sheet
    c) Pedigree sheet d) None of the above
106. The individual selection is practiced for-
    a) High heritable traits b) Low heritable traits
    c) Sex limited traits d) All of the above
107. Individual selection criteria is not practiced for which of the following traits-
    a) Carcass traits b) Growth traits
    c) Production traits d) Disease resistance traits
108. Which of the following selection criteria will be effective for sex limited traits?
    a) Individual selection b) Pedigree selection
    c) Progeny testing selection d) Sib selection
109. Progeny testing is the basis of choice for selection of breeding-
    a) Females b) Males
    c) Heifers d) Calves

110. The selection based on the use of high density SNPs genotyping to predict the breeding value is-
 a) Gene selection b) Genomic selection
 c) Mass selection d) Gene editing

111. Which path of genetic improvement of farm animal is most efficient-
 a) Sire producing bull b) Sire producing cow
 c) Dam producing bull d) Dam producing cow

112. Which path of genetic improvement of farm animal is least efficient-
 a) Sire producing bull b) Sire producing cow
 c) Dam producing bull d) Dam producing cow

113. In traditional method of breeding, the contribution share in genetic improvement by Sire is about-
 a) 33% b) 50%
 c) 66% d) 75%

114. Reciprocal recurrent selection is used to improve the-
 a) GCA b) SCA
 c) Both GCA and SCA d) None of the above

115. What type of gene action possessed in general combining ability?
 a) Additive b) Non-additive
 c) Both 'a' and 'b' d) None of the above

116. The final goal of the selection is-
 a) Change in gene frequency b) Creation of new genes
 c) Change in the variation d) None of the above

117. Minimum number of daughters per bull for progeny testing is-
 a) 1 b) 5
 c) 10 d) 15

118. The changes are observed in which the following due to Inbreeding practices?
 a) Gene frequency b) Genotype frequency
 c) Both of the above d) None of the above

119. Which among the following is not a cause of heterosis?
 a) Dominance b) Overdominance
 c) Epistasis d) Additive gene action

120. The amount of heterosis is depend upon the –
 a) Difference of gene frequency among the populations
 b) Dominance deviation
 c) Both 'a' and 'b'
 d) None of the above

121. The value of heterosis in F2 generation is how much time of heterosis in F_1 generation?
 a) 1 b) 2
 c) ½ d) None of the above

122. Maintaining hybrid vigour in cow herds is accomplished through-
  a) Rotational crossing b) Grading up
  c) Inbreeding depression d) Top crossing
123. Rotational crossing is preferred in-
  a) Swine breeding b) Cattle breeding
  c) Buffalo breeding d) None of the above
124. The breeding value of a individual is equal to-
  a) Equal to transmitting ability b) Twice to transmitting ability
  c) Half to transmitting ability d) quarter to transmitting ability
125. The most effective criteria of selection is-
  a) Mass selection b) Ancestral selection
  c) Progeny testing d) None of the above
126. The fraction of the population that manifests genetic death is-
  a) Genetic linkage b) Genetic load
  c) Genetic sterility d) Genetic drift
127. The contribution of offspring to the next generation is known as-
  a) Adoptive value b) Fitness
  c) Selective value d) All of the above
128. Among the following, which traits usually show low heritability?
  a) Anatomical traits b) Reproductive traits
  c) Production traits d) None of the above
129. Selection index is a numerical score assigning to the individual to estimates its-
  a) Phenotypic value b) Genotypic value
  c) Breeding value d) All of the above
130. The emergence of ancestral characteristics after several generations is known as-
  a) Prepotency b) Expressivity
  c) Atavism d) Mutation
131. Ability of an individual tp stamp its characteristics on its progeny-
  a) Prepotency b) Breeding value
  c) Response to selection d) None of the above
132. When the response to selection is ceased, the population is said to be as-
  a) Selection limit b) Selection pressure
  c) Selection load d) Selection intensity
133. A highly inbred strain is use as tester for non inbred population in-
  a) Recurrent selection b) Reciprocal recurrent selection
  c) Both 'a' and 'b' d) None of the above
134. The term genetic slippage is given by-
  a) Hull b) Lerner
  c) Shull d) Dickerson

135. The term Heterosis is given by-
   a) Hull   b) Lerner
   c) Shull   d) Dickerson

136. Resemblance among relative serves as the foundation for estimating the-
   a) Heritability   b) Repeatability
   c) Genetic correlation   d) Regression coefficient

137. Conservation includes-
   a) Preservation only   b) Improvement only
   c) Both 'a' & 'b'   d) None of the above

Answer Key

1	d	2	b	3	b	4	c	5	c	6	a	7	b
8	b	9	b	10	d	11	c	12	d	13	c	14	d
15	d	16	b	17	b	18	a	19	c	20	b	21	c
22	a	23	b	24	b	25	a	26	c	27	c	28	d
29	c	30	d	31	a	32	a	33	d	34	c	35	a
36	d	37	b	38	a	39	a	40	d	41	c	42	b
43	c	44	b	45	b	46	a	47	b	48	a	49	a
50	c	51	a	52	c	53	a	54	c	55	a	56	b
57	a	58	c	59	b	60	a	61	c	62	b	63	a
64	a	65	b	66	c	67	d	68	a	69	b	70	c
71	c	72	a	73	c	74	a	75	a	76	a	77	a
78	d	79	a	80	a	81	d	82	a	83	b	84	c
85	a	86	b	87	c	88	c	89	a	90	a	91	c
92	d	93	b	94	a	95	b	96	d	97	c	98	a
99	b	100	d	101	c	102	a	103	a	104	b	105	c
106	a	107	a	108	d	109	b	110	b	111	a	112	d
113	c	114	c	115	a	116	a	117	c	118	b	119	b
120	c	121	c	122	a	123	a	124	b	125	c	126	c
127	d	128	b	129	c	130	c	131	a	132	a	133	a
134	d	135	c	136	a	137	c						

15

Production of Bio-fuel from Animal Fat

D.N. Singh[1]*, Ranjana Kumari[1], and M.M. Islam[2]

[1]*Bihar Veterinary College, BASU, Patna*

[2]*VASERU, Kamdhenu University, Ramna Muvada, Gujarat*

Introduction

The agro-food & slaughter house animal by-product industry generates large amounts of waste that contribute to environmental contamination and leads to pollution. Animal by-product production, as part of the meat and poultry processing chain, is huge. Animal fat waste constitutes some of the most relevant waste and the treatment of such waste is quite costly because environmental regulations are quite strict. Fossil fuels remain the main source of primary energy accounting for over 80 % of worldwide energy consumption. The continuous consumption of non-renewable resources is leading to their fast depletion while causing the accumulation of CO_2 and other greenhouse gases (GHGs) in the atmosphere. Also, energy demands are expected to rise by over 25 % by 2040, which claims for a shift toward the use of renewable and carbon-neutral fuels to ensure environmental and economic sustainability.

About millions animals (cattle, sheep, pigs and goats) and poultry (mainly chickens and turkeys) were slaughtered various parts of countries. Such a high number of slaughtered animals produces enormous amounts of waste animal residue including fats that need to be treated to reduce pollution or recycled to give them some added value. Such fats include beef tallow extracted from rendering fatty tissue of cattle, mutton tallow from rendering sheep, pork lard from rendering pigs and chicken fat from rendering feathers, blood, skin, offal and trims for conversion into bio-diesel.

Bio-diesel constitutes a valid renewable source of energy because it is biodegradable, non-toxic and has a good combustion emission profile and can be blended up to 20% with fossil diesel for its use in many countries. Biodiesel has attracted an increased attention worldwide. Beside many advantages of biodiesel over diesel fuel, such as: renewability, ready availability, portability, lower sulfur and aromatic content, higher efficiency, higher cetane number, better emission profile and safer handling [1], the high cost of bio-diesel production is the main reason for its limited commercial application. Furthermore, up to 70% of the total cost of biodiesel majorly depends on the cost of the raw materials used, which can be reduced using animal fat waste because they are cheaper than vegetable oil waste. In fact, 6% of total feedstock corresponded to animal fat in 2019. Transesterification with alkaline catalysis is still preferred at industrial plants producing biodiesel. Recent developments in heterogeneous catalysts that can be easily recovered, regenerated and reused, as well as immobilized lipases with increased stability and resistance to alcohol denaturation, are promising for future industrial use. Biodiesel also contributes to sustainability by reducing the carbon footprint due to lower CO_2 emission compared to fossil diesel fuel. CO_2 is one of the most relevant gases because it contributes up to 72% of greenhouse gases. Biodiesel from animal fat achieves nearly 80% fossil CO_2 reduction in comparison to 30% for soya. In addition, the emission of polycyclic aromatic hydrocarbons is 75–90% lower than in conventional diesel, whereas total unburned hydrocarbon is 90% lower, emissions of sulfur and CO are also reduced to a greater extent. The International Energy Agency reported that bioenergy must increase up to 25% until 2025 and continue to grow, and is estimated to reach 30% of the world's road transport fuel mix by 2050.

Biodiesel is made up of monoalkyl esters of long-chain fatty acids that are made from oil with the help of an acid, base, or enzyme catalyst. The most practical method for manufacturing biodiesel on a large scale has been determined to be acid and base catalyzed processes. As a result, the current study utilizes WAF as a feedstock for biodiesel synthesis, utilizing acid and base catalysts, and compares the resulting biodiesel to commercial diesel. The biodiesel to be sold in the market, must meet certain quality specifications. In the United States, biodiesel must meet the American Society for Testing and Materials (ASTM) requirements for biodiesel fuel in its D 6751 standard. The standard in Europe is defined by EN14214.

Multiple Choice Questions (MCQ)

1. Bio fuel is generally made-up of

   a) Beef tallow b) Pork lard

   c) Chicken fat d) All of these

2. The major advantages of bio fuel preparation from animal fat is

   a) High cloud point b) Cheaper & Economic

   c) Lower CO_2 emission d) All of these

3. The cloud point for biodiesel made from beef tallow and pork lard is ranges from

   a) 30 to 40°F b) 35 to 50°F

   c) 55 to 60°F d) 60 to 65°F

4. The flash point for biodiesel is about

   a) 50°F b) 100°F

   c) 150°F d) 200°F

5. The bio-diesel falls under the category of National Fire Protection Association codes

   a) Hazardous, short chain fatty acid

   b) Non-hazardous, short chain fatty acid

   c) Hazardous, long chain fatty acid

   d) Non-hazardous long chain fatty acid

6. The major constraints of bio-diesel made from animal fat is

   a) Containing high free fatty acids b) High production cost

   c) Difficult purification process d) All of these

7. The latest steps for removal of glycerol as well as other impurities like residual catalyst, unconverted fats, and soap from animal fat is
   a) Oxidation & dehydration
   b) Rendering & carbonization
   c) Refining, Trans easternization & Purification
   d) Peroxidation
8. The World's largest biodiesel producer and, on an energy basis (represents nearly 75% of the total transport biofuels market) is
   a) European Union
   b) Eurasian Economic Union
   c) African Union
   d) Kuwait Trade Union Federation
9. The highest acceptable kinematic viscosity for biodiesel as per standard for the European market ranges between
   a) 1.0 to 2.0 mm^2/s
   b) 3.5 to 5.0 mm^2/s
   c) 5.0 to 7.5 mm^2/s
   d) 7.5 to 8.5 mm^2/s
10. Which type of animal fat used to produce biodiesel fuel
   a) Animal fat with low cetane number
   b) Animal fat with high cetane number
   c) Animal fat with no cetane numbe
   d) None of these
11. Which technique is reliable for removing the Sulphur level in biodiesel produced from animal fat
   a) Pyrolysis
   b) Micro emulsion
   c) Vaccum distillation
   d) All of these
12 Which animal fat suitable for biofuel production
   a) Milk fat
   b) Tallow
   c) Fish fat
   d) Marine oil
13. Fatty acids that separate from glycerol during hydrolysis are known as
   a) Non-saturated fatty acid
   b) Saturated fatty acid
   c) Free fatty acid
   d) Waste animal fat
14. Which biofuels help to reduce the negative effects of the currently developing energy criris
   a) Ethanol based biofuel
   b) Methanol based biofuel
   c) Glycerol based biofuel
   d) None of these
15. Sulphur contain in beef tallow
   a) 25 PPM
   b) 50 PPM
   c) 75 PPM
   d) 100 PPM
16. Pork lard consist how much percentage of saturated fatty acid
   a) 20 %
   b) 40 %
   c) 60 %
   d) 80 %

17. Which test to determine cetane number of biodiesel sample
    a) Acid Number test b) Copper strip test
    c) ASTM test d) Catalyst test
18. Which reaction is the most commercially used in method of biofuel synthesis
    a) Transesterification b) Transformation
    c) Catalytic reaction d) All of these
19. Bio-diesel made from beef tallow and pork lard has a cloud point
    a) 35-40 °F b) 55- 60 °F
    c) 65-70 °F d) 75-80 °F
20. Jojoba oil is prepared from waste from
    a) Animal slaughter house b) Fish Industry
    c) Poultry industry d) Agro-industry
21. Biofuels made from
    a) Algae b) Corn
    c) Biological ingredients d) Agro-industry by-product
22. Which of the following is not the potential bio-fuel
    a) Hydrogen fuel cells b) Gasoline
    c) Algae bio-diesel d) None of these
23. ....can be utilized as a source of bio-diesel
    a) Animal Skin b) Animal Teeth
    c) Animal bone d) Animal fat
24. Which of the following is not a biofuel
    a) Ethanol b) Methanol
    c) Natural gas d) Butanol
25. With B20 biodiesel, what does the "20" indicate the percentage of?
    a) Biodiesel Fuel b) Standard Fuel
    c) Energy d) All of these
26. Which one is also called a biogas
    a) Bio-butanol b) Bio-diesel
    c) Bio-ethanol d) Bio-methane
27. Function of pre-treatment of raw animal fat is
    a) Remove impurities and water of the raw material
    b) Smooth the process
    c) Safety consideration
    d) Reduce the cost of processing
28. What is a by-product of producing biodiesel?
    a) Salt b) Glycerine
    c) Methanol d) Polymer

29. Waste materials from bio-diesel production is

a) Gas b) Water
c) Oil d) Energy

30. Beef tallow and pork lard are typically containing how much sum of myristic, palmitic and stearic acids

a) 20 % b) 40 %
c) 60 % d) 80 %

31. Chicken fat consist how much percentage of saturated fatty acid

a) 20 % b) 30 %
c) 40 % d) 60 %

32. Standard Method for Determination of Biodiesel and Triglyceride Content in Diesel by using

a) FTIR Transmission Method b) Mid Infrared Spectroscopy
c) Both a & b d) Spectroscopic method

33. National Policy on bio-fuels was first released in

a) 2009 b) 2010
c) 2011 d) 2015

34. Biodiesel from animal fats tends to produce

a) Smaller increase in NOx b) Higher increase in NOx
c) Lower Organic acid d) Lower oxygen

35. Bioethanol is mixed with ________ to prepare transport fuel

a) Oil b) Petrol
c) Kerosene d) Diesel

36. By-products generated during the rectification of bioethanol is utilized as

a) Sheep feed b) Cow feed
c) Dog feed d) Pig feed

37. In bio-methane, the percentage of carbon dioxide is

a) 55-60 b) 35-45
c) 30-40 d) 32-43

38. Production of bioethanol is through fermentation of ________ and starch components

a) Alcohol b) Sugar
c) Milk d) Acid

39. Improved cetane number and high flash point is characteristic feature of

a) Kerosine b) Petroleum Diesel
c) Bio-diesel d) Petrol

40. The major significance of bio-diesel is reducing the emission of

a) Sulphur b) CO
c) CO_2 d) All of these

41. Biodiesel contributes to sustainability by reducing the carbon footprint due to lower
 a) Sulphur b) NOX
 c) CO_2 d) All of these

42. Biodiesel from animal fat reduces nearly ---------------% fossil CO_2 reduction.
 a) 20 b) 40
 c) 50 d) 80

43. Global biodiesel production is expected to reach about .... by 2024
 a) 18 billion litres b) 25 billion litres
 c) 39 billion litres d) 80 billion litres

44. Tick the correct statement about the bio-diesel
 a) Biodiesel has a higher oxygen content
 b) Biodiesel has a higher the carbon to hydrogen ratio is also lower
 c) Higher content of sulphur, hydrocarbon and carbon monoxide
 d) All of the above

45. Tick the correct statement about the bio-diesel production
 a) Nearly 81% of caul and lung fat and 26% of cod and kidney, knob and channel fat from cattle are destined for biodiesel production.
 b) In the case of sheep fats, 88% of caul fat, 43.3% of lung fat and 67.1% of knob and channel fat are destined for biodiesel production
 c) Both a & b
 d) Nearly 90% of caul and lung fat and 28% of cod and kidney, knob and channel fat from cattle & Sheep are destined for biodiesel production

46. The cetane number reflects .... characteristics of the fuel
 a) Purity
 b) Ignition
 c) Both a & b
 d) Nearly 90% of caul and lung fat and 28% of cod and kidney, knob and channel fat from cattle & Sheep are destined for biodiesel production

47. Biodiesel from animal fats compare to fossils fuel tends to produce
 a) Lower NO_X b) Higher NO_X
 c) Lower CO_2 d) Both a and c

48. B100 (pure biodiesel) made from animal fat should only be used in
 a) Warm climate. b) Cold climate
 c) Sub-tropical climate d) Temperate climate

49. Biodiesel from animal fats that provides better safety during transport and storage due to high flash point
 a) 120 °C b) 130 °C
 c) 140 °C d) 150 °C

50. The saturated fatty acids in animal fats should contribute to for biodiesel due to
    a) Lower oxidative stability
    b) Higher oxidative stability
    c) Lower esterification ability
    d) Higher esterification ability
51. Non-edible feedstocks have recently increased and used as alternatives to vegetable oils in the production of biodiscl
    a) Animal fat wastes (AFWs)
    b) Animal protein waste (APWs)
    c) Animal Blood waste (ABWs)
    d) None of these
52. New emerging techniques for the production of biodiesel from animal fat
    a) Ultrasound-assisted (UA)
    b) Microwave-assisted (MA)
    c) ATT technique
    d) Both a and c
53. Animal fat obtained from leather industry fleshing wastes were used to produce
    a) Methyl ester
    b) Ethyl ester
    c) Propyl ester
    d) All of these
54. Animal fats are generally formed of a mixture of
    a) Triglycerides and Water
    b) Proteins and water
    c) Diverse minerals
    d) Triglycerides, proteins, water and minerals
55. Which catalysts used for biodiesel production from waste animal fat
    a) H_2SO_4
    b) KOH
    c) Cao
    d) Both a and b
56. Which nano catalysts used in transesterification process for biodiesel production from chicken fat.
    a) Cao
    b) Mgo
    c) Cao/$CuFe_2O_4$
    d) $CuFe_2O_4$
57. Global warming can be reduced by use of
    a) Green manuring
    b) Bio-diesel
    c) Vermicomposting
    d) All of these
58. Biodiesel is made up of
    a) Cyclo Mono-alkyl alkane
    b) Mono-alkyl esters of long-chain fatty acids
    c) Cyclo Mono-alkyl aldehyde
    d) Mono-alkyl ethers
59. The cloud point (CP) of biodiesel samples are determined according to
    a) ASTM D2500-91
    b) ASTM D97-96
    c) Vermicomposting
    d) All of these
60. The pour point (PP) of biodiesel samples are determined according to
    a) ASTM D2500-91
    b) ASTM D97-96
    c) ASTM D3500-205
    d) ASTM D99-97

61. The HHVs of biodiesel samples are measured in a bomb calorimeter according to the

a) ASTM D 91 standard method b) ASTM D 91 standard method

c) ASTM D2015 standard method d) ASTM D99-97

62. Measures the ignition delay and utilizes a constant volume combustion chamber with direct fuel injection into heated, compressed air for the estimation of

a) Cloud Point b) Pour point

c) HHV d) Cetane number

63. The density of the biodiesel is about

a) 0.8326 g/l b) 0.9415 g/l

c) 1.0121 g/l d) 2.012 g/l

64. The viscosity of the biodiesel is about

a) 0.82 mm^2/sec b) 1.42 mm^2/sec

c) 6.024 mm^2/sec d) 8.35 mm^2/sec

65. The acid number of the biodiesel was .... petro-diesel (0.35) but it does not harm the engine parts.

a) Almost Equal b) Little higher

c) Little Lower d) Significantly lower

66. The acid number of the biodiesel (0.497 mg KOH/g) was a little higher than that of petro-diesel (0.35) but it does not harm the engine parts.

a) 0.82 mm^2/sec b) 1.42 mm^2/sec

c) 6.024 mm^2/sec d) 8.35 mm^2/sec

67. The calorific value of the generated biodiesel should be in the range of

a) 10.24 MJ/Kg b) 20.84 MJ/Kg

c) 40.21 MJ/Kg d) 45.21 MJ/Kg

68. .... catalysts were employed in biodiesel production from WAF by the transesterification method

a) H_2SO_4 and KOH b) H_2SO_4 and NaOH

c) HNO_3 and NaOH d) HCl and KOH

69. ....is the most commonly used as alcohol reactants to produce biodiesel from vegetable oils and animal fats is

a) Methanol b) Ethanol

c) Propanol d) Acetyl Alcohol

70. Methanol is more frequently used as alcohol reactants to produce biodiesel from vegetable oils and animal fats is mainly due to

a) Cheaper b) Easily available

c) Fast reactive d) All of these

71. The nano-catalyst during the transesterification process was successfully assayed for biodiesel production from chicken fat is

a) $CuO/Ca(OH)_2$ b) $CaO/CuFe_2O_4$

c) Manganese Dioxide d) Hydrogen peroxide

72. The brake specific fuel of biodiesel from animal fat was ....than fossil diesel

a) 10% lower
b) 15% higher
c) 26% higher
d) 35% lower

73. The brake thermal efficiency of bio-diesel is about..................than

a) 4% lower
b) 10% lower
c) 11% higher
d) 25% higher

74. The more active catalyst responsible for bio-diesel production is

a) Acid catalyst
b) Basic catalyst
c) Aldehyde catalyst
d) Carboxyl catalyst

75. The advantages of biodiesel over normal diesel is

a) Emitting low amounts of SOx
b) Improving lubricity
c) Reducing engine damage
d) All of these

76. .... is an important indicator for fuel production that defines the lowest temperature at which the vapors of the material ignite.

a) Cloud point
b) Break point
c) Acid number
d) Flash point

77. The minimum values of the cetane number for biodiesel dictated by ASTM D6751 and EN 14214 standards are

a) 24 and 46
b) 36 and 53
c) 47 and 51
d) 49 and 59

78. The process of separation of fat from the protein fraction of animal fat is termed as

a) Wet rendering
b) Dry rendering
c) Esterification
d) Emulsification

79. Biodiesel is produced through reaction of a fat with a short-chain alcohol in the presence of a catalyst is termed as

a) Wet rendering
b) Dry rendering
c) Esterification
d) Transesterification

80. Biodiesel has a ....

a) Higher oxygen content
b) Lower Carbon to Hydrogen ration
c) Both a & b
d) Non-biodegradable.

81. ....can be utilized for bio-diesel production

a) Animal skin
b) Animal fat
c) Animal Teeth
d) Animal bone

82. Ethanol refers to any bio-fuel made from

a) Grass
b) Corn
c) Plant Carbohydrates
d) Leaves

83. What is the primary source of biodiesel production among the world is

a) Soybeans b) Plant oil

c) Animal Fat d) None of these

84. What is the basic production method of biodiesel?

a) Saponification b) Hydrogenation

c) De-hydrogenation d) Esterification

85. What is the blend ratio of biodiesel with conventional fossil fuel?

a) 20% b) 30%

c) 50% d) 85%

86. What are the advantages of biodiesel over fossil fuels?

a) Easy to oxidize b) Can clog engine

c) High cost d) All of the above

87. Which techniques exist to reduce the potentially high viscosity of biofuels made from animal fats

a) Micro-emulsions b) Pyrolysis

c) Alcoholysis d) All of these

88. Waste animal fats obtained from meat processing industries, tanneries, and slaughterhouses are used to biofuel synthesis due to

a) Renewable nature, b) Good calorific value

c) Zero corrosivity d) All of these

89. The biodiesel production with high yield (96%) can be achieved from

a) Beef tallow b) Pork lard

c) Chicken fat d) All of these

90. Absolute ethanol was found to be better than absolute methanol for processing restaurants fat to biodiesel due to

a) Catalyst activity b) Cheaper

c) Lower viscosity d) All of these

91. __________ is made by combining alcohol with vegetable oil, animal fat or recycled cooking grease.

a) Biodiesel b) Biomass

c) Bioelectricity d) Syngas

92. Which alcohol reactants to produce biodiesel from animal fats

a) Methanol b) Ethanol

c) Both a and b d) Propanol

93. Other short-chain alcohols can used as an alternative in biofuel formation

a) Ethanol b) Isopropanol

c) Methanol d) Propanol

94. Which Process of waste leather tanning to produce biodiesel under supercritical conditions.

a) Methanolysis b) Hydrolysis

c) Electrolysis d) None of these

95. Mixing biomass with fossil fuels in conventional power plants is referred to as ___________

a) Agitation b) Infuse

c) Co-firingt d) Interbreed

96. Which gas can be chemically converted into other fuels or products, burned in a conventional boiler, or used instead of natural gas in gas turbine?

a) Freon b) Natural gas

c) Syngas d) Noble gas

97. What type of fire system is used in Bio power?

a) Hand firing b) Mechanical stoke firing

c) Direct firing d) Indirect firing

98. The saturated fatty acids have high cetane number with values..................

a) <20 b) <40

c) <50 d) >60

99. Biodiesel made from animal fat has a high cloud point due to

a) Highly saturated fatty acids b) Low saturated fatty acid

c) High saponification value d) Low saponification value

100. The word ASTM stands for ....

a) American State Testing Mills

b) American Saturated Testing Meat

c) American Society for Testing and Materials

d) Anglo-Static Mines & materials

Answer Key

1	d	2	d	3	c	4	d	5	b	6	b	7	c
8	a	9	b	10	b	11	c	12	b	13	c	14	a
15	d	16	b	17	c	18	a	19	b	20	b	21	c
22	a	23	d	24	c	25	a	26	d	27	a	28	b
29	b	30	b	31	b	32	b	33	a	34	a	35	b
36	c	37	c	38	b	39	b	40	d	41	c	42	d
43	c	44	a	45	c	46	b	47	d	48	a	49	d
50	b	51	a	52	d	53	a	54	d	55	d	56	c
57	b	58	b	59	a	60	b	61	c	62	a	63	a
64	d	65	b	66	d	67	c	68	a	69	a	70	d
71	b	72	c	73	a	74	a	75	d	76	d	77	c
78	a	79	d	80	c	81	b	82	c	83	c	84	d
85	a	86	a	87	d	88	d	89	a	90	c	91	a
92	c	93	b	94	a	95	c	96	c	97	c	98	d
99	a	100	c										

16

Entrepreneur Development Through Livestock Farming

Mastanbi Shaik

Department of Veterinary and Animal Husbandry Extension Education, College of Veterinary Science, Garividi-535101, Andhra Pradesh, India

Introduction

Livestock sector is an important subsector of the agriculture of Indian economy. It forms an important livelihood activity for most of the farmers, supporting agriculture in the form of critical inputs, contributing to the household, supplementing incomes, offering employment opportunities, and finally it acts as a supplementary and complementary enterprise. Livestock plays a vital role in the economic development of the country. Livestock Sector has continuously been growing and contributed 4.90% (at constant prices) of total GVA (Gross Value Added) in 2020-21 (Annual Report, 2021-2022). India ranks first among the world's milk producing nations, achieving an annual production of 230.58 million tonnes of milk and with per capita availability of 459 gms/day during the year 2022-23 (Annual Report, 2022-2023). In India, livestock population includes cattle (193.46 million), buffalo (109.85 million), sheep (74.26 million) and goat (148.88 million) (20th Livestock Census, 2019).

The rapidly expanding demand for livestock products offers an opportunity as well as a challenge to livestock production. The livestock sector is moving towards specialization with the increasing involvement of big farmers and investors. Support services including livestock related technical skills and science-based information need to be in place to make use of livestock entrepreneurship as a viable career option in the emerging interest of marginalized rural populations. The lack of access to land, livestock resources and good marketing opportunities for some cultivators stand in the way of a more successful diversification of livestock activities. Livestock farming has been one of the most important value-adding farming systems adopted in different countries.

Entrepreneurship through livestock rearing help the entrepreneurs to manage their own enterprises and becomes economically self sufficient. The entrepreneurs are known for their special characteristics which make them entrepreneur. An entrepreneur may not posses all characteristics such as Self-Confident, Task oriented, Risk bearer, innovator, etc. There is no sex discrimination in becoming entrepreneur, males and females are equally competent to become entrepreneur in the livestock sector. And also an entrepreneur possesses information seeking behavior and is always lookout for relevant current information related to the product, process, market etc. He also procures and utilize the available resources judiciously and develop good network of relationships with the persons, agencies, organizations connected with the enterprise.

Livestock entrepreneurship impact is positive on improving livelihood and the level of income of weaker section of rural society, particularly landless laborers, and small and marginal farmers. Entrepreneurship is now understood to be the catalyst for industrialization and economic growth. By investing the necessary time and effort, taking on the corresponding financial, psychological, and social risks, and reaping the ensuing rewards of a financial nature, personal satisfaction, and independence of decision-making, livestock entrepreneurship is defined as the process of creating something new with value. The cattle business owner is motivated to engage in farming since it raises living standards, generates decent revenue, and elevates one's social and economic standing. By entering the sheep farming industry, the livestock entrepreneur developed decision-making abilities, self-assurance, inventiveness, risk-taking prowess, tenacity, enthusiasm for success, leadership, and optimism.

Livestock-based entrepreneurship offers numerous benefits, including income generation, food security, and improved access to healthcare and education. Furthermore, entrepreneurship and self-employment through livestock provide livelihood sustainability by while incorporating innovative approaches for increased productivity and profitability. However, realizing the full potential of entrepreneurship and self-employment through livestock requires concerted efforts from various stakeholders. Governments, non-governmental organizations, and development agencies must collaborate to provide adequate support, including training, financial resources, and market linkages.

The Indian government has recognized the potential of livestock entrepreneurship in driving rural development, improving livelihoods, and ensuring food security. One prominent initiative is the National Livestock Mission (NLM), launched in 2014, which aims to enhance livestock productivity, promote entrepreneurship, and provide sustainable livelihood opportunities. Under the NLM, financial assistance is provided to individuals, self-help groups, and cooperatives for activities such as breed improvement, feed and fodder development, skill training, and capacity building. This scheme plays a crucial role in empowering farmers and entrepreneurs to adopt modern livestock management practices and increase their income levels.

The Prime Minister's Employment Generation Programme (PMEGP) is another important scheme that supports livestock entrepreneurship. It aims to generate sustainable employment opportunities in rural and urban areas by providing financial assistance for setting up micro-enterprises, including livestock-based businesses. By offering loans and subsidies, PMEGP enables aspiring entrepreneurs to establish their ventures, create jobs, and contribute to economic growth.

In conclusion, the Indian government's schemes to promote livestock entrepreneurship demonstrate a commitment to rural development, poverty alleviation, and economic growth. By offering financial assistance, technical support, and capacity building, these initiatives empower individuals, especially marginal farmers and unemployed youth, to venture into livestock-based businesses.

1. The Word "Entrepreneur" is derived from
   a) Dutch
   b) Spanish
   c) French
   d) Italian

2. The word "Entreprendre" means
   a) o create or to make anything b) to run or nurture everything
   c) to build or to make nothing d) to undertake or to do something
3. The Word Entrepreneur first used by
   a) Remo Disouza b) Radison Bernard
   c) Robert Downey d) Richard Cantillon
4. According to Marx, Entrepreneur is termed as
   a) Ectoparasite b) Self Parasite
   c) Ecto and Endo Parasite d) Social Parasite
5. Which of the following are not a characteristic of Entrepreneur
   a) Self-Confident b) Task oriented
   c) Risk bearer d) Fun oriented
6. A framework within which decision concerning what to produce, how much to produce, where to produce are taken by an entrepreneur is called as
   a) Surprise b) SunRise
   c) Enterprise d) Expertise
7. A person who is interested in salary but not in taking risk is
   a) Entrepreneur b) Manager
   c) Manipulator d) Modern Thinker
8. Entrepreneurs who are conservative or orthodox in outlook are
   a) Plane Entrepreneurs b) Flying Entrepreneurs
   c) Drone Entrepreneurs d) Air Entrepreneurs
9. Entrepreneurs who prefer to set up their business individually
   a) Polo operator b) Null operator
   c) Full operator d) Solo operator
10. Entrepreneurs that are very much skeptical in their approach in adopting or innovating new technology in their enterprise are
    a) Fabian Entrepreneurs b) Asian Entrepreneurs
    c) Australian Entrepreneurs d) European Entrepreneurs
11. A Person who takes active interest in establishing new enterprises but never stay in that business for a long time is
    a) Personal Entrepreneur b) Professional Entrepreneur
    c) People Entrepreneur d) Public Entrepreneur
12. Entrepreneurs who are traditional /stereotype in their approach are
    a) Jazz Entrepreneurs b) Rock Entrepreneurs
    c) Classical Entrepreneurs d) Musical Entrepreneurs
13. An individual who takes responsibility of creating innovation of any kind from within the organization is
    a) Interpreneur b) Intrapreneur
    c) Infrapreneur d) Indipreneur

14. Entrepreneurs who produce goods and services in accordance with changing needs of the time and adopt the changes very quickly are:
    a) Metal Entrepreneurs
    b) Medieval Entrepreneurs
    c) Mundane Entrepreneurs
    d) Modern Entrepreneurs
15. Entrepreneurs who believe in their own performance while undertaking business activities are
    a) Imperfect Entrepreneurs
    b) Improper Entrepreneurs
    c) Pure Entrepreneurs
    d) Impure Entrepreneurs
16. Entrepreneurs who primarily involve in research and development activities are called as
    a) Incubators
    b) Incinerators
    c) Incorporators
    d) Inventors
17. Entrepreneurs who explore opportunities to purchase the existing units which may be seized or are in running condition are called as
    a) Buyers
    b) Butchers
    c) Boxers
    d) Bearers
18. Entrepreneurs who do not possess any family business background before hand are called as
    a) Best generation entrepreneurs
    b) First generation entrepreneurs
    c) Last generation entrepreneurs
    d) Must generation entrepreneurs
19. Entrepreneur who leaves the venture when it reaches the final stage of venture creation and looks for a new opportunity to create another one is
    a) Modern Entrepreneur
    b) Torch Entrepreneur
    c) Meta Entrepreneur
    d) Mobile Entrepreneur
20. Theory of Religious belief in Entrepreneurship was proposed by
    a) Roger
    b) Carter
    c) Weber
    d) Parker
21. Theory of Entrepreneurial Supply was proposed by
    a) Tehran
    b) Gibran
    c) Cullinan
    d) Cochran
22. Theory of Social Change was proposed by
    a) Vegan
    b) Megan
    c) Reagan
    d) Hagen
23. Theory of group level pattern of entrepreneurship was proposed by
    a) Young
    b) Old
    c) Strong
    d) Weak
24. Central feature of Weberian theory of Entrepreneurship is
    a) Catholic ethic and spirit of communism
    b) Protestant ethic and spirit of Capitalism
    c) Pentecost ethic and spirit of Marxism
    d) Christian ethic and spirit of Radicalism

25. Theory of Entrepreneurial Supply emphasizes over
    a) Cultural value, role expectation and social sanctions
    b) Modern value, Scale expectation and spiritual sanctions
    c) Liberal Value, School Expectation and Sensual sanctions
    d) Primary value, Academic expectation and Psychological sanctions
26. Theory of innovation was proposed by
    a) Sinister b) Scholar
    c) Skimmer d) Schumpter
27. Theory of X-efficiency was proposed by
    a) Sebastian b) Leibenstein
    c) Mark Twain d) Mid Vayne
28. Theory of Achievement was proposed by
    a) Richard gere b) Rober John
    c) David McClelland d) Martin Rutherford
29. Theory of Profit was proposed by
    a) Knight b) Daniel
    c) Craig d) Johnson
30. Theory of Market Equilibrium was proposed by
    a) Jack b) Hayek
    c) Rack d) Flock.
31. Conceptual model of entrepreneurship was proposed by
    a) Van Den Ban b) Manouver
    c) Haze D'Connor d) John J Kao
32. Integrated model of Entrepreneurship was developed by
    a) Al Hafiz Syed b) Al Abu Baqar
    c) Abdul Imtiaz d) Abdul Aziz Mahmud
33. Conceptual model of entrepreneurship is also known as the ECO analysis framework. "ECO" stands for
    a) Entrepreneurship, Complexity and Organization
    b) Enterprise, Credibility and Obligation
    c) Excellence, Casualty and Orchestration
    d) Entrepreneurship, Creativity and Organization
34. EMT - Lab associated with
    a) Excellency development b) Eco-friendly development
    c) Enterprise development d) Entrepreneurship Development
35. Entrepreneurship Development cycle includes
    a) Signatory, Sustainability and Superficial phases
    b) Superiority, Susceptibility and Serological phases
    c) Stimulatory, Support and Sustaining phases
    d) Sincerity, Survivability and Signatory Phases

36. NSTEDB Stands for
    a) National Sustainability and Tutorial Excellency Development Board
    b) National Science and Technology Entrepreneurship Development Board
    c) National Social and Technical Ecological Development Board
    d) National Science and Technology Endurance Development Board
37. EDII stands for
    a) Enterprise Development Institute of India
    b) Excellence Development Institute of India
    c) Entrepreneurial Development Institute of India
    d) Entrepreneurship Development Institute of India
38. MANAGE stands for
    a) Managing Agriculture and Nature Governing Institute
    b) Material and Nature Governing Institute of India
    c) National Institute of Agricultural Extension Management
    d) National Institute of Agronomy and Extension Management
39. "KVIC" stands for
    a) Krishi Vigyan Industrial Corporation
    b) Khadi and Village Industry Commission
    c) Krishi Vigyan Innovation Commission
    d) Khadi and Village Innovation Corporation
40. "NIESBUD" stands for
    a) National Institute forEndurance, Sustainability, Business Development
    b) National Institute for Entrepreneurship, Sustainability, Business Development
    c) National Institute for Entrepreneurship and Small Business Development
    d) National Institute for Enterprise, Successfull Business Development
41. SIDO stands for
    a) Small Innovation Development Organization
    b) Successful Information Development Organization
    c) Small Industry Development Organization
    d) Successful Innovation Development Organization
42. Staffing demands defining the
    a) Work Force   b) Promotion and Remuneration
    c) Both a & b   d) None of the above
43. Amidst Challenges towards opportunities, leading the entrepreneurial unit involves
    a) Addressing the desire of Individuals /group
    b) Addressing the attitude and behavior of individuals /group
    c) Both a & b
    d) None of the above

44. Measuring and correcting the activities of staff to assure that events conform to plan is called

a) Organising b) Leading
c) Controlling d) Staffing

45. A Conscious search for the solutions, secking information about the problems whocj arise during the entrepreneurial process is called as

a) Incubation b) Idea generation
c) Preparation d) Initiation

46. A process of mental fermentation which allows the entrepreneur to collect and assimilate further relevant information and develop clarity of thinking is called

a) Idea generation b) Initiation
c) Incubation d) Preparation

47. Which of the following is not considered in Entrepreneurial project Identification

a) Availability of Market b) Availability of critical inputs
c) Availability of loyal people d) Availability of skills

48. Which of the following is not a positive outcome from Entrepreneurship development

a) Optimum utilization of resources and facilities and value addition to products and services
b) Developing capability of men and women to cope up with the impact of globalization
c) Critical analysis of the warships and ware houses
d) New and unexplored fields of activity may be the subject matter for Entrepreneurship development

49. IDBI stands for

a) Indian Development Bank of Innovation
b) Innovative Development Bank of India
c) Incredible Development Bank of India
d) Industrial Development Bank of India

50. ICICI stands for

a) Industrial Credit and Investment Corporation of India
b) Industrial Cash and Investment Corporation of India
c) Indian Cash and Industry Corporation of India
d) Intellectual Credit and Industry Corporation of India

51. Which of the following is not a characteristic of an entrepreneur

a) Self Confidence b) Achievement motivation
c) Short term Involvement d) Risk taking

52. "EXIM" in Exim Bank stands for

a) Exponential Industrial Maintenance Bank of India
b) Entrepreneurial Innovation Bank of India
c) Existential Bank of India
d) Export - Import Bank of India

53. "SEZs" stand for
   a) Special Entrepreneurship Zones
   b) Sensitive Enterprises Zones
   c) Superlative Educational Zones
   d) Special Economic Zones
54. Stay in an Orchard or Plantation, experiencing the rural lifestyle and taking part in local cuisine is called as
   a) Rural Tourism
   b) Local Tourism
   c) Land Tourism
   d) Farm Tourism
55. According to Singh (2007), which of the following are Socio-personal constraints perceived by Rural Entrepreneurs
   a) High level of Education
   b) High level of Persistent Knowledge about innovations
   c) Both a & b
   d) None of the above
56. Publicity, awareness creation and motivational campaigns are included in which of the following phases of REDP
   a) Training phase
   b) Post Training phase
   c) Pre-training phase
   d) Proper training phase
57. Which of the following problems are particularly encountered by women entrepreneurs
   a) Problems of marketing
   b) Limited mobility
   c) Lack of Risk bearing capacity
   d) All the above
58. According to Singhal and Rogers (2001), India needs entrepreneurs who believe in
   a) Making money and doing business at the same time
   b) Doing business and part time work at the same time
   c) Making entrepreneurs and helping their business at the same time
   d) Making money and doing good at the same time
59. NABARD stands for
   a) National Bank for Agripreneurs and Rural Development
   b) National Bank for Associations and Rural Development
   c) National Bank for Agriculture and Rural Development
   d) National Bank for Agronomy and Rural Development
60. Which of the following are strengths of Indian Dairy Industry
   a) Demand Profile - Optimistic
   b) Availability of Raw material - Abundant
   c) Margins - reasonable, even on packed liquid milk
   d) All the above
61. Which of the following subsidies are available as Government incentives to Entrepreneurs
   a) Export Subsidy
   b) Tax subsidy
   c) Excise duty Exemption
   d) All the above

62. Following services are provided by Venture Capitalists
    a) Personal Assistance
    b) Professional Assistance
    c) Political Assistance
    d) Financial Assistance
63 The entrepreneur has to transform knowledge into action to create an
    a) Educational Institution
    b) Excise duty exemption
    c) Enterprise
    d) Excellence
64. Venture capital is provided to the ventures considering the following characteristics
    a) Personality of Entrepreneurs
    b) Management Characteristics of entrepreneurs
    c) Experience of the Entrepreneurs
    d) All the above
65. Commercial support to new ideas and for the introduction and adaptation of new technologies is involved in
    a) Agribusiness centres
    b) Agriclinics
    c) Stock market financing
    d) Venture capital financing
66. Acquisition or buy out financing has the following objectives
    a) Acquisition of another business
    b) Management buyout financing
    c) Turn around financing
    d) All the above
67. Important value added services provided by the venture capitalists are
    a) Planning and decision making for the investor company
    b) Access to market and Technology
    c) Creation of new markets
    d) All the above
68. Venture capital financing wherein the stage when the finance is required for the expanded activities of the venture
    a) Early bird financing
    b) First stage financing
    c) Managemental financing
    d) Expansion financing
69. The objectives for the development of entrepreneurship in the New Industrial Policy 1991 were:
    a) Development of the capital market
    b) Dismantling of regulatory system
    c) Spread industrialization to backward areas
    d) All the above
70. "WCED" stands for
    a) Women and Child Entrepreneurship Development
    b) Working Capital Entrepreneurs Development
    c) Women Corporate Entrepreneur Development
    d) Wadhani Centre for Entrepreneurship Development

71. Which of the following are State Level Entrepreneurship Training Institutions
    a) Institute of Entrepreneurship Development
    b) Centre of Entrepreneurship Development
    c) Centre of Entrepreneurship and Management Development
    d) All the above
72. The foundation set up in 1993 to create wealth for the nation through innovations in resource management and capacity building of the people
    a) Moracco foundation
    b) Morarji Desai Foundation
    c) Marcopolo Foundation
    d) Morarka Foundation
73. Which of the following are Central Finance Institutions
    a) Industrial Development Bank of India
    b) Industrial Finance Corporation of India
    c) Industrial Credit and Investment Corporation of India
    d) All the above
74. Exploration of new markets is an essential component of ____policy
    a) TAXIM
    b) MAXIM
    c) EXAM
    d) EXIM
75. Which of the following are threats in Indian Dairy Industry according to Sur (2007)
    a) Environment norms and energy costs
    b) Need for immediate implementation of foof safety norms
    c) Milk Vendors
    d) All the above
76. Which of the following are Weaknesses of Indian Dairy Industry
    a) Perishability
    b) Logistics of Procurement
    c) Need for Cold Chain
    d) All the above
77. Which of the following parameters is not considered in judging the quality of a fresh produce
    a) Appearance
    b) Texture
    c) Flavor
    d) Price
78. Process associated with increasing economic openness, growing economic interdependence among the nations and deepening economic integration globally is called as
    a) Sustainable Development
    b) Entrepreneurship Development
    c) Market Extension
    d) Globalization
79. Agripreneurship is required because
    a) To reduce malnutrition
    b) Increaing demand for organic/quality food
    c) Willingness of the private sector to enter into Agribusiness
    d) All the above

80. Entrepreneur is an innovator with potentialities of doing things in a new way according to
   a) John Muller
   b) Ivan Pavlov
   c) Joseph Schumpter
   d) Jack Munich

81. General Characteristics of Entrepreneurs are
   a) Commitment and Determination
   b) Leadership
   c) Tolerance of risk, ambiguity and Uncertainty
   d) All the above

82. _____ is one who organizes, operates and assumes the risk in a business venture in an expectation of making a profit
   a) Agripreneur
   b) Intrapreneur
   c) Extrapreneur
   d) Entrepreneur

83. Which of the following factors are responsible for Entrepreneurship according to Amarnath and Samuel (2008)
   a) Religious, Social and Cultural factors
   b) Psychological factors
   c) Economic policies of the Government
   d) All the above

84. Psychological factor which inhibit promotion of entrepreneurship
   a) Security orientation
   b) Conformity and Compliance
   c) High need for affiliation
   d) All the above

85. According to Bahal (2008), entrepreneurship is a process of change comprising which of the following behavioral components
   a) Identification, Evaluation and Exploitation of an opportunity
   b) Management of a new or transformed organization
   c) Creation of value through successful exploitation of new Idea
   d) All the above

86. Addressing the desire, attitude and behavior of Individual and groups amidst Challenges towards opportunities is called as
   a) Controlling
   b) Staffing
   c) Leading
   d) Organizing

87. What are the steps in putting an enterprise in to Action
   a) Arrangement of credit
   b) Supervising and guiding the Entrepreneurs
   c) Assistance to the Entrepreneur in Marketing and Networking
   d) All the above

88. In Indian context, development of new female entrepreneurs should have the following prerequisites
   a) Pre marital exposure to Entrepreneurial activities
   b) Support from the spouse, relatives and friends
   c) Financial Assistance and facilities for loans
   d) All the above

89. _____ model emphasizes minimal Government intervention in the economy as the best way to maintain incentives for entrepreneurial behavior
a) Positive market
b) International market
c) Collective market
d) Free market

90. Factors which may be considered for entrepreneurial project identification are
a) Availability of market
b) Availability of critical inputs
c) Availability of Technology
d) All the above

91. Strengths of an organization are:
a) Availability of necessary infrastructure
b) Good location
c) Skilled manpower
d) All the above

92. Weakness of an organization are
a) Inadequate infrastructure
b) Lack of effective coordination
c) Outdated Technology
d) All the above

93. Threats of an organization are
a) Changing customer tastes and preferences
b) Rejection by the market
c) Prolonged economic depressions
d) All the above

94. Opportunities of an Organization are
a) Favorable Government Policies
b) Availability of appropriate technology
c) Presence of favorable Cultural environment
d) All the above

95. Which of the following facilities and incentives provided by government for Entrepreneurial Development
a) Quick approval of Project Reports
b) Establishment of Science and technology entrepreneurs park
c) Government subsidy to tribal and rural areas to encourage industries and exports
d) All the above

96. _______ parks will help create backward linkages with farmers and processors and also provide forward linkages by processors and the markets
a) Agri parks
b) Product parks
c) Tourist parks
d) Food parks

97. The key economic features of Globalization are
a) Growth in trade
b) Foreign direct investment
c) Global competition
d) All the above

98. Positive outcome from Entrepreneurship Development
a) It generates more income and employment
b) New products and services may be created in process
c) Optima utilization of resources and facilities and value addition to products and services
d) All the above

99. Certain principles of managing competition, the entrepreneur should adopt are
   a) Spotting early opportunities
   b) Developing a deeper understanding of the customer
   c) Identifying current trends which would shape the future
   d) All the above

100. Defining the Workforce, utilization of manpower, appointment, promotion and remuneration is called as
   a) Leading
   b) Controlling
   c) Organising
   d) Staffing

101. A need of which the people are not aware of at present, but may be brought to the level of felt need is called as
   a) Unsatisfied need
   b) Unwanted need
   c) Unfelt need
   d) Unusual need

102. A strategic fit or match which is a crucial criterion for the success of an entrepreneurial project is
   a) Enterprise - Efficiency
   b) Endurance - Entrepreneur
   c) Excellence - Enterprise
   d) Enterprise - Entrepreneur

103. An Individual who takes the responsibility of Controlling and Administering the Organization
   a) Organizer
   b) Entrepreneur
   c) Manager
   d) Administrator

104. _____ is the specific tool of an entrepreneur
   a) Knife
   b) Intention
   c) Introspection
   d) Innovation

105. An economic agent who unites all means of production such as land, labor and the capital thus produces a product
   a) RAW Agent
   b) Entrepreneur
   c) Organizer
   d) Innovator

106. An Individual who searches for change, responds to it and exploit opportunities
   a) Moderator
   b) Modulator
   c) Manifester
   d) Entrepreneur

107. ___ is a means of a dynamic process of creating progressive asset
   a) Membership
   b) Workmanship
   c) Statesmanship
   d) Entrepreneurship

108. Stage at which organization of business is very simple and farmers has to do most of the work by themselves
   a) Nourishment
   b) Establishment
   c) Statement
   d) Judgment

109. PRODIP stands for
   a) Production, Development, Integration and Profiting
   b) Production, Design, Intervention and Politicizing
   c) Product development Design Intervention and Packaging
   d) Product, Design, Institution and Profiting
110. PPP mode means
   a) Profit, Pioneer and Placement mode
   b) Public, Proprietor and Procurement mode
   c) Public Private Partnership mode
   d) Progress, Process and Partnership mode
111. MSMEs stands for
   a) Moderate, Small and Maximum Entrepreneurs
   b) Modern, Sufficient and Minimum Enterprises
   c) Micro, Small and Medium enterprises
   d) Massive, Small and Micro Enterprises
112. RIF stands for
   a) Rural information Fund
   b) Rural Innovation Fund
   c) Rural Institution Fund
   d) Rural Infrastructure Fund
113. SFAC stands for
   a) Society of farmers and Agriculture Corporation
   b) Small Farmers Agri Business Consortium
   c) Society of Farmers and Agribusiness Consortium
   d) Small Farmers Agriculture Cooperation
114. SIDBI stands for
   a) Small Industries Development Bank of India
   b) Small Industries Development Board of India
   c) Small Scale Industries Development Bank of India
   d) Small Farmers and Industries Development Bank of India
115. NIF stands for
   a) National Infrastructure Fund
   b) National Innovation Fund
   c) National Information Fund
   d) National Incubation Fund
116. NRDC stands for
   a) National Research and Development Corporation
   b) National Research and Declaration Corporation
   c) National Rice and Dal Corporation
   d) National Ratification and Declaration Corporation

117. NIFTEM stands for
   a) National Institute of Food Technology Entrepreneurship and Management
   b) National Institute of Fruit Technology and Entrepreneurship and Management
   c) National Institute of Floral Technology Entrepreneurship and Management
   d) National Institute of Feed Technology Entrepreneurship and Management
118. ABI Centres stands for
   a) Agriculture and Board Incubation Centers
   b) Agriculture Scientist Board innovation Centers
   c) Agri and Aqua Business Innovation Centers
   d) Agri Business Centres
119. ICAR stands for
   a) Indian Council of Aqua Research
   b) Indian Centre of Agriculture Research
   c) Indian Council of Agricultural Research
   d) Indian Council of Agronomy Research
120. MAITRI stands for
   a) Multipurpose AI Technician in Rural India
   b) Multipurpose Artificial Intelligence Technicians in Rural India
   c) Multipurpose All Industries Technicians in Rural India
   d) Multipurpose Available Informal Technicians in Rural India
121. NLM stands for
   a) National Livestock Entrepreneurs Module
   b) National Liberal Mission
   c) National Low cost Mission
   d) National Livestock Mission
122. National Award introduced by AH Department in 2022 is
   a) Gokul Ratna Award b) Gopal Ratna Award
   c) Gopi Ratna Award d) Gehlot Ratna Award
123. The submissions of NLM Scheme are
   a) Breed Development of Livestock and Poultry
   b) Feed and Fodder Development
   c) Extension and Innovation
   d) All the above
124. SELF stands for
   a) State Entrepreneurship of Livestock and Fisheries
   b) Self Entrepreneurship of Livestock Farmers
   c) Self-Employment in Livestock farming
   d) Self Enterprise in Livestock Farms

125. NPDD stands for
   a) National Programme for Departmental Discussions
   b) National Programme for Dairying and Development
   c) National Programme for Dairy Development
   d) National Programme for Dairy and Departments
126. KCC stands for
   a) Kisan Common Care   b) Kisan Care Circular
   c) Kisan Credibility Care   d) Kisan Credit Card
127. AHIDF stands for
   a) Animal Husbandry Institution Dairy and Fisheries
   b) Animal Husbandry Infrastructure for Dairy and Fisheries
   c) Animal Husbandry Intelligence for Dairying and Fisheries
   d) Animal Husbandry Infrastructure Development Fund
128. RGM stands for
   a) Rural Guarantee Mission   b) Rashtriya Gram Module
   c) Rural Garv Model   d) Rashtriya Gokul Mission
129. NADCP stands for
   a) National Animal Husbandry Dairying Cooperative Programme
   b) National Animal and Dairy Cooperative Programme
   c) National Animal Disease Control Programme
   d) National Animal Disease Conservation Programme
130. FPOs stands for
   a) Farmer Production Organization   b) Farmer Plan Organization
   c) Farmer Products Outlets   d) Farmer Producer Organizations
131. National Livestock Mission aims towards
   a) Employment Generation   b) Entrepreneurship Development
   c) Increase in Per Animal Productivity   d) All the above
132. The Mission Objectives of NLM Scheme are
   a) Increase in Production of Meat, Egg, Goat Milk, Wool and Fodder
   b) Promoting Risk Management measures including Livestock Insurance
   c) Capacity Building of State Functionaries and Livestock Owner through strengthened Extension Machinery
   d) All the above
133. NAFED stands for
   a) National Agricultural Cooperative Marketing Federation of India
   b) National Agricultural Farmers Entrepreneurship Development
   c) National Aquaculture Farmers Educational Development
   d) National Agriculture and Farms Establishment and Development

134. NDDB stands for
   a) National Dairying and Departmental Board National
   b) Development and Discussion Board
   c) National Dairy Development Board
   d) National and District Development Board

135. JLGs stands for
   a) Joint Livestock Groups
   b) Joint Livestock Gaurantees
   c) Joint Liability Groups
   d) Joint Leverage Groups

136. NCDC stands for
   a) National Corporation for Dairy Coooperatives
   b) National Council for Dairy Coooperatives
   c) National Cooperative Development Corporation
   d) National Council for Development of Cooperatives

137. MoFAHD stands for
   a) Ministry of Farmers of Animal Husbandry Department
   b) Ministry of Fisheries and Animal Husbandry Department
   c) Ministry of Fisheries, Agriculture and Human Resource Development
   d) Ministry of Fisheries, Animal Husbandry and Dairying

138. SMILE in Andhra Pradesh stands for
   a) State Management Institute of Livestock Entrepreneurship
   b) State Membership of Institutional Livestock Entrepreneurs
   c) Society for Modern Intelligence in Livestock Entrepreneurship
   d) Society for Management of Indigenous Livestock Entrepreneurs

139. Objectives of Sub-Mission on Innovation and Extension of NLM Scheme are
   a) To carry out Extension Activities for Propagating the Various Activities taking olace in the Livestock sector
   b) To carry out the work of Livestock Insurance
   c) To encourage persons, Institution and State Governments to bring innovations for the sector
   d) All the above

140. Objectives of Entrepreneurship activities in feed and fodder of NLM scheme are
   a) Promoting, Developing and Disseminating forage technologies through frintline technology demonstrations
   b) To make available quality fodder with affordable prices at the local level
   c) To encourage the fodder production by the local farmers for supplying to these entrepreneurs. Thus use the fodder as acash crop.
   d) All the above

141. The Objectives of Promoting Piggery Entrepreneurship through NLM scheme are
   a) To substitute import dependency in pork and start export of pork and pork products
   b) Spreading scientific awareness about scientific pig rearing practices, nutrition, disease prevention etc
   c) Creation of forward and backward linkages in the Piggery sector
   d) All the above

142. A process that focuses on supporting innivative, early stage enterprises that have high potential for growth and to become competitive by serving, enriching or linking to farm produces is called as
   a) Agribusiness installation   b) Agribusiness instrumentation
   c) Agribusiness inauguration   d) Agribusiness incubation

143. A person who is not directly involved in production or processing, but, provides the input support, credit linkage and output linkage for establishment of venture is called as
   a) Moderator   b) Facilitator
   c) Inducer   d) Innovator

144. NSIC stands for
   a) National Small Industries Corporation
   b) National Special Innovations Corporation
   c) National Scientific Institutes Corporation
   d) National Social Individuals Corporation

145. RGUMY stands for
   a) Rajiv Gandhi Udyamimitra Yojana
   b) Rajiv Gandhi Uniform Management Yojana
   c) Rajiv Gandhi Union Ministries Yojana
   d) Rajiv Gandhi Unicorn Management Yojana

146. The points which must be considered for prospective Entrepreneurship
   a) Guidance and Consultation
   b) Addressing or Solution to the Problem
   c) Effective Execution
   d) All the above

147. The development of a farm enterprise as a business occurs in the following stages
   a) Establishment   b) Survival
   c) Maturity   d) All the above

148. An entrepreneur to be successful need to have certain qualities which are
   a) Courage to risk   b) Hard worker and Stress bearer
   c) Innovative Skill   d) All the above

149. DEDS stands for
   a) Dairy Entrepreneurship Development Scheme
   b) Dairy Entrepreneurs Discussion Scheme
   c) Development of Entrepreneurs in Dairying Scheme
   d) Dairy Enablers and Development Scheme

150. NEISBUD is located at
   a) Bengaluru
   b) Chennai
   c) Noida
   d) Hyderabad

Answer Key

1	c	2	d	3	d	4	d	5	d	6	c	7	b
8	c	9	d	10	a	11	b	12	c	13	b	14	d
15	c	16	d	17	a	18	b	19	d	20	c	21	d
22	d	23	a	24	b	25	a	26	d	27	b	28	c
29	a	30	b	31	d	32	d	33	d	34	d	35	c
36	b	37	d	38	c	39	b	40	c	41	c	42	c
43	c	44	c	45	c	46	c	47	c	48	c	49	d
50	a	51	c	52	d	53	d	54	d	55	d	56	c
57	d	58	d	59	c	60	d	61	d	62	d	63	c
64	d	65	d	66	d	67	d	68	d	69	d	70	d
71	d	72	d	73	d	74	d	75	d	76	d	77	d
78	d	79	d	80	c	81	d	82	d	83	d	84	d
85	d	86	c	87	d	88	d	89	d	90	d	91	d
92	d	93	d	94	d	95	d	96	d	97	d	98	d
99	d	100	d	101	c	102	d	103	c	104	d	105	c
106	d	107	d	108	b	109	c	110	c	111	c	112	d
113	b	114	b	115	b	116	a	117	a	118	d	119	c
120	a	121	d	122	b	123	d	124	c	125	c	126	d
127	d	128	d	129	c	130	d	131	d	132	d	133	a
134	c	135	c	136	c	137	d	138	a	139	d	140	d
141	d	142	d	143	b	144	a	145	a	146	d	147	d
148	d	149	a	150	c								

17

Genetic Marker and Herd Evaluation

Monoshree Sarma[1], Jayanthi K.V.[2], Surita Majumder[3], Mrinmoyee Sarma[4], Safeeda Sultana Begum[5], and Farida Rahman[1]

[1]*Department of Veterinary Pharmacology and Toxicology, Institute of Veterinary Science and Animal Husbandry, Siksha 'O' Anusandhan, Bhubaneswar, Odisha*

[2]*Department of Animal Genetics and Breeding, Veterinary College Hebbal, KVAFSU Bangalore, Karnataka*

[3]*Department of Animal Genetics and Breeding, Institute of Veterinary Science and Animal Husbandry, Siksha 'O' Anusandhan, Bhubaneswar, Odisha*

[4]*Department of Veterinary Public Health and Epidemiology, Institute of Veterinary Science and Animal Husbandry, Siksha 'O' Anusandhan, Bhubaneswar, Odisha*

[5]*Department of Veterinary Medicine, COVAS, Kishanjganj, BASU, Patna, Bihar*

Introduction

Genetic Marker

Genetic characterization using DNA markers is a cutting edge technology that makes it possible to study animal variability at basic level. A genetic marker can be any stable and inherited variation which is measurable or detectable by a suitable method and can be used subsequently to detect the presence of a specific genotype or phenotype other than itself, which otherwise is non-measurable of very difficult to detect. Such variations exist at morphology, chromosome, biochemistry or DNA levels that can serve as genetic markers. Molecular markers are the markers that reveal variations at the DNA sequence level.

The polymorphisms observed at the DNA sequence has many applications which include percentage determination, genetic distance estimation and evolution, determination of individual identity, identification of disease carrier (heterozygous) animals, determination of twin zygosity and freemartinism, gene mapping, marker assisted selection (MAS), sex determination, DNA fingerprinting and transgenic breeding.

Gene mapping is a tool to identify the genes responsible for specific traits. The genetic map is constructed from linkage relationship based on the frequency of meiotic exchange (amount of recombination) among linked traits. Genetic map helps in tracking the genes responsible for traits and thus show the relative orders and distances between loci of the chromosomes.

Marker assisted selection (MAS) is an important biotechnological method that helps in indirect selection of superior breeding stock. It greatly depends on identification of associations between the genetic markers and the linked quantitative trait loci (QTL) with useful effects. The association between the markers and quantitative trait loci and marker is guided by the difference between the markers and target traits. However, the MAS is of use in case of traits with low heritability and when the genetic variance is more explained by the marker than the economic trait.

DNA fingerprinting is the process of characterization of one or more rare features of an individuals' genome (hereditary make up) by developing the DNA fragment band (alleles) patterns. It is beneficial in individual identification, pedigree analysis and percentage verification, zygosity testing (twins), sex determination, conservation of genetic resources (identification of genetic relatedness), demographic studies (estimation of individual and population homozygosity, effective population size, population sub division, relatedness, social organization and kin selection), identification of loci controlling quanitative traits or disease resistance, pathogen identification, detection of source of tissues, particularly in meat industry to avoid adulteration, detection of somatic mutation or cancer, taxonomical tool and quality control of cell banks.

With the help of transgenesis, now it is possible to alter the genetic composition of an individual. Transgenesis is a technique that puts a single functional gene or clusters of genes into the chromosomal DNA with the use of genetic engineering. It involves introduction of foreign DNA into the genome of an animal so that all the cells of an animal including germ cells are genetically changed.

Random Amplified Polymorphic DNA (RAPD) is a form of molecular technique which is of great use in DNA polymorphism analysis with high level of detectable polymorphism. It makes use or Polymerase Chain Reaction or PCR.

Herd Evaluation

Evaluation is a process of placing a group of dairy cows in a sequential order from most to least desirable based on milk production and yield. It also involves examination of the disease profile of animals. Prior to evaluation, it is imperative to study and understand the objectives and goals of each individual animal involved in the farm. It is vital to ensure that the herd evaluations are carried out in a consistent manner so as to be thorough and efficient to check the opportunity for missing something important. Once a herd's examination is performed, the data being collected is interpreted by an expertise veterinarian to interpret all the findings in context of veterinarian's clinical observation.

MCQs

1. Genetic markers are
   a) Physically evaluated traits   b) Biochemical markers
   c) Molecular markers   d) All the above
2. Molecular markers are also known as
   a) DNA markers   b) Physical markers
   c) Biochemical markers   d) None of the above
3. Which among this is Hybridization based molecular marker
   a) RAPD   b) RFLP
   c) AFLP   d) SNP

4. PCR based DNA markers include
   a) RAPD
   b) SSR
   c) AFLP
   d) All of the above
5. AFLP is
   a) PCR based marker
   b) Hybridization based marker
   c) Sequencing based marker
   d) None of the above
6. SSR is
   a) PCR based marker
   b) Non-PCR marker
   c) Hybridization based marker
   d) Sequencing based marker
7. RFLP is
   a) PCR based marker
   b) Non-PCR marker
   c) Hybridization based marker
   d) Both b & c
8. Example of DNA chip & sequencing based DNA marker
   a) RAPD
   b) SSR
   c) AFLP
   d) SNP
9. Genetic markers are DNA sequences with known locations on the genome that are used to:
   a) Track genetic variation in populations
   b) Encode proteins
   c) Identify genes responsible for diseases
   d) Diagnose infectious disease
10. Which of the following is NOT a type of genetic marker?
   a) Restriction Fragment Length Polymorphism (RFLP)
   b) Single Nucleotide Polymorphism (SNP)
   c) Short Tandem Repeat (STR)
   d) DNA ligase
11. Genetic markers are commonly used in which scientific field?
   a) Meteorology
   b) Astrobiology
   c) Geology
   d) Genetics and genomics
12. Single Nucleotide Polymorphisms (SNPs) are variations in a single nucleotide base. They are useful for:
   a) Tracking evolutionary relationships between species
   b) Identifying genes involved in rare genetic disorders
   c) Diagnosing infectious diseases
   d) Encoding proteins in the cytoplasm
13. Short Tandem Repeats (STRs) are composed of repeating sequences of DNA They are commonly used in:
   a) Paternity testing and forensic analysis
   b) DNA replication
   c) Protein synthesis
   d) RNA transcription

14. Restriction Fragment Length Polymorphisms (RFLPs) are variations in the length of DNA fragments caused by:
    a) Mutations in protein-coding regions
    b) Differences in restriction enzyme recognition sites
    c) Changes in gene expression
    d) DNA repair mechanisms
15. Amplified Fragment Length Polymorphism (AFLP) is a genetic marker technique based on:
    a) Observing chromosome structures
    b) PCR (Polymerase Chain Reaction) amplification of specific DNA fragments
    c) Cloning of genes
    d) Sequencing entire genomes
16. Genetic markers are used in genome-wide association studies (GWAS) to:
    a) Study RNA splicing
    b) Analyze ancient DNA
    c) Study gene regulation
    d) Identify genes associated with diseases or traits
17. Microsatellites are short DNA sequences with tandem repeats. They are used as genetic markers due to their:
    a) Association with transcription factors
    b) High mutation rate and polymorphism
    c) Role in DNA replication
    d) Ability to encode proteins
18. Which of the following is an example of a genetic marker used in human identity testing and forensics?
    a) RNA interference (RNAi)
    b) Polymerase Chain Reaction (PCR)
    c) Variable Number Tandem Repeat (VNTR)
    d) DNA polymerase
19. SNP markers are generally one of the following type
    a) Biallelic b) Triallelic
    c) Tetrallelic d) Multiallelic
20. RFLP markers are one of the following type
    a) Dominant type b) Codominant type
    c) Both of these d) None of these
21. Silver staining is used in one among the following
    a) PCR-RFLP b) RFLP
    c) SSCP d) All of these

22. SSCP stands for one of the following
    a) Single sustained controlled polymorphism
    b) Single strand conformation polymorphism
    c) Single strand controlled polymorphism
    d) All of these
23. DAF molecular markers are acronym for one of the following
    a) DNA amplification fragmentation
    b) DNA amplification fingerprinting
    c) Dominant amplification and fragmentation
    d) All of these
24. No prior knowledge of DNA sequence is required in one of the following markers
    a) RFLP b) RAPD
    c) AFLP d) Microsatellite
25. Adapter is useful for the analysis of which of the following
    a) RFLP b) RAPD
    c) AFLP d) Microsatellite
26. Which of the following is analogically correct
    a) AFLP= RFLP+PCR b) RFLP= AFLP+PCR
    c) RAPD= RFLP+PCR d) RFLP= RAPD+PCR
27. RFLP was proposed by Bostein *et al.*
    a) Bostein *et al.* b) Goldstein
    c) Morgan d) All of them
28. The Animal model
    a) Simultaneously evaluates cows and sires using all their ancestor relationship
    b) Evaluates cows using all their ancestor relationship
    c) Evaluates sires using all their family relationship
    d) None
29. Mixed model equation (MME)were developed by
    a) R.A. Fisher b) A.C.Aitken
    c) Henderson d) All of them
30. Micro-satellite was coined by
    a) Litt & Luty b) Morgan
    c) Goldstein d) Schlotterer
31. Marker is a piece of
    a) DNA molecule that is associated with a certain trait of a organism
    b) Gene that is associated with a trait
    c) Sequence that linked with a trait
    d) None

32. Animals are selected based on structural & numerical variations
    a) Chromosomal Markers b) Biochemical Markers
    c) Molecular Marker d) Morphological Marker
33. Animals are selected based on pigmentation
    a) Chromosomal Markers b) Biochemical Markers
    c) Molecular Marker d) Morphological Marker
34. Animals are selected based on biochemical properties
    a) Chromosomal Markers b) Biochemical Markers
    c) Molecular Marker d) Morphological Marker
35. RFLP (Restriction fragment length polymorphisms) are detected by
    a) Cutting genomic RNA with restriction enzymes
    b) Cutting genomic DNA with restriction enzymes
    c) Cutting genomic DNA
    d) None
36. RFLP & DFP (DNA fingerprinting) are
    a) Micro-satellite markers
    b) Hybridization based DNA markers
    c) PCR based DNA markers
    d) Hybridization & PCR based DNA markers
37. AFLP, SNP, PCR-RFLP, RAPD are
    a) Micro-satellite markers
    b) Hybridization based DNA markers
    c) PCR based DNA markers
    d) Hybridization & PCR based DNA markers
38. Minisatellites are
    a) 10-12 bp b) 1-6 bp fragments
    c) 20-30 d) None
39. 2 types of DNA array-based technology
    a) cDNA microarrays
    b) cDNA microarrays& oligonucleotide microarrays
    c) Oligonucleotide microarrays
    d) Both
40. Mount hope index is also known as
    a) Yaap's index b) Krishnan index
    c) Intermediate index d) None
41. Corrected daughter average index
    a) Yaap's index b) Krishnan index
    c) Both d) None

42. ____________ Choice of marker for the genetic characterization of breed (by FAO & NBAGR)
    a) Micro-satellite markers
    b) Hybridization based DNA markers
    c) Minisatellites
    d) All of these
43. RAPD-PCR has been developed as a powerful tool for fingerprinting the
    a) Genotypes b) Gene
    c) Phenotypes d) All of these
44. Simple daughter average
    a) 1932 b) 1967
    c) 1905 d) None
45. Sire model
    a) To predict the sire breeding value on the basis of progeny's performance
    b) Predict the sire breeding value on the basis of family performance
    c) Predict the dam breeding value on the basis of pedigree performance
    d) None
46. Contemporary daughter Av. Index
    a) Yaap b) Krishnan *et al.*
    c) Sunderasan *et al.* d) None
47. Micro-satellite markers are also known as
    a) STR, SSR, SSLP b) STR & SSLP
    c) RAPD d) None
48. LINEs are
    a) More than 1000 times in the genome
    b) Less than 1000 times in the genome
    c) More than 1lakh times in the genome
    d) Less than 1lakh times in the genome
49. To predict the breeding value of all animals in the pedigree
    a) Sire model b) Animal model
    c) Repeatability model d) All of these
50. SINEs & LINEs are type of
    a) Interspersed repetitive elements b) Tandem repeats
    c) Short tandem repeats d) All of these
51. SINEs & LINEs are
    a) 20 % of mammalian DNA b) 10% of mammalian DNA
    c) 5% of mammalian DNA d) None
52. HendersonEstimated Breeding Value by using
    a) MME b) MGSM
    c) BLUP d) BLUE

53. Intermediate index
  a) Yaap's index b) Krishnan index
  c) both d) None
54. To predict the breeding value of the animals with repeated records
  a) Sire model b) Animal model
  c) Repeatability model d) All of these
55. Simplest genetic evaluation of dairy cattle under BLUP
  a) Sire model b) Animal model
  c) Repeatability model d) All of these
56. MGSM is
  a) Maternal grand sib model b) Maternal grand sire model
  c) Mega grand sire model d) None
57. RFLP was proposed by Bostein *et al.*
  a) Bostein *et al.* b) Goldstein
  c) Morgan d) All of them
58. The Animal model
  a) Simultaneously evaluates cows and sires using all their ancestor relationship
  b) Evaluates cows using all their ancestor relationship
  c) Evaluates sires using all their family relationship
  d) None
59. Mixed model equation (MME)were developed by
  a) R.A. Fisher b) A.C.Aitken
  c) Henderson d) All of them
60. Micro-satellite was coined by
  a) Litt & Luty a) Morgan
  b) Goldstein c) Schlotterer
61. What is the term used to describe the product of realised heritability and selection differential?
  a) Accuracy of selection b) Intensity of selection
  c) Response to selection d) Limit of selection
62. The sib selection is a type of
  a) Progeny selection b) Pedigree selection
  c) Family selection d) Individual selection
63. Individual selection and pedigree selection are more effective when the heritability of a trait is
  a) High b) Low
  c) Medium d) None

64. Family selection and Progeny selection are more effective when the heritability of a trait is
    a) High b) Low
    c) Medium d) None
65. Which exotic breeds of pig is used for upgradation of local breeds?
    a) Berkshire b) Landrace
    c) LWY d) MWY
66. Which exotic breed of cattle is used for upgradation of local breeds?
    a) Jersey b) HF
    c) Brown Swiss d) All of the above
67. Most effective aid to selection for improving sex limited traits is
    a) Progeny selection b) Family selection
    c) Pedigree selection d) Individual selection
68. Genetic correlation between two traits is due to which of the following reasons?
    a) Heterozygosity b) Pleiotropy
    c) Linkage d) All of the above
69. Contribution of offspring to the next generation is known as
    a) Fitness b) Selective value
    c) Adaptive value d) All of the above
70. The genetic correlation between milk yield and fat yield is generally
    a) Positive and High b) Positive and Low
    c) Negative and High d) Negative and Low
71. The ratio of response to selection to selection differential is termed as
    a) Realised heritability b) Heritability in narrow sense
    c) Heritability in broader sense d) None of the above
72. Genetic gain per year depends on
    a) Calving interval b) Generation interval
    c) Calving index d) Lactation period
73. "Resemblance between relatives" is the basis of estimation of
    a) Heritability b) Repeatability
    c) Genetic correlation d) Both (a) and (b)
74. Repeatability is generally estimated by
    a) BLUP b) Regression
    c) Intra class correlation d) Half sib correlation
75. Pleiotropy is
    a) Transient cause of genetic correlation
    b) Permanent cause of genetic correlation
    c) Increase homozygosity
    d) Increase heterozygosity

76. Linkage is
   a) Transient cause of genetic correlation
   b) Permanent cause of genetic correlation
   c) Increase homozygosity
   d) Increase heterozygosity
77. Best way to increase heritability
   a) Providing uniform environment b) Increasing inbreeding
   c) Increasing homozygosity d) All of the above
78. In ONBS (Open Nuclear Breeding System), Sire is selected on the basis of
   a) Progeny testing b) Sibling test
   c) Individual selection d) Pedigree selection
79. Breeding policy adopted for Buffalo improvement in India
   a) Grading up b) Selective Breeding
   c) Both (a) and (b) d) Crossbreeding
80. Selective breeding falls under
   a) Progeny testing program b) Crossbreeding
   c) Both d) None
81. Maintenance of hybrid vigour in cattle herd is done by
   a) Grading up b) Inbreeding
   c) Top crossing d) Rotational crossing
82. The process that increases the frequency of desirable genes without introducing new genes
   a) Inbreeding b) Outbreeding
   c) Selection d) None
83. Most recent and best method of sire evaluation is
   a) BLUP b) Contemporary index
   c) Equi-parent index d) None
84. If a trait is largely controlled by environment, then h2 estimate will be
   a) Low b) High
   c) Medium d) None
85. Systemic process/force operates in
   a) Small population b) Large population
   c) Both d) None
86. Breeding policy adopted for increasing milk production of non-descript cattle is
   a) Inbreeding b) Crossbreeding
   c) Grading up d) Line breeding
87. Means deviation of progeny from its population mean is known as
   a) Transmitting ability b) Breeding value
   c) Adaptive value d) None of the above

88. Heritability is a property of
   a) Population b) Trait
   c) Environment d) All of the above
89. Non Additive Gene Action includes
   a) Dominance b) Incomplete dominance
   c) Over dominance d) All of the above
90. Random fluctuation in general frequency in small population is known as
   a) Genetic drift b) Genetic load
   c) Genetic death d) None
91. Progeny testing
   a) Increases generation interval b) Reduces genetic gain per year
   c) Estimated Breeding Value d) All of the above
92. Progeny testing is used for the selection of
   a) Dam b) Sire
   c) Son d) Daughter
93. Outcrossing within a herd by use of selected sires
   a) Top crossing b) Selective breeding
   c) Inter se mating d) Grading up
94. Half of the herd is
   a) Sire b) Dam
   c) Son d) Daughter
95. Transient genetic correlation between two traits is due to
   a) Linkage b) Pleiotropy
   c) Both d) None
96. Chief determiner of resemblance between relatives
   a) Non Additive Gene Action b) Additive Genetic Action
   c) Pleiotropy d) Linkage
97. The percentage of individuals with a given genotype that expresses the expected genotype is known as
   a) Epistasis b) Expressivity
   c) Penetrance d) Recessive
98. The Global Data Bank for Animal Genetic Resources is functioning at
   a) FAO, Rome b) OIE, France
   c) NBAGR, Karnal d) None
99. Concept on ONBS was given by
   a) Wright b) Kempthorn
   c) Kunningham d) None of these
100. Formula for coefficient of relationship was given by?
   a) R.A. Fisher b) S.W. Wright
   c) Kunningham d) None of them

101. RH mapping stands for?
   a) Random b) Radiation
   c) Rotational d) None of these
102. The effects of natural selection may be countered by?
   a) Gene flow b) Genetic drift
   c) Mutation d) Inbreeding
103. Which of the following is a property of molecular markers?
   a) Detect variation at DNA sequence level
   b) Not dependent on sex limited and age dependent
   c) Not influenced by environment
   d) All of these
104. To prepare clones representing expressed genes from a eukaryotic cell, you would mix total cellular mRNA with?
   a) Reverse transcriptase b) RNA polymerase
   c) DNA polymerase d) Integrase
105. What is the function of dideoxynucleotides in Sanger DNA sequencing??
   a) They act as primer for DNA polymerase
   b) They act as primers for reverse transcriptase
   c) They cut the sequenced DNA at specific sites
   d) They stop synthesis at a specific site, so the base at that site can be determined
106. System of mating in which 3 breeds are crossed in rotational manner
   a) Criss cross b) 3 way rotational crossing
   c) Triple crossing d) 3 way cross
107. Heritability is a property of
   a) Population b) Trait
   c) Environment d) All of the above
108. Transient genetic correlation between two traits is due to
   a) Linkage b) Pleiotropy
   c) Both d) None
109. RH mapping stands for?
   a) Random b) Radiation
   c) Rotational d) None of these
110. The Global Data Bank for Animal Genetic Resources is functioning at
   a) FAO, Rome b) OIE, France
   c) NBAGR, Karnal d) None
111. DNA has how many parts?
   a) Two b) Three
   c) Four d) None of the above
112. What are the two parts of DNA?
   a) Coding part b) Non-coding part
   c) Both (a) and (b) d) Neither (a) not (b)

113. Which part of DNA is known as 'junk' DNA?
   a) Coding part
   b) Non-coding part
   c) Both (a) and (b)
   d) Neither (a) not (b)

114. Thank coding part of DNA is about
   a) 90%
   b) 50%
   c) 20%
   d) 5%

115. Which part of DNA has lesser variability among individuals?
   a) Coding part
   b) Non-coding part
   c) Both (a) and (b)
   d) Neither (a) not (b)

116. The accumulation of mutations creates genetic variability within
   a) Coding part
   b) Non-coding part
   c) Both (a) and (b)
   d) Neither (a) not (b)

117. Which part of DNA leads to a high level of polymorphism?
   a) Coding part
   b) Non-coding part
   c) Both (a) and (b)
   d) Neither (a) not (b)

118. Which of the following is a method for determining polymorphism?
   a) Site directed polymorphism
   b) Anonymous polymorphism
   c) Both (a) and (b)
   d) None of the above

119. Which method is used to reveal arbitrary polymorphism?
   a) Site directed polymorphism
   b) Anonymous polymorphism
   c) Both (a) and (b)
   d) None of the above

120. Pertaining to minisatellite, which of the following is true
   a) It is 1-5 bp long
   b) It is 10-20 bp long
   c) It is 15-60 bp long
   d) None of the above

121. What is the full form of VNTR
   a) Variable numbers of Tandem Repeats
   b) Variable numbers of Tandem Results
   c) Visible number of Tandem Results
   d) None of the above

122. What are the applications of molecular markers?
   a) Sex determination
   b) Transgenic breeding
   c) Individual identity
   d) All of the above

123. What is the full form of MAAP?
   a) Multiple Amplitude Autonomous Profiling
   b) Multiple Arbitrary Amplicon Polymorphism
   c) Multiple Arbitrary Amplicon Profiling
   d) Multiple Arbitrary Amplicon Polymorphism

124. What is the full form of AFLP?
   a) Amplified Filament length polymorphism
   b) Amplified Fragment length polymorphism
   c) Amplified Fragment length Profiling
   d) Amplified Filament length Profiling
125. What is the full form of RAPD?
   a) Rapid Amplified Polymorphic DNA
   b) Rapid Arbitrary Polymorphic DNA
   c) Random Amplified Polymorphic DNA
   d) Random Arbitrary Polymorphic DNA
126. Which of the following is a approach of sexing?
   a) Enzyme activity method b) H-Y antigen detection
   c) Karyotyping d) All of the above
127. The term microsatellite was coined by
   a) George and Hung b) Tomar
   c) Litt and Luty d) Kary Mullis
128. Variable Number of Tandom Repeats (VNTR) can be examined by
   a) Northern Blotting b) Southern Blotting
   c) Western Blotting d) None of the above
129. What is the full form of PAGE?
   a) Picture acrylamide gel electrophoresis
   b) Poly acrylamide gel electrophoresis
   c) Poly amplified gel electrophoresis
   d) Picture amplified gel electrophoresis
130. Microsatellite is also known as
   a) Simple sequence repeat b) Short tandem repeat
   c) Sequence tagged microsatellite repeat d) All of the above
131. Sire evaluation by BLUP method is given by
   a) Henderson b) Lush
   c) Harvey d) Bakewell
132. In open nucleus breeding system, the replacement female of nucleus are generated from
   a) Cooperating herds b) Nucleus herd
   c) Both (a) and (b) d) None
133. Close herd is
   a) No male transferred to outside
   b) Male selected & used within the same herd
   c) Both (a) and (b)
   d) No female transferred from outside

134. PT is a
   a) Method of selection of sires
   b) Method of selection of dams
   c) Method of selection of progenies
   d) Method of selection of family
135. Improvement of human race
   a) Eugenics
   b) Heredity
   c) Euphenics
   d) Epigenetics
136. In RRS,
   a) Parent in each generation selected on the performance of sires
   b) Parent in each generation selected on the performance of progenies
   c) Parent in each generation selected on the performance of dam
   d) All
137. ONBS concept given by
   a) Kempthorn
   b) Wright
   c) Kunningham
   d) All
138. GCA is
   a) Caused by Non-Additive gene effect
   b) Caused by Additive gene effect
   c) Both (a) & b)
   d) None
139. Objectives of AICRP on goat
   a) Increase the production of meat
   b) Increase the production of fiber
   c) Increase the production of milk
   d) All of the above
140. Dam Selection by
   a) Reproduction problem
   b) EBV
   c) MPPA
   d) All
141. Kadaknath poultry blood is darker
   a) due to melanin
   b) due to carotene
   c) due to anthocyanin
   d) due to xanthophylls
142. HU (Haugh Unit) is related to
   a) Albumen
   b) Yolk
   c) Egg shell
   d) All
143. Diallel cross in case of
   a) Swine
   b) Poultry
   c) Both (a) and (b)
   d) All
144. No of CPDO working in India for poultry
   a) 4
   b) 7
   c) 8
   d) 15
145. The widest possible kind of out breeding is
   a) Top crossing
   b) Species hybridization
   c) In breeding
   d) Line breeding
146. Founder effect is
   a) Genetic drift
   b) Selection
   c) Mutation
   d) Migration

147. Hen Feathering in poultry is controlled by
   a) Sex limited gene
   b) Sex influenced gene
   c) both (a) & (b)
   d) None

148. Random mating is
   a) Out breeding
   b) Pan mixia
   c) both (a) & (b)
   d) None

149. By cross breeding
   a) New breeds can be evolved
   b) Composite breeds can be evolved
   c) Both (a) & (b)
   d) None

150. Rotational crossing
   a) Crossbreeding with a sequence of three or more breeds
   b) Crossbreeding
   c) Both (a) & b)
   d) None

Answer Key

1	d	2	a	3	b	4	d	5	a	6	a	7	
8	d	9	a	10	d	11	d	12	b	13	a	14	b
15	b	16	d	17	b	18	c	19	a	20	b	21	d
22	b	23	b	24	b	25	c	26	a	27	a	28	a
29	c	30	a	31	a	32	a	33	d	34	b	35	b
36	b	37	c	38	a	39	b	40	a	41	b	42	a
43	a	44	a	45	a	46	c	47	a	48	a	49	b
50	a	51	a	52	a	53	a	54	c	55	a	56	b
57	a	58	a	59	c	60	a	61	c	62	c	63	a
64	b	65	c	66	a	67	a	68	d	69	d	70	c
71	a	72	b	73	a	74	c	75	b	76	a	77	a
78	b	79	c	80	a	81	d	82	a	83	a	84	a
85	c	86	b	87	a	88	d	89	d	90	a	91	d
92	b	93	b	94	a	95	a	96	b	97	c	98	a
99	c	100	c	101	c	102	a	103	d	104	a	105	d
106	b	107	d	108	a	109	c	110	a	111	a	112	c
113	b	114	d	115	a	116	b	117	b	118	c	119	b
120	c	121	a	122	d	123	c	124	b	125	c	126	d
127	c	128	b	129	b	130	d	131	a	132	c	133	b
134	a	135	a	136	b	137	c	138	b	139	d	140	d
141	a	142	a	143	b	144	a	145	b	146	a	147	b
148	b	149	a	150	a								

18

Management of Animal Well-being for Meat Quality

Tadung Taku

Department of Animal Husbandry, Rajiv Gandhi University, Rono Hills, Doimuk Arunachal Pradesh

Introduction

Animal flesh when consumed as food is known as meat. Meat was introduced into man's diet early on during Stone Age when they were hunter and gatherer. Humans seem evolved to a meat diet based on the structure of teeth and the unsophisticated nature of our digestive system. Presently man used many varieties of animals' species for producing meat however domesticated cattle, goat, sheep, buffalo, pig and poultry continue to be major contributor of meat to the ever increasing human population. Meat is one of the best and major sources of protein for human, meat protein content all the essential amino acid in required quantity and is easily assimilated by human guts. Fat is essential for development of flavor; at least the bare minimum is desire. Besides this it also has all the other crucial nutrients in smaller amount. The essential elements of good quality meat are firm texture, moderate fat content, tender, good flavour, juiciness and normal meat odor, and to produce such meat it require proper care and management of meat animal. Hence, right and efficient management is to be given to the animals for producing better meat quality. Management broadly includes selection of genetically superior animals, providing sufficient housing, protection from adverse climatic condition, supply of fresh feed and fodder, culling of unproductive animal, daily care and management and control of diseases

Selection

Choosing of genetically superior male and female to produce next generation is known as selection. The animals chosen for selection should be free from disease, healthy, possess high growth rate, noted mothering ability and carcass quality. Selection is necessary since there are genetics influences on meat quality as they incorporate characters from both the parent in the offspring. While selection equal due must be given to both the parents as each contributes half of the genetic makeup of the offspring and has a significant impact on how well their progeny fare. For meat production it's important to select those parents with high daily weight gain and dressing percentage. Carcass with high fat content is not desirable; with proper selection, we can lower the total amount of fat in animal carcass.

Housing

House is the place where animal spend most of their time and it protect them from adverse climatic condition and predators thus, profoundly impacting their performance hence, they should be provide adequate space to move around freely and other facilities to keep them comfort. The facilities includes adequate lighting and ventilation for fresh air, easily accessible fresh and clean water, not too smooth or too rough dry floor for rest and so on. Avoid overcrowding to prevent unhygienic condition and stress as it can consequent in reducing animal muscle growth. The house should be designed and construct as per the requirement of the animal and climate and topographic condition of the region. The direction, height, wide, and site of the house need to be properly followed as per the recommendation while constructing house for should maximum comfort.

Feeding and management

The feed that is fed to the animal is be properly balanced with all vital nutrients like fats, carbohydrates, proteins, minerals and vitamins, in adequate proportion and amount and contain low anti-nutritional factors for optimum growth and production. Feed management aids in producing desire type of meat as per our requirement, solid meat and their fat firm and white can be produce from Corn-fed swine. The essential principle for feeding an animal is first they are to be segregate on the basis of their physiological status. Feeding of growing and fattening animal for meat requires high energy and protein diet with sufficient minerals and vitamins, for the appropriate growth of muscles and other protein tissues. To obtained lean meat, high protein with low energy content ration is offer to the animal. The feeds of the animal are to be change gradually since the animal's health suffers when the feed is abruptly changed, also maintain regular feeding schedule. Animals dislike food that is dirty, dusty and mouldy, or tainted with manure or urine thus offer clean and fresh ration. Castration of male animal is effective way to remove taint odour and accelerate muscle growth

Disease control

Disease refers to any detrimental departure from an animal's normal structural or functional condition, it is typically accompanied by specific signs and symptoms. The biggest risks to the meat industry today are diseases, parasitic infestation, which not only lowers the amount of meat that can be produced but also has a negative impact on its quality. The animal suffering any disease stop gaining weight and rise cost of meat production especially if they suffer from chronic wasting disease like Tuberculosis. Thus initiative should be taken to prevent disease among animals; this can be attain by improving the living condition of the animals with optimum feed, floor space, clean and hygiene house and regular grooming of healthy animal. The house should get enough sunlight and fresh air, regularly disinfect with disinfectant such as chlorine, fresh lime and formalin. Prevent entry of unknown person and animal in the farm premises, quarantine and isolation of disease animal and vaccination against common prevailing disease.

Handling of live animal before slaughter

Handling of live animal before slaughter is gaining more important day by day. Animal not handle properly before slaughter will negatively impact quality of carcass and meat. Animals are transported from their shed to slaughter house in the market, this bring stress in animals, especially at the time loading and unloading, during transportation enough space, ventilation must be provided to all animals, so the animals are free of any injury and health related issue. Animal must spend sufficient time at lairage before slaughter, about 24 hours to get enough rest. Pale, soft, and exudative (PSE) meat in pigs and dark, firm, and dry (DFD) meat in cattle are the most widely known effects of subpar preslaughter handling of animal.

Multiple Choice Questions

1. What is the term used to describe the fat breakdown of fatty acids and glycerol in muscle tissue, resulting in lower pH and higher temperature after slaughter?

   a) Lipolysis b) Lipogenesis
   c) Lipid peroxidation d) Lipid synthesis

2. What is the term used to describe the meat ability to retain water during cooking or storage, which affects its juiciness, tenderness, and appearance?

   a) Water-holding capacity b) Water activity
   c) Water potential d) Water content

3. What s the name of the quality assurance program that includes animal welfare audits and is widely used in the meat industry?

   a) HACCP (Hazard Analysis & Critical Control Points)
   b) ISO (International Organization for Standardization)
   c) GMP (Good Manufacturing Practice)
   d) GAP (Good Agricultural Practice)

4. What is the name of the undesirable meat condition that is characterized by high pH and low temperature after slaughter, resulting in poor color, texture, water-holding capacity, and shelf life?

   a) Dark cutting meat b) PSE meat
   c) DFD meat d) RSE meat

5. What are some of the behavioral changes that occur in stressed animals before slaughter, indicating poor animal welfare and reducing meat quality?

   a) Increased vocalization, aggression, escape attempts, falls, slips, injuries, and mortality
   b) Decreased vocalization, aggression, escape attempts, falls, slips, injuries, and mortality
   c) Increased rest time, positive reinforcement, gentle voice commands, slow movements
   d) Decreased rest time, positive reinforcement, gentle voice commands, slow movements

6. What are some of the management methods that can enhance animal welfare and meat quality before slaughter?

   a) Selecting animals with suitable genetics for meat production and stress resistance
   b) Providing animals with adequate nutrition, health care, and environmental enrichment on the farm
   c) Planning transportation carefully to avoid long distances, durations, delays, overcrowding, mixing of unfamiliar animals, extreme weather conditions
   d) All of above

7. Which of the following factors does not influence meat quality?
   a) Genetics b) Nutrition
   c) Environment d) Packaging
8. What is the term used to describe animals physical & mental state, which can be affected by stress, pain, fear, and discomfort?
   a) Animal welfare b) Animal well being
   c) Animal health d) Animal behavior
9. What are the three main sources of stress for animals before slaughter?
   a) Transportation, handling, and stunning
   b) Nutrition, health care, and enrichment
   c) Genetics, metabolism, and blood flow
   d) Temperature, humidity, and noise
10. What is the name of the undesirable meat condition that is characterized by low pH and high temperature after slaughter, resulting in poor color, texture, water-holding capacity, and shelf life?
   a) Dark cutting meat b) PSE meat
   c) DFD meat d) RSE meat
11. What are the two hormones that are released in increased amounts in stressed animals, affecting the metabolism of muscle tissue and the distribution of blood flow?
   a) Insulin and glucagon b) Testosterone and estrogen
   c) Catecholamines and cortisol d) Thyroxine and calcitonin
12. Cross striated myofibrils embedded fibre are called
   a) Sarcomere b) Sarcoplasm
   c) Endomysium d) Epimysium
13. What are some of the factors that can cause stress and reduce well-being in animals during transport?
   a) Mixing with unfamiliar animals
   b) Exposure to extreme temperatures and humidity
   c) Vibration and noise
   d) All of above
14. Which of the following is a not consequence of stress on meat quality?
   a) PSE meat b) DFD meat
   c) Cold shortening and thaw rigor d) High fat content
15. Each myofibrils is about _____ thick improve well-being in animals before slaughter?
   a) 1 μ diameter b) 2 μ diameter
   c) 1.5 μ diameter d) 2.5 μ diameter

16. Muscle fibres are usually
    a) 10 to 100 μ diameter
    b) 10 to 1000 μ diameter
    c) 10 to 90 μ diameter
    d) 10 to 110 μ diameter
17. The factor that does not affect the tenderness of meat is.
    a) Muscle type and fibre characteristics
    b) Connective tissue and fat content
    c) Post-mortem ageing and proteolysis
    d) Regular exercise
18. The method that is not used for measuring the tenderness of meat?
    a) Shear force and compression tests
    b) Sensory evaluation for consumer preference
    c) Sarcomere length and collagen solubility
    d) Protein percentage in meat.
19. Which tissue serves as the major supportive elements of the animal body? Species and breed differences
    a) Connective tissue
    b) Collagen
    c) Elastin
    d) Recticulin
20. Elastin do not hydrolyses upon ________________ process What are some of the methods used to measure the colour of meat?
    a) Frying
    b) Boiling
    c) Steaming
    d) Braising
21. The water-holding capacity of meat is not affected by
    a) pH and ionic strength
    b) Protein denaturation and aggregation
    c) Drip & cooking loss
    d) Myoglobin content
22. Meat lipids are predominantly __________ in nature.
    a) Saturated
    b) Unsaturated
    c) Polyunsaturated
    d) Monounsaturated
23. Which of the following is not responsible for legal and regulatory frameworks that govern animal welfare and meat production?
    a) International and national standards and guidelines
    b) Codes of practice and quality assurance schemes
    c) Animal welfare audits and inspections
    d) Food safety and standard and authority of India
24. Mostly found saturated fatty acid in meat is
    a) Palmitic and stearic acid
    b) Oleic acid
    c) Linolenic acid
    d) Linoleic acid
25. Decline in meat pH starts during first few hours after slaughter is
    a) 5 to 6 hours
    b) 6 to 7 hours
    c) 3 to 4 hours
    d) 8 to 9 hours

26. Which of the following is not recommendations for improving animal welfare and meat quality?
    a) Adopting a holistic and multidisciplinary approach
    b) Implementing continuous improvement and feedback loops
36. ___________ is recommended for tough cut of meat What are the benefits of improving animal welfare for meat quality?
    a) Heat cooking b) Moist heat cooking
    c) Broiling d) Sauteing
37. The _____ of an animal before slaughter can affect its meat quality by influencing the rate and extent of post-mortem acidification.
    a) Age b) Breed
    c) Stress d) Weight
38. The _____ of meat is its ability of water retention during application by external forces such as cutting, heating, grinding or pressing.
    a) Water activity b) Water-holding capacity
    c) Moisture content d) Hydration state
39. The _____ of meat is force requiring to cut or shear standardized piece of meat across the muscle fibers.
    a) Toughness b) Tenderness
    c) Shear force d) Texture
40. The _____ of meat is degree of pinkness or redness of the meat, mainly determined by amount and chemical state of pigment myoglobin.
    a) Hue b) Color
    c) Chroma d) Value
41. The _____ of meat is process of improving meat tenderness by aging it in controlled conditions of temperature and humidity for a period of time.
    a) Maturation b) Conditioning
    c) Marination d) Tenderization
42. The _____ of meat is measure of its juiciness, influenced by amount of intramuscular fat, water-holding capacity, and cooking method.
    a) Flavor b) Succulence
    c) Palatability d) Aroma
43. The _____ of meat is sensory perception of its taste and smell, which is affected by the animal's diet, age, sex, breed, and post-mortem conditions.
    a) Flavor b) Succulence
    c) Palatability d) Aroma
44. The _____ of meat is measure of its overall acceptability to the consumer, which is determined by the combination of tenderness, juiciness, and flavor.
    a) Flavor b) Succulence
    c) Palatability d) Aroma

45. The _____ of meat is process of adding salt, water, and other ingredients to meat to improve its flavor, juiciness, and shelf-life.

a) Curing b) Smoking
c) Injection d) Marination

46. The _____ of meat is process of exposing meat to smoke of burning wood or other materials to impart flavor, color, and preservative effects.

a) Curing b) Smoking
c) Injection d) Marination

47. Rigor mortis is

a) The process of muscle conversion into meat after slaughter.
b) The process of breaking down muscle glycogen into lactic acid after slaughter
c) The process of relaxing the muscle fibers and restoring the extensibility of meat after rigor mortis.
d) The process of improving meat tenderness by aging it under controlled temperature and humidity for a period of time.

48. Post-mortem acidification is

a) The process of muscle conversion to meat after slaughter.
b) The process of breaking down muscle glycogen into lactic acid after slaughter
c) The process of relaxing the muscle fibers and restoring the extensibility of meat after rigor mortis.
d) The process of improving meat tenderness by aging it under controlled temperature and humidity for a period of time.

49. Resolution of rigor is

a) The process of muscle conversion to meat after slaughter.
b) The process of breaking down muscle glycogen into lactic acid after slaughter
c) The process of relaxing the muscle fibers and restoring the extensibility of meat after rigor mortis.
d) The process of improving meat tenderness by aging it under controlled temperature and humidity for a period of time.

50. Tenderization is

a) The process of muscle conversion to meat after slaughter.
b) The process of breaking down muscle glycogen into lactic acid after slaughter
c) The process of relaxing the muscle fibers and restoring the extensibility of meat after rigor mortis.
d) The process of improving meat tenderness by aging it under controlled temperature and humidity for a period of time.

51. What is the name of the enzyme that catalyzes the breakdown of muscle glycogen into lactic acid after slaughter?

a) Glycogen synthase b) Glycogen phosphorylase
c) Lactate dehydrogenase d) Pyruvate kinase

52. What is the name of the protein that binds to myoglobin and oxygen in muscle and regulates the oxygen supply to the mitochondria?

a) Hemoglobin b) Myosin

c) Myoglobin d) Myoglobin reductase

53. What is the name of the connective tissue surrounding the entire muscle and separates it from other muscles and tissues?

a) Epimysium b) Perimysium

c) Endomysium d) Sarcolemma

54. What is the name of the process that involves the use of mechanical, electrical, or ultrasound treatments to disrupt the muscle structure and increase the tenderness of meat?

a) Tenderization b) Stimulation

c) Intervention d) Activation

55. What is the name of the quality defect in pork that is characterized by a pale, soft & exudative appearance of the meat, caused by a rapid post-mortem pH decline and high muscle temperature?

a) DFD pork b) PSE pork

c) Acid, tough and watery (ATW) pork d) Pale, tough and dry (PTD) pork

56. What is the name of the enzyme that catalyzes the breakdown of muscle proteins by enzymes after slaughter?

a) Protease b) Peptidase

c) Calpain d) Cathepsin

57. What is the name of the protein that forms the thin filaments of the muscle sarcomere and interacts with myosin to produce contraction?

a) Actin b) Tropomyosin

c) Troponin d) Titin

58. What is the name of the connective tissue surrounding muscle fascicles and contains blood vessels and nerves?

a) Epimysium b) Perimysium

c) Endomysium d) Sarcolemma

59. What is the name of the process that involves the use of high pressure to disrupt the muscle structure and increase the tenderness of meat?

a) Hydrostatic pressure b) Ultrahigh pressure

c) Hydrodynamic pressure d) Ultrasonic pressure

60. What is the name of the quality defect in beef that is characterized by a dark, firm & dry appearance of the meat, caused by a high post-mortem pH and low glycogen content?

a) DFD beef b) PSE beef

c) Acid, tough and watery (ATW) beef d) Pale, tough and dry (PTD) beef

61. The _____ of meat is measure of its electrical conductivity, which is related to its water-holding capacity, pH, and drip loss.
    a) Impedance
    b) Resistance
    c) Capacitance
    d) Inductance
62. The _____ of meat is sensory perception of its aroma, influenced by volatile compounds produced by the animal's diet, metabolism, and post-mortem reactions.
    a) Flavor
    b) Succulence
    c) Palatability
    d) Odor
63. The _____ of meat is measure of its firmness, cohesiveness, springiness, and chewiness, which are affected by the muscle fiber type, connective tissue, fat, and cooking method.
    a) Texture
    b) Structure
    c) Consistency
    d) Quality
64. The _____ of meat is process of applying heat to meat to induce physical and chemical changes that affect its flavor, color, texture, and safety.
    a) Cooking
    b) Heating
    c) Roasting
    d) Baking
65. The _____ of meat is process of adding enzymes, bacteria, fungi, or other microorganisms to meat to modify its flavor, texture, and shelf-life.
    a) Fermentation
    b) Digestion
    c) Decomposition
    d) spoilage
66. Marbling is
    a) The amount of fat deposited between muscle fibers
    b) The contraction of muscle fibers due to carcasses rapid chilling
    c) The release of water from frozen meat during thawing
    d) The toughening of meat due to freezing & thawing
67. Cold shortening is
    a) The amount of fat deposited between muscle fibers
    b) The contraction of muscle fibers due to carcasses rapid chilling
    c) The release of water from frozen meat during thawing
    d) The toughening of meat due to thawing & freezing
68. Thaw rigor is
    a) The amount of fat deposited between muscle fibers
    b) The contraction of muscle fibers due to carcasses rapid chilling
    c) The release of water from frozen meat during thawing
    d) The toughening of meat due to thawing & freezing
69. Drip loss is
    a) The amount of fat deposited between muscle fibers
    b) The contraction of muscle fibers due to carcasses rapid chilling
    c) The release of water from frozen meat during thawing
    d) The toughening of meat due to thawing & freezing

70. Which of the following is not one of the three Rs principles of humane animal research?
    a) Replacement b) Reduction
    c) Refinement d) Replication
71. Which of the following is an example of a positive indicator of animal welfare?
    a) Cortisol level b) Body condition score
    c) Play behaviour d) Heart rate
72. Which of the following is a legal requirement for farm animal welfare in UK?
    a) Providing animals with adequate space and ventilation
    b) Providing animals with environmental enrichment
    c) Providing animals with organic feed
    d) Providing animals with access to natural light
73. Which of the following is a benefit of improved farm animal welfare for the consumers?
    a) Lower price of animal products
    b) Higher quality and safety of animal products
    c) Higher availability and variety of animal products
    d) Higher ethical and moral satisfaction
74. Which of the following is not a challenge or barrier to implementing animal welfare standards and practices?
    a) Lack of scientific knowledge and evidence
    b) Lack of public awareness and education
    c) Lack of economic incentives and resources
    d) Lack of enough number of slaughter house
75. Meat spoilage mold and yeast can grow upto a water activity of What are the three main aspects of animal well-being that affect meat quality?
    a) 0.99 b) 0.91
    c) 0.86 d) 0.76
76. What is the main cause of DFD meat in cattle?
    a) High glycogen and low pH in the muscle
    b) Low glycogen and high pH in the muscle
    c) Low glycogen and low pH in the muscle
    d) High glycogen and high pH in the muscle
77. What is the main effect of electrical stimulation in meat quality?
    a) It accelerates rigor mortis onset & tenderizes the meat
    b) It delays rigor mortis onset & toughens the meat
    c) It accelerates rigor mortis onset & toughens the meat
    d) It delays rigor mortis onset & tenderizes the meat

78. The functional unit of myofibril is.
   a) Sarcoma
   b) Sarcomere
   c) Dark band
   d) I - band
79. What are the main methods of improving the colour and flavour of meat?
   a) Curing, smoking, and marinating
   b) Freezing, thawing, and cooking
   c) Aging, tenderizing, and trimming
   d) Irradiation, canning, and chilling
80. What is the term used to describe addition of salt, nitrite, and other ingredients to meat to enhance its colour and flavour?
   a) Curing
   b) Smoking
   c) Marinating
   d) Coating
81. What is the main benefit of ageing meat for a period of time under controlled conditions?
   a) It reduces the microbial load and spoilage of meat
   b) It increases water-holding capacity & juiciness of meat
   c) It enhances the tenderness and flavour of meat by the action of endogenous enzymes
   d) It improves the colour and appearance of meat by oxymyoglobin formation
82. What is the main cause of PSE meat in pigs?
   a) High glycogen and low pH in the muscle
   b) Low glycogen and high pH in the muscle
   c) High glycogen and high pH in the muscle
   d) Low glycogen and low pH in the muscle
83. Which of the following serve as a carrier of oxygen to the muscle fibres? What is the main effect of packaging meat using different materials and methods, such as vacuum, modified atmosphere, and active packaging?
   a) Haemoglobin
   b) Metmyoglobin
   c) Oxymyoglobin
   d) Myoglobin
84. Bacon is generally processed from ______part of the body.
   a) Pork belly
   b) Pork rib
   c) Pork shoulder
   d) Pork head

Fill in the Blank Questions

1. Well-being of animal is a complex and multidimensional concept that involves the ________, __________, and ________ of animals.
2. The main aspects of animal well-being that affect meat quality are __, __, and __.
3. The main cause of DFD meat is depletion of __________ in the muscle due to stress or starvation before slaughter.
4. The main technique that improves meat tenderness by increasing the activity of proteolytic enzymes is ___________.

5. The ________ is the principal muscle tissue in meat.
6. The process of converting muscle to meat after slaughter is called ____________.
7. The amount of fat deposited between muscle fibers is called __________.
8. The contraction of muscle fibers due to carcasses rapid chilling is called ___________.
9. The release of water from frozen meat during thawing is called _________.
10. The oxidation of unsaturated fatty acids due to exposure to air, light or heat is called ____________.
11. Meat quality is influenced by many factors, such as __________, nutrition, environment, and processing.
12. Animal well-being refers to physical and mental state of animal, which can be affected by _________, pain, fear, and discomfort.
13. The main sources of stress for animals before slaughter are __________, handling, and stunning.
14. Transportation involves moving animals from the farm to the __________, which can expose them to changes in temperature, humidity, ventilation, noise, vibration, and social mixing.
15. Handling involves moving animals within the slaughterhouse, which can involve the use of electric prods, whips, sticks, or other devices that can cause _________, or fear.
16. Stunning involves rendering animals ____________ before slaughter, which can be done by electrical, mechanical and gas methods.
17. Some of the physiological changes that occur in stressed animals are increased heart rate, blood pressure, respiration rate, body temperature, and blood _________ levels.
18. These changes can lead to glycogen depletion in muscle tissue, which results in lower ____________ and higher temperature after slaughter.
19. Low pH and high temperature cause protein denaturation and water loss in meat, resulting in ___________ meat.
20. PSE meat is undesirable because it has poor color, texture, water-holding capacity, and _____________ life.
21. Another physiological change occurring in stressed animals is increased release of __ (adrenaline and noradrenaline) and cortisol (a stress hormone).
22. These hormones can affect the metabolism of muscle tissue and the distribution of blood __________.
23. High levels of catecholamines can cause glycogenolysis (breakdown of glycogen) and glycolysis (conversion of glucose to lactate) in muscle tissue, resulting in higher pH and lower temperature after slaughter. High levels of cortisol can cause lipolysis (breakdown of fat) and proteolysis (breakdown of protein) in muscle tissue, resulting in lower pH and higher temperature after slaughter. High pH and low temperature can cause protein aggregation and water retention in meat, resulting in _________ meat.

24. Animal welfare is concerned with ___________, __________, and ___________ of animals.
25. The ___________ animal welfare approach focuses on subjective experiences of animals, such as pain, pleasure, fear, and frustration.
26. The __________ animal welfare approach focuses on the natural behaviour and preferences of animals, such as social, foraging, and nesting.
27. The __________ animal welfare approach focuses on the biological functioning and adaptation of animals, such as growth, reproduction, and immunity.
28. The ___________ is a widely used tool for assessing animal welfare on farms, based on 4 principles and 12 criteria.

True or False questions

1. T/F: Animal well-being refers to physical and chemical state of an animal, which can be affected by stress, pain, fear, and discomfort.
2. T/F: Poor animal well-being can have positive consequences for meat quality, such as PSE meat in pigs and poultry, dark cutting meat in cattle and sheep, and reduced tenderness, juiciness & flavor in all species.
3. T/F: The main sources of stress for animals before slaughter are transportation, handling, and stunning.
4. T/F: Transportation involves moving animals from the farm to the slaughterhouse, which can expose them to changes in temperature, humidity, ventilation, noise, vibration, and social mixing.
5. T/F: Handling involves moving animals within the slaughterhouse, which can involve the use of electric prods, whips, sticks, or other devices that can cause pain or fear.
6. T/F: Stunning involves rendering animals conscious before slaughter, which can be done by electrical, mechanical & gas methods.
7. T/F: Some of the physiological changes that occur in stressed animals are increased heart rate, blood pressure, respiration rate, body temperature, and blood lactate levels.
8. T/F: These changes can lead to glycogen depletion in muscle tissue, which results in higher pH and lower temperature after slaughter.
9. T/F: Low pH and high temperature cause protein denaturation and water loss in meat, resulting in PSE meat.
10. T/F: PSE meat is desirable because it has good color, texture, water-holding capacity, and shelf life.
11. T/F: Another physiological change occurring in stressed animals is increased release of catecholamines (adrenaline and noradrenaline) and cortisol (a stress hormone).
12. T/F: These hormones can affect the metabolism of muscle tissue and the distribution of blood flow.
13. T/F: High levels of catecholamines can cause glycogenolysis (breakdown of glycogen) and glycolysis (conversion of glucose to lactate) in muscle tissue, resulting in higher pH and lower temperature after slaughter.

14. T/F: High cortisol level can cause lipolysis (breakdown of fat) and proteolysis (breakdown of protein) in muscle tissue, resulting in lower pH and higher temperature after slaughter.
15. T/F: High pH and low temperature can cause protein aggregation and water retention in meat, resulting in dark cutting meat.
16. T/F: Dark cutting meat is desirable because it has good color, texture, water-holding capacity, and shelf life.
17. Animal well-being is the same as animal welfare. T/F
18. Stress can affect both the animal and the meat quality. T/F
19. Stunning is not necessary for animal welfare and meat quality. T/F
20. Meat colour is determined by the amount of fat in the muscle. T/F
21. Water-holding capacity is inversely related to drip & cooking loss. T/F
22. Meat quality is influenced by both pre-slaughter and post-slaughter factors. (True/False)
23. The pH of meat is inversely related to its water-holding capacity. (True/False)
24. Meat tenderness is determined by the amount of intramuscular fat. (True/False)
25. The color of meat is determined by the amount of chemical state of the pigment hemoglobin. (True/False)
26. The palatability of meat is mainly determined by the combination of tenderness, juiciness, and flavor. (True/False)
27. Water-holding capacity of meat is directly related to its juiciness and succulence. (True/False)
28. Meat tenderness is inversely related to the amount and type of connective tissue. (True/False)
29. The color of meat is mainly determined by the amount and chemical state of the pigment myoglobin. (True/False)
30. The palatability of meat is influenced by the animal's diet, age, sex, breed, and post-mortem conditions. (True/False)
31. The curing of meat is done by adding salt, water, and other ingredients to meat to improve its flavor, juiciness, and shelf-life. (True/False)
32. The water-holding capacity of meat is directly related to its juiciness and succulence. (True/False)
33. Meat tenderness is inversely related to the amount and type of connective tissue. (True/False)
34. The color of meat is determined by the amount of chemical state of the pigment myoglobin. (True/False)
35. Palatability of meat is influenced by animal's diet, age, sex, breed, and post-mortem conditions. (True/False)
36. The curing of meat is done by adding salt, water, and other ingredients to meat to improve its flavor, juiciness, and shelf-life. (True/False)
37. Animal welfare is the same as animal rights. T/F

38. Animal welfare is improved by providing animals with adequate housing, food, water, and health care. T/F
39. Animal welfare is measured by using only one approach or method T/F
40. Animal welfare can affect the quality and safety of meat products. T/F
41. Animal welfare is enhanced by genetic selection for desirable traits. T/F

Answer Key

1	a	2	a	3	a	4	a	5	a	6	d	7	d
8	b	9	a	10	b	11	c	12	b	13	d	14	d
15	a	16	a	17	d	18	d	19	a	20	b	21	d
22	a	23	d	24	a	25	a	26	d	27	b	28	d
29	b	30	b	31	a	32	a	33	b	34	d	35	d
36	b	37	c	38	b	39	c	40	b	41	d	42	b
43	a	44	c	45	a	46	b	47	c	48	b	49	a
50	d	51	b	52	c	53	a	54	c	55	b	56	c
57	a	58	b	59	b	60	a	61	a	62	d	63	a
64	a	65	a	66	a	67	b	68	d	69	c	70	d
71	c	72	a	73	b	74	d	75	c	76	b	77	a
78	b	79	a	80	a	81	c	82	a	83	d	84	a

19

Selection of Male for Genetic Improvement

Monoshree Sarma[1], Mrinmoyee Sarma[2], Surita Majumder[3], Safeeda Sultana Begum[4], and Farida Rahman[1]

[1]*Department of Veterinary Pharmacology and Toxicology, Institute of Veterinary Science and Animal Husbandry, Siksha 'O' Anusandhan, Bhubaneswar, Odisha*

[2]*Department of Veterinary Public Health and Epidemiology, Institute of Veterinary Science and Animal Husbandry, Siksha 'O' Anusandhan, Bhubaneswar, Odisha*

[3]*Department of Animal Genetics and Breeding, Institute of Veterinary Science and Animal Husbandry, Siksha 'O' Anusandhan, Bhubaneswar, Odisha*

[4]*Department of Veterinary Medicine, COVAS, Kishanjganj, BASU, Patna, Bihar*

[5]*Department of Veterinary Pharmacology and Toxicology, College of Veterinary Science, Khanapara, Guwahati, Assam*

Introduction

Selection of sire

Selection is a phenomenon of giving preference to certain individuals in a population to reproduce over other individuals that are deprived of the opportunity to reproduce. In common parlance, it is the process to choose individuals from the herd that are going to produce the next generation and influence the performance of the herd. Performance of a herd is guided by the genes of the parents. In a herd, males give rise to more off springs and hence selection of males is an opportunity to boost cattle husbandry. The contribution of males to the inheritance of polygenic traits is equal with that of females. Hence, it is central to pay equal emphasis while selecting males and females. Selection of sire is more important than dam selection due to numerous reasons. The first reason is that a sire produces more numbers of progenies compared to one dam. Since a sire is called "half the herd", it determines the performance of the herd. Modern initiatives like artificial insemination and frozen semen technology has further extended the use of sire and highlights the importance of sire selection. Artificial insemination has allowed the superior traits to reach different corners of the globe and this has benefitted the present generation at large. Frozen semen technology together with artificial insemination is milestone to the field of genetics and breeding. It is now possible to preserve the superior traits even beyond the lifetime of bull.

Methods of male selection

As sires cannot be selected on the basis of their performance, hence they are selected based on different basis like pedigree and progeny. At the outset preliminary selection of male is done based on breed characteristics, physical defect, body growth and health, maturity age, testicles, libido, semen production and quality as well as freezability of semen. Pertaining to pedigree selection, the expected predicted difference is calculated on the basis of dam's performance. The final selection is done on the basis of progeny. Pedigree and progeny testing are of immense help when it comes to selecting a male. Sex-limited traits which indicate the economic performance are often expressed in females, for e.g., mil yield, lactation length, egg production etc. In such cases its pedigree and progeny give information on the performance of the male. A male can be evaluated and selected based on the performance of its pedigree, progeny and collateral relatives. Pedigree refers to the list or record of ancestors in the past few generations of the individual. The ancestors are parents, grandparents, great grandparents, etc the estimated breeding value (E.B.V) is determined for the particular male individual on the basis of performance of its pedigree. Pedigree records give first hand information and are less costly. With respect to progeny selection, the results are expressed in the form of an index which is the index of genetic worth of the sire and such an index is known as sire index. Sire index represents a numerical value which is indicative of the production ability of the sire.

Constraints in Sire evaluation

Albeit, sire evaluation is a tedious process and brings it with many constraints. Certain factors which hinder sire evaluation are population size, infrastructure and generation interval. Since in a country like India, most of the herds are small sized owing to financial difficulties, the opportunity of genetic improvement is less as genetic improvement heavily relies on the population size. Genetic improvement is unlikely in a herd of small size. Another problem which needs attention is that farmers are generally uneducated and do not properly maintains records. Record keeping is poor and often unreliable. Therefore, it is the need of the hour to train the livestock farmers on how to maintain records properly and efficiently. Another factor that hinders sire evaluation is generation interval. Cattles and buffaloes generally have long generation interval owing to slow growth rate, delayed maturity and poor breeding efficiency. However, this can improved with use of young bulls, heifer and improving the plane of nutrition and management. Use of part lactation records is of immense help when in comes to improving the sire at a young age. Bull disposal is another criterion that impacts sire evaluation. A great number of sires are not served and remain idle for years between test mating to the time progeny testing results are available. Keeping bulls idle for long time incurs economic loss. Some die or becomes infertile. However, this problem is addressed to a great extent by the use of frozen semen technology.

MCQs

1. The progeny of an individual is the index of
   a) Father's genetic worth b) Parent's genetic worth
   c) Mother's genetic worth d) All of the above
2. Different genes are transmitted by a parent to its different progenies due to segregation of genes during gamete formation and the probability to receive exactly the same set of genes by its progenies is very low for polygenic traits. The segregation is called
   a) Darwin's error b) Lush's error
   c) Mendelian's error d) None of the above

3. .... is 'half the herd'

a) Sire b) Dam

c) Calf d) None of the above.

4. Which of the following has extended the extensive use of sire in many herds?

a) Artificial Insemination b) Frozen Semen technology

c) Both b(a)band (b d) Natural breeding

5. As a result of higher intensity of selection in case of males, the selection differential is ....

a) Negligible b) Lesser

c) Constant d) Larger

6. Sire selection is important in which of the following?

a) Grading up programme b) Crossbreeding programme

c) Inheritance of polygenic traits d) All of the above

7. What are the steps in 'Sire selection' in chronological order

a) Selection of young bull based on pedigree- preliminary or phenotypic selection – sire evaluation based on progeny performance

b) Preliminary or phenotypic selection – selection of young bull based on pedigree- sire evaluation based on progeny performance

c) Sire evaluation based on progeny performance – selection of young bull based on pedigree- preliminary or phenotypic selection

d) Preliminary or phenotypic selection –sire evaluation based on pedigree- selection of young bull based on pedigree.

8. Determination of Expected Predicted Difference (EPdD) is an important part in which step?

a) Selection of female based on progeny testing

b) Selection of male based on progeny testing

c) Selection of males based on pedigree

d) Preliminary selection of males

9. Examining the males for breed characteristics, any physical defect, body growth and health, maturity age, testicles, libido, semen production and quality as well as freezability of semen is an important criterion in which step?

a) Selection of male based on pedigree b) Preliminary selection of males

c) Progeny testing d) None of the above

10. which of the following if NOT a problem in sire evaluation?

a) Population size b) Infrastructure

c) Generation interval d) None of the above

11. The genetic improvement is less in a herd of

a) Small size b) Very large size

c) Large size d) Medium size

12. Which of the following is NOT a reason for very long generation interval in dairy cattle and buffaloes?

    a) Early puberty
    b) Delayed maturity
    c) Slow growth rate
    d) Poor breeding efficiency

13. The generation interval can be reduced by-

    a) Using part lactation record
    b) Avoid using young Bull
    c) Improving the plane of nutrition
    d) Using heifers

14. What is bull disposal ?

    a) Collection of Semen and freezing them before disposing the bull
    b) Properly disposing the carcass of diseased bull to prevent spread of disease
    c) Disposing the remaining of the bull with the carcass
    d) Disposing the bull after natural breeding

15. The anticipated performance of the female at subsequent age is known as

    a) Expected Breeding Value (EBV)
    b) Most Probable Producing Ability (MPPA)
    c) Expected Producing Ability (EPA)
    d) Probable Breeding Value (PBV)

16. Most Probable Producing Ability (MPPA) concept was given by

    a) Lush in 1945
    b) Lush in 1955
    c) Mendel in 1945
    d) Mendel in 1955

17. Which of the method is NOT a multi trait selection method for females?

    a) Tandem selection
    b) Independent Culling Level method
    c) Selection Index method
    d) Progeny testing method

18. Which are the traits that can be measured in living animals

    a) Slaughter trait
    b) Longevity
    c) Milk production
    d) Lifetime production

19. The traits for which individual selection cannot be applied are

    a) Sex limited traits
    b) Slaughter traits
    c) Longevity
    d) All of the above

20. The estimation of breeding value (B.V.) of an individual based on ancestors performance (parents and grand parents) is known as

    a) Family selection
    b) Pedigree selection
    c) Progeny selection
    d) Individual selection

21. The estimation of breeding value (B.V.) of an individual based on collateral relatives is known as

    a) Family selection
    b) Pedigree selection
    c) Progeny selection
    d) Individual selection

22. The source of information based on which the breeding value of the individual is estimated is called as
    a) Basis of selection
    b) Aids to selection
    c) Criteria of selection
    d) All of the above
23. The selection of an animal at the second stage based on the breeding value of the animals which is the final selection is called as
    a) Genetic selection
    b) Phenotypic selection
    c) Natural selection
    d) Individual selection
24. Who found the genetic variability in the occurrence of certain diseases in Murrah Buffalo?
    a) Tomar
    b) Lush
    c) Mendel
    d) Briles
25. Which of the following is the method to identify and select the individual for differences in resistance
    a) Occurrence of disease under normal environmental conditions
    b) Inoculation of animals with pathogen causing the disease
    c) Use of indicators of resistance
    d) All of the above
26. Who elaborated the efficiency of individual selection and family selection on the basis of the incidence of the disease
    a) Briles
    b) Tomar
27. With reference to selection and breeding for disease resistance, the individual selection is less effective when
    a) The proportion of resistant individual is very low, but the family selection is more effective.
    b) The proportion of resistant individual is very high and the family selection is more effective
    c) The proportion of resistant individual is very low and the family selection is less effective
    d) The proportion of resistant individual is very high, but the family selection is less effective.
28. The smallest unit of selection is
    a) Genotype
    b) Family
    c) Individual
    d) Herd
29. Which of the following is NOT true in case of individual selection??
    a) It minimises the environmental effects
    b) Not applicable to sex limited traits
    c) Not effective for traits with low heritability
    d) It does not allow a great selection differential
30. The phenotypic value is a poor indicator of B.V. if
    a) h^2 is low
    b) h^2 is high
    c) h^2 is moderate
    d) None of the above

31. Individual selection is not suitable for selecting a male because
    a) The most important economic characters are sex limited
    b) Have low heritability estimates
    c) Genetic interval is shorter
    d) Both (a) and (b).
32. Which of the following are aids to individual selection?
    a) Additional records
    b) Most probable Producing ability (MPPA)
    c) Use of part records
    d) All of the above
33. Which of the following is NOT true with respect to 'addition records' ?
    a) It involves less cost
    b) It increases the generation interval
    c) The selection differential is reduced
    d) None of the above
34. Tandem selection is practiced for how many traits?
    a) Multiple trait
    b) Two trait at a time
    c) One trait at a time
    d) All of the above
35. Which of the following is NOT true for tandem method of selection?
    a) It is less efficient than other methods
    b) It requires more time for improvement
    c) This method does not depend on the genetic correlation among the traits under selection
    d) None of the above
36. Which of the following statements pertaining to tandem selection are correct?
    a) A desirable genetic association would lead improvement in other trait while selection is made for one trait.
    b) The low genetic correlation will decrease the efficiency of this method because there will be no correlated response in other trait.
    c) An undesirable genetic correlation between two trait results in a decrease in the other trait, would neutralize the genetic progress made in any one trait.
    d) All of the above
37. Independent Culling Level is practiced for how many traits?
    a) One trait at a time
    b) Two trait at a time
    c) Two or more trait at a time
    d) None of the above
38. In which type of selection, an animal is rejected despite of it being exceptionally good in one trait but little poor in another trait?
    a) Tandem selection
    b) Independent culling level selection method
    c) Total score or selection index
    d) None of the above

39. Which of the following is NOT true for Independent Culling Level?
    a) Selection of more than one trait
    b) Less emphasis to early expressed traits
    c) No compensation for other trait
    d) Culling at early age
40. What is the relationship between intensity of selection and number of traits?
    a) The intensity of selection is reduced with increase in number of traits
    b) The intensity of selection is increased with increase in number of traits
    c) The intensity of selection is not affected by increase in number of traits
    d) None of the above
41. Which of the following is NOT true for Total score or selection index method?
    a) It is an index of the net merit of an animal for many traits
    b) Each trait is weighted by a score and these scores for individual traits are summed to a total score for each animal
    c) Superiority in some traits can make up deficiency in others
    d) Culling levels are rigid
42. Which method permit extra merit in one trait to off set slight defects in another
    a) Tandem
    b) Independent Culling Level
    c) Both (a) and (b)
    d) Selection Index
43. Which of the following is NOT true for Total Score Method?
    a) Superior genotypes are saved for breeding
    b) It involves the technique of discriminant function
    c) The same intensity of selection is expected to give the same proportionate improvement for each trait
    d) The traits are correlated with each other to which the index gives appropriate consideration
44. The technique of discriminant function was originally developed by
    a) Fisher in 1936
    b) Smith in 1936
    c) Hazel in 1943
    d) None of the above
45. What is the requirements to construct selection index?
    a) The economic value or the relative net economic importance of each of the trait
    b) The genetic and phenotypic variances of all traits
    c) The phenotypic and genetic covariances among all traits
    d) All of the above
46. Which of the following is a economic traits for a dairy cattle
    a) Resistance to disease
    b) Body weight
    c) Height of animal
    d) Age at first calving

47. Which of the following is NOT taken into account while calculating Age at First Calving
    a) Expenditure on feed and fodder fed per day per head
    b) Labour and miscellaneous charges
    c) Both (a) and (b)
    d) Medicine charges
48. With reference to economic trait, one standard unit is equal to
    a) 100 percent standard deviation of the trait
    b) 10 percent standard deviation of the trait
    c) 1 percent standard deviation of the trait
    d) None of the above
49. What are the steps in construction of selection index?
    a) Estimation of partial regression coefficients- selection index- Estimation of genetic and economic parameters
    b) Estimation of partial regression coefficients – Estimation of genetic and economic parameters – Selection Index
    c) Estimation of genetic and economic parameters – Estimation of partial regression coefficients – Selection Index
    d) None of the above
50. The method of Restricted Selection Index was developed by
    a) Young and Finney
    b) Kempthrone and Nordskog
    c) Hazel and Lush
    d) None of the above
51. Which of the following is NOT an assumption in constructing Restricted Selection Index?
    a) Relative weights are known without error
    b) Relative economic weights remain constant over the range of variation likely to occur for the different traits
    c) Genetic and phenotypic variances are known without error
    d) The traits under consideration are non- heritable
52. Which of the following is NOT true for pedigree selection
    a) It is helpful in multistage selection
    b) Useful for sex-limited traits
    c) It introduces non random biases
    d) It is costly
53. The accuracy of pedigree selection is low because of –
    a) The different possibilities of combinations resulting from segregation of genes
    b) It is not possible to predict as to which half of the dam's genes are transmitted to the offspring because of the halving process and sampling nature of inheritance
    c) The different environmental conditions prevail at the time of taking records of ancestors and the individual
    d) All of the above

54. The accuracy of selection based on one Half-sib is
   a) 0.25 h b) 0.50 h
   c) 0.75 h d) 1.00 h
55. The accuracy of selection based on one Full-sib is
   a) 0.25 h b) 0.50 h
   c) 0.75 h d) 1.00 h
56. What is the relationship between accuracy OS sib selection and h^2
   a) The accuracy of sib selection decreases along with increase in h^2
   b) The accuracy of sib selection increases along with increase in h^2
   c) The accuracy of sib selection is not affected by h^2
   d) None of the above
57. Sire index is calculated on basis of performance of
   a) Individual b) Family
   c) Sib d) Progeny
58. Which among the following is the objective of calculation of sire indices?
   a) To provide the estimate of the breeding value (genetic worth)of the sire
   b) To rank the sires in order of their genetic merit for use in genetic improvement programs.
   c) Both (a) and (b)
   d) None of the above
59. Which of the following is the method used for indexing of sires
   a) Simple daughter average index
   b) Daughter-dam comparison method
   c) Herd-mate comparison method
   d) All of the above
60. Equi-parent index is valid only if
   a) h2 = 1.00 b) h2 = 0.75
   c) h2 = 0.50 d) h2 = 0.25
61. Simple Daughter Average Index was proposed by?
   a) Edward b) Lush
   c) Tomar d) Henderson
62. Equi- parent index was first used for the selection of
   a) Boar b) Sire
   c) Cock d) Ram
63. Equi-parent index was first proposed by?
   a) Edward b) Lush
   c) Hansson d) Henderson

64. With reference to the equi parent index, Daughter' s average is equal to
   a) Sire's Breeding Value/ 2
   b) Dam's Breeding Value/2
   c) (Sire's Breeding Value+ Dam's Breeding Value)/2
   d) None of the above

65. With reference to equi parent index , sire's breeding value or sire's index is equal to
   a) (2× Dam's average) – (Daughter's average)
   b) (2× Daughter's average) – (Dam's average)
   c) 2× (Daughter's average – Dam's average)
   d) None of the above

66. Which of the following is NOT true with respect to simple daughter average index?
   a) Useful for predicting the performance of future daughters of the sire born to dams of the same genetic level as those used for producing current daughters
   b) The variable numbers of daughters available for different sires are not taken into consideration
   c) The future daughters will be reared and tested under similar environmental conditions as the current daughters
   d) It takes into consideration heritability of the trait

67. Equi parent index is also known as?
   a) Intermediate Index b) Mount Hope Index
   c) Hanson Yapp's index d) All of the above

68. Which one of the following is a problem of equi parent index?
   a) The dams and daughters may be seldom used under similar environmental conditions
   b) Equi-parent index is valid only if the trait is assumed to be completely heritable
   c) The index does not take into account the variable numbers of daughters available for different sires.
   d) All of the above

69. The herd- mate comparison method of sire evaluation is also known as
   a) Intermediate Index
   b) Contemporary daughter average index
   c) Hanson Yapp's index
   d) Mount Hope Index

70. The herd-mate comparison method of sire evaluation is credited to
   a) Edward b) Lush
   c) Hansson d) Henderson

71. The herd-mate comparison method of sire evaluation compares
   a) The production of bull's daughters with their counterparts in the same herd in different year
   b) The production of bull's daughters with their counterparts in different herd in same year
   c) The production of bull's daughters with their counterparts in the same herd in same year
   d) The production of bull's daughters with their counterparts in the different herd in different year
72. The term 'herd mate refers to
   a) All the daughters of all other sires which had calved in the same month or preceding or succeeding one month
   b) All the daughters of all other sires which had calved in the same month or preceding or succeeding two months
   c) All the daughters of all other sires which had calved in the same month or preceding or succeeding three months
   d) All the daughters of all other sires which had calved in the same month or preceding or succeeding six months
73. The average performance of the herd mates is based on
   a) 13 months moving average in the year
   b) 7 months moving average in the year
   c) 5 months moving average in the year
   d) 3 months moving average in the year
74. What is the condition of modified herd-mate comparison method??
   a) A bull must have 5 daughters with herd- mates for the first time
   b) A bull must have 10 daughters with herd-mates for the first time
   c) A bull must have 15 daughters with herd-mates for the first time
   d) A bull must have 20 daughters with herd-mates for the first time
75. The literary meaning of 'tandem' is
   a) All at a time
   b) Two or more at a time
   c) One after the other
   d) None of the above
76. The scope of genetic improvement is greatest through
   a) Selection of males
   b) Selection of females
   c) Both (a) and (b)
   d) None of the above
77. Which of the following is the best for selection of cock?
   a) Sib selection
   b) Combined selection
   c) Both (a) and (b)
   d) Progeny testing
78. Which of the following is a general consideration in Breeding Program?
   a) Development Policy
   b) Production environment and systems including market conditions
   c) Infrastructure
   d) All of the above

79. Which of the following is a genetic consideration in Breeding Program?
    a) Choice of foundation stock(s)
    b) Trait measurement
    c) Dissemination of genetic improvement
    d) All of the above

80. Which of the following is NOT acomponent of the genetic improvement program under Net Work/ AICRP?
    a) Non- nominated matings
    b) Selection of test bulls
    c) Test mating program
    d) Freezing and storage of semen of test bulls

81. Which of the following is a progeny testing under Organized Herds?
    a) Single – herd progeny testing
    b) Associated – herd progeny testing
    c) Both (a) and (b)
    d) None of the above

82. Which program has lower accuracy in progeny testing program?
    a) Single- herd progeny testing
    b) Associated- herd Progeny testing
    c) Multi-herd progeny testing
    d) None of the above

83. Which of the following is a salient feature of field progeny testing program?
    a) Selection of operational area
    b) Animal identification and performance recording
    c) Data storage, analysis and breeding value evaluation
    d) All of the above

84. Which of the following has published a manual for implementing a field progeny testing program?
    a) National Dairy Research Institute, Karnal
    b) National Dairy Development Board
    c) Central Institute of Research on Buffalo, Hissar
    d) National Institute of Animal Health

85. The decision on introduction/ migration or within herd improvement rest on which of the following factor?
    a) Performance of the herd
    b) Genetic variability
    c) Heterotic Effect
    d) All of the above

86. Which is the best method for multi trait selection?
    a) Index selection
    b) Independent culling level
    c) Tandem
    d) All of the above

87. Selection alone is not sufficient when the genetic variation
    a) Of additive type is important
    b) Non-additive type is important
    c) Both additive and non additive has equal importance
    d) None of the above

88. Individual selection is advocated for which traits
   a) Traits with high heritability
   b) Expressed in both sexes
   c) Both (a) and (b)
   d) Neither (a) not (b)
89. The genetic improvement by selection in a generation is a function of which of the following
   a) Generation interval
   b) Accuracy of selection
   c) Selection pressure
   d) All of the above
90. The formulation of breeding plan involves:
   a) To decide the type of production required
   b) The choice of breed as a foundation stock
   c) To take a decision whether genetic improvement within herd/flock is possible or introduction of superior genes from outside is required
   d) All of the above
91. Individual selection is not suitable for which traits?
   a) Traits with high heritability
   b) Expressed in both sexes
   c) Both (a) and (b)
   d) Neither (a) not (b)
92. Which of the following is a feature of National Cattle Breeding Policy?
   a) Selective breeding in indigenous breeds
   b) Crossbreeding of non-descript low producers with exotic breeds stabilizing 50-75% exotic inheritance
   c) Conservation of endangered indigenous breeds
   d) All of the above
93. The indigenous breeds of animals in India have poor production potential for the reason of
   a) Improper breeding policies
   b) Inadequate nutrition
   c) Lack of health coverage
   d) All of the above
94. Which of the following is a situation for use of indirect selection?
   a) When measurement of trait is difficult and expensive
   b) Inability to apply high selection intensity
   c) When direct selection increases generation interval
   d) All of the above
95. What is breeding value?
   a) It is additive
   b) No additive
   c) Product
   d) None of the above
96. Breeding plan involves
   a) Selection system
   b) Mating system
   c) Both (a) and (b)
   d) None of the above
97. What is panmixia?
   a) Random mating
   b) Non- random mating
   c) Positive assortative mating
   d) Negative assortative mating

98. Which of the following is a advantage of random mating?
   a) Simple and inexpensive
   b) Useful in genetic evaluation
   c) Serves as benchmark for comparing the genetic consequences of other systems of mating
   d) All of the above

99. Genetic improvement of livestock involves:
   a) Choice of parents (selection)
   b) Choice of mates (mating system)
   c) Both (a) and (b)
   d) Neither (a) not (b)

100. What is not true with respect to milk yield?
   a) It is economically most important
   b) It is not heritable
   c) It is accurately measurable
   d) None of the above

101. What is the heritability of milk yield?
   a) 0.25
   b) 0.50
   c) 0.75
   d) 0.10

102. National Cooperative Dairy Herd Improvement Program is a program of
   a) USA
   b) India
   c) UK
   d) Australia

103. In a breeding herd, if not weaned, milk yield is recorded from which day??
   a) 1st
   b) 3rd
   c) 5th
   d) 10th

104. In a breeding herd, if weaned, milk yield is recorded from which day?
   a) 1st
   b) 3rd
   c) 5th
   d) 10th

105. What is the 'days to reach peak yield' in case of dairy cow?
   a) 30-40 days
   b) 50-60 days
   c) 60-70 days
   d) 70-80 days

106. The process of crossing of a large number of individuals with a tester line is known as
   a) Crossbreeding
   b) Recurrent selection
   c) Reciprocal recurrent selection
   d) All of the above

107. What is the full form of NAGA?
   a) Non Acquiring Genetic Aggregation
   b) Non Additive Genetic Aggregation
   c) Non Additive Gene action
   d) Non Acquiring Gene action

108. In which process randomly selected individuals from each each of the two non inbred strains are progeny tested in crosses with each other?
   a) Crossbreeding
   b) Recurrent selection
   c) Reciprocal recurrent selection
   d) All of the above

109. What is the full form of GCA?
   a) Gross Compatibility Assessment
   b) General Combining Ability
   c) Gross Computing Ability
   d) None of the above

110. What is the full form of SCA?
   a) Specific Combining Ability
   b) Specific Compatibility Assessment
   c) Specific Computing Ability
   d) None of the above

111. Which of the following factors reduces the net response to selection?
   a) Heritability
   b) Selection differential
   c) Population size
   d) All of the above

112. What is the relationship between the numbers of genes affecting a character and magnitude of their effect?
   a) Inverse
   b) Direct
   c) Variable
   d) None of the above

113. What is the relationship between the numbers of genes affecting a character and response to selection?
   a) Inverse
   b) Direct
   c) Variable
   d) None of the above

114. Which of the following is a reason of failure to respond in the presence of genetic variance?
   a) Over dominance genetic action
   b) Low frequency of recessive genes
   c) Linkage
   d) All of the above

115. Out crossing can be done in which of the following way?
   a) Crossing of two selected strains at limit
   b) Crossing of selected strain at limit to an unselected strain
   c) Both (a) and (b)
   d) None of the above

116. The effects of mutagenic agents are
   a) Selective
   b) Random
   c) Seldom selective
   d) None of the above

117. Which of the following is a salient feature of field progeny testing program?
   a) Selection of operational area
   b) Animal identification and performance recording
   c) Data storage, analysis and breeding value evaluation
   d) All of the above

118. Which of the following is a collateral relative?
   a) Full sib b) Uncle
   c) Nephew d) All of the above
119. Which of the following is not a collateral relative?
   a) Mother b) Full sib
   c) Half sib d) Nephew
120. Which of the following is progeny?
   a) Son b) Daughter
   c) Both (a) and (b) d) None of the above
121. The most effective method of selection
   a) Mass selection b) Pedigree selection
   c) Progeny testing d) Selection index
122. Quantitative traits shows
   a) Continuous variation b) Discontinuous variation
   c) Both a and b d) None of the above
123. 2 way selections is also called as
   a) Centripetal selection b) Disruptive selection
   c) Balanced selection d) None of the above
124. Stabilizing selection is also known as
   a) Centipetal selection b) Unifying selection
   c) Balanced selection d) All of these
125. 1 way selection is also called as
   a) Centipetal selection b) Unifying selection
   c) Balanced selection d) Directional selection
126. Positive assortative mating is an example of
   a) Random mating b) Inbreeding
   c) Mating of dwarf sire to dwarf dam d) Directional selection
127. Jersey of goat
   a) Alpine b) Saanen
   c) Anglo Nubian d) All of these
128. Excellent chevon production
   a) Jamunapari b) Beetal
   c) Barbari d) Black Bengal
129. Best dairy goat in India
   a) Jamunapari b) Sirohi
   c) Pantja d) Barbari
130. Mildest form of out breeding is
   a) Crossbreeding b) Out crossing
   c) Close breeding d) Criss crossing

131. Sire evaluation by BLUP method is given by
    a) Henderson   b) Lush
    c) Harvey   d) Bakewell

132. In open nucleus breeding system, the replacement female of nucleus are generated from
    a) Cooperating herds   b) Nucleus herd
    c) Both (a) and (b)   d) None

133. Close herd is
    a) No male transferred to outside
    b) Male selected & used within the same herd
    c) Both (a) and (b)
    d) No female transferred from outside

134. PT is a
    a) Method of selection of sires   b) Method of selection of dams
    c) Method of selection of progeniesT   d) Method of selection of family

135. Improvement of human race
    a) Eugenics   b) Heredity
    c) Euphenics   d) Epigenetics

136. In RRS,
    a) Parent in each generation selected on the performance of sires
    b) Parent in each generation selected on the performance of progenies
    c) Parent in each generation selected on the performance of dam
    d) All

137. ONBS cocept given by
    a) Kempthorn   b) Wright
    c) Kunningham   d) All

138. GCA is
    a) Caused by Non-Additive gene effect   b) Caused by Additive gene effect
    c) Both (a) & b)   d) None

139. Objectives of AICRP on goat
    a) Increase the production of meat   b) Increase the production of fiber
    c) Increase the production of milk   d) All of the above

140. Dam Selection by
    a) Reproduction problem   b) EBV
    c) MPPA   d) All

141. Kadaknath poultry blood is darker
    a) Due to melanin   b) Due tocarotene
    c) Due toanthocyanin   d) Due to xanthophylls

142. HU (Haugh Unit) is related to
   a) Albumen
   b) Yolk
   c) Egg shell
   d) All

143. Diallel cross in case of
   a) Swine
   b) Poultry
   c) Both (a) and b)
   d) All

144. No of CPDO working in India for poultry
   a) 4
   b) 7
   c) 8
   d) 15

145. The widest possible kind of out breeding is
   a) Top crossing
   b) Species hybridization
   c) In breeding
   d) Line breeding

146. Founder effect is
   a) Genetic drift
   b) Selection
   c) Mutation
   d) Migration

147. Hen Feathering in poultry is controlled by
   a) Sex limited gene
   b) Sex influenced gene
   c) Both (a) & (b)
   d) None

148. Random mating is
   a) Out breeding
   b) Pan mixia
   c) Both (a) &(b)
   d) None

149. By cross breeding
   a) New breeds can be evolved
   b) Composite breeds can be evolved
   c) Both (a) & (b)
   d) None

150. Rotational crossing
   a) Crossbreeding with a sequence of three or more breeds
   b) Crossbreeding
   c) Both (a) & b)
   d) None

Answer Key

1	b	2	c	3	a	4	c	5	d	6	d	7	a
8	c	9	b	10	d	11	a	12	a	13	b	14	a
15	c	16	a	17	d	18	c	19	d	20	b	21	a
22	d	23	a	24	a	25	d	26	d	27	a	28	c
29	d	30	a	31	d	32	d	33	a	34	c	35	c
36	d	37	c	38	b	39	b	40	a	41	d	42	d
43	c	44	a	45	d	46	d	47	d	48	c	49	c
50	b	51	d	52	d	53	d	54	a	55	b	56	a

57	d	58	c	59	d	60	a	61	a	62	c	63	c
64	c	65	b	66	d	67	d	68	d	69	b	70	d
71	c	72	b	73	c	74	b	75	c	76	a	77	c
78	d	79	d	80	a	81	c	82	c	83	d	84	b
85	d	86	a	87	b	88	c	89	d	90	d	91	d
92	d	93	d	94	d	95	a	96	c	97	a	98	d
99	c	100	b	101	a	102	a	103	c	104	a	105	b
106	b	107	c	108	c	109	b	110	a	111	d	112	a
113	b	114	d	115	c	116	b	117	d	118	d	119	a
120	c	121	d	122	a	123	b	124	d	125	d	126	c
127	c	128	d	129	a	130	b	131	a	132	c	133	b
134	a	135	a	136	b	137	c	138	b	139	d	140	d
141	a	142	a	143	b	144	a	145	b	146	a	147	b
148	b	149	a	150	a								

20

Feed and Fodder

Anuradha Kumari, Utkarsh Kumar Tripathi, Manish Kumar and Anshuman Kumar

Faculty of Veterinary and Animal Sciences, IAS, RGSC, Banaras Hindu University Varanasi, Uttar Pradesh

Introduction

Current status of feed and fodder availability in India

Globally India ranks 1st in terms of total livestock (535.78 million) and buffalo population in the world (109.85 million), 2nd in cattle (192.49 million), goat (148.88 million) and 3rd in sheep population. So, the availability of adequate quantity and quality feed and fodder resources for livestock is essential for improving livestock productivity. Grazing lands and fodder cultivation areas are gradually dwindling either due to degradation or restriction for livestock grazing. Total area under fodder cultivation is around 8.4 mha (5.23%) which is almost static for the past two decades. Even though feed and fodder availability has improved in the last decade still gap exists with demand and availability of fodder during lean periods and abnormal weather conditions like droughts/floods. At present, India faces a net deficit of 35.6% green fodder (GF), 10.95% dry crop residues and 44% concentrate feeds. In India, open forest cover is around 29 million hectares (mha), which can be further utilized for growing fodder trees without affecting standing trees, mostly as an under-storey on the partially shaded ground

Area under fodder production

Sorghum (2.6 M ha) and Egyptian clover (1.9 M ha) account for roughly 54% of the total cultivated fodder area in the kharif and *rabi* seasons, respectively. Farmers are growing grasses and legumes including hybrid Napier, guinea grass, paragrass, velvet bean, stylo, etc in many areas. Farmers with small ruminants, in particular, pick tree-top fodders in times of scarcity.

Availability of data (2000-01) on grazing resources shows that forests contribute about 69.41 mha (22.70%) followed by fallow lands (8.1%), barren uncultivable wasteland (6.30%), cultivable wastelands (4.50%), permanent grazing lands (3.60%) and fallow land other than current fallows (3.30%) and total common property resources other than forests (17.70%). Thus, sizeable amount of fodder demand can be fulfilled through vast grasslands and rangelands.

Importance of forage crops

Fodders crops are cultivated plant species that are utilized as livestock feed. Fodder refers mostly the crops which are harvested and used for stall feeding. Forage may be defined as the vegetative matter, fresh or preserved, utilized as feed for animals. Forage crops include grasses, legumes, crucifers and other crops cultivated and used in the form of hay, pasture, fodder and silage

Characteristics of fodder crops

- Quick re growth and short duration.
- Profuse foliage and heavy yield of fodders.
- Should have high palatability and nutritive value.
- Should be adaptable to various agro-climatic conditions and different soils.
- Resistance to diseases and pests and safe to feed at all stages of its growth without any deleterious effect on animal health and growth.

Plant sources of animal feed

- **Straw:** Means the dried remnant of a crop from which the seed has been threshed. The term is most commonly used to wheat, oats, barely, rice etc.
- **Husks (Hulls):** Husks are available in bulk in the milling industry like rice milling, solvent extraction plants for groundnut oil and corn oil, groundnut husks, maize husks etc. They are of low density and are unpalatable.
- **Hay:** Conserved of high-quality forages by drying is termed as hay.
- **Silage:** Conservation of green fodders under anaerobic conditions in the green form is called ensiling and the conserved green fodder is called silage.
- **Stovers:** Stovers are the byproducts after harvesting the grains (maize, jowar, millets etc. .
- **Grasses:** All grasses belonging to the family of plants, gramineae comprising 450 genera and more than 6000 species distributed throughout the world. Grasses include all the cultivated cereal feed crops. Grasses considerably vary in their habbits, size and habitat. Some grasses are annuals, while others are perennials. When plants dries up after flowering and seeding in the course of a single season, it is termed as annual, but when new shoots and older ones ending in inflorescence and found mixed in the same plant, it is termed perennial.

Forages are classified based on various features

On the basis of season of cultivation

- Kharif (June - September) Eg. Cowpea, Cluster bean, Field bean, Bajra, Sorghum, Maize
- Rabi (October -Dec/Jan) Eg. Berseem, Lucerne, Oats, Barley
- Summer (April - June) Eg. Cowpea, Cluster bean, Field bean, Bajra, Sorghum, Maize

On the basis of nutrient density in the dry matter

- **Non –maintenance -** Eg. Wheat straw, Rice straw, Ragi straw, Maize and Sorghum stover, Jungle hay, cereal forages harvested at advanced maturity
- **Maintenance** - Eg. Sorghum, Maize, Bajra, Hybrid napier, Para grass and all grasses
- **Production** - Maize, Oats, Barley, Sorghum Root crops etc. (Low protein) and Berseem, Lucerne, Cowpea, Subabool and all Legumes (High protein)

On the basis of plant family and duration of the crop

- Generally fodders are grouped as those belong to the plant family Leguminacea and those not. It is called legume fodders and non-legume fodders. Each category has annuals and perennials.
- **Legumes** - Eg
- *Annual :* Berseem, Cowpea
- *Perennial :* Stylo, Desmanthes
- **Non-legumes** - Eg.
- *Annual :* Fodder Maize, Sorghum
- *Perennial :* Hybrid Napier grass, Para grass

1. International fed classification proposed by
   a) Antoine laoisier b) Crampton and Harris
   c) Wolff-Lehmann d) M.Babcock
2. How many is groups in international feed classes?
   a) 5 b) 6
   c) 7 d) 8
3. International feed classes also known as
   a) NRC classification b) ARC classification
   c) ICAR classification d) BARC classification
4. Feed stuff is classified into roughage and concentrate based on
   a) Crude protein content b) Crude fiber content
   c) Water content d) NFE content
5. Productive type roughage has
   a) Below 3% DCP b) More than 3% DCP
   c) About 3-5% DCP d) More than 5% DCP
6. Cereal fodder is classified under
   a) Maintenance type of roughage b) Productive type of roughage
   c) Non maintenance type of roughage d) None of these
7. Product that contains more than 35% cell wall in their dry state are classified as
   a) Forage b) Concentrate
   c) Fodder d) Husk
8. Feedstuff that contains less than 18% crude fiber are classified as
   a) Forage b) Roughages
   c) Fodder d) Concentrate
9. Product obtained by drying in the sun or shed is termed as
   a) Hay b) Straw
   c) Fodder d) Stover
10. In hay moisture content of the product is not more than....................%
    a) 12-14 b) 14-16
    c) 16-18 d) 18-20

11. By product leftover after harvesting, threshing and removal of the grain from cereal and millet is

    a) Hay b) Straw
    c) Fodder d) Stover

12. Stalks and leaves of millet crop left over after separating the grains is known as

    a) Bagasse b) Straw
    c) Roughages d) Stover

13 Dry outer covering of grains is

    a) Bagasse b) Hull
    c) Husk d) Shells

14. Which one is not a legumes pasture

    a) Stylosantheshamata b) Cenchrus ciliaris
    c) Butterfly pea d) Siratro

15. Pasture when cut and fed to animal in its own stall is known as

    a) Controlled grazing b) Zero grazing
    c) Rotational grazing d) Deferred grazing

16. Which one is kharif fodder crop

    a) Oats b) Lucerne
    c) Berseem d) Cow pea

17. Rabi fodder crop

    a) Jowar b) Maize
    c) Oats d) Sunhemp

18. Fodder grass

    a) Babul b) Subabul
    c) Sesbania d) Sudan

19. Fodder tree

    a) Napier b) Guinea
    c) Rhodes d) Glyricidia

20. To be classified as a protein feed stuff, the protein content should be...

    a) Less than 18% b) More than 18%
    c) Less than 20% d) More than 20%

21. Energy feed

    a) Cereal grains b) Mill by products
    c) Nuts and roots d) All of the above

22. Hydraulic pressure method of oil extraction from seed is also known as

    a) Ghani process b) Expeller process
    c) Solvent extraction process d) Soiling process

23. Fat content of cake processed by solvent extraction process

    a) less than 1% b) 6%
    c) 8% d) 10%

24. Which one is correct
   a) Meal having more protein content
   b) Meal having higher fat content
   c) Cake having more protein content
   d) Cake having less fat content
25. Stage at which 1/10 to 2/3 of the plants are in bloom is called
   a) Early bloom stage
   b) Mid bloom stage
   c) Full bloom stage
   d) Late bloom stage
26. Leguminous fodder
   a) Sorghum
   b) Maize
   c) Lucerne
   d) Sudan
27. Fodder is not primary feed for which animal?
   a) Cow
   b) Pig
   c) Goat
   d) Buffalo
28. ICAR-Indian Grassland and Fodder Research Institute (IGFRI), located at
   a) Alamadhi, Chennai
   b) Jhansi, M.P
   c) Hissar, Hariyana
   d) Hassarghata, Bangalore
29. Leguminous fodder is
   a) High in fiber
   b) High in fat
   c) High in protein
   d) High in calcium
30. Silage is
   a) Sun dried fodder
   b) Succulent, fermented and preserved dried fodder
   c) Succulent, fermented and preserved green fodder
   d) Succulent, fermented and preserved dried hay
31 Urea is good source of which mineral for crops
   a) Nitrogen
   b) Potassium
   c) Phosphorus
   d) Calcium
32. Pusagiant napier grass and paddy straw contains the metal- binding substances called
   a) Phosphates
   b) Carbonates
   c) Oxalates
   d) Sulphates
33. Crops are not good for silage making
   a) CHO rich fodder
   b) Leguminous fodder
   c) Cereals
   d) All
34. A silage containing animal organic waste (poultry dropping, swine excreta is called
   a) Haylage
   b) Wastelage
   c) Brown silage
   d) Bad silage
35. Under intensive production system feeding constitute about
   a) 50 % of the expenditure on livestock production
   b) 60 % of the expenditure on livestock production
   c) 70 % of the expenditure on livestock production
   d) 80 % of the expenditure on livestock production

36. Major crop residue available in India is
 a) Paddy straw b) Wheat straw
 c) Sugar can bagasse d) Husk
37. DCP content of paddy straw is
 a) 0 b) 1
 c) 2 d) 3
38. Area under cultivated fodder accounts for only .... of the total cultivated land
 a) 4% b) 8.4 %
 c) 15% d) 22.7%
39. Currently country is facing deficiency of green fodder around
 a) 35.6% b) 10.95%
 c) 44% d) 25
40. Losses of nutrients in hay making due to...............
 a) By shattering b) Losses in fermentation
 c) By leaching d) All the above
41. Russian giant is a variety of
 a) Soya bean b) Leucerne
 c) Cowpea d) Cluster bean
42. Which type silo common in India?
 a) Bunker silo b) Tower silo
 c) Trench silo d) Pit silo
43. DCP % of leguminous fodder is
 a) 1 b) 3
 c) 5 d) 7
44. DCP % of non-leguminous fodder is
 a) 1 b) 3
 c) 5 d) 7
45. Non leguminous fodder crop
 a) Clovers b) Medics
 c) Crotalaria d) Teosinte
46. Not a member of crotalaria fodder crop
 a) Sunhemp b) Lobia
 c) Sudan d) Kudzu vine
47. Cereal fodder
 a) Para b) Sudan
 c) Bajra d) Napier
48. Hybrid napier is cross of Napier with
 a) Sorghum b) Oat
 c) Bajra d) Maize

49. Scientific name of Napier grass
    a) Brachianamutica
    b) Panicum maximum
    c) Pennisetum purpureum
    d) Panicum antidotale
50. Scientific name of sudan grass
    a) Brachianamutica
    b) Chloris gayana
    c) Sorghum vulgare
    d) Panicum antidotale
51. Hariali grass
    a) Kolukattain grass
    b) Dhub grass
    c) Giant star grass
    d) Masel grass
52 Introduced grass
    a) Sewan grass
    b) Deenabandhu grass
    c) Marvel grass
    d) Anjan grass
53. Pennisetum pedicellatum is
    a) Deenabandhu grass
    b) Napier grass
    c) Guinea grass
    d) Para grass
54. As per BIS specification the minimum crude protein % in grade I compound feed is
    a) 18
    b) 20
    c) 22
    d) 24
55. Fodder production and utilization depend on the
    a) Cropping pattern
    b) Climate
    c) Socioeconomic condition
    d) All the above
56. The ICAR-National Institute of Animal Nutrition and Physiology (NIANP) located at
    a) Chennai
    b) Hyderabad
    c) Bangalore
    d) New Delhi
57. Sweet clover is
    a) Shaftal
    b) Senji
    c) Berseem
    d) Lobia
58. Makchari
    a) Sorghum
    b) Pearl millet
    c) Teosinte
    d) Barley
59. Wheat straw is main crop residue in
    a) Arid ecosystem
    b) Irrigated ecosystem
    c) Rain fed ecosystem
    d) Hill and mountain area
60. Major concentrate ingredient in India ?
    a) Bran
    b) Chunnies
    c) Oil cakes
    d) Husks
61. Of the total available concentrate ingredients major portion is utilized in
    a) Large ruminant production
    b) Small ruminant production
    c) Poultry sector
    d) Aquaculture

62. The area under cultivated fodder

a) 2.6 million ha b) 1.9 million ha
c) 5.6 million ha d) 8.4 million ha

63. Area under forest in India

a) 4.4% b) 8.0%
c) 22.7% d) 33%

64. Plant species that are cultivated and harvested for feeding the animals is

a) Silage b) Hay
c) Fodder d) Forage

65. Among kharif crop which one occupy the maximum cultivated fodder crop area

a) Sorghum b) Maize
c) Bajra d) Jawar

66. Among rabi crop which one occupy the maximum cultivated fodder crop area

a) Berseem b) Senji
c) Sarson d) Safflower

67. Not a cultivated fodder tree

a) Glyricedia b) Subabul
c) Orchard d) Sesbania

68. Tree leaves are deficient in

a) Ca b) P
c) Both d) None

69. The green forage that are cut and fed in fresh condition to the animals termed as

a) Hay making b) Silage making
c) Haylage d) Soiling of crop

70. Moisture content of silage

a) 50-55% b) 60-65%
c) 70-75% d) 90-95%

71. Cereals are deficient in

a) Ca b) P
c) Vit-D d) All

72. Ph of very good silage

a) 3.5 -4.2 b) 4.2-4.5
c) 4.5-4.8 d) >4.8

73. Best crop for silage making

a) Maize b) Bajra
c) Oat d) Sorghum

74. Dhurrin (a precursor for HCN) present particularly in the early stages of

a) Bajra b) Barley
c) Sorghum d) Maize

75. Brix value term related
   a) Urea b) Molasses
   c) Silage d) Fat

76. Tamarind seed hulls contains
   a) Lignin b) Tanin
   c) Ricin d) Mowrin

77. Top feed resources includes
   a) Paddy straw b) Grass
   c) Tree fodder d) Cereal fodder

78. Poor silage have
   a) High butyric acid content b) Low pH
   c) Bad smell d) Lactic acid fermenting bacterial

79. Subabul leaves contain anti nutritional factor
   a) Tannin b) Mimosine
   c) Gossypol d) Cydopropenoids

80. Brewers grains is a good source of
   a) Protein and vitamins B b) Fiber and minerals
   c) Energy and minerals d) Energy and calcium

81. Green forage in the ration helps to meet out
   a) Carotene requirement b) Vitamin D requirement
   c) Vitamin B_{12} requirement d) Calcium requirement

82. Tubers are rich in
   a) Protein b) Fat
   c) Carbohydrate d) Fiber

83. Cow grazing on young leguminous fodder leads to
   a) Bloat b) Acidosis
   c) Ketosis d) Milk fever

84. Cereal grains are essentially
   a) Fat concentrate b) Carbohydrate concentrate
   c) Fiber concentrate d) Protein concentrate

85. According to BIS the concentrate mixture for dairy cattle should contain
   a) Minimum CP of 16% b) Minimum CP of 18%
   c) Minimum CP of 20% d) None of the above

86. Roughages are classified into succulent or dry based on its
   a) Crude fiber content b) Moisture content
   c) Crude protein content d) Fat content

87. The biological value of phosphorus in cereals and brans is less because presence of
   a) Phytate b) Oxalate
   c) Sulphate d) Chlorides

88. The bulkiness of a feed is due to
 a) High crude fiber content b) High crude protein content
 c) High fat content d) High ash content
89. MP chari is variety of
 a) Jawar b) Maize
 c) Teosinte d) Bajra
90. Fodder can be cultivated in water logged area
 a) NB-21 b) Para grass
 c) Guinea grass d) Anjan grass
91. NB-21 is high yielding variety developed by crossing of
 a) Napier and sorghum b) Napier and bajra
 c) Para and napier d) Napier and berley
92. Non leguminous annual fodder crop
 a) Oat b) Para grass
 c) Napier grass d) Anjan grass
93. Non leguminous perennial fodder crop
 a) Maize b) Bajra
 c) Napier d) Sorghum
94. Leguminous annual fodder crop
 a) Lucern b) Siratro
 c) Kudju d) Cow pea
95. Leguminous perennial fodder crop
 a) Cow pea b) Berseem
 c) Guar d) Stylo
96. Tree fodder having maximum protein content
 a) Alianthusexcelsa b) Azardiracht indica
 c) Leucaena leucocephala d) Jharberi
97. Grazing land occupied by perennial pasture or by self-seeding annual plants, which remains unploughed for a number of years
 a) Permanent pasture b) Rotation pasture
 c) Supplemental pasture d) Annual pasture
98. Type of natural pasture
 a) Range b) Wood land pasture
 c) Brush pasture d) All of the above
99. How many types of grass cover distributed in country
 a) 3 b) 4
 c) 5 d) 6
100. Grass cover type of mountain region is
 a) Sehima-Dichanthium type b) Temperate Alpine type
 c) Themeda-Arundinella type d) Phragmites-Saccharum Imperata type

101. Carrying capacity of semi -arid area is
  a) 0.2 ACU/ha b) 0.5 ACU/ha
  c) 1 ACU/ha d) 10 ACU/ha
102. Land on which different types of edible grasses and other plant grow for grazing livestock known as
  a) Ranches b) Pasture
  c) Fallow land d) Forest
103. How many types of grass cover distributed in plains
  a) 3 b) 4
  c) 5 d) 6
104. Area wise largest grass land cover of country
  a) Sehima-Dichanthium type
  b) Temperate Alpine type
  c) Themeda-Arundinella type
  d) Phragmites-Saccharum Imperata type
105. Quality of grass land with respect of utility for the livestock is best
  a) Dichanthium-Cenchrus-Lasiurus type
  b) Temperate Alpine type
  c) Themeda-Arundinella type
  d) Phragmites-Saccharum Imperata type
106. Consequences of over grazing
  a) Soil erosion b) Desertification
  c) Spread of unpalatable weeds d) All of the above
107. System of grazing in which the most productive animals graza first, followed by second best and so on known as
  a) Zero grazing b) Deferred grazing
  c) Hohenheim system d) Controlled continuous grazing
108. In western countries a hectare pasture is apportioned for grazing by
  a) 1 to 2 adult bovine in year b) 15 to 20 adult bovine in year
  c) 50 to 100 adult bovine in year d) > 100 adult bovine in year
109. System of grazing in which limiting the no of animals on a area of grass land on a continuous basis
  a) Controlled continuous grazing b) Deferred grazing
  c) Hohenheim system d) Rotational grazing
110. System of grazing, which stop grazing in the most vulnerable season
  a) Controlled continuous grazing b) Deferred grazing
  c) Hohenheim system d) Rotational grazing
111. Grazing land management is done by
  a) Pasture cultivation b) Reseeding
  c) User charges d) All of the these

112. Grass farming in forest of horticulture plantation enclosures is known as
   a) Silvipasture b) Dryland farming
   c) Plantation farming d) Mixed farming
113. Farm equipment used to smoothen the soil after ploughing
   a) Driller b) Combines
   c) Harrow d) Plough
114. Tree leaves are rich of
   a) Protein and Phosphorus b) Protein and magnesium
   c) Carbohydrate and calcium d) Protein and calcium
115. Water hyacinth when fed fresh to cattle leads to
   a) Tetany b) Diuresis
   c) Hypoxia d) Edema
116. Toxic principle present in mahua cake is
   a) Phenols b) Cyanides
   c) Maurine d) Tanins
117. Select the correct statement
   a) Fruit waste rich in proteins
   b) Vegetable waste rich in protein
   c) Fruit waste rich in either exract
   d) Vegetable waste rich in carbohydrate
118. Toxic symptom of urea toxicity occurs when, rumen ammonia level elevated to
   a) 20 mg/100ml b) 40 mg/100ml
   c) 80 mg/100ml d) 120 mg/100ml
119. Addition of which mineral is required when urea is supplemented in feed
   a) Nitrogen b) Calcium
   c) Sulphur d) Copper
120. The nitrogen fixing fodder tree
   a) Babul b) Neem
   c) Subabul d) Acacia
121. Fodder grass tolerate shade
   a) Para grass b) Pennisetum grass
   c) Guinea grass d) Rhodes grass
122. Lucerne is a ………. fodder crop:
   a) Annual b) Biennial
   c) Perennial d) All of these
123. Napier cannot withstand
   a) Water logging b) Saline soils
   c) Frost d) All of these

124. Fodder maize may be intercropped with
a) Lucerne
b) Berseem
c) Fodder cowpea
d) None of these

125. Kent, is popular variety of
a) Oat
b) Bajar
c) Barley
d) Maize

126. Most important cultivated species of Oat is
a) Avena sativa
b) Avena byzantine
c) Avena abyssisica
d) Avena brewis

127. Rhizobium species used for treating lucerne seeds
a) Rhizobium meliloti
b) Rhizobium trofolli
c) Bradyrhizobium japonicum
d) Rhizobium leguminosarum

128. Cluster bean is used as
a) Fodder
b) Feed
c) Vegetable
d) All of these

129. King of Forage crop.
a) Berseem
b) Lucerne
c) Oat
d) Sorghum

130. Queen of forage crop.
a) Berseem
b) Lucerne
c) Maize
d) Sorghum

131. Elephant Grass
a) Deenabandhu grass
b) Napier grass
c) Guinea grass
d) Para grass

132. Fodder that tolerates waterlogged condition
a) Deenabandhu grass
b) Napier grass
c) Guinea grass
d) Para grass

133. Para grass also known as
a) Dina grass
b) Buffalo grass
c) Hariali grass
d) Elephant grass

134. Causes of pasture deterioration of pastures is
a) Over grazing
b) Bad drainage
c) Depletion of soil fertility
d) All of these

135. Soil suitable for berseem cultivation is
a) Heavy soil
b) Sandy loam
c) Clay loam
d) Black soil

136. Dominant grass species found in India, called as Anjan grass is
a) Guinea grass
b) Stylosanthes
c) Cenchrus
d) Haryali grass

137. Major weed found in berseem is
   a) Chicory b) Orobanche
   c) Cuscuta d) Striga
138. Forage having C_4 type of photosynthesis
   a) Temperate grass b) Temperate legumes
   c) Tropical grasses d) Tropical legumes
139. Select the incorrect statement
   a) Lignin is higher in steam than leaves
   b) Lignin is higher in leaves than steam
   c) As plant mature lignin content increases
   d) Tropical climate stimulates more lignin production than temperate
140. In well preserved silage the fermentation losses should not exceed
   a) 0.1 to 1 % of the energy b) 0.3 to 3% of the energy
   c) 0.5 to 5 % of the energy d) 10 to 15 % of the energy
141. Meskawi is popular variety
   a) Cow pea b) Berseem
   c) Alfa-alfa d) Guar
142. One of the best drought and heat resistant fodder crops of the world
   a) Teosinte b) Jowar
   c) Para grass d) Maize
143. Low moisture silage
   a) Haylage b) Wastelage
   c) Brown silage d) Bad silage
144. Ideal leguminous crop for hay making
   a) Berseem b) Cow pea
   c) Clovers d) Lucerne
145. Form of storing hay
   a) Chopped hay b) Petteting
   c) Wafering d) All of these
146. Fibrous residue of the cane stalk left after crushing and extraction of the juice
   a) Molasses b) Bran
   c) Meals d) Bagasse
147. Not a correct guide line regarding urea feeding
   a) Calf are ill equipped to utilize
   b) Urea should not exceed 3 % of the total ration
   c) Urea should not be more than 3 % of a concentrate
   d) Urea should nor exceed one third of the total crude protein equivalent

148. The precipitated impurities contained in the cane juice, after removal by filtration is called

a) Pressmud
b) Bagasse
c) Molasses
d) Cane tops

149. The final effluent obtained in the preparation of sugar by repeated crystallization is

a) Pressmud
b) Bagasse
c) Molasses
d) Filter mud

150 Kharif season

a) June-September
b) October-Dec/Jan
c) April-June
d) July-October

Answer Key

1	b	2	d	3	a	4	b	5	d	6	a	7	a
8	d	9	a	10	a	11	b	12	d	13	c	14	b
15	b	16	d	17	c	18	d	19	d	20	d	21	d
22	a	23	a	24	a	25	b	26	c	27	b	28	b
29	c	30	c	31	a	32	c	33	b	34	b	35	c
36	a	37	a	38	a	39	a	40	d	41	c	42	d
43	b	44	a	45	d	46	c	47	c	48	c	49	c
50	c	51	b	52	b	53	a	54	c	55	d	56	c
57	b	58	c	59	a	60	c	61	c	62	d	63	c
64	c	65	a	66	a	67	c	68	b	69	d	70	b
71	a	72	a	73	a	74	c	75	b	76	b	77	c
78	a	79	b	80	a	81	a	82	c	83	a	84	b
85	c	86	b	87	a	88	a	89	a	90	b	91	b
92	a	93	c	94	d	95	d	96	c	97	a	98	d
99	c	100	b	101	c	102	b	103	b	104	a	105	b
106	d	107	c	108	a	109	a	110	b	111	d	112	a
113	c	114	d	115	b	116	c	117	b	118	c	119	c
120	c	121	c	122	c	123	d	124	c	125	a	126	a
127	a	128	d	129	a	130	b	131	b	132	d	133	b
134	d	135	c	136	c	137	a	138	c	139	b	140	c
141	b	142	b	143	a	144	d	145	d	146	d	147	b
148	a	149	c	150	a								

21

General Reproduction and Reproductive Performance of Animals

***Nikita Singh*[1], *Rajesh Kumar*[1], *Bhoopendra Singh*[1], and *Pramod Kumar*[2]**

[1]*Department of Veterinary Gynaecology and Obstetrics, College of Veterinary Science and Animal Husbandry, Acharya Narendra Deva University of Agriculture and Technology, Kumarganj, Ayodhya, Uttar Pradesh*

[2]*Department of Veterinary Physiology and Biochemistry, College of Veterinary Science and Animal Husbandry, Acharya Narendra Deva University of Agriculture and Technology, Kumarganj, Ayodhya, Uttar Pradesh*

Introduction

The study of general reproduction and reproductive performance in animals is a vast and intricate field that spans across various species, habitats, and biological systems. Reproduction is a fundamental biological process that ensures the continuity of life across generations. It involves a series of complex physiological and behavioural events, from mating and fertilization to gestation and birth. The general reproduction and reproductive performance in domesticated animals is a fascinating and complex field that has significant implications for various aspects of human society, including agriculture, pet ownership, and conservation efforts. Domesticated animals encompass a wide range of species, from farm animals such as cows and chickens to pets like dogs and cats, and even animals kept for conservation or recreational purposes, such as horses and certain bird species. Each of these species has unique reproductive systems and cycles, and understanding these is crucial for effective management and care. For instance, the gestation period for dogs is typically around two months, while for horses, it's closer to a year. Similarly, some birds, like parrots, may lay eggs only once or twice a year, while others, like chickens, can lay almost daily. Reproductive performance in domesticated animals is not just about the ability to produce offspring but also about the health, longevity, and quality of the offspring produced. Factors such as fertility, litter or clutch size, birth weight, survival rate, and growth rate are all important indicators of reproductive performance. Poor reproductive performance can lead to a range of issues, from economic losses in a farming context to the potential extinction of endangered species in a conservation context. Advancements in reproductive technologies, such as artificial insemination, embryo transfer, and even cloning, have revolutionized the field of animal reproduction. These technologies allow for improved genetic selection, increased productivity, and the preservation of endangered species. However, they also raise ethical and welfare considerations that must be carefully navigated. Furthermore, reproductive performance is influenced by a multitude of factors, including nutrition, health status, age, genetics, and environmental conditions. For example, stress, disease, or poor nutrition can all negatively impact reproductive function, leading to infertility or reduced fertility. Therefore, proper management and care practices are essential to ensuring optimal reproductive performance. In conclusion, the study of general reproduction and reproductive performance in domesticated animals is a complex and multifaceted field that plays a vital role in various aspects of human society. It requires a deep understanding of the biological processes involved in reproduction, as well as the various factors that can influence reproductive performance. As such, it remains an area of ongoing research and development with the potential to significantly impact our world.

1. What is the gestation period of stallion.
   a) 340 days b) 290 days
   c) 310 days d) 380 days
2. Which type of Placenta Present in Elephant.
   a) Zonary b) Cotyledonary
   c) Diffuse d) Discoidal
3. Sperm Abnormalities should not exceed?
   a) 10 b) 5-10
   c) 20 d) 1
4. Non-penetrating type of Cryoprotective used in semen dilution.
   a) Albumin b) DMSO
   c) Glycerol d) Fructose
5. Placentophagy is commonly noticed in?
   a) Cow b) Bitch
   c) Mare d) Sow
6. Ring womb condition is commonly found in.
   a) Cattle b) Mare
   c) Goat d) Dog
7. Foal heat occurs after how many days of foaling?
   a) 2-4 b) 15-20
   c) 12-15 d) None
8. Analogue of GnRH?
   a) Receptal b) Folligen
   c) Mephipristone d) Chorulone
9. Which Hormone used in superovulation?
   a) LH b) FSH
   c) PMSG d) both b and c
10. Dose rate of bromocriptine?
    a) 0.2 mg b) 0.3mg
    c) 5 mg d) 0.1mg
11. Time of Ovulation in cattle.
    a) 12 hrs after end of estrum b) Diestrus
    c) 12 hrs before onset of estrus d) All of the above

12. Which is not estrogen?
    a) Stilbesterol b) Progynon
    c) Estradiol benzoate d) Estrumate
13. Abortion caused by the vibriosis is due to?
    a) *C.fetus* b) Mycotic
    c) Brucella abortus d) None
14. Early embryonic death is suspected from?
    a) Long estrus cycle b) Short estrus cycle
    c) Intense estrus d) None
15. Which of the following enzymes involved during the process of Ovulation in cows.
    a) Lipase b) Hyoluronidase
    c) Collegenase d) Estrase
16. Which of following is dopamine agonists?
    a) Estrogen b) Duraprogen
    c) Chorulone d) Bromocriptine
17. Transuterine migration of conceptus is noticed in which species?
    a) Cow b) Sheep
    c) Sow d) Mare
18. Waxing of teat occur in which animal?
    a) Mare b) Cow
    c) Dog d) Sow
19. Common type of tumor of penis of Bull?
    a) TVT b) Squamous cell carcinoma
    c) Teratoma d) Transmissible fibroma pilloma
20. Aspermia denotes?
    a) Non volume b) Zero Sperm
    c) Decreased sperm. d) Increase sperm
21. Terminal part of penis contains spines?
    a) Dog b) Cat
    c) Camel d) Giraffe
22. Gynaecomastia is caused due to?
    a) Seminoma b) Leydig cell tumor
    c) Sertoli cell tumor d) All
23. Conception rate of cattle in India by AI is about?
    a) 40% b) 70%
    c) 80% d) 50%
24. Impotentiagenerandi disorder of Bull?
    a) No sex drive b) Testicular degeneration
    c) Low fertility d) Epididymitis

25. The tight coiling of sperm over mid piece is known?
   a) Diadem effect b) Cork screw
   c) Dag defect d) Knobbed
26. MRP of mare in days?
   a) 14 days b) 17 days
   c) 16 days d) 11 days
27. Secretion of ampulla in horse?
   a) Inositol b) Ergothioneine
   c) Fructose d) All
28. Function of Inositol in pig?
   a) Motility of sperm b) pH balance
   c) Improve concentration d) Osmotic balance
29. Highest concentration of sperm is found in?
   a) Pig b) Buck
   c) Bull d) Poultry
30. Fossa glandis is found in?
   a) Stallion b) Dog
   c) Bull d) Pig
31. Urethral process is found in-
   a) Pig b) Dog
   c) Ram d) stallion
32. Colliculisseminalis is part of-
   a) Bladder b) Urethra
   c) Epididymis d) Cowper gland
33. Match the following

List A	List B
a) Estrogen	1. 17-Carbon
b) Progesterone	2. 18-Carbon
c) Testosterone	3. 19-Carbon
d) Prostaglandin	4. 20-Carbon

   a) (a) -1, (b)-4, (c) -3,(d)-2 b) (a) -3,(b)-1, (c) -4,(d)-1
   c) (a) -2,(b)-1, (c) -4,(d)-3 d) (a) -1,(b)-2, (c) -3,(d)-4
34. Mach the following

List A	List B
a) Almond shape	1. Bitch
b) Kidney shape	2. Sow
c) Mulberry shape	3. Mare
d) Oval shape	4. Cow

   a) (a) -1,(b)-4, (c) -3,(d)-2 b) (a) -2,(b)-1, (c) -4,(d)-1
   c) (a) -3,(b)-2, c) -1,(d)-4 d) (a) -4,(b)-3, (c) -2,(d)-1

35. Mach the following

List A	List B
a) Inhibin	1. Increase FSH
b) Relaxin	2. Decrease FSH
c) PGF2 alpha	3. Dilate cervix
d) Follistatin	4. Uterine contraction

a) (a) -1,(b)-4, (c) -2,(d)-3
b) (a) -2,(b)-3, (c) -4,(d)-1
c) (a) -3,(b)-2, (c) -1,(d)-4
d) (a) -4,(b)-1, (c) -3,(d)-2

36. Mach the following

List A	List B
a) Bicarnuate	I. Mare
b) Bipartite	II. Human female
c) Simplex	III. Rabbit
d) Duplex	IV. Cow

a) (a) -4,(b)-1, c) -2,(d)-3
b) (a) -3,(b)-2, c) -1,(d)-4
c) (a) -2,(b)-3, c) -4,(d)-1
d) (a) -1,(b)-4, c) -3,(d)-2

37. Mach the following

List A	List B
a) GnRH	I. Pseudopregnancy
b) LH	II. Stimulate release of LH& FSH
c) Prolactin	III. Leydig cell
d) FSH	IV. Regulate spermiogenesis

a) (a) -2,(b)-4, c) -1,(d)-3
b) (a) -3,(b)-2, c) -4,(d)-1
c) (a) -2,(b)-3, c) -1,(d)-4
d) (a) -1,(b)-4, c) -3,(d)-2

38. Mach the following

List A	List B
a) ECG	1. Endometrial Cup
b) HCG	2. FSH like
c) PMSG	3. Spermatogonia
d) Testosterone	4. LH like

a) (a) -2,(b)-4, (c) -1,(d)-3
b) (a) -1,(b)-3, (c) -4,(d)-2
c) (a) -1,(b)-2, (c) -3,(d)-4
d) (a) -4,(b)-1, (c) -2,(d)-3

39. Mach the following

List A	List B
a) Prostaglandin	1. Pregnancy maintaining
b) Progesterone	2. milk ejaculatory
c) Estrogen	3. Lysis of CL
d) Oxytocin	4. Heat detection

a) (a) -2,(b)-4,(c) -1,(d)-3
b) (a) -1,(b)-3, (c) -4,(d)-2
c) (a) -3,(b)-2, (c) -4,(d)-1
d) (a) -2,(b)-1, (c) -3,(d)-4

40. Mach the following

List A - Animal	List B- Fertile life of sperm
a) Sow	1. 1-2 days
b) Cattle	2. 3-5 days
c) Horse	3. 1-3 days
d) Goat	4. 1-2 days
e) Sheep	5. 1-2 days

a) (a) -3,(b)-5, (c) -2,(d)-4,(e)-1
b) (a) -2,(b)-3, (c) -4,(d)-1,(e)-5
c) (a) -3,(b)-2, (c) -1,(d)-4,(e)-5
d) (a) -4,(b)-1, (c) -3,(d)-2,(e)-5

41. Mach the following

List A- Animal	List B- Fertile life of ovum
a) Horse	1. 6-8hrs
b) Sow	2. 8-12 hrs
c) Goat	3. 1 day
d) Sheep	4. 1 day
e) Cattle	5. 1 day

(1) (a) -1,(b)-2, c) -4,(d)-5,(e)-3
(2) (a) -2,(b)-3, c) -4,(d)-1,(e)-5
(3) (a) -3,(b)-2, c) -1,(d)-4,(e)-5
(4) (a) -4,(b)-1, c) -2,(d)-3,(e)-5

42. The first cloned sheep 'Dolly' was created through which of these techniques?

a) Nuclear transfer
b) Gene transfer
c) Germinal cell transfer
d) Somatic cell transfer

43. Lactose found in milk is a disaccharide composed of

a) Glucose and glucose
b) Glucose and fructose
c) Maltose and glucose
d) Galactose and glucose

44. The lightest body weighed goat is-

a) Beetal
b) Barbari
c) Jamnapari
d) Toggenburg

45. This method is carried out for the castration of male pigs

a) Burdizzo
b) Hot iron
c) Knife
d) Elastrator

46. The chemical nature of Estrogen is
    a) Amino acid
    b) Protein
    c) Fatty acid
    d) Steroid
47. Strip cup is used
    a) Just after milking
    b) Just before milking
    c) At the middle of milking
    d) Anytime during milking
48. Female Hen has a following set of chromosomes
    a) Xx
    b) Xw
    c) Zz
    d) Zy
49. Terminology used for the high per cent of abnormal sperms
    a) Teratozoospermia
    b) Aspermia
    c) Asthenozoospermia
    d) Necrozoospermia
50. Effect of novelty of stimulus females reduces refractory period in males is known as-
    a) Balling up effect
    b) Coolidge effect
    c) Bruce effect
    d) Pederasty
51. Testosterone is secreted by which cell-
    a) Islets cells
    b) Sertoli cells
    c) Brunner's gland
    d) Leydig cell
52. Erythritol sugar plays important role in pathogenesis of-
    a) Clostridium spp.
    b) Brucella spp.
    c) Bacillus spp.
    d) Corynebacterium spp.
53. Oxytocin is secreted by the:
    a) Adenohypophysis
    b) Neurohypophysis
    c) Zona glomerulosa
    d) Pars intermedia
54. Which of the following animal presents ovulation fossa on its ovary?
    a) Cow
    b) Mare
    c) Bitch
    d) Doe
55. Vibriosis in a herd can best be diagnosed by-
    a) Serum agglutination test
    b) Vaginal mucus agglutination test
    c) Milk ring test
    d) Rose Bengal plate test
56. Induction of estrus by premature regression of the corpus luteum can be done by using-
    a) PRID
    b) GnRH
    c) $PGF2\alpha$
    d) HCG
57. Under which of the following conditions animal is acyclic
    a) Delayed ovulation
    b) Silent heat
    c) Anovulation
    d) None of the above
58. Time of ovulation in a cow is-
    a) 12-24 hrs before the end of estrum
    b) 30-40 hrs after the end of estrum
    c) About the last day of estrum
    d) 10-12 hrs after the end of estrum

59. Yellowish or whitish, thick, opaque uterine secretion nourishing the ovum and embryo is called-
   a) Lochia b) Yolk sac
   c) Uterine milk d) Oviductal fluid
60. Length of diestrus period of estrus cycle in bovine is
   a) 10 days b) 13 days
   c) 18 days d) 15 days
61. Shortest period of estrous cycle is–
   a) Estrus b) Procesturs
   c) Metestrus d) Diestrus
62. Prostaglandin, fructose and ascorbic acid are secreated by-
   a) Seminal vesicles b) Prostate
   c) Cowper gland d) Epididymis
63. Study of male reproductive system is known as
   a) Gynaecology b) Andrology
   c) Reproductive physiology d) All
64. Split heat & foal heat is common in-
   a) Cattle b) Buffalo
   c) Mare d) Sheep
65. The hormone responsible for the growth of duct system of mammary gland
   a) Estrogen b) Progesterone
   c) Both d) None
66. Which of the following is spontaneous ovulator
   a) She - camel b) Rabbit
   c) Cat d) Cattle
67. Sperm reservoir in cow,ewe and doe is
   a) Vagina b) Cervix
   c) Uterus d) Utero- tubal junction
68. The site of fertilization in cattle is
   a) Ampullary - isthmic junction b) Ampulla
   c) Isthmus d) Uterus
69. Best season for total sperm production in the bull is
   a) Rainy b) Summer
   c) Autumn d) Winter
70. Post-coital pyometra in cattle is caused by
   a) Leptospira b) Listeria
   c) Trichomonas d) Campylobacter
71. Semen collection should be done during..... for best results
   a) Morning before feeling b) Morning after feeding
   c) Evening before feeling d) Evening after feeding

72. The second stage of parturition is characterized by....
    a) Dilation of the cervix
    b) Expulsion of fetal membrane
    c) Involution of uterus
    d) Delivery of the newborn
73. Gestation period of Sow is
    a) 114 days
    b) 110 days
    c) 105 days
    d) 100 days
74. Gestation period of Rabbit is...
    a) 45 days
    b) 30 days
    c) 35 days
    d) 50 days
75. Cocking of the tail is the method of pregnancy diagnosis in...
    a) Mare
    b) Sow
    c) She- camel
    d) Cattle
76. Trichomonas foetus causes Abortion in cattle during ...... trimester of pregnancy.
    a) 1st
    b) 2nd
    c) 3rd
    d) None
77. MRP in sow is due to ...?
    a) Luteal Estrogen
    b) Embryonic Estrogen
    c) Placental lactogen
    d) All
78. Most confirmatory sign of heat in cow...?
    a) Restlessness
    b) Bellowing
    c) Vulvar discharge
    d) Stand still on mounting
79. Age of Bull for maximum semen output should be....?
    a) 3-4 years
    b) 5-8 years
    c) 2-3 years
    d) 8-10 years
80. In case of bovine gestation,the period of foetus is started from -
    a) 13th day onwards
    b) 45th day onwards
    c) 30th day onwards
    d) 60th day onwards
81. Corpus luteum size is smaller than follicle size in which animal -
    a) Cow
    b) Bitch
    c) Mare
    d) Sow
82. Which type of placenta is found in camel?
    a) Syndesmochoreal
    b) Endotheliochorial
    c) Epitheliochorial
    d) Haemochorial
83. Zonary and endotheliochoreal type of placenta is found in?
    a) Cow
    b) Bitch
    c) Camel
    d) Elephant
84. Shape of cotyledons in cow is?
    a) Concave
    b) Convex
    c) Both
    d) None

85. Presence of placentomes is positive sign of pregnancy?
   a) True b) False
   c) Both d) None
86. Slipping of fetal membrane during pregnancy diagnosis is detected during which period?
   a) 90 days b) 60 days
   c) 120 days d) 35-45 days
87. Which type of mummification is common in domestic animal?
   a) Papyraceous type b) Haematic type
   c) Both d) None
88. Time require to complete a cycle of spermatogenesis in boar?
   a) 45 days b) 6 days
   c) 9 days d) 24 days
89. Descend of testes in buck occurs at?
   a) 90 days b) 75 days
   c) 85 days d) 150 days
90. Intrapreputial urination is found in?
   a) Dog b) Ruminants
   c) Both b and d d) Swine
91. Musculo cavernous type of penis is found in?
   a) Equine b) Canine
   c) Feline d) All of these
92. Interferon tau for MRP is responsible in which animal?
   a) Cow b) Sow
   c) Mare d) Bitch
93. Which amongst the following is responsible for MRP in pig?
   a) Progesterone b) Estrogen
   c) Inter uterine migration d) Prostaglandin
94. Which type of CL is present during pregnancy?
   a) Corpus albicans b) Corpus luteum Verum
   c) Corpus luteum haemorrhagicum d) Corpus luteum
95. Degenerating CL is known as?
   a) Corpus luteum Verum b) Corpus albicans
   c) Corpus luteum haemorrhagicum d) Corpus luteum
96. Ferguson reflex is due to which hormone?
   a) Estrogen b) Progesterone
   c) Oxytocin d) Prostaglandin
97. Flehmen reaction/response is absent in which animal?
   a) Cow b) Pig
   c) Dog d) Mare

98. T-shape uterus is found in which animal?
   a) Bitch b) Pig
   c) Mare d) Cow
99. How many days of estrous cycle is present in sheep?
   a) 21 days b) 17 days
   c) 14 days d) 20 days
100. Androgen binding protein is secreted from?
   a) Interstitial cell b) Sertoli cell
   c) Peg cell d) Both a and b
101. inhibin inhibits which hormone?
   a) LH b) FSH
   c) Oxytocin d) Estrogen
102. In which animal pheromones is secreted from saliva?
   a) Dog b) Fox
   c) Pig d) Poultry
103. Expulsion of dead foetus at completion of gestation period is known as?
   a) Abortion b) Still birth
   c) Pre-mature birth d) Eutocia
104. in ageing female early embryonic mortality may occurs due to?
   a) Hormonal imbalance b) Poor egg quality
   c) High rise of temperature d) None
105. Uetention of foetal membrane and necrotic placentitis is common in abortion due to?
   a) Trichomoniasis b) Vibriosis
   c) Trucellosis d) B and C
106. uterine involution is very fast in which domestic animal?
   a) Dog b) Mare
   c) Doe d) Sow
107. Uterine torsion is more common in bovine due to?
   a) Cornual pregnancy
   b) Attachment of ligaments
   c) Typical pattern of lying down and getting up
   d) All
108. when second conception occurs in uterus already containing atleast one live foetus is known as?
   a) Superfoetation b) Superfecundation
   c) Telephony d) Multiple pregnancy
109. Retention of testes in stallion is known as?
   a) Rig b) Rigling
   c) Original d) All of the above

110. Testes descend in dog?
   a) 12-15 days before birth
   b) 12-15 days after birth
   c) 2-5 days after birth
   d) 2-5 days before birth
111. greenish colour ejaculate indicates infection of which organism?
   a) Pseudomonas aerogenosa
   b) Staphylococcus aureus
   c) Tricomonas foetus
   d) All
112. Percentage of glycerol as cryoprotectant?
   a) 7
   b) 14
   c) 21
   d) 28
113. Hypospadia is?
   a) Urethra opens dorsally
   b) Urethra opens with prepucial cavity
   c) Congenital condition
   d) Both b and c
114. Which hormone is responsible for development of accessory corpus luteum in mare?
   a) HCG
   b) PMSG
   c) Estrogen
   d) Progesterone
115. antigonadotropin hormone is secreted from which gland?
   a) Pituitary gland
   b) Hypothalamus
   c) Pineal gland
   d) Prostate gland
116. which type of placenta is present in elephant?
   a) Zonary
   b) Cotyledonary
   c) Diffuse
   d) Discoidal
117. which enzyme is responsible for converting of progesterone to estrogen at the time of parturition?
   a) 17-alpha hydroxylase
   b) 17-beta hydroxylase
   c) 14-alpha hydroxylase
   d) 1-beta hydroxylase
118. bloated bull frog like calf present in which type of complexity of pregnancy?
   a) Hydramnion
   b) Hydrallantois
   c) Hydrocephalus
   d) Tumefaction
119. Swiss cheese type of endometrium is seen in which type of cyst?
   a) Follicular
   b) Luteal
   c) Cystic corpora lutea
   d) None
120. which spermicidal agent is present in milk?
   a) Lecithin
   b) Lactenin
   c) Phospholipid
   d) Cholesterol
121. what should be the minimum concentration of sperm in semen straw for AI.
   a) 10 million
   b) 20 million
   c) 30 million
   d) 5 million

122. Which method is best for milking.
   a) Striping b) Fisting
   c) Full hand milking d) Both b and c
123. Pro-estrous bleeding is found in?
   a) Mare b) Bitch
   c) Cow d) Sow
124. Metestrous bleeding is found in?
   a) Cattle b) Mare
   c) Bitch d) Camel
125. Which phase of estrous cycle is absent in bitch?
   a) Esrtus b) Proetrus
   c) Metestrus d) Diestrus
126. Which animal is short day breeder?
   a) Sheep b) Dog
   c) Cattle d) Camel
127. what is the concentration of French mini straw.
   a) 0.25 ml b) 0.5 ml
   c) 0.2 ml d) 0.1 ml
128. Bulbourethral gland is absent in?
   a) Cow b) Mare
   c) Dog d) Cat
129. Pulsation at base of penis is noticed during ejaculation in?
   a) Dog b) Stallion
   c) Bull d) Boar
130. Sperm remain alive in epididymis for how many days?
   a) 2-3 days b) 4 -5 days
   c) 1-2 days d) 7 days
131. Puberty in Stallion, Cow, Ramand Sow is respectively.
   a) 18 months,10-12 months, 7-8 months,4-8 months
   b) 4-8 months, 10-12 months, 7-8 months, 18 months
   c) 10-12 months, 4-8 months, 18 months, 7-8 months
   d) 4-8 months, 7-8 months, 10-12 months, 18 months
132. Average life span of goat.
   a) 10 years b) 12 years
   c) 16 years d) 20 years
133. What is the term used for ram castrated after service.
   a) Seggy b) Wedder
   c) Bleating d) Gimmer
134. Os-penis is present in...?
   a) Dog b) Cat
   c) Goat d) Camel

135. Statement-(A) :Pseudopregnancy occur in bitch due to prolactin.
Statement-(B): Pseudopregnancy occur in cat due to progesterone.
a) A is true B is false
b) A is true and B correctly explains it.
c) Both A and B true
d) Both A and B false

136. fructose is absent in semen of which animal?
a) Sow b) Mare
c) Bitch d) Cow

137. yellow colour of semen is due to which pigment?
a) Carotene b) Xanthene
c) Riboflavin d) Pectin

138. full form of TRIS?
a) Triamine methyl hydroxy methane b) Hydroxymethyltriaminomethane
c) Triamine ethyl hydroxy ethane d) Hydroxy ethyl triamino ethane

139. knobbed defect show which type of sperm defect?
a) Defect in head b) Defect in mid piece
c) Defect in tail d) None

140. carbon dioxide bubble formation is found in which type of room temperature dilutor?
a) Coconut milk extender b) Illani's variable temperature
c) Millovanov's method d) Cornell university extender

141. pre scrotal sigmoid flexure is present in?
a) Dog b) Pig
c) Cow d) Sheep

142. sigmoid flexure is absent in?
a) Dog b) Cow
c) Sheep d) Pig

143. horizontal orientation of testes is present in?
a) Dog b) Stallion
c) Bull d) Sheep

144. mediastinum testes and rete testes are absent in?
a) Cow b) Stallion
c) Dog d) Sow

145. Half-life of oxytocin is?
a) 10 days b) 5 days
c) 2 minute d) 4 minute

146. Half-life of PMSG is directly proportional to-
a) Sialic acid content b) Prostaglandin
c) Ascorbic acid d) Carnitine

147. PMSG is secreted from
   a) Chorionic girdle b) Endometrial cup
   c) Both d) None

148. What is estrous cycle?
   a) Phase between two mid estrous
   b) Phase between diestrous to proestrous
   c) Phase between two estrous
   d) Phase between proestrous to estrous

149. Temperature of liquid nitrogen is.
   a) (-79) Degree celcius b) (-196) Degree Fahrenheit
   c) (-196) Degree celcius d) (-79) Degree fahrenheit

150. Calf should get first colostrum within how much time after calving.
   a) 2 hours b) 4 hours
   c) 6 hours c) 1/2 hours

Answer Key

1	a	2	a	3	c	4	a	5	b	6	c	7	c
8	a	9	d	10	b	11	a	12	d	13	a	14	a
15	c	16	d	17	d	18	a	19	d	20	a	21	b
22	c	23	a	24	a	25	c	26		27	b	28	d
29	d	30	a	31	c	32	b	33	d	34	d	35	b
36	a	37	a	38	a	39	a	40	a	41	a	42	a
43	d	44	a	45	c	46	d	47	a	48	d	49	a
50	b	51	d	52	b	53	b	54	b	55	b	56	c
57	d	58	d	59	c	60	b	61	a	62	a	63	b
64	c	65	a	66	c	67	b	68	a	69	b	70	c
71	a	72	d	73	a	74	c	75	d	76	a	77	b
78	d	79	b	80	b	81	c	82	c	83	b	84	b
85	a	86	a	87	a	88	c	89	b	90	c	91	d
92	a	93	b	94	b	95	b	96	c	97	b	98	c
99	b	100	b	101	b	102	c	103	b	104	a	105	c
106	d	107	d	108	a	109	d	110	c	111	a	112	b
113	d	114	b	115	c	116	a	117	a	118	b	119	a
120	b	121	a	122	d	123	b	124	a	125	c	126	a
127	a	128	c	129	b	130	b	131	a	132	b	133	a
134	a	135	c	136	c	137	c	138	b	139	a	140	b
141	b	142	b	143	b	144	b	145	c	146	a	147	b
148	c	149	c	150	a								

22

Biotechnological and Genomic Approaches in Breeding of Animals

Monoshree Sarma[1*], Vidya M.K[2], Mrinmoyee Sarma[3], Safeeda Sultana Begum[4], and Farida Rahman[4]

[1]*Department of Veterinary Pharmacology and Toxicology, Institute of Veterinary Science and Animal Husbandry, Siksha 'O' Anusandhan, Bhubaneswar, Odisha*

[2]*Department of Veterinary Physiology and Biochemistry, Veterinary College Hassan, KVAFSU, Hassan, Karnataka*

[3]*Department of Veterinary Public Health and Epidemiology, Institute of Veterinary Science and Animal Husbandry, Siksha 'O' Anusandhan, Bhubaneswar, Odisha*

[4]*Department of Veterinary Medicine, COVAS, Kishanjganj, BASU, Patna, Bihar*

Introduction

The Convention on Biotechnology has defined biotechnology as "any technological application that uses biological systems, living organisms or derivatives thereof, to make or modify products or process for specific use".

The global food requirement is increasing with growing population, so the productivity gap could be filled by improving genetic health. Animal breeding focuses on genetic improvement through biotechnological and genomic approaches. Genetic progress is influenced by the type of biotechnology such as selection accuracy, genetic interval, intensity of selection, genetic variance. It helps to improve animal production, treatment of genetic disorders, production of transgenic animals resistant to diseases, vaccine production and also to maintain genetic diversity for endangered species. Genomic selection is a type of marker assisted selection. It improves the genetic gain by decreasing genetic interval and improving reliability. These novel approaches have high potential in animal breeding, if executed judiciously may provide practical benefits to mankind.

The magnitude of genetic improvement of livestock species is determined by the genetic variation in population and by the methods to exploit the genetic variability. A lot of genetic improvement has been brought about by performance recording and crossbreeding programs involved in different traditional breeding programmes.

Biotechnology has paved the way for genetic improvement by contributing at large to increase reproductive efficiency, global transport and multiplication of genetic material and conservation of valuable genetic material. Cutting edge technologies in the field of genetics are artificial insemination, embryo transfer, embryo production and preservation, semen and embryo sexing, embryo splitting and cloning.

Artificial insemination and frozen semen technology has led dissemination of superior germplasm by widespread use of outstanding males, introduction of new genetic material by importing semen instead of live animals, progeny testing under different environment so as to increase the rate and efficiency of selection and reduction in spreading the sexually transmitted diseases. Frozen semen has the advantage of being used even after the death of sire.

Embryo transfer technology involves superovulation, estrus synchronization, artificial insemination, embryo recovery, embryo transfer and sometimes cryopreservation and micro manipulation of embryos. It has helped in rapid multiplication of rare genotypes, rapid improvement in livestock, control of sexually transmitted diseases and animal conservation programme.

In vitro production (IVP) of embryos involves several steps: Collection of immature oocytes- maturation of oocytes- sperm capacitation- *in vitro* fertilization- culture of embryos- embryo sexing- freezing and transfer to the uterus. Embryo cryopreservation is of immense help in preserving endangered or unique genotype so as to propagate such genotype at faster rate. Embryo splitting is a technological breakthrough where the embryo is divided into two halves to have two embryos or into one quarter to get four embryos or sometimes to get sixteen embryos from single embryo. The objective is to get numerous offspring from a given donor. It is clanged to the idea of increasing the intensities of selection.

Embryo transfer technology is successfully adopted in our country India. APAU Tirupati is the first to produce Embryo Transfer calf (cattle) in 1986. In India, embryo transfer technology got a wing with the initiation of National Service and Technology Project on Embryo transfer technology in 1987. It was operated by Department of Biotechnology with National Dairy Development Board (NDDB) as the lead implementing agency and Sabarmati Ashram, Bidaj as the main Embryo transfer laboratory.

In recent time, biotechnology has revolutionised the fiend of genetics and breeding. Recent advances include genome analysis and manipulation of genome. Genome analysis involves study of chromosomal karyotyping, chromosomal aberrations and genetic characterization of population to identify the variations in blood group, biochemical polymorphism and manipulation of genome. DNA polymorphism can be identified by two methods: (a) site directed polymorphism and (b) anonymous polymorphism.

Random Amplified Polymorphic DNA (RAPD) is a form of variation that is useful in DNA polymorphism analysis with high level of detectable polymorphism. It is a type of polymorphic DNA that is produced by random amplification with PCR. For this purpose, a randomly designed single primer is used.

Another important technique in the field of biotechnology is DNA fingerprinting. The characterization of one or more rare feature of an individuals' genome (hereditary make up) by developing the DNA fragment band (alleles) pattern is called as DNA fingerprinting or DNA identification analysis or identity testing or DNA profiling/typing or genotyping. It involves a series of steps: isolation of DNA, digestion of DNA by restriction endonucleases, electrophoretic separation of different fragments, transfer of DNA on nylon membrane, probe labelling, and hybridization of labelled probe DNA, autoradiography, analysis and interpretation of band patterns. The application of DNA fingerprinting (DFP) include individual identification, pedigree analysis and percentage verification, zygosity testing, sex determination, conservation of genetic resources, demographic studies, identification of loci controlling quantitative traits or disease resistance, pathogen identification, detection of source of tissue particularly in meat industry to check adulteration, detection of somatic mutation or cancer, taxonomical tool and quality control of cell banks.

Manipulation of gene involves transgenesis, cloning, etc. transgenesis involves isolation of gene of interest on a strand of DNA, cutting of DNA at specific points by restriction enzymes and joinng the cut DNA with a vector which may be a virus or plasmid. The gene of interest is carried by the vector into the organism that will produce the protein. Cloning involves fusion of donor cell to an oocyte or zygote following its enucleation.

MCQs

1. What is the full form of RAPD?
   a) Rapidly amplified polymorphic DNA
   b) Random amplified polymorphic DNA
   c) Random amplified polymeric DNA
   d) Rapidly annealed polymorphic DNA
2. Micro array technology can be used for
   a) Gene expression analysis b) DNA sequencing
   c) Both a and b d) None of the above
3. ______ is the biological processes of mRNA degradation induced by complimentary sequences double standard small interfering rna and suppression of target gene expression
   a) DNA sequencing b) r DNA technology
   c) RNA interference d) Marker assisted selection
4. Marker assisted selection uses ____ to define the genetic makeup and predict the performance of the animal
   a) DNA marker b) RFLP
   c) RNA marker d) SNP
5. Which of the following statement is true about dna markers
   a) Relatively difficult to assay b) Affected by the environment
   c) Highly heritable d) All the above
6. Which is the earliest form of dna marker use to build up the first true genomic map
   a) RFLP b) AFLP
   c) RAPD d) SNP
7. When was RFLP technique invented
   a) 1981 b) 1999
   c) 1975 d) 1984
8. Use of microsattelite in livestock sector
   a) Disease diagnostic b) Forensic analysis
   c) Marker assisted technique d) All of the above

9. ____ is a noble web resources based candidate gene identification approach
   a) GWAS
   b) DigiCGA
   c) Computer facilitated candidate gene approach
   d) Both b and c
10. Which of the following are application software or online tools for prioritizing candidate genes
   a) GFSST b) ENDEARVOUR
   c) POCUS d) All of the above
11 . Steps in genome scan approach
   Phenotyping trates of resource population 2.design and construction of resource population 3. Selection of genetic markers 4. Construction of linkage maps 5.genotyping of population for selected markers 6. Statistical analysis of the phenotypic and genotypic data derived from resource population
   a) 1-2-3-4-5-6 b) 2-1-3-5-4-6
   c) 2-6-1-4-3-5 d) 1-6-5-4-2-3
12 . Which of the following are the most well known methods that have been adopted in develop and developing livestock production
   a) Transgenic animal and cloning
   b) Transgenic animals and artificial insemination
   c) Cloning and embryo transfer
   d) Artificial insemination and embryo transfer
13. Purpose of producing transgenic animal include producing better breed lines
   a) To reduce susceptible disease b) For less carcas
   c) Increase milk production d) Both a and c
14. which of the following is the most common method to creats transgenic animals
   a) Pronuclear micro injection
   b) Transgenic somatic cell nuclear transfer
   c) None of the above
   d) All of the above
15 . Which is the first transgenic animal produce using pronuclear micro injection
   a) Transgenic sheep b) Transgenic cattle
   c) Transgenic pig d) Transgenic mice
16. _____ is an alternative technique using natural ability of Spermatozoa as a vector to transfer exogenous vector in to the cell at fertilization
   a) GIFT b) SMGT
   c) ET d) AI
17. who is the first person to introduce SMGT
   a) Duszewska1 et al b) Venkatesh
   c) Levitrano et al d) Zani

18. Name of the first animal develop by cloning technology
    a) Mira _ goat
    b) Cumuline _ mouse
    c) Dolly _ sheep
    d) Prometea _ horse
19. Which of the following statement is not true about genomic selection
    a) Young bulls can be genotype early in life and breeding values computed
    b) Can be use to select young bulls to be progeny tested, thereby reducing cost
    c) Higher accuracy of about 60-80 % for young bulls above parent average
    d) Reduction in generation interval
20. In which of the following animal first embryo transfer has been done?
    a) Rabbit
    b) Rat
    c) Sheep
    d) Cattle
21. Which of the following media is used for maturation of oocytes
    a) DMEM
    b) TCM-199
    c) Ham's F-10
    d) Both b and c
22. Which technique holds promise in future for conservation of endangered species?
    a) Intraspecies cloning techniques
    b) Interspecies cloning techniques
    c) IVF
    d) Both a and b
23. In Intracytoplasmic Sperm Injection (ICSI) the sperm is injected in
    a) Nucleoplasm
    b) Cytoplasm
    c) Perivitelline space
    d) None
24. Who is regarded as the father of tissue culture?
    a) Harrison
    b) Arnold
    c) Ross
    d) Roux
25. Vero cell line is obtained from Kidney cells of
    a) African green monkey
    b) Chinese hamster
    c) Calf
    d) Swine
26. Which was the first restriction enzyme to be discovered?
    a) AluI
    b) HinfI
    c) HindII
    d) HindIII
27. Which of the following is not true about retrotransposons.?
    a) Retrovirus like elements
    b) Have gag and pol genes but lack env genes
    c) Ty elements and copia elements are retrotransposons
    d) Found in prokaryotes only
28. In HMC cloning technique which enzyme is commonly used for digesting zona pellucid?
    a) Trypsin
    b) Pepsin
    c) Pronase
    d) Hyaluronidase

29. Hybridoma is a cell formed by fusion of?
    a) Plasma cell with a plasma cell of another species
    b) T cell with myeloma cell
    c) Macrophage with myeloma cell
    d) Plasma cell with myeloma cell
30. Inbreeding is carried out in animal husbandry because
    a) Increase vigour b) Improves breed
    c) Increase homozygosity d) None of these
31. Chromosomes may be isolated from metaphase cells by
    a) Hypertonic lysis b) Hypotonic lyis
    c) Either (a) or (b) d) Isotonic lysis
32. Which protein has been produced generating a transgenic sheep that is used for replacement therapy for individual at risk from emphysema
    a) Plasminogen activator b) Antitrypsin
    c) Casein d) Amyloid precursor protein
33. The response to selection increases when
    a) Properties of individual selected increases
    b) Proportion of individual selected decreases
    c) Heritability of trait is low
    d) None of the above
34. The heritability of character in narrow sense will be more when it is controlled by
    a) Gene with non additive effective b) Gene with additive effects
    c) Both (a) and (b) d) None of the above
35. The precision of heritability estimates is known by its
    a) Standard error b) Magnitude
    c) Method estimation d) Deviation
36. Plasmids are used as cloning vectors for which of following reason
    a) Can be multiplied in culture
    b) Self replication in bacterial cell
    c) Can be multiplied in laboratories with help of enzymes
    d) Duplicate freely outside bacterial cells
37. A foreign DNA and plasmid cut same by restriction endonuclease can be joined to recombinant plasmid using
    a) Taq polymerase b) Polymerase 3
    c) Ligase d) Eco R 1
38. The technique used in animal biotechnology for rapid multiplication and production of animals with desirable genotype is
    a) Protoplast fusion and embryo transfer
    b) Hybrid selection and embryo transfer
    c) *In vitro* fertilization and embryo transfer
    d) All of these

39. Technique for transferring foreign DNA into a host organism DNA is known as
    a) Blotting technique
    b) Recombinant DNA technology
    c) Gene cloning technique
    d) PCR technique
40. Which of the following statement is /all always true about process of cloning
    1. It is possible only in animal
    2. It is results in exact replication of cell, a living part or anorganism
    3. It results in large number of off springs
    a) A & B
    b) Only B
    c) B & C
    d) Only A
41. Specific biomolecules which show easily detectable difference among different strains of species or different species termed as
    a) DNA finger printing
    b) Molecular markers
    c) Molecular scissors
    d) RFLP
42. All statements are true regarding RFLP & RAPD except
    a) RAPD is quick method compared to RFLP
    b) PFLP is more reliable than RAPD
    c) Species specific primer are required for RAPD
    d) Radioactive probe are not required for RAPD
43. The variant fragment that distinguish one individual from another is called?
    a) Variant fragment
    b) Marking fragment
    c) Differing fragment
    d) All of these
44. The resemblance b/w offspring and parents provide the basis for
    a) Discrete breeding
    b) Inbreeding
    c) Random
    d) Selection breeding
45. Faster rate of genetic improvement can be achieved in
    a) Dairy cattle for milk production
    b) Sheep for lamb production
    c) Pig for litter size
    d) Broilers for growth rate
46. Difference b/w genotype and breeding value of particular genotype is
    a) Dominance deviation
    b) No dominance
    c) Direct dominance
    d) None of the above
47. Transplantation of tissue from one end to other of same species is known as
    a) Antro transplantation
    b) Allogenic
    c) Xeno transplantation
    d) Isogenic
48. transplantation of tissue from one end to other of different species is
    a) Autotransplantation
    b) Allogenjc
    c) Xenotransplantation
    d) Isogenic
49. Transgenic animals are used to study what is the form of --------gene
    a) Foreign
    b) Regular
    c) Same
    d) Old

50. 95% transgenic animals are
   a) Sheep b) Rabbits
   c) Pigs d) Mice
51. Genetic gain per year is increased by
   a) Increasing generation interval b) Decreasing generation interval
   c) Constant generation interval d) Eliminating generation interval
52. Selection of single tract at a time is known as
   a) Tandom selection b) Receprocal recurrent selection
   c) Mass selection d) None
53. Young are unable to produce argimine due to artificial breeding is called
   a) Moratorium b) Argininemia
   c) Originaemia d) None
54. All of the following is used in co culture system for growth of oocytes except
   a) Buffalo oviduct cells b) Rpf
   c) Cancerous cells d) Rabbit oviduct cells
55. In the 1 st transgenic animal experience gene from wats was cloned in to mice
   a) Somatotropin b) Metallothiomim
   c) Plasmogen d) Vasolatin
56. Term cytogene coined by
   a) Batson b) Suffon
   c) Morgan d) Chaffon
57. The improvement method suggested forimprovement of Sahiwal cattle and niliravi buffalo in pakistans breeding policy
   a) Through genetic selection b) Dvpmnt of gene pool
   c) Establishment of farmers co operative d) aAl of the above
58. MOET is referred to
   a) Most embryo transferred b) Mother of elite goat
   c) Multiple ovulation and embryo transfer d) None of these
59. Breeding value is defined as
   a) The value of an individual as a parent
   b) The value of progeny
   c) The value of an individual as a parent and value of offspring as producer
   d) All
60. The most extensively used bred for cross breeding is
   a) Nili ravi b) Kundi
   c) Sahiwal d) Dajal
61. The development of young one outside the body of Female parent is called
   a) Ectogenesis b) Ectopic pregnancy
   c) *In vitro* fertilization d) All of the above

62. Ectogenesis is normaly used in
   a) Sheep and Goat
   b) Fishes and frog
   c) Dog and cat
   d) None of the above
63 Amniocentesis is a technique use to
   a) Diagnose the birth defect in fetus
   b) To determine the sex of the fetus
   c) Both a and b
   d) None of the above
64. Invitro maturation of oocyte consist of
   a) TCM -199 supplemented with FSH, LH and estradiol
   b) TCM-199 supplement with PGFalpha
   c) TCM-199 supplemented with GnRH
   d) All of the above
65. Transgenic technology is used in studying the
   a) Expression of certain gene
   b) Genetics basis of disease
   c) Immunological and oncological events
   d) All of the above
66. All of the following are used for capacitation except
   a) Bovine serum albumin
   b) Heparin
   c) EDTA
   d) Caggeine
67. Commonly used hormone for superovulation is
   a) Pregnant mare serum gonadotropins (PMSG)
   b) Follicular stimulating hormone
   c) Both of the above
   d) None of the above
68. The best extender commonly used for semen dilution is
   a) Citric acid whey
   b) Egg yolk citrate
   c) Krebs riager phosphate buffer
   d) TRIS buffer
69. Use of single nucleotide polymorphism (SNP) markers will leads to
   a) Greater thermotolerance in high producing dairy breeds
   b) Greater thermotolerance in low producing dairy breeds
   c) Both of the above
   d) None of the above
70. The reaction norm (RM) model and multiple trait model used widely to estimate
   a) Genetics components of heat tolerance in dairy cattle
   b) Genetics components of heat tolerance in breeding cattle
   c) Genetics components of heat tolerance in domestic animal
   d) All of the above

71. Which is the major animal considered as a xenotransplant donor to humans
    a) Monkey b) Pig
    c) Dog d) Cat
72. Transgenic goat have been used to produce which of the following protein that is used for dissolving blood clots.
    a) Amyloid precursor protein
    b) Alfa anti trypsin (AAT)
    c) Casein
    d) A variant of human tissue type plasminogen activator.
73. Which of the following is a contribution of Reproductive Biotechnology?
    a) Reproductive efficiency
    b) Global transport and multiplication of genetic material
    c) Conservation of unique genetic material
    d) All of the above
74. Artificial Insemination (A.I.) has played a pivotal role in which of the following?
    a) Dissemination of superior germplasm
    b) Introduction of new genetic material
    c) Progeny testing under different environments
    d) All of the above
75. AICRP on poultry breeding was started in the year
    a) 1970 b) 1971
    c) 1972 d) 1973
76. Project Directorate of Poultry is located at
    a) Izzatnagar b) Hyderabad
    c) Delhi d) Chennai
77. National Institute of Animal Biotechnology is located in
    a) Hyderabad b) Mumbai
    c) Jorhat d) Delhi
78. Project Directorate on Cattle is located at
    a) Raipur b) Jhansi
    c) Meerut d) Murshidabad
79. Institutional Centre including field testing of Nili Ravi Buffaloes is at
    a) GAU junagarh b) CIRB substation Nabha
    c) IGFRI Jhansi d) MPKV Kolhapur
80. Institutional Centre including field testing of Murrah is at
    a) NDUAT Faizabad b) AAU Khanapara
    c) LRS Vallabhnagaar d) BRS, Angaru
81. Institutional Centre including field testing ofSurti is at
    a) NDUAT Faizabad b) AAU Khanapara
    c) LRS Vallabhnagaar d) BRS, Angaru

82. Institutional Centre including field testing of Godavari is at
   a) NDUAT Faizabad b) AAU Khanapara
   c) LRS Vallabhnagaar d) BRS, Angaru
83. Institutional Centre including field testing of Swamp is at
   a) NDUAT Faizabad b) AAU Khanapara
   c) LRS Vallabhnagaar d) BRS, Angaru
84. First Millitary Dairy Farm (MDF) in India was started at
   a) Bombay b) Chennai
   c) Hyderabad d) Allahabad
85. Key Village Scheme was launched in the year
   a) 1950 b) 1951
   c) 1952 d) 1953
86. Which of the following is a progeny testing scheme??
   a) Single Herd P.T. Scheme b) Associated Herd P.T. Scheme
   c) Field P.T. Scheme d) All of the above
87. Integrated Cattle Development Program was started in which year??
   a) 1963 b) 1964
   c) 1965 d) 1966
88. International convention on registration of cattle was held in?
   a) Switzerland b) Milan
   c) Rome d) Geneva
89. Open Nucleus Breeding Scheme is also known as
   a) Contract Breeding Scheme b) Community Breeding Scheme
   c) Cooperative Breeding Scheme d) All of the above
90. Which of the following is a variant of MOET nucleus scheme?
   a) Juvenile MOET b) Adult MOET
   c) Hybrid MOET d) All of the above
91. An ad-hoc committee on Sheep Breeding Policy was constituted by Government of India in which year?
   a) 1968 b) 1969
   c) 1970 d) 1971
92. When was AICRP on Goat transformed to Network Project?
   a) 1970 b) 1980
   c) 1990 d) 2000
93. Which of the following is NOT a advantage of embryo transfer technology
   a) Parental sex determination
   b) Twinning rate can be decreased
   c) Rapid multiplication of rare genotype
   d) Low cost in transporting embryos instead of living animals which also require quarantine

94. Which of the following is the sequential arrangement of the steps in in vitro production ?
   a) Collection of immature oocytes- maturation of oocytes- sperm capacitation – *in vitro* fertilization – culture of embryos- embryo sexing
   b) Collection of immature oocytes- maturation of oocytes-embryo sexing- culture of embryo- sperm capacitation – in vitro fertilization
   c) Collection of immature oocytes-maturation of oocytes- sperm capacitation – *in vitro* fertilization – embryo sexing – culture of embryos
   d) None of the above

95. Which of the following is true for Embryo transfer?
   a) Donors need no hormonal stimulation
   b) Nearly 30% animals do not produce viable embryos
   c) Prepuberal donors can be used
   d) Infertile animals can be used

96. Which of the following is true for in vitro production of embryos?
   a) Good information is required on reproductive status
   b) Prepuberal donors cannot be used
   c) Oocytes of same donor cannot be fertilized individually with semen of any Bull
   d) Aspiration of follicles can be done twice a week over a long period

97. With respect to Embryo transfer how many sires are used on a donor at one time?
   a) Only one b) Two
   c) Three d) Many

98. Sperm capacitation is done by using
   a) Serratopeptidase b) Insulin
   c) Heparin d) All of the above

99. With respect to Embryo transfer technology which of the following is true?
   a) Pregnant donors upto third month of pregnancy can be used
   b) Non- pregnant donors are used
   c) Pregnant donors upto six month of pregnancy can be used
   d) Pregnant donors in last trimester of pregnancy are used

100. With respect to Embryo technology, flushing can be repeated after how many months?
   a) 2 months b) 3 months
   c) 6 months d) None of the above

101. The aim of embryo splitting is
   a) To obtain greater number of offspring from many donor
   b) To obtain one offspring from many donors
   c) To obtain greater number of offspring from a given donor
   d) None of the above

102. The survival rate of split embryo is

a) Same b) Less

c) More d) Cannot say

103. Which Institute has produced the first Embryo Transfer (E.T.) calf (Cattle)

a) National Dairy Research Institute, Karnal

b) APAU, Tirupati

c) The National Institute of Immunology

d) Sabarmati Ashram Gaushala, Bidaj

104. Which Institute has produced the first Embryo Transfer (E.T.) Buffalo Calf (Cattle)

a) National Dairy Research Institute, Karnal

b) APAU, Tirupati

c) The National Institute of Immunology

d) Sabarmati Ashram Gaushala, Bidaj

105. In which year Government of India initiated the National Service and Technology Project on E.T.T.?

a) 1987 b) 1988

c) 1989 d) 1990

106. Which is the lead implementing agency of National Service and Technology Project on E.T.T.?

a) National Dairy Research Institute, Karnal

b) APAU, Tirupati

c) The National Institute of Immunology

d) Dept. Of Biotechnology , NDDB

107. Which is the main E.T. laboratory of National Service and Technology Project on E.T.T.

a) National Dairy Research Institute, Karnal

b) APAU, Tirupathi

c) The National Institute of Immunology

d) Sabarmati Ashram Gaushala, Bidaj

108. How many collaborating centres are there in National Service and Technology Project on E.T.T.?

a) Three b) Four

c) Six d) Five

109. Which of the following is not a collaborating centre of National Service and Technology Project on E.T.T.?

a) APAU, Tirupati

b) IVRI Izzatnagar

c) National Institute of Immunology, New Delhi

d) Central Frozen Semen Production and Training Institute, Hessarghatta

110. Genome analysis include
  a) Chromosomal karyotyping b) Chromosomal aberration
  c) Genetic characterization of population d) All of the above
111. DNA has how many parts?
  a) Two b) Three
  c) Four d) None of the above
112. What are the two parts of DNA?
  a) Coding part b) Non-coding part
  c) Both (a) and (b) d) Neither (a) not (b)
113. Which part of DNA is known as 'junk' DNA?
  a) Coding part b) Non-coding part
  c) Both (a) and (b) d) Neither (a) not (b)
114. Thank coding part of DNA is about
  a) 90% b) 50%
  c) 20% d) 5%
115. Which part of DNA has lesser variability among individuals?
  a) Coding part b) Non-coding part
  c) Both (a) and (b) d) Neither (a) not (b)
116. The accumulation of mutations creates genetic variability within
  a) Coding part b) Non-coding part
  c) Both (a) and (b) d) Neither (a) not (b)
117. Which part of DNA leads to a high level of polymorphism?
  a) Coding part b) Non-coding part
  c) Both (a) and (b) d) Neither (a) not (b)
118. Which of the following is a method for determining polymorphism?
  a) Site directed polymorphism b) Anonymous polymorphism
  c) Both (a) and (b) d) None of the above
119. Which method is used to reveal arbitrary polymorphism?
  a) Site directed polymorphism b) Anonymous polymorphism
  c) Both (a) and (b) d) None of the above
120. Pertaining to minisatellite, which of the following is true
  a) It is 1-5 bp long b) It is 10-20 bp long
  c) It is 15-60 bp long d) None of the above
121. What is the full form of VNTR
  a) Variable numbers of Tandem Repeats
  b) Variable numbers of Tandem Results
  c) Visible number of Tandem Results
  d) None of the above

122. What are the applications of molecular markers?
a) Sex determination
b) Transgenic breeding
c) Individual identity
d) All of the above

123. What is the full form of MAAP?
a) Multiple Amplitude Autonomous Profiling
b) Multiple Arbitrary Amplicon Polymorphism
c) Multiple Arbitrary Amplicon Profiling
d) Multiple Arbitrary Amplicon Polymorphism

124. What is the full form of AFLP?
a) Amplified Filament length polymorphism
b) Amplified Fragment length polymorphism
c) Amplified Fragment length Profiling
d) Amplified Filament length Profiling

125. What is the full form of RAPD?
a) Rapid Amplified Polymorphic DNA
b) Rapid Arbitrary Polymorphic DNA
c) Random Amplified Polymorphic DNA
d) Random Arbitrary Polymorphic DNA

126. Which of the following is a approach of sexing?
a) Enzyme activity method
b) H-Y antigen detection
c) Karyotyping
d) All of the above

127. The term microsatellite was coined by
a) George and Hung
b) Tomar
c) Littand Luty
d) KaryMullis

128. Variable Number of Tandom Repeats (VNTR) can be examined by
a) Northern Blotting
b) Southern Blotting
c) Western Blotting
d) None of the above

129. What is the full form of PAGE?
a) Picture acrylamide gel electrophoresis
b) Poly acrylamide gel electrophoresis
c) Poly amplified gel electrophoresis
d) Picture amplified gel electrophoresis

130. Microsatellite is also known as
a) Simple sequence repeat
b) Short tandem repeat
c) Sequence tagged microsatellite repeat
d) All of the above

131. PCR was invented by
a) George and Hung
b) Tomar
c) Litt and Luty
d) Kary Mullis

132. What is the full form of FISH?
   a) Fluorescence in situ hybridization
   b) Fluorescence integrated site hybridization
   c) Fluorescence integrated segment hybridization
   d) None of the above
133. Which of the following is the correct sequence for DNA fingerprinting?
   a) Isolation of DNA- Digestion of DNA by restriction endonuclease- probe labelling – hybridization of labelled probe- electrophoresis separation of different fragments – transfer of DNA on nylon membrane – autoradiography- analysis and interpretation
   b) Isolation of DNA- Digestion of DNA by restriction endonuclease- autoradiography- probe labelling – hybridization of labelled probe- electrophoresis separation of different fragments – transfer of DNA on nylon membrane - analysis and interpretation
   c) Isolation of DNA- Digestion of DNA by restriction endonuclease- electrophoresis separation of different fragments – transfer of DNA on nylon membrane -probe labelling – hybridization of labelled probe- – autoradiography- analysis and interpretation
   d) All of the above
134. Which of the following is an application of DNA fingerprinting?
   a) Individual identification
   b) Pedigree analysis and percentage verification
   c) Zygosity testing
   d) All of the above
135. Transgenesis is applied first on which animal?
   a) Rat b) Mice
   c) Rabbit d) Birds
136. Which of the following is a promise of cloning technology?
   a) Cloning of a proven valuable animal b) Simpler and effective means
   c) To increase population size d) All of the above
137. Transgenesis was first introduced by
   a) Litt and Luty b) George and Hung
   c) Gorden and Ruddle d) KaryMulis
138. Transgenesis was first introduced in the year
   a) 1982 b) 1983
   c) 1984 d) 1985
139. Which of the following is an application of DNA fingerprinting?
   a) Taxonomical tool b) Quality control of cell banks
   c) Pathogen identification d) All of the above

140. PCR was invented in which year?
  a) 1983 b) 1984
  c) 1985 d) 1986

141. Central Frozen Semen Production and Training Institute is located in which state?
  a) Karnataka b) Tamil Nadu
  c) Kerala d) Maharashtra

142. Embryo transfer technology involves
  a) Superovulation b) Artificial Insemination
  c) Embryo recovery d) All of the above

143. Which cultural media is prefered for maturation of oocyte
  a) TCM 192 b) TCM 199
  c) TCM 182 d) TCM 189

144. The genetic improvement by selection in a generation is the function of which of the following?
  a) Variability in the trait under selection b) Heritability
  c) Population size d) All of the above

145. In which of the following techniques a foreign genetic is introduced into the animal?
  a) Cloning b) Transgenesis
  c) Marker assisted selection d) All of the above

Answer Key

1	b	2	c	3	c	4	a	5	c	6	a	7	d
8	d	9	d	10	d	11	b	12	d	13	d	14	d
15	d	16	b	17	c	18	c	19	c	20	a	21	b
22	b	23	b	24	c	25	a	26	c	27	d	28	c
29	c	30	c	31	b	32	b	33	a	34	b	35	a
36	b	37	c	38	c	39	b	40	c	41	b	42	c
43	b	44	d	45	b	46	a	47	b	48	c	49	a
50	d	51	b	52	a	53	c	54	c	55	d	56	b
57	d	58	c	59	a	60	c	61	a	62	b	63	c
64	a	65	d	66	b	67	c	68	b	69	a	70	a
71	b	72	d	73	d	74	d	75	b	76	b	77	a
78	c	79	b	80	a	81	c	82	d	83	b	84	d
85	b	86	d	87	d	88	c	89	c	90	d	91	c
92	c	93	b	94	a	95	b	96	d	97	a	98	c
99	b	100	a	101	c	102	b	103	b	104	d	105	a
106	d	107	d	108	b	109	a	110	d	111	a	112	c
113	b	114	d	115	a	116	b	117	b	118	c	119	b
120	c	121	a	122	d	123	c	124	b	125	c	126	d

127	c	128	b	129	b	130	d	131	d	132	a	133	c
134	d	135	b	136	d	137	c	138	a	139	d	140	c
141	a	142	d	143	b	144	d	145	b	146			

23

Care and Management of Newborn

Priya[1], Rachana Sharma[1], Vivek Sahu[2], and Shwetambri Jamwal[1]

[1] *College of Veterinary Science, Rampura Phul- GADVASU, Ludhiana, Punjab*

[2] *College of Veterinary Science, GADVASU, Ludhiana, Punjab*

Introduction

Care and management of calf

- Begins before its birth.
- Good dairy herds are raised rather than purchased.
- Dam should be dried 6-8 weeks before expected calving and should be fed well.
- Underfed dam will give weak and small calves.

Steps of calf management

1. **Removal of mucous**
   - Immediately after birth: removal of mucous or phlegm from nostril, mouth, eyes & ears for normal breathing.
   - Rub and dry the calf with a dry cloth or gunny bag
   - If cow not licking: sprinkle a little common salt on calf's body.
   - If calf does not start breathing: Provide artificial respiration by:
   - Compressing and relaxing the chest with hands
   - Swinging
   - Inserting twig in nostril
2. **Ligation of naval cord**
   - Cutting of naval cord: ligate-2.5cm & cutting-1cm below.
   - 0.5% Tr. Iodine or boric acid or any antiseptic on stump for 2-3 days
3. **Removal of wet bedding from pen: clean & dry stall.**
4. **Weighing of czalf**
5. **Cleaning of cow's udder & teat (preferably with chlorine solution) and dry.**
6. **Calf attempts to stand within half to one hour. Help too weak calves to nurse.**

7. Colostrum feeding

- Colostrum is rich source of gamma globulins (antibodies), vitamins and minerals
- Colostrum Temp.: 99ºF-102ºF
- Colostrum feeding: first 3-5 days.
- Whole milk: after 5 days
- Feed the total amount of milk at 3 or 4 equal intervals up to the age of 7 days and then twice daily
- Quantity of colostrum: 10 % of body weight.
- Overfeeding: calf scour/diarrhoea

Advantage of colostrum feeding

1. Transfer of passive immunity

- Gamma globulins
- Permeability of intestinal mucosa is higher during initial 24 hrs after birth.

2. Laxative action

- Colostrum acts as laxative due to higher dry matter content as compare to milk,
- Easy passage of first faeces (meconium)
- Prevent the chances of gastrointestinal tract infection

3. Nutritious Food

- Colostrum is highly nutritious food available to newly born young ones at birth.
- In absence of colostrum: ½-1 lit. skimmed milk + 2 eggs + 5 ml castor oil (Artificial colostrum)
- Rumen development in calf completes around 3 months.

Feeding schedule of calf

Age in days	Feed
1-4	Colostrum @1/10 BW
5-15	Whole milk @ 1/10 BW
16-30	Whole or skimmed milk @ 1/20 BW + 100g milk replacer + small green legume hay or fodder
31-60	Whole or skimmed milk @ 1/20 BW + 500g milk replacer + little or more green legume hay or fodder
61-90	Whole or skimmed milk @ 1/20 BW + 0.75 kg – 1 kg milk replacer + more green legume hay or fodder
Above 90	Ad libitum green fodder

- **Calf starter:** High energy & high protein concentrate mixture consisting of ground farm grains, protein feeds, minerals, vitamins and antibiotics. Should contain 16 to 21 % CP.
- 2nd week to 90 days

- **Milk replacer:** This is an easy approach to feed pre-ruminant stock; milk replacers are just milk substitutes. Constitutes up to 25% protein, 10%–15% stabilised high-quality fat, and at least 50% spray-dried skim milk powder. For each kg of decrease in milk, 200 gm of milk replacer should be added.
- A minimum of two litres of milk with milk replacer must be given to calves each day. The combination is diluted six to eight times with warm water and provided in liquid form.
- **Antibiotic feeding:** Between the fourth day and three to four months, aureomycin feeding at a dosage of 80 mg per calf per day improves appetite, increases growth rate by 10 to 30%, smoothes the coat of hair, and reduces the incidence of calf scours.

Commom Terms for New Born of Different Species

	Cattle	Buffalo	Goat	Sheep	Pig	Camel	Horse
Young male	Bull calf	Buffalo bull calf	Buckling or male kid	Ram lamb or Tup lamb	Boarling	Tordia (< 4yr of age)	Colt
Young female	Heifer calf	Buffalo heifer calf	Goatling	Ewe lamb or Gimmer lamb	Gilt	Tordi (< 4yr of age)	Filly

Feeding schedule for kids of different ages

Age (days)	Approximate live wt. (kg)	Milk (litre)	Starter ration (20-24 % DCP; 70 % TDN)	Green fodder (gm)
Birth to 5	1.5 – 2.0	Colostrum	---------------	----------------
5-30	2.0- 3.0	0.3 – 0.5	Small quantity	Small quantity
	3.0 - 5.0	0.4 – 0.5	50-100	Do
60-90	5.0 – 7.5	0.35 -.0.5	100-150	250
90-120	7.5 – 10.0	-----------	200-250	500

Care and management of piglet

1. Make sure new born piglet get colostrum on time. Sow should suckle piglets 8 to 10 times initially in 24 hours period.
2. **Feeding pre-starter pigs**: First feed for the pigs weaned before 3 weeks of age i.e. 1-3 weeks of age and is supposed to replace milk known as milk replacer. Each pig consumes 1.5 to 2 kg of pre-starter ration during this period.
3. After about a week, the piglets begin nibbling at their food, and in two to three weeks, they begin to eat.
4. **Nutritional anemia in piglet** (3-6 weeks of age): Because placental transfer and iron transfer into sow's milk are poor, the newborn pig's iron reserve for hemoglobin synthesis is restricte d) A newborn pig needs between 5 and 10 milligrams of iron each day. Nevertheless, the liver of a newborn pig contains only around 50 mg of iron. Piglets will start to show symptoms of labored breathing known as thumps, get

dull and tired, become lethargic, have a rough coat, and be lean and weak. Piglets are given 1 milliliter of iron dextran injection, which contains 100–150 mg of iron, on the 4th and 14th day of their age to prevent nutritional anemia.

5. Piglets aged three to eight weeks are given starter ration, commonly referred to as creep feed) It consists of the practice of feeding piglets in a separate enclosure known as the creep, who also nurse from their mother, highly digestible concentrate feed that contains 22% protein and 3500 kcal/kg DM of digestible energy.
6. Newborn pigs lack a well-developed thermoregulatory system.
7. The piglets' lowest critical temperature is 34° C.
8. The best method for reviving a cold pig is to submerge its entire body—apart from its head—in warm water for a brief period of time.
9. Piglets' eight tiny tusk-like teeth, known as needle/wolf teeth (one canine and one incisor on each side), should be clipped as soon as possible after birth using a sterile/ disinfected tooth cutting pliers.

1. In dairy cattle, licking of the new born calf can be induced by
   a) Sprinkling common salt on calf's body
   b) Sprinkling sand on calf's body
   c) Sprinkling common salt on cattle's body
   d) Sprinkling sand on cattle's body
2. Pressing and relaxing alternatively the chest wall of calf's body are the means of
   a) Disinfection c) Colostrum feeding
   b) Artificial respiration d) Management
3. The distance at which navel cord should be tied away from a calf's body is
   a) 7 cm c) 10 cm
   b) 1 cm d) 2.5 cm
4. The navel cord of new born should be cut about ....cm below the ligature
   a) 1 0c) 5
   b) 4 d) 10
5. Antiseptics should be applied to the stump for at least
   a) 2-3 days c) 1 day
   b) 10 days d) 15 days
6. After birth, after how much time new born calf should get up?
   a) 10 minute c) 45 minute
   b) 30 minute d) 60 minute
7. After birth, within how much time colostrum feeding should be practiced?
   a) 4 hr c) 1 hr
   b) 6 hr d) 8 hr
8. How much quantity of colostrum needed by a calf daily?
   a) 2 litres c) 1 litre
   b) 6 litres d) 3-4 litres

9. Daily feeding of colostrum should be divided in how many feeds or parts?
   a) 2 c) 9
   b) 3-4 d) 7
10. The primary function of colostrum feeding is to
   a) Fortify disease resistance c) Pass meconium
   b) Help in artificial respiration d) Helps in standing of calf
11. Mortality rate is higher in
   a) Buffalo calves c) None of the above
   b) Cow calves d) Both of the above
12. Among buffalo calves, mortality rate is higher in
   a) Male calves c) Equal in both
   b) Female calves d) None of the above
13. In cattle, mortality rate is higher in
   a) Male calves c) Equal in both
   b) Female calves d) None of the above
14. High calf mortality (60 percent) is relatively observed during the first
   a) 3 months of age c) 1 year of age
   b) 6 months of age d) 2 year of age
15. Within half to one hour of parturition, first colostrum feeding should be given at a rate of
   a) 3-5 per cent c) 10 per cent
   b) 6-8 per cent d) 15 per cent
16. The main predisposing cause for diarrhea by E.coli is
   a) Toxemia c) Dehydration
   b) Septicemia d) Dysbacteriosis
17. The important cause of mortality among calves is
   a) Pneumonia c) Gastro-enteritis
   b) Pyosepticemia d) Acquired diseases
18. The main predisposing cause for parasitic diarrhea in calves is
   a) Giardia b) *Ascaris vitulorum*
   c) Amoeba d) Cryptosporidia
19. What should be given to newly purchased calves to quench their thirst on arrival at farm?
   a) Adlibiltum drinking water c) Artificial colostrum
   b) 10-15 per cent glucose solution d) 3-5 percent glucose solution
20. Among sugars, neonatal calves are able to utilize
   a) Lactose c) Sucrose
   b) Glucose d) Both a and b
21. Overfeeding of sugars like sucrose and starch to calves will result in proliferation of
   a) Lipolytic bacteria c) Asaccharolytic bacteria
   b) Saccharolytic bacteria d) Proteolytic bacteria

22. For prevention of excess proliferation of saccharolytic bacteria, lactose or glucose should not be given not more than ----------g/day
    a) 200 c) 1000
    b) 500 d) 1500
23. Disbudding in cattle calves is done at an age of
    a) 1 week c) 3 week
    b) 2 week d) 4 week
24. Disbudding in buffalo calves is done at an age of
    a) 1 week c) 3 week
    b) 2 week d) 4 week
25. Disbudding in goat kids is done at an age of
    a) 1 week c) 3 week
    b) 2 week d) 4 week
26. Chemicals used for disbudding are
    a) Caustic potash c) Sodium Hydroxide
    b) Caustic soda d) Both a and b
27. In mechanical method of disbudding, material used is
    a) Caustic soda c) Elastrator
    b) Saw d) Hot iron disbudder
28. The temperature of electrical disbudder should be
    a) 540^0 C c) 240^0 C
    b) 100^0 C d) 1000^0 C
29. The equipment used for dehorning of younger animals is
    a) Saw c) Chemicals
    b) Clippers d) Disbudder
30. The equipment used for dehorning of adult animals is
    a) Saw c) Chemicals
    b) Clippers d) Disbudder
31. The time of application for electric disbudder should be
    a) 2 sec c) 2 min
    b) 8-10 sec d) 5 min
32. The castration age for male calves is
    a) 1 year c) 2-3 weeks
    b) 8-10 weeks d) None of above
33. The most prevalent vice among calves is
    a) Tongue rolling c) Licking
    b) Head rubbing d) None of above
34. New born of goat is
    a) Calf c) Kid
    b) Colt d) Foal

35. New born of pig is
 a) Calf
 b) Colt
 c) Piglet
 d) Foal

36. Newborn of horse is
 a) Calf
 b) Colt
 c) Kid
 d) Foal

37. One calf (0-3 months) is considered as
 a) 0.2 ALU (Adult Livestock Unit)
 b) 0.4 ALU
 c) 0.6 ALU
 d) 1.0 ALU

38. Milking done before calving is called as
 a) Stripping
 b) Waxing
 c) Prenating
 d) None of the above

39. The average birth weight in medium breeds of buffalo calves is
 a) 10-20 kg
 b) 20-30 kg
 c) 30-40 kg
 d) 50 kg

40. The average birth weight in large breeds of buffalo calves is
 a) 10-20 kg
 b) 20-30 kg
 c) 30-40 kg
 d) 50 kg

41. Calving in buffalo most commonly occurs during
 a) March to April
 b) August to October
 c) July to January
 d) February to March

42. Vitamin absent in new born calf is
 a) a
 b) d
 c) c
 d) e

43. The most common viral cause of diarrhea in calves and lambs is
 a) Rotavirus
 b) Coronavirus
 c) Torovirus
 d) None of above

44. Quantity of colostrum to be fed as per cent of body weight during 15-30 mnts of life
 a) 5-8
 b) 10
 c) 15
 d) 20

45. Quantity of colostrum to be fed as per cent of body weight during 10-12 hrs of life
 a) 5-8
 b) 10
 c) 15
 d) 20

46. Quantity of colostrum to be fed as per cent of body weight during 2nd and 3rd day of life
 a) 5-8
 b) 10
 c) 15
 d) 20

47. Period of suckling allowed for calves a day after their birth
 a) 5-minute; 4-5 times
 b) 2-minute; 2 times
 c) 10-minute; 4-5 times
 d) 20-minute; 10 times

48. Consumption of excessive colostrum by calves may result in
a) Scours
b) Impaction
c) Tympany
d) None of above

.49. Colostrum is a highly fortified source of nutrients having --------times protein of normal milk
a) 2
b) 4
c) 7
d) 11

50. Colostrum is a highly fortified source of nutrients having --------times total solids of normal milk
a) 2
b) 4
c) 7
d) 11

51. Lactose content (%) of colostrum is
a) 4.80
b) 21.00
c) 28.00
d) 2.50

52. Total solids content (%) of colostrum is
a) 4.80
b) 21.00
c) 28.00
d) 2.50

53. Total protein content (%) of colostrum is
a) 4.80
b) 21.00
c) 28.00
d) 2.50

54. The quantity and quality of γ-globulins in colostrum is increased by
a) Vaccination of dry cows
b) Isolation of dry cows
c) Improved feeding
d) None of the above

55. Colostrum of mature cows is of higher quality than that produced by heifers.
a) True
b) False
c) Can't say
d)

56. Globulins (%) present in colostrum is
a) 15
b) 5
c) 20
d) 30

57. Vitamin absent in new born calf is
a) a
b) d
c) c
d) e

58. In Indian condition, calf mortality (Per cent) under 1 year of age is
a) 10-15
b) 20-30
c) 40-50
d) <5

59. Ideally calf mortality in dairy farms should be less than
a) 10%
b) 15%
c) 18%
d) 8%

60. Housing of calves in individual boxes should be done at least up to age of
a) 3 month
b) 1 month
c) 5 month
d) 6 month

61. Separation of female and male calves should be done at an age of
   a) 1 month c) 3 month
   b) 6 month d) 12 month
62. Milk of which type of animal is higher in fat (%)
   a) Zebu c) Crossbred
   b) Exotic d) Both b and c
63. Addition of aureomycin to calf starter should be done at the rate of
   a) 40 mg/animal/day c) 120 mg/animal/day
   b) 80 mg/animal/day d) 200 mg/animal/day
64. Hay should be fed to calves at age of
   a) Birth c) 14th day
   b) 30th day d) 60th day
65. In place of whole milk, skim milk can be given at an age of
   a) 14th day c) 60th day
   b) 30th day d) 90th day
66. In case of using skim milk as a substitution, complete stoppage of feeding whole milk is done at an age of
   a) 14th day c) 60th day
   b) 30th day d) 90th day
67. How much milk replacer is substituted for 1 kg reduction in milk feeding?
   a) 100 gm c) 500 gm
   b) 200 gm d) 1000 gm
68. After birth, colostrum should be ideally fed within
   a) 30 minutes c) 6 hr
   b) 1 hr d) 12 hr
69. Quantity of colostrum to be daily fed to a newborn calf up to 3 days
   a) 5 kg c) 7 kg
   b) 1 kg d) 2-3 kg
70. How much time (hrs.) after birth intact antibodies are absorbed by intestine of newborn calf?
   a) 12 c) 48
   b) 24 d) 72
71. How much total milk and skim milk is required for raising one calf?
   a) 300 kg and 100 kg c) 100-150 kg and 250-300 kg
   b) 50 kg and 100 kg d) None of above
72. Calf starter should contain how much TDN%
   a) 60 c) 75
   b) 90 d) 50
73. Calf starter should contain how much DCP%
   a) 14-16 c) 10
   b) 23-25 d) 35

74. Main component of a milk replacer is
    a) Castor oil
    b) Grains
    c) Skim milk powder
    d) Egg
75. The ratio at which milk replacer is mixed with hot water
    a) 1:4
    b) 1:6
    c) 1:10
    d) 1:8
76. Amount of which component is restricted/limited in partial milk replacer
    a) Wheat
    b) Skim milk powder
    c) Fish meal
    d) Linseed meal
77. First dry concentrate mixture fed to calf is called as
    a) Creep feed
    b) Calf starter
    c) Hay
    d) Milk replacer
78. First dry concentrate mixture fed to piglet is called as
    a) Creep fee
    b) Calf starter
    c) Hay
    d) Milk replacer
79. How much quantity of milk should be given with milk replacer?
    a) 6L
    b) 8L
    c) 4L
    d) 2L
80. An enzyme present in bovine colostrum which prevents digestion of antibodies
    a) Protease inhibitor
    b) Lipase inhibitor
    c) Trypsin inhibitor
    d) All of above
81. Age of calf at which silage feeding can be done
    a) Birth
    b) 1 month
    c) >3 month
    d) 2 month
82. Calf should be dewormed first at an age of
    a) 10-15 days
    b) 2 month
    c) 6 month
    d) 1 year
83. Vaccination of calf should be done at an age of
    a) 1 month
    b) 2 month
    c) 3 month
    d) 6 month
84. Male calves castrated at an early age is known as
    a) Steer
    b) Bullock
    c) Teaser
    d) None of above
85. Male calves castrated after attaining maturity is known as
    a) Steer
    b) Bullock
    c) Teaser
    d) None of above
86. Vaccination of goat kids should be done at an age of
    a) 1 month
    b) 2 month
    c) 3 month
    d) 6 month
87. Vaccination of piglet should be done at an age of
    a) 1 month
    b) 2 month
    c) 3 month
    d) 6 month

88. Optimum age of castration of male calves by Burdizzo castrator is
   a) Birth c) 4-6 month
   b) 1 month d) 12 month
89. Species which are not able to convert glucose to fat are
   a) Cattle c) Horse
   b) Pig d) None of above
90. Animal identification should be performed
   a) 2 month c) 6 month
   b) Soon after birth d) 12 month
91. Birth weight of goat kid is
   a) 20 kg c) 10 kg
   b) 2-3 kg d) 1-2 kg
92. Birth weight of piglet is
   a) 20 kg c) 10 kg
   b) 2-3 kg d) 1-2 kg
93. The ideal size of brand number for cattle is
   a) 2.5 cm c) 10 cm
   b) 7.5 cm d) 20 cm
94. Heating of brand during hot branding should be done till
   a) Bright white c) Bright red
   b) Warm d) Slightly warm
95. Cutting of naval cord after birth should be done leaving a stump of
   a) 5 cm c) 10 cm
   b) 7 cm d) 2 cm
96. Application of brand should be done for how much time during hot branding
   a) 1 sec c) 7 sec
   b) 3 sec d) 10 sec
97. Immunoglobulins present in higher amount in colostrum
   a) Ig G c) Ig E
   b) Ig d) Ig M
98. One livestock unit (A.L.U) is equivalent to
   a) 200 kg c) 500 kg
   b) 300 kg d) 700 kg
99. Coagulation of colostrum occurs due to high amount of
   a) Casein c) Albumin
   b) Fat d) Carotene
100. Part of stomach fully developed in newborn calf
   a) Reticulum c) Omasum
   b) Rumen d) Abomasum
101. Calf raising is the most economical by which method?
   a) Natural method c) Conventional method
   b) Weaning method d) Non-conventional

102. Feeding of milk replacer to calves is practiced at an age of
   a) 30-40 day c) Birth
   b) 15 day d) 90 day

103. For every 10 to 12 kg body weight, how much milk is required to be fed to calf per day?
   a) 2 kg c) 1 kg
   b) 3kg d) 4 kg

104. Calf scours occurs to young calves due to
   a) Overfeeding of milk c) Skim milk feeding
   b) High far percentage of milk d) Both a and b

105. How much per cent increase in growth rate is resulted due to aureomycin feeding to calves?
   a) 10-30 c) 50
   b) 5-10 d) 75

106. Per cent of Stabilized high quality fat incorporated in milk replacer
   a) 10-15 c) 25
   b) 50 d) 75

107. Minimum amount (%) of spray dried skim milk powder incorporated in milk replacer
   a) 10-15 c) 25
   b) 50 d) 75

108. Calf shed should be located with respect to milking barn
   a) Away c) Some distance
   b) Near d) None of above

109. Weaning age of lambs is
   a) 3 months c) 5 month
   b) 1 month d) 6-7 month

110. Weaning age of piglet is
   a) 3 months c) 2 month
   b) 1 month d) 6-7 month

111. Before feeding to lambs, grains should be cracked up to --------weeks of age
   a) 6 c) 12
   b) 3 d) 16

112. Number of lambs/kids housed per shed from weaning up to attaining maturity
   a) 25 c) 100
   b) 50 d) 75

113. In pig, average litter size at birth
   a) 8-10 c) 5
   b) 10-12 d) 15-17

114. In pig, average litter size at weaning
   a) 8-10 c) 5
   b) 10-12 d) 15-17

115. In gilts, average litter weight at weaning
 a) 120 kg c) 100 kg
 b) 150 kg d) 200 kg

116. In sows, average litter weight at weaning
 a) 120 kg c) 100 kg
 b) 150 kg d) 200 kg

117. Desirable number of functional teats in mother for adequate nutrition of baby pigs
 a) 14-16 c) 8-10
 b) 10-12 d) 5-7

118. Phase 1 of suckling by piglets lasts for
 a) 120 seconds c) 20-60 seconds
 b) 5 seconds d) 10 seconds

119. Phase 2 of suckling by piglets lasts for
 a) 120 seconds c) 20-60 seconds
 b) 30-40 seconds d) 10 seconds

120. Phase 3 of suckling by piglets lasts for
 a) 120 seconds c) 20-60 seconds
 b) 30-40 seconds d) 10 seconds

121. Each piglet swallow how much ml of milk during each suckling
 a) 40-80 c) 150
 b) 20 d) 200

122. Immediately after birth, teat order is seen in
 a) Cattle c) Pig
 b) Goat d) Buffalo

23. Orphan pigs can be raised by which method?
 a) Cross-fostering c) Use of sow milk replacer
 b) Use of cow milk d) All of the above

124. Transfer of orphan pigs to a sow with surplus teat should be done within how many days of farrowing?
 a) 3 c) 7
 b) 5 d) 9

125. Which is an important management practice for equalization of litter size?
 a) Cross-fostering c) Early weaning
 b) Split weaning d) None of above

126. For acceptance of orphan pig by sow, they should be soiled with
 a) Soil c) Common salt
 b) Placental fluid of sow d) None of above

127. Amount of milk consumed by each piglet per day
 a) 100 ml c) 750 ml
 b) 300-500 ml d) 1000 ml

128. Best substitute for sow's milk
   a) Cow's milk
   b) Buffalo's milk
   c) Goat's milk
   d) None of above
129. Composition of sow's milk replacer
   a) 1 egg yolk + 1/2 ltr of cow milk
   b) 1 whole egg + 1 ltr of buffalo milk
   c) 2 egg yolk + 1 ltr of cow milk
   d) 1 egg yolk + 1 ltr of cow milk
130. Quantity of ferrous sulphate added to sow's milk replacer
   a) 1/2th teaspoon
   b) 1/4th teaspoon
   c) 1/8th teaspoon
   d) 1/6th teaspoon
131. Best substitute for sow's milk
   a) Cow's milk
   b) Butter milk
   c) Sweet skim milk
   d) All of the above
132. Piglets jostling for position on the udder is comprised by
   a) Phase 1 of suckling
   b) Phase 2 of suckling
   c) Phase 3 of suckling
   d) None of above
133. Nosing and butting the udder is comprised by
   a) Phase 1 of suckling
   b) Phase 2 of suckling
   c) Phase 3 of suckling
   d) None of above
134. Milk suckling by piglets is comprised by
   a) Phase 1 of suckling
   b) Phase 2 of suckling
   c) Phase 3 of suckling
   d) None of above
135. Almost 61.33 % of total death of piglets occurs in
   a) 1st week
   b) 2nd week
   c) 3rd week
   d) 4th week
136. The major causes of piglet mortality are
   a) Agalactia)
   b) Pneumonia)
   c) Gastroenteritis
   d) All of above
137. Permanent removal of part of litter during a certain period before complete weaning is called as
   a) Split weaning
   b) Fractionated weaning
   c) Early weaning
   d) Both a and b
138. Lactational anoestrum is a prominent feature in
   a) Cattle
   b) Buffalo
   c) Swine
   d) None of above
139. Early weaning in pigs is done at an age of
   a) 3 to 6 weeks
   b) 8 weeks
   c) 12 weeks
   d) 16 weeks
140. Nibbling at food by piglets is observed at which age?
   a) 2 week
   b) 1 week
   c) 3 week
   d) 4 week

141. Consumption of feed by piglets is observed at which age?
a) 2 week
b) 1 week
c) 3 week
d) 4 week

142. First feed for pigs weaned before 3 weeks of age
a) Grower ration
b) Finisher ration
c) Pre-starter ration
d) Starter ration

143. Nutritional anemia is the most common in
a) Piglet
b) Kids
c) Lambs
d) Calves

144. Daily requirement of iron (mg) by newborn pig is
a) 20 mg
b) 5-10mg
c) 30 mg
d) 50 mg

145. Laboured breathing shown by piglets due to nutritional anemia is called as
a) Thumps
b) Heaves
c) Hoven
d) None of above

146. Kidding interval is on an average?
a) 5 month
b) 12 month
c) 7-7.5 month
d) 15 month

147. Digestibility coefficient (%) of goat milk is
a) 70
b) 85
c) 60
d) 50

148. Time taken by lamb/kid to get up after birth
a) 1hr
b) 2hr
c) Immediately
d) 3hr

149. The characteristic of glossy kid skin is seen in
a) Jamunapari
b) Black Bengal
c) Beetal
d) Jakhrana

150. Birth weight of kids from crossbred goats is
a) 3-3.5 kg
b) 2 kg
c) 1-1.5 kg
d) 5-5.5 kg

151. Lamb produced out of season is called as
a) Spring lamb
b) Hot house lamb
c) Ester lamb
d) None of above

152. Lighter lamb of 10-12 kg is called as
a) Spring lamb
b) Hot house lamb
c) Ester lamb
d) None of above

153. Recording of birth weight of lamb/kid should be done
a) Before colostrum feeding
b) After colostrum feeding
c) 12 hr after birth
d) 2 day after birth

154. The common type of infection seen in kids of up to 30 days of age is
a) Chlamydia
b) *E.coli*
c) Coccidia
d) Giardia

155. Kid of up to 3 months of age requires how much covered floor space (m^2)
   a) 0.5 c) 1.0
   b) 0.75 d) 0.2-0.25

156. The critical temperature of newborn pig is
   a) 20°C b) 25°C
   c) 30°C d) 35°C

157. Calf of up to 2 months of age requires how much covered floor space (m^2)
   a) 0.5 c) 1.0
   b) 0.75 d) 2.0

158. The highest fat and protein content is found in colostrum of which livestock species?
   a) Ewe c) Doe
   b) Cow d) Sow

159. Crude protein content (%) present in creep fee d)
   a) 20-25 c) 25-30
   b) 30-35 d) 15-20

160. A device by which only piglets are allowed access to creep feed
   a) Farrowing crate c) Rail
   b) Creep d) None of above

161. Creep feed is also known as
   a) Pig starter ration c) Pre-starter ration
   b) Pre-weaning feed) d) Both a and b

162. Starting and ending age of offering creep feed to piglet is
   a) 2nd week and 8th week c) 3rd and 8th week
   b) 4th and 8th week d) 4th and 6th week

163. Causes of piglet anemia are
   a) Rapid growth rate of piglet
   b) Inefficient iron transfer into sow's milk
   c) Poor placental transfer of iron
   d) All of the above

164. Needle teeth in piglet are
   a) Canine and 3rd incisor c) Incisor
   b) Canine d) Premolar

165. In piglet, corner incisor teeth are called as
   a) Tusk c) Wolf teeth
   b) Needle teeth d) All of the above

166. Pair of needle teeth present in piglet
   a) 2 pair c) 1 pair
   b) 4 pair d) 3 pair

167. Young one of which livestock species is the most immature at time of birth?
   a) Calf c) Kid
   b) Foal d) Piglet

168. Age for cutting of needle teeth in piglet is
   a) 1-3 days
   b) 7 days
   c) 10 days
   d) 14 days
169. Iron dextran injection is administered to piglets on which days?
   a) 2nd and 10th days
   b) 4th and 14th days
   c) 5th and 20th days
   d) 10th and 25th days
170. Piglets are prevented from crushing by mother using
   a) Guard rail
   b) Vaccination
   c) Iron administration
   d) None of above
171. Guard rails are kept at what height from floor?
   a) 12-15 inch
   b) 8-10 inch
   c) 4-6 inch
   d) 15-20 inch
172. Traditional weaning age of piglet is
   a) 4 week
   b) 12 week
   c) 8 week
   d) 16 week
173. Device in farrowing pen installed to provide space to piglets and to prevent them from crushing
   a) Guard rail
   b) Creep
   c) Farrowing crate
   d) Hobble
174. Thermoregulatory mechanism in piglet is
   a) Fully developed
   b) Absent
   c) Same as cattle
   d) Poor developed
175. Brooder temperature for new born pigs should be maintained at
   a) 50°F
   b) 60°F
   c) 80°F
   d) 70°F
176. Immunoglobulins ingested by piglet at birth decline rapidly after first week of life and fall below protective levels by
   a) 5 days
   b) 8 days
   c) 14 days
   d) 21 days
177. Identify the one which is done with a baby piglet with in the first couple of days
   a) Tail docking
   b) Needle teeth clipping
   c) Ear notching
   d) All

Answer Key

1	a	2	b	3	d	4	a	5	a	6	a	7	b
8	d	9	b	10	a	11	a	12	a	13	b	14	a
15	b	16	d	17	c	18	b	19	d	20	d	21	b
22	a	23	b	24	a	25	c	26	c	27	d	28	C
29	c	30	c	31	b	32	b	33	a	34	b	35	a
36	b	37	c	38	c	39	b	40	c	41	b	42	c
43	b	44	d	45	b	46	a	47	b	48	c	49	a

50	d	51	b	52	a	53	c	54	c	55	d	56	b
57	d	58	c	59	a	60	c	61	a	62	b	63	c
64	a	65	d	66	b	67	c	68	b	69	a	70	a
71	b	72	c	73	c	74	c	75	b	76	b	77	a
78	c	79	b	80	a	81	c	82	d	83	b	84	d
85	b	86	d	87	d	88	c	89	c	90	d	91	c
92	c	93	b	94	a	95	b	96	b	97	d	98	c
99	b	100	a	101	c	102	b	103	b	104	d	105	a
106	d	107	d	108	b	109	a	110	d	111	a	112	c
113	b	114	d	115	a	116	b	117	b	118	c	119	b
120	c	121	a	122	d	123	c	124	b	125	c	126	d
127	c	128	b	129	b	130	d	131	d	132	a	133	c
134	d	135	b	136	d	137	c	138	a	139	d	140	c
141	a	142	d	143	b	144	d	145	b				

24

Raising of Animals

Parag Acharya, and Tanmoy Rana

[1]RRTTS, Bhawanipatna, Odisha University Agriculture and Technology (OUAT) Bhubaneswar, Odisha

[2]Department of Veterinary Clinical Complex, West Bengal University of Animal & Fishery Sciences, Kolkata, West Bengal

Introduction

Raising healthy and productive animals is a cornerstone of successful livestock farming. Whether the goal is milk production, meat, draught power or breeding, the foundation of a thriving animal enterprise lies in appropriate general management and feeding practices that consider the animal's stage of growth, reproductive status and work requirements. Each class of animal—calves, heifers, pregnant and lactating females, dry animals, bulls and working animals—has unique physiological needs that must be addressed through specialized care and nutrition.

Modern animal husbandry aims not just at higher productivity but also at ensuring animal welfare, sustainability and profitability. Scientific and stage-specific practices improve the animals' lifetime performance and reduce mortality, disease incidence and reproductive failure. In this context, proper rearing practices are not merely a routine, but a strategic necessity.

The calf represents the future of the herd. Ensuring its survival, growth and development is crucial for long-term productivity. Calf rearing begins immediately after birth with colostrum feeding, which must be administered within the first 2–4 hours. Colostrum provides immunity, energy and nutrients essential for survival in the first days of life. Calves must be housed in clean, dry and ventilated environments. They should be protected from drafts, heat stress and infections. Feeding practices transition from whole milk or milk replacers to calf starter feed by 2–3 weeks of age. Proper deworming, vaccination and sanitation must be part of the management plan.

Nutritionally, the focus is on supplying high-quality protein, energy and minerals to support rapid growth and organ development. Calves must have access to clean water and be gradually introduced to green fodder. The rearing practices followed at this stage determine future milk yield, reproductive performance and overall health.

Once the calf is weaned, it transitions into the heifer phase. This period is marked by skeletal growth, muscle development and the onset of puberty. The goal during heifer rearing is to achieve optimal body weight and condition for first calving at around 24–30 months. Management must include adequate space for exercise, regular health check-ups and strategic feeding. Overfeeding may result in excessive fat deposition in the udder, while underfeeding can delay puberty and reduce future productivity.

Heifers require diets containing balanced protein, energy, vitamins (especially A and D), and trace minerals like calcium, phosphorus, and zinc to support bone development and hormonal balance. Introducing mineral mixture supplementation early helps prevent reproductive issues later. The management of this group must also involve proper record-keeping, heat detection and preparation for breeding. Sound heifer rearing is central to achieving higher lifetime productivity in female animals.

Pregnancy marks a high-demand phase in a female animal's lifecycle. During gestation, especially in the last trimester, nutrient demands increase significantly due to rapid foetal growth and preparation for lactation. Proper feeding ensures the health of both the dam and the developing foetus. Management must focus on stress reduction, disease prevention, and physical comfort. Pregnant animals should not be overworked or subjected to rough handling. Regular veterinary supervision is critical for monitoring the health of the uterus, udder and overall metabolism.

The feed should be energy-dense, with emphasis on protein, calcium, phosphorus, selenium and iodine. Special care must be taken to avoid mineral imbalances, which could lead to issues like retained placenta or milk fever. Providing clean water, shade, comfortable bedding and a quiet environment ensures that pregnant animals remain healthy and can successfully deliver strong, viable offspring. Lactating animals are the productive core of a dairy operation. During this phase, they require maximum nutrient intake to sustain milk production and maintain body condition. The risk of metabolic diseases like ketosis, acidosis, and mastitis is also highest during this period.

Management practices should include frequent and hygienic milking, clean housing, foot care and health monitoring. Feeding must meet the energy and protein demands of milk production. Lactating animals typically require 2.5–3.5% of their body weight in dry matter daily. Their diets should include high-quality roughages (green fodder, silage), concentrates rich in energy and bypass protein and balanced mineral mixtures. Water is critical; an animal producing 10 liters of milk may need 50–100 liters of water daily.

Environmental comfort, stress-free milking and routine disease control ensure sustained production. Lactating animals must also be gradually transitioned into dry periods to prepare for the next reproductive cycle. The dry period—usually 60 days before calving—is essential for udder tissue regeneration and foetal growth. This phase should not be neglected, as its mismanagement can lead to poor milk yield in the subsequent lactation. Dry animals must be separated from the lactating group and housed comfortably. Feeding should avoid excessive energy that could lead to obesity or fatty liver disease. Diets must be fibre-rich and low in calcium during the early dry phase, with calcium increased 1–2 weeks before calving to prevent milk fever. Proper hoof trimming, deworming, vaccination and teat sealing may be required during this phase. The dry period is an opportunity to restore animal health, prepare the body for calving, and prevent postpartum complications.

Bulls contribute 50% of the genetic makeup of a herd, making their care and management vitally important. Bulls must be handled with respect and caution. Their housing should be separate, secure and spacious, allowing for exercise and safety. Feeding must aim to maintain optimal body condition—neither too thin nor obese—as both extremes reduce libido and semen quality. Their diet should be rich in protein, energy, vitamin E and trace minerals like zinc and selenium, which are crucial for sperm production.

Routine grooming, hoof trimming, parasite control and regular semen evaluation must be part of their schedule. Bulls also need psychological enrichment, such as social interaction and physical activity, to prevent aggressive or destructive behaviour. In many parts of the world, bullocks, donkeys and other animals are still widely used for agricultural and transportation work. These animals require special attention during peak workload seasons.

Working animals burn a significant amount of energy and must be fed accordingly. Diets must be high in digestible carbohydrates (like grains) along with fibrous feeds. Adequate salt and water are essential. Post-work feeding should be carefully planned to replenish energy and electrolyte loss. Animal-friendly yoking systems, soft harnesses and rest periods are key to preventing injury. Hoof care and skin inspections should be carried out regularly. Overworking or underfeeding leads to premature exhaustion, illness and poor work performance.

1. Colostrum is fed at .... of calf's body weight.
   a) 5 % b) 10%
   c) 15% d) None of the above
2. Calf should get first colostrum................. hr after calving ?
   a) 2 hr b) 4 hr
   c) 6 hr d) Anytime
3. The first faecal material voids from the calf after consuming colostrums is known as
   a) Muconium b) Phlegm
   c) Mucous d) All
4. The daily allowance of milk for young calves during first few weeks should be....... of body weight.
   a) $1/5^{th}$ b) $1/10^{th}$
   c) $1/20^{th}$ d) $1/25^{th}$
5. The immunity provided by colostrums to calf is
   a) Active b) Lacto-Globulin
   c) Passive d) Serum Proteins
6. Advantage of weaning in calf-
   a) Proper recording of cow's milk production
   b) Milking without calf: more hygienic & sanitary
   c) Both a and b
   d) Only a
7. Calf starter is-
   a) It is high energy and low protein concentrate mixture.
   b) It can be given to calves from 2nd week to 90 days of age
   c) Only b is correct
   d) Both a and b are correct

8. Pick the correct one
   a) Month of calving and difficulties at time of calving can influence total milk production in one lactation.
   b) In certain farms an arbitrary amount of 450 liters was added to lactation yield to account of portion consumed by calf.
   c) Older cow seem to show a greater increase in milk yield when subjected to more frequent milking
   d) Both a and b are correct
9. Rumen in buffalo calf develops by the age of
   a) 1 month b) 2 months
   c) 3 months d) 4 months
10. Most labour intensive dairy farm operation is:
   a) Feeding b) Cleaning
   c) Milking d) Harvesting
11. Disbudding in buffalo calf should be carried out by the age of
   a) 1 weeks b) 2 weeks
   c) 3 weeks d) 4 weeks
12. Disbudding in cattle calf should be carried out by the age of
   a) 2 weeks b) 1 weeks
   c) 3 weeks d) 4 weeks
13. Disbudding in kid should be carried out by the age of
   a) 2 weeks b) 1 weeks
   c) 3 weeks d) 4 weeks
14. Which of the following is not correct?
   a) Tagging in calves is generally done at 6 months of age.
   b) Branding in calves is preferred after one year of age.
   c) Supernumerary teats are removed at around one or two days of age.
   d) None of the above.
15. Which of the following is correct?
   a) Calf should be housed in individual pen for 3 months of age.
   b) After six months, male and female calf should be housed separately.
   c) Only a is correct.
   d) Both a & b are correct.
16. If the caving rate of a dairy farm is 80 % then inter calving period will be
   a) 12 months b) 15 months
   c) 18 months d) 21 months
17. Approximate number of calving pens required for dairy unit of 100 cows.
   a) 3-4 b) 7-8
   c) 15-16 d) 17-18

18. Early weaning of calves results in shorter
    a) Lactation Length
    b) Dry Period
    c) Service Period
    d) Gestation Period
19. Chemical caustic potash is used for
    a) Castration
    b) Weaning
    c) Breeding
    d) Disbudding
20. Removal of undesirable stock from the herd is known as
    a) Culling
    b) Quarantine
    c) Isolation
    d) Weaning
21. Optimum age of first service in buffalo heifer is
    a) 24-30 months
    b) 30-36 months
    c) 36-42 months
    d) 42-46 months
22. Which is true?
    a) Sexual maturity is occurrence of first estrous in female animal where as, stage of attaining full reproductive capacity is puberty.
    b) Puberty is occurrence of first estrous in female animal, where as stage of attaining full reproductive capacity is sexual maturity.
    c) Larger breeds of particular breed attain puberty earlier than smaller breeds.
    d) Season has no influence on puberty.
23. Which of the following is correct regarding rearing of heifer?
    a) Heifer of exotic cattle mature later than the zebu breed breeds
    b) Body weight of at first service should be around 60 % of mature body weight.
    c) De-worming should be carried out at every 3 months interval.
    d) Only b and c are correct.
24. Best behavioral sign of heat/estrous in cattle
    a) Bellowing
    b) Mounts on other cows
    c) Stands to be mounted
    d) Sniffing
25. Pregnant animals should be transferred to calving pen ....weeks prior to calving:
    a) 2 week
    b) 4 week
    c) 6 week
    d) 8 week
26. Pregnancy diagnosis should be done in cow at ....days after last insemination,
    a) 20-45 days
    b) 45- 60 days
    c) 60 -90 days
    d) 90-120 days
27. Removal of milk partially from 'udder' of cows before calving is known as
    a) Incomplete milking
    b) Intermittent milking
    c) Pre-netting
    d) Complete cessation
28. Challenge feeding is usually carried
    a) Before Calving
    b) After 15 days of calving
    c) At breeding
    d) At drying

29. In a ideal dairy herd the ratio between Milch: Dry cow is
    a) 1:1 b) 2:1
    c) 4:1 d) 8:1
30. Body condition score of cows at the time of calving should be around
    a) 1.5-2.0 b) 2.0-2.5
    c) 2.5-3.0 d) 3.5-4.0
31. The period between - date of calving and date of successful conception is known as-
    a) Dry period b) Service period
    c) Lactation period d) None
32. Which of the following is correct regarding milking of cows?
    a) 10 -15 % more milk can be produced when cows are milked thrice than twice.
    b) Wet hand milking is preferred than dry hand milking.
    c) Only a is correct
    d) Both a & b are correct
33. Average time required for milking of a dairy cow
    a) 5-7 minutes b) 10-12 minutes
    c) 12-14 minutes d) 15-17 minutes
34. Which of the following method should be avoided for milking of cows?
    a) Full hand b) Knuckling
    c) Stripping d) None
35. Thumb rule for feeding one kg of concentrate to lactating buffalo for every ....litres of milk
    a) 1.0 kg b) 1.5 kg
    c) 2.0 kg d) 3.0 kg
36. Placenta is normally expelled within ....hour after calving in cattle.
    a) 1-2 hour b) 2- 4 hour
    c) 4- 8 hour d) 8-10 hour
37. Dairy cow attains peak milk yield .... weeks after lactation ?
    a) 1-2 b) 2-4
    c) 4-6 d) 6-8
38. Ideal udder of cattle should be ....shaped
    a) Conical b) Bowl
    c) Ball d) Wedge
39. Which of the following term is related with nutrient reserve of the show animal?
    a) Blanketing b) Trimming
    c) Conditioning d) Drying
40. ....is given maximum weightage during selection of milch cow.
    a) Conformation b) Dairy Character
    c) Body capacity d) Udder

41. Strong front and rear udder attachment should be evident as......respectively.
 a) Acute, shallow b) Shallow, distinct cleft
 c) Distinct cleft, acute d) Distinct cleft, flat

42. After machine milking, left out milk is removed by
 a) Fisting b) Knuckling
 c) Stripping d) None

43. The cow should be milked from .... side.
 a) Left b) Right
 c) Either side d) None

44. One milker is sufficient for twice a day milking of .... Buffaloes.
 a) 6 b) 10
 c) 18 d) 24

45. How many cows can be milked by a single milker through hand & machine milking?
 a) 5 & 10 b) 12 & 20
 c) 18 & 30 d) None of the above

46. Shaeffer's formula is used for the determination of .... in cattle.
 a) Age b) Body weight
 c) Both of the above d) None of the above

47. Age of cattle can be determined by using .... formula.
 a) 2 + number of horn ring b) 3 + number of horn ring
 c) 4 + number of horn ring d) 5 + number of horn ring

48. What should be the ideal replacement rate dairy cattle and buffalo for maintaining efficiency of production?
 a) 5 % b) 10 %
 c) 20 % d) 30 %

49. What is the ideal voluntary period (days) for breeding in cross bred cows?
 a) 45 b) 60
 c) 70 d) 90

50. Sexual maturity in dairy animal is mostly influenced by
 a) Body weight b) Age
 c) Genetics d) All of the above

51. What should be the ideal ratio of cows and buffaloes in milk to that of dry in a farm at any time throughout the year for maximum production of milk?
 a) 65 : 35 in buffaloes and 75:25 in cross bred cows
 b) 50: 50 in buffaloes and 60:40 in cross bred cows
 c) 75 : 25 in buffaloes and 65:35 in cross bred cows
 d) 60: 40 in buffaloes and 50:50 in cross bred cows

52. Which of the following is not a method of drying off?
 a) Incomplete milking b) Intermittent milking
 c) Pre-netting d) Complete cessation

53. For cattle, feed efficiency for weight gain is maximum during-
   a) Dry period b) Late lactation
   c) Transition period d) None
54. Which of the following is true regarding 'Dry cow therapy'?
   a) It's a therapy to prevent mastitis after drying off.
   b) Teats are sealed after infusing suitable antibiotic in these.
   c) Only a is correct
   d) Both a & b are correct.
55. Which of the following is/are advantage of 'Dry period'?
   a) It prepares the mammary system for next lactation
   b) For optimum supply of nutrients for foetus development
   c) Making body nutrient reserve for the next lactation
   d) All of the above
56. Castration of male calf should be preferably done at ....years of age
   a) 3 months b) 6 months
   c) 1 year d) 2 year
57. Selection of bulls for breeding purposes starts at around ....months of age.
   a) 3 months b) 6 months
   c) 1 year d) 2 year
58. Training of bull for semen collection for A.I., starts at around ....months of age.
   a) 3 months b) 6 months
   c) 12 months d) 18 months
59. The optimum number of services per conception for cattle and buffalo should be...... & ....respectively.
   a) 1.7, 1.5 b) 1.5, 1.7
   c) 2.1, 3 .1 d) 5.1, 7.1
60. Ringing of bull is preferably done at around ....months of age.
   a) 3-6 b) 9-12
   c) 18-24 d) 24-30
61. Which of the following is correct regarding raising of bull?
   a) Daily exercise improves quality of semen.
   b) Semen should not be collected more than 2-3 times per week.
   c) Bull should be housed separately.
   d) All are correct.
62. Ideal working age for indigenous bullock is
   a) 1 year b) 2 year
   c) 4 year d) 6 year

63. For a bullock 'normal work' is considered as-
   a) 6 hrs of carting or 4 hrs of ploughing
   b) 8 hrs of carting or 6 hrs of ploughing
   c) 4 hrs of carting or 2 hrs of ploughing
   d) 2 hrs of carting or 1 hrs of ploughing
64. For a bullock 'heavy work' is considered as-
   a) 6 hrs of carting or 4 hrs of ploughing
   b) 8 hrs of carting or 6 hrs of ploughing
   c) 4 hrs of carting or 2 hrs of ploughing
   d) 2 hrs of carting or 1 hrs of ploughing
65. In case of ewe, feeding of extra concentrate 2-3 weeks prior to breeding season is known as
   a) Flushing b) Steaming up
   c) Challenge feeding d) None
66. Castration of buckling should be preferably done at.......................
   a) 1-2 months b) 2-4 months
   c) 6- 10 months d) 6 months
67. Optimum weaning age for goat is-
   a) 30 days b) 60 days
   c) 90 days d) 120 days
68. What is/are the purpose of identification in sheep and goat ?
   a) To maintain records of animals.
   b) For proper feeding and better management
   c) For insurance and to establish the ownership
   d) All of the above
69. Which of the following is correct regarding 'castration' of goat
   a) The preferable age of castration of male goat is 2-4 months.
   b) Castration helps in attaining faster growth rate
   c) It improves meat and skin quality as well as dressing percentage
   d) All are correct
70. Dry matter requirement for maintenance purpose in goat is
   a) 2.5 % to 3.0% of body weight
   b) 3.0 % to 3.5 % of body weight
   c) 3.5 % to 4.5 % of body weight
   d) 4.5 % to 5 % of body weight
71. CP and TDN requirement for young kid is
   a) 15-20 % and 60 % TDN on dry matter basis
   b) 20-24% CP and 72% TDN on dry matter basis
   c) 10-15% CP and 50 % TDN on dry matter basis
   d) 16-18 % and 60-65 % TDN on dry matter basis

72. CP and TDN requirement for growing kid/lamb is
    a) 16-18 % and 60-65 % TDN on dry matter basis
    b) 20-24% CP and 72% TDN on dry matter basis
    c) 10-15% CP and 50 % TDN on dry matter basis
    d) 30-40 % CP and 80 % TDN on dry matter basis
73. CP and TDN requirement for finisher ration is
    a) 16-18 % and 60-65 % TDN on dry matter basis
    b) 20-24% CP and 72% TDN on dry matter basis
    c) 10-12% CP and 60-65 % TDN on dry matter basis
    d) 30-40 % CP and 80 % TDN on dry matter basis
74. Which of the following pair is not matched properly?
    a) Tagging- shearing of wool from neck, belly and sheath region
    b) Eyeing- clipping of excess wool around the eyes
    c) Ringing- shearing of wool from neck, belly and sheath region
    d) Flushing: Feeding extra grain
75. Weaning weight of kids should be ....times of birth weight as a rule of thumb
    a) 1.5 b) 2.0
    c) 3.0 d) 5.0
76. Ideal characteristics for selection of fattening lamb/kid should be
    a) Higher birth weight b) Higher ADG
    c) Higher FCE d) All of these
77. Removal of wool around the sheath of ram is known as
    a) Eyeing b) Tupping
    c) Ringing d) Docking
78. Age of puberty in gilt at organized pig farm should be around (months)
    a) 6-7 b) 9-10
    c) 12-13 d) 14-15
79. Castration of male pig should be preferably done at..................
    a) 1-2 weeks b) 2-3 weeks
    c) 3-4 weeks d) 4-5 weeks
80. Maximum age of weaning (weeks) of piglets is
    a) 1 b) 2
    c) 4 d) 8
81. Piglets can be weaned at the earliest by
    a) 21 days b) 45 days
    c) 35 days d) 56 days
82. The length of estrous cycle in gilts and sows varies from ......to......days
    a) 12-18 b) 18- 24
    c) 24- 36 d) 10-12

83. Piglet possess .... number of needle teeth at the time of birth.

a) 4 b) 8

c) 6 d) 2

84. Which of the following is correct regarding selection breeding sow?

a) Litter size > 8 b) Good temperament

c) 12 functional teats d) All are correct

85. Sows for breeding should be selected after performance of at least ...... litter.

a) 1 b) 2

c) 3 d) 4

86. The breeding ratio of Boar: Sow should be

a) 1: 10 b) 1: 15

c) 1:20 d) 1:30

87. Duration of estrous cycle in Gilt is........... days.

a) 1-2 b) 2-3

c) 3-4 d) 4-5

88. Duration of estrous cycle in Sow is........... days.

a) 1 b) 2

c) 3 d) 4

89. Time of ovulation in sow is ....

a) 24-48 hrs after the onset of estrous

b) 24-48 hrs before the onset of estrous

c) At the end of estrous

d) None of the above

90. Behavioural sign of heat in sow is –

a) Characteristic grunting or roaring sound

b) Frequent urination, reduced appetite, restlessness

c) Pricking of ears

d) All of the above

91. .... is the first full proof method of heat detection in sow ?

a) Standing reflex : immobility on back pressure

b) Pricking of ears

c) Mounting over other females

d) All of the above

92. Which of the following is correct regarding time of mating/A.I. in sows ?

a) 10-12 hrs before ovulation.

b) Double service at an interval of 8-10 hrs.

c) AI: 1st : 24 hrs, 2nd : 36 hrs after onset of heat.

d) All are correct

93. Average semen volume per ejaculate of boar is................ ml.
   a) 50 - 100   b) 100- 200
   c) 200 -300   d) 300-500
94. Average sperm concentration in boar semen is .... million/ml.
   a) 150   b) 250
   c) 350   d) 450
95. Full form of MMA in pig is-
   a) Mastitis Metritis Anaemia   b) Mastitis Metritis Agalactia
   c) Malfunction Moribound Animal   d) None of the above
96. Needle teeth in piglet should be clipped ....days after farrowing.
   a) 1st or 2nd   b) 3rd – 4th
   c) 5th -6th   d) 7th-8th
97. .... is the common method for identification in pigs.
   a) Tagging   b) Branding
   c) Ear notching   d) All
98. . ... chemical is used for temporary identification in piglets.
   a) KI   b) $Ag NO_3$
   c) NaCl   d) Methylene Blue
99. Which of the following is correct regarding 'Piglet anemia'?
   a) It is more common on pucca floor.
   b) Iron dextran @100-150 mg is given on 4th and 14th days to prevent it.
   c) Only a is correct.
   d) Both a and b are correct.
100. Which of the following is correct regarding raising of boar?
   a) Service by boar below 1 yr: once daily.
   b) Service by boar above 1 yr: twice daily, but maximum 5-7 services / week.
   c) Used for breeding till 6-8 years.
   d) All are correct .
101. Which of the following animal has highest dressing percentage?
   a) Cattle   b) Buffalo
   c) Pig   d) Goat
102. Permanent dental formula of cattle is –
   a) 2 (I 3/3, C 0/0, PM 3/3, M 0/0)   b) 2 (I 3/3, C 0/0, PM 3/3, M 3/3)
   c) 2 (I 3/3, C 1/1, PM 3/3, M 3/3)   d) 2 (I 3/3, C 0/0, PM 4/3, M 3/3)
103. Permanent dental formula of pig is –
   a) 2 (I 3/3, C 0/0, PM 3/3, M 0/0)   b) 2 (I 3/3, C 0/0, PM 3/3, M 3/3)
   c) 2 (I 3/3, C 1/1, PM 4/4, M 3/3)   d) 2 (I 3/3, C 1/1, PM 3/3, M 3/3)
104. Permanent dental formula of Male horse is –
   a) 2 (I 3/3, C 0/0, PM 3/3, M 0/0)   b) 2 (I 3/3, C 0/0, PM 3/3, M 3/3)
   c) 2 (I 3/3, C 1/1, PM 3or 4/3, M 3/3)   d) 2 (I 3/3, C 0/0, PM 3or 4/3, M 3/3)

105. Permanent dental formula of Female horse is -
a) 2 (I 3/3, C 0/0, PM 3/3, M 0/0)
b) 2 (I 3/3, C 0/0, PM 3/3, M 3/3)
c) 2 (I 3/3, C 1/1, PM 3or 4/3, M 3/3)
d) 2 (I 3/3, C 0/0, PM 3or 4/3, M 3/3)

106. Dental star of horse appear at the age of .... in incisor, intermediate & corner respectively.
a) 2, 3, 4
b) 4, 5, 6
c) 6, 7, 8
d) 8, 9, 10

107. Galvayne's groove in horse appear at the age of-
a) 10
b) 15
c) 20
d) 25

108. An attempt to look an old mouth horse look younger is known as -
a) Bridling
b) Bishoping
c) Gelding
d) Culling

109. Which of the following is wrong?
a) Puberty age of mare occurs at around 6-7 months of age.
b) Mares are seasonally polyestrous.
c) Estrus duration of mare is 5-7days.
d) The average gestation period of mare is 340 days.

110. Duration of estrous cycle in mare is........ days.
a) 15-17
b) 21-23
c) 25-30
d) None

111. Foal heat/Dhaman appears .... days after foaling ?
a) 1-2
b) 9-11
c) 15-16
d) 20-25

112. .... Is the most prominent sign of heat in mare?
a) Frequent urination
b) Winking of clitoris
c) Vaginal discharge
d) All

113. The normal weaning period of foal is –
a) 3 months
b) 6 months
c) 9 months
d) 1 year

114. .... is a prominent sign of foaling in case of mare?
a) Frequent urination
b) Winking of clitoris
c) Waxing of teat
d) All

115. Advantage of hot shoeing over cold shoeing is –
a) Lesser fitting time
b) Exact juxtaposition between hoof and iron
c) Only a is correct
d) Both a & b are correct.

116. Most commonly used grain for horse is
a) Maize
b) Oat
c) Sorghum
d) Bajra

117. Most common body colour of horse is-
 a) Bay b) Brown
 c) Black d) White
118. Which of the following is correct regarding protein requirement of horse?
 a) New born foal – 20 % b) Weaning – 14 %
 c) Mature horse – 10 % d) All are correct
119. Which of the following statement is correct?
 a) Horses can tolerate urea as high as 4%
 b) Lysine is an important amino acid for younger horses
 c) Feeding excessive protein to working horse is detrimental
 d) All are correct
120. The ideal Stallion: Mare ratio for breeding is-
 a) 1: 10-20 b) 1: 30-40
 c) 1: 40-50 d) 1:50-60
121. The average semen volume per ejaculate in stallion is .... ml
 a) 20-30 b) 70- 80
 c) 50- 150 d) 350-500
122. Which of the following is correct regarding 'dimension of stall' for horses?
 a) Stallion - 14' X 14' b) Brood mare - 16' X 16'
 c) Foaling box- 24' X 24' d) All are correct
123. Biting vice is more common in –
 a) Stallion b) Mare
 c) Brood mare d) Equally seen in all
124. Eating food too fast without adequate chewing in case of horse is known as-
 a) Bolting b) Weaving
 c) Sucking d) None
125. Which of the following is a vice in horse?
 a) Coprophagia b) Biting
 c) Bolting d) All
126. Which of the following method is used for casting of horse?
 a) Reuff's method b) Side-line method
 c) By using twitch d) Both b & c
127. Which of the following method is used for casting of cattle?
 a) Reuff's method b) Side-line method
 c) Burley method d) Both a & c
128. Which of the following method is used for casting of pig?
 a) Reuff's method b) Side-line method
 c) Burley method d) By pig catcher
129. A period of strong sexual activity in male camels is known as -
 a) Thoot b) Rut
 c) Musth d) All

130. Induced ovulation occurs in -

a) Camel b) Rabbit

c) Cat d) All

131. In male camel soft palate protrudes .... during sexual excitement.

a) Dulaa b) Pole gland

c) Rutt d) All

132. Which of the following is correct?

a) Dulaa is present in both sexes, but much more developed in entire males

b) Majority of male camels display the dulaa at the right side of the mouth

c) Bactrian camel does not have a dulaa

d) All are correct

133. Cocking of tail is a method of pregnancy diagnosis in –

a) Camel b) Cattle

c) Goat d) Pig

134. Hutch is term used for housing of .... species.

a) Camel b) Rabbit

c) Goat d) Pig

135. Portion controlled feeding is recommended regimen for growing –

a) Camel b) Rabbit

c) Goat d) Dog

136. Young one of mice is usually weaned at the age of

a) 7-14 days b) 21-28 days

c) 35-42 days d) 56-63 days

137. Among small laboratory animals, cheek pouch is present in .... species.

a) Mouse b) Hamster

c) Rat d) Guinea pig

138. Which of the following laboratory animal is not a rodent?

a) Mouse b) Rat

c) Rabbit d) Guinea Pig

139. The best choice of method of mating in rabbits is-

a) Harem system b) Colony mating

c) Monogamous pair system d) Hand mating

140. Vitamin C is essential in the diet of ....laboratory animal.

a) Rat b) Mice

c) Hamster d) Guinea Pig

141. ....oil is most extensively fed to horses.

a) Castor oil b) Linseed oil

c) Cotton seed oil d) Sunflower oil

142. Breeding in camel generally takes place during-
   a) Winter b) Spring
   c) Summer d) Autumn
143. Adaptive feature of yak for cold climate is -
   a) Large rumen b) Small scrotum
   c) Fetal hemoglobin d) All
144. The gestation period in camels is-
   a) 285 days b) 390 days
   c) 330 days d) 310 days
145. Permanent dental formula of rabbit:
   a) I 1/1, C 0/0, PM 3/3, M 0/0 X 2 b) I 2/1, C 0/0, PM 3/2, M 3/3 X 2
   c) I 0/4, C 0/0, PM 3/3, M 0/3 X 2 d) I 0/0, C 0/0, PM 3/3, M 0/3 X 2
146. Gestation period in guinea pig:
   a) 65-72 days b) 30-32 days
   c) 50-60 days d) 40-45 days
147. The male: female breeding ratio in commercial rabbit units should be:
   a) 1: 20 b) 1: 10
   c) 1: 04 d) 1: 15
148. Act of parturition in cat is called
   a) Whelping b) Queening
   c) Kindling d) Kidding
149. Act of parturition in dog is called
   a) Whelping b) Queening
   c) Kindling d) Kidding
150. Estrous cycle in mice-
   a) 14-18 days b) 4- 6 days
   c) 1-2 days d) 10-12 days
151. Which of the following lab animal practices coprophagy ?
   a) Rabbit b) Guinea pig
   c) Mouse d) Both a & b
152. Pellets of...........mm diameter and ....mm length are preferable in rabbit feeding.
   a) 1-2 mm & 5-7 mm b) 2-3 & 7-9 mm
   c) 3-4 mm & 10-15 mm d) 5-10 mm & 15-20 mm

Answer Key

1	b	2	d	3	a	4	b	5	c	6	c	7	c
8	d	9	c	10	c	11	a	12	a	13	c	14	c
15	d	16	b	17	b	18	d	19	d	20	a	21	b

22	b	23	d	24	c	25	a	26	b	27	c	28	a
29	b	30	d	31	b	32	c	33	a	34	b	35	c
36	c	37	c	38	b	39	c	40	d	41	b	42	c
43	a	44	c	45	b	46	b	47	a	48	c	49	a
50	a	51	a	52	c	53	b	54	d	55	d	56	c
57	b	58	d	59	b	60	b	61	d	62	c	63	a
64	b	65	a	66	b	67	d	68	d	69	d	70	a
71	b	72	a	73	c	74	a	75	c	76	d	77	c
78	a	79	c	80	d	81	a	82	b	83	b	84	d
85	b	86	a	87	a	88	c	89	a	90	d	91	a
92	d	93	d	94	b	95	b	96	a	97	c	98	b
99	d	100	d	101	c	102	b	103	c	104	c	105	d
106	d	107	d	108	a	109	b	110	a	111	b	112	b
113	b	114	b	115	c	116	d	117	b	118	a	119	d
120	d	121	b	122	c	123	d	124	a	125	a	126	d
127	d	128	d	129	d	130	d	131	d	132	a	133	d
134	a	135	b	136	b	137	b	138	c	139	d	140	d
141	b	142	a	143	b	144	a	145	b	146	a	147	b
148	b	149	a	150	b	151	d	152	c				

25

Colostrum Management and Its Importance

***Priya*[1], *Rachana Sharma*[1], *Vivek Sahu*[2], *and Anand Prakash*[1]**

[1]*College of Veterinary Science, Rampura Phul-GADVASU, Ludhiana, Punjab*

[2]*College of Veterinary Science, GADVASU, Ludhiana, Punjab*

Introduction

Colostrum feeding

- Colostrum is rich source of gamma globulins (antibodies), vitamins and minerals
- Colostrum Temp.: 99°F-102°F
- Colostrum feeding: first 3-5 days.
- Whole milk: after 5 days
- Feed the total amount of milk at 3 or 4 equal intervals up to the age of 7 days and then twice daily
- Quantity of colostrum: 10 % of body weight.
- Overfeeding: calf scour/diarrhea.
- Around 0.5% of a cow's yearly milk production is made up of colostrum.
- After birth, the amount of immunoglobulins that can be absorbed from colostrum drops by 1/3 as soon as 6 hours, by 2/3 after 12 hours, and an intestinal barrier forms after 24 hours.
- Colostrum must be given in sufficient amounts to the newborn calf because during the first 24 hours after parturition, the permeability of the stomach and the concentration of immunoglobulins drop sharply.
- Cow colostrum must meet minimum requirements for both immunological and bacteriological characteristics: >50 g/l of IgG and <100,000 cfu/ml for the total plate count

Chemical constituents of colostrum

1. Carbohydrate

Lactose: Found in low concentrations in colostrum, lactose reacts negatively with other components like fat, protein, and ash. In colostrum, lactose concentrations as low as 1.2% have been documented)Within seven days of giving birth, the lactose concentration returns to normal. Approximately half of the osmotic pressure in milk is caused by lactose.

Oligosaccharides: Other sugars found in milk in trace levels include glucose, fructose, glucosamine, galactosamine, N-acetylneuraminic acid, and oligosaccharides, which are carbohydrates made up of three to ten monosaccharides covalently linked by glycosidic bonds. Lactose is the only sugar found in milk. The two main kinds of oligosaccharides are neutral and acidic)Whereas acidic oligosaccharides have one or more negatively charged N-acetylneuraminic acid (sialic acid)residues, neutral oligosaccharides, also known as galacto-oligosaccharides (GOS), do not contain any charged carbohydrate residues. Colostrum has an oligosaccharide content of between 0.7 and 1.2 g. mL−1. In cow colostrum, 40 oligosaccharides have been found thus far.

Protein

- Colostrum has a higher casein concentration than milk. Increased amounts of IgG, IgA, and IgM are present in colostrum, and 70–80% of the protein in colostrum is composed of immunoglobulins.
- The majority of the Igs in colostrum are made up of IgG1, which is followed by IgM, IgA, and IgG2.
- Compared to mature milk, colostrum has larger quantities of beta-lactoglobulin (β-lg) and alpha-lactalbumin (α-la). Colostrum has a four-fold higher ratio of β-lg/α-la than mature milk.
- Colostrum has a higher concentration of bovine serum albumin (2.63 mg.mL−1 BSa)than milk. A cationic glycoprotein of mammalian origin that binds iron, lactoferrin is essential to the mammary gland's defense mechanism. The usual range of lactoferrin content in colostrum is 1.5 to 5mg.mL−1.

A total of 29 minor proteins were identified in colostrum and milk, of which several were observed only in colostrum, i.e. fibrinogen β-chain, chitinase 3-like 1, α-antitrypsin, complement C3 α-chain, gelsolin.

2. **Growth factors**: Epidermal growth factor (EGF), betacellulin (BT c) , insulin-like growth factor I (IGF-I), IGF-II, transforming growth factor-β1 (TGF-β1), TGF-β2, fibroblast growth factor 1 and 2 (FGF1 and FGF2), and platelet-derived growth factor (PGDF) are the primary growth factors found in colostrum and milk. Mature milk has less than 10 μg.L−1 of each IGF-I and IGF-II, while colostrum has concentrations of 50 to 2000 μg.L−1 and 200–600 μg.L−1, respectively.
3. **Lipids**: Colostrum often has a higher fat content than milk, however this isn't always the case. Colostrum contains low amounts of stearic acid, oleic acid, and short-chain fatty acids (C4–C10), which rise with time. Colostrum has high concentrations of long-chain fatty acids because cows near parturition have negative energy balances, which induce adipose tissue fatty acids to be mobilized and integrated into milk fat.
4. **Minerals**: Citrates, phosphates, and chlorides of H+, K+, Na+, Mg2+, and Ca2+ are among the mineral constituents, also known as milk salts. These ions can be found in solution or as colloidal species that have complexed with the caseins. Milk is saturated with respect to calcium and phosphate ions, which exist in a dynamic equilibrium between serum and colloidal forms.
5. **Enzymes:** There are about seventy native enzymes known to exist in milk, and they come from four main sources: blood plasma, cytoplasm of secretory cells, milk fat globule membrane (MFGM), and somatic cells. Generally speaking, colostrum has more enzymes than milk.

- Antioxidant enzymes: One member of the peroxidase family, lactoperoxidase (LPO), catalyses the oxidation of thiocynates in the presence of hydrogen peroxide, producing intermediate compounds with a variety of antibacterial properties. The LPO content of colostrum ranges from 13 to 30 mg.L−1, in contrast to milk's 11–45 mg.L−1.Proteinases: Plasmin, a serine protease derived from plasminogen, is the principal indigenous proteinase in milk whose concentration is higher in colostrum than that in milk.
- Lipases and esterase: The main naturally occurring lipase in milk is called lipoprotein lipase (LPL). Mammary LPL activity rises noticeably before delivery and stays elevated during lactation. A number of phosphatases are also found in milk, the two main ones being acid and alkaline phosphatase. In addition to these enzymes, colostrum also contains lysozymes, γ-glutamyl transferase (γ-GT), and nucleases.

6. **Nucleotides and Nucleosides**: The non-protein-nitrogen (NPN) fraction of milk contains nucleotides and nucleosides, which are found in sub-milligram amounts per litre.
7. **Cytokines:** A broad class of proteins, peptides, or glycoproteins known as cytokines, can have significant biological effects at very low quantities (10 to 1000 pg.mL−1). These consist of interleukins (IL), interferons (INF), and tumour necrosis factors (TNF). Colostrum has higher quantities of TNF-α, INF-γ, IL-1β, IL-6, and IL-1ra than milk.

Advantage of colostrum feeding

1. Transfer of passive immunity

- Gamma globulins
- Permeability of intestinal mucosa is higher during initial 24 hrs after birth.

2. Laxative action:

- Colostrum acts as laxative due to higher dry matter content as compare to milk,
- Easy passage of first faeces (meconium)
- Prevent the chances of gastrointestinal tract infection

3. Nutritious Food

- Colostrum is highly nutritious food available to newly born young ones at birth.
- In absence of colostrum: ½-1 lit. skimmed milk + 2 eggs + 5 ml castor oil (Artificial colostrum)

4. Thermoregulation

Composition of chemical constituents (in range; g/kg) of colostrum of different livestock species

Species	Fat	Protein	Lactose
Cattle	34-38	125-135	30-32
Goat	87-92	75-85	24-26
Horse	6-8	185-195	45-47
Pig	70-74	175-185	23-25
Sheep	122-126	125-135	32-36
Rabbit	45-49	130-140	14-18
Dog	76-78	135-140	25-30

1. How much energy is provided by cow milk fat?
   a) 9 Kcal/gm c) 15 Kcal/gm
   b) 4 Kcal/gm d) 20 Kcal/gm
2. Which of the following is not true for cow milk?
   a) Good source of iron c) Good source of calcium
   b) Good source of vitamin d) Both a and b
3. How much blood passes through udder for production of 1 liter of milk?
   a) 10-20 Liter c) 400-500 mL
   b) 400-500 Liter d) 1 Liter
4. Milk component absent in colostrum in comparison to cow milk
   a) High lactose c) High protein
   b) High fat d) All the above
5. Amino acid which is the most predominant in cow milk is
   a) Cysteine c) Lysine
   b) Leucine d) Isoleucine
6. The constituent (%) present in higher amount in colostrum of dairy cows is
   a) Total solids c) Fat
   b) Total protein d) Lactose
7. Colostrum is a highly fortified source of nutrients having --------times protein of normal milk
   a) 2 c) 7
   b) 4 d) 11
8. Colostrum is a highly fortified source of nutrients having --------times total solids of normal milk
   a) 2 c) 7
   b) 4 d) 11
9. Lactose content (%) of cow colostrum is
   a) 4.80 c) 28.00
   b) 21.00 d) 2.50

10. Total solids content (%) of cow colostrum is

a) 4.80 c) 28.00

b) 21.00 d) 2.50

11. Total protein content (%) of cow colostrum is

a) 4.80 c) 28.00

b) 21.00 d) 2.50

12. The quantity and quality of γ-globulins in colostrum is increased by

a) Vaccination of dry cows c) Improved feeding

b) Isolation of dry cows d) None of the above

13. Colostrum of mature cows is of higher quality than that produced by heifers.

a) True c) Can't say

b) False d)

14. Globulins (%) present in colostrum of dairy cows is

a) 15 c) 20

b) 5 d) 30

15. Vitamin absent in new born calf is

a) a c) c

b) d d) e

16. Quantity of colostrum to be fed as per cent of body weight during 15-30 mnts of life

a) 5-8 c) 15

b) 10 d) 20

17. Quantity of colostrum to be fed as per cent of body weight during 10-12 hrs of life

a) 5-8 c) 15

b) 10 d) 20

18. Quantity of colostrum to be fed as per cent of body weight during 2nd and 3rd day of life

a) 5-8 c) 15

b) 10 d) 20

19. Period of suckling allowed for calves a day after their birth

a) 5-minute; 4-5 times c) 10-minute; 4-5 times

b) 2-minute; 2 times d) 20-minute; 10 times

20. Consumption of excessive colostrum by calves may result in

a) Scours c) Tympany

b) Impaction d) None of above

21. Amount of immunoglobulin absorbed by calves into their blood depends on

a) Amount of colostrum fed c) Both a and b

b) Age of calves d) None of above

22. Calves receiving 2 liters colostrum absorbed ---------times than those fed 1 liter
    a) 2
    b) 4
    c) 6
    d) 1/2
23. Calves receiving 2 liters colostrum absorbed ---------times than those fed 1/2 liter
    a) 2
    b) 4
    c) 6
    d) 1/2
24. After birth, within how much time colostrum feeding should be practiced?
    a) 4 hr
    b) 6 hr
    c) 1 hr
    d) 8 hr
25. How much quantity of colostrum needed by a calf daily?
    a) 2 litres
    b) 6 litres
    c) 1 litre
    d) 3-4 litres
26. Daily feeding of colostrum should be divided in how many feeds or parts?
    a) 2
    b) 3-4
    c) 10
    d) 7
27. The primary function of colostrum feeding is to
    a) Fortify disease resistance
    b) Help in artificial respiration
    c) Pass meconium
    d) Helps in standing of calf
28. Ash content (%) of colostrum is
    a) 1.60
    b) 0.50
    c) 3.0
    d) 6.0
29. Second dose of colostrum feeding should be done in approx. -----------hours
    a) 4-5
    b) 10-12
    c) 24
    d) 48
30. Quantity of colostrum to be daily fed to a newborn calf up to 3 days
    a) 5 kg
    b) 1 kg
    c) 7 kg
    d) 2-3 kg
31. How much time (hrs.) after birth intact antibodies are absorbed by intestine of newborn calf?
    a) 12
    b) 24
    c) 48
    d) 72
32. An enzyme present in bovine colostrum which prevents digestion of antibodies
    a) Protease inhibitor
    b) Lipase inhibitor
    c) Trypsin inhibitor
    d) All of above
33. Age of calf at which silage feeding can be done
    a) Birth
    b) 1 month
    c) >3 month
    d) 2 month
34. Immunoglobulins present in higher amount in colostrum
    a) Ig G
    b) Iga)
    c) Ig E
    d) Ig M

35. Coagulation of colostrum occurs due to high amount of
    a) Casein
    b) Fat
    c) Albumin
    d) Carotene
36. The highest fat and protein content is found in colostrum of which livestock species?
    a) Ewe
    b) Cow
    c) Doe
    d) Sow
37. Failure of passive immunity in calves is seen if serum IgG concentration falls below
    a) 10 g/L
    b) 20 g/L
    c) 30 g/L
    d) 40 g/L
38. A mixture of lacteal secretions and constituents of blood serum, most notably Ig and other serum proteins, which accumulate in the mammary gland during the prepartum dry period is
    a) Whole milk
    b) Colostrum
    c) Milk replacer
    d) None of above
39. IgG accounts for approximately -------------- of the total Ig in colostrum
    a) 85-90%
    b) 5%
    c) 7-10%
    d) 25-50%
40. IgA account for approximately -------------of the total Ig in colostrum
    a) 85-90%
    b) 5%
    c) 7-10%
    d) 25-50%
41. IgM account for approximately ----------of the total Ig in colostrum
    a) 85-90%
    b) 5%
    c) 7-10%
    d) 25-50%
42. IgG1 accounts for --------of the total IgG in bovine colostrum
    a) 80-90%
    b) 5%
    c) 7-10%
    d) 25-50%
43. Mean bovine colostral concentration of IgG is
    a) 75-80 g/L
    b) 4.0-4.4 g/L
    c) 4.9-5.3 g/L
    d) 10-15 g/L
44. Mean bovine colostral concentration of IgA is
    a) 75-80 g/L
    b) 4.0-4.4 g/L
    c) 4.9-5.3 g/L
    d) 10-15 g/L
45. Mean bovine colostral concentration of IgM is
    a) 75-80 g/L
    b) 4.0-4.4 g/L
    c) 4.9-5.3 g/L
    d) 10-15 g/L
46. The rate of decay of colostral antibodies from calf's circulation can be influenced by
    a) Active viral infections
    b) Age of calf
    c) Vaccination
    d) All of the above

47. Nonnutritive factors found in increased levels in colostrum include
    a) Hormones c) Nonspecific antimicrobial factors
    b) Cytokines d) All of the above
48. Trypsin inhibitor is found how many times in colostrum than in milk?
    a) 25 c) 100
    b) 75 d) 50
49. Growth factors in bovine colostrum include
    a) TGF beta-2 c) Growth hormone
    b) Insulin d) All of the above
50. A minimum amount of IgG needs to be delivered to the calf shortly after birth
    a) 150-200 c) 75
    b) 100 d) 50
51. Quality of colostrum produced by cows ---------with their age
    a) Decreases c) Remains same
    b) Increases d) None of above
52. Cows with excessively short dry periods (<21 days) produce colostrum with
    a) Lower IgG concentration c) Both a and b
    b) Lower colostrum yields d) None of above
53. Instruments which are used to measure colostrum quality
    a) Colostrometer c) Both a and b
    b) Brix refractometer d) None of above
54. Unique ability of the neonatal enterocyte to non-selectively absorb intact large molecules, such as Ig is known as
    a) Open gut c) Selective absorption
    b) Discriminate absorption d) Gut closure
55. Process playing a major role during open gut is
    a) Pinocytosis c) Phagocytosis
    b) Endocytosis d) None of above
56. Decrease in the absorption of Ig across the intestinal epithelium linearly with time from birth to completely close at approximately 24 hours is termed as
    a) Open gut c) Selective absorption
    b) Discriminate absorption d) Gut closure
57. High bacteria levels in colostrum, particularly coliform bacteria, may result in
    a) Binding free Ig in the gut lumen c) Interfere passive Ig transfer
    b) Block direct uptake d) All of the above
58. Decreased colostral Ig absorption in the first 12 hours has been reported in calves with
    a) Postnatal respiratory acidosis c) Hypoxia
    b) Hypothermia) d) All of the above
59. Colostral Ig absorption may be improved by
    a) Warming the calves c) Presence of dam
    b) Drying calves d) All of the above

60. Colostrum feeding after the gut closure may result in
    a) Stimulation GIT development by bioactive compounds
    c) Both a and b
    b) Local GIT protection
    d) None of above
61. Total plate count in fresh/raw colostrum should be less than
    a) 200,000 cfu/mL c) 300,000 cfu/mL
    b) 150,000 cfu/mL d) 100,000 cfu/mL
62. Total coliform count in fresh/raw colostrum should be less than
    a) 10,000 cfu/mL c) 30,000 cfu/mL
    b) 20,000 cfu/mL d) 40,000 cfu/mL
63. Colostrum contamination can be reduced by
    a) Cleaning and sanitizing udders
    c) Clean, sanitized storage equipment
    b) Use of clean bucket
    d) All of the above
64. Period of collection within which colostrum should be frozen /refrigerated)
    a) 1 hour c) 12 hour
    b) 6 hour d) 24 hour
65. Frozen colostrum can be stored for up to
    a) 2 year c) 3 year
    b) 1 year d) 5 year
66. Gold standard for evaluating passive transfer in calves is
    a) Radial immunodiffusion (RId)assay c) AGIT
    b) CFT d) Western blot
67. Advantages of feeding heat treated (HT) colostrum are
    a) Improved efficiency of IgG absorption c) Reduce diarrhea
    b) Enhanced GIT colonization d) All of the above
68. Minimum total plate count levels in HT colostrum should be
    a) 30,000 cfu/mL c) 20,000 cfu/mL
    b) 40,000 cfu/mL d) 50,000 cfu/mL
69. Minimum coliform count levels in HT colostrum should be
    a) 200 cfu/mL c) 300 cfu/mL
    b) 100 cfu/mL d) 500 cfu/mL
70. The most important management factor in determining calf health and survival is
    a) Colostrum management c) Summer management
    b) Health management d) Winter management
71. Starting period of ruminant colostrogenesis is
    a) Last months of pregnancy c) Last days of pregnancy
    b) Last weeks of pregnancy d) Post-calving

72. End period of ruminant colostrogenesis is
  a) Last months of pregnancy c) Last days of pregnancy
  b) Last weeks of pregnancy d) Post-calving
73. The most variable component of colostrum is
  a) Fat c) Ash
  b) Protein d) Total solids
74. Bovine colostrum contains ------------ g/L proteins
  a) 30-200 c) 10-30
  b) 100-500 d) 500-800
75. The high protein content of colostrum is mainly due to
  a) Bioactive compounds c) Hormones
  b) Immunoglobulins d) Growth regulators
76. Bioactive compounds present in colostrum are
  a) Lactoferrin c) Growth factors
  b) Lysozyme d) All of the above
77. Antigenic glycopeptides are present in colostrum of which species?
  a) Buffalo c) Human
  b) Cow d) All of the above
78. Macrophage-activating oligosaccharides are present in colostrum of which species?
  a) Buffalo c) Human
  b) Cow d) All of the above
79. Decrease in minerals of ruminant colostrum is seen after how many days of calving?
  a) 3 c) 7
  b) 5 d) 9
80. Functions of colostrum feeding to neonates are
  a) Laxative c) Immunoprotection
  b) Thermoregulation d) All of the above
81. Colostrometer measures which parameter of colostrum?
  a) Fat content c) Specific gravity
  b) Direct Ig concentration d) None of above
82. Colostrometer uses a color scale to calibrate Ig concentration in
  a) mg/mL c) mg/L
  b) g/mL d) µg/mL
83. Concentration of Ig present in colostrum tested green on use of color scale of colostrometer?
  a) > 10 mg/mL c) > 30 mg/mL
  b) > 20 mg/mL d) > 50 mg/mL

84. Concentration of Ig present in colostrum tested yellow on use of color scale of colostrometer?

a) <20 mg/mL
b) 20-50 mg/mL
c) > 100 mg/mL
d) > 50 mg/mL

85. Concentration of Ig present in colostrum tested red on use of color scale of colostrometer?

a) <20 mg/mL
b) 20-50 mg/mL
c) > 100 mg/mL
d) > 50 mg/mL

86. Brix value of 22% for colostrum shows --------Ig concentration

a) 10 mg/mL
b) 20 mg/mL
c) 30 mg/mL
d) 50 mg/mL

87. Passive immunity transfer in calves is affected by

a) Respiratory acidosis of new born
b) Time of colostrum intake
c) Presence of mother
d) All of the above

88. The onset of immunocompetence (active immunity) occurs after how much age of calves?

a) 1 week
b) 2 week
c) 3 week
d) 4 week

89. Milk produced on 2nd and 3rd day after calving is known as

a) Colostrum
b) Transition milk
c) Whole milk
d) None of above

90. Freezing and thawing of colostrum destroy which component of colostrum?

a) RBCs
b) Fat
c) Leukocytes
d) Ash

91. Flash-frozen colostrum is produced by using

a) Plastic bags
b) HM-HDPE
c) Perflouroalkoxy bags
d) None of above

92. Colostrum pasteurization can eliminate many pathogens like present in colostrum including

a) Mycobacterium paratuberculosis
b) Salmonella spp.
c) Mycoplasma ssp.
d) All of the above

93. Additives to Colostrum are

a) Potassium isobutyrate (KI
b) sodium bicarbonate
c) Se (Na-selenite)
d) All of the above

94. The most abundant peptide found in bovine colostrum whey proteins

a) β-lactoglobulin
b) α-lactoglobulin
c) Lactoperoxidase
d) Lactoferrin

95. The most abundant carbohydrate in bovine colostrum is

a) Sucrose
b) Lactose
c) Fructose
d) Ribose

96. The most abundant phosphoprotein in bovine colostrum is
   a) Caseins
   b) Whey proteins
   c) β-lactoglobulin
   d) α-lactoglobulin
97. Dietary oligosaccharides content in bovine colostrum is
   a) 1g/L
   b) 5g/L
   c) 10g/L
   d) 20g/L
98. The bovine colostrum lipid profile is characterized by around 65–75% of
   a) Monounsaturated fatty acids
   b) Polyunsaturated fatty acids
   c) Saturated fatty acids
   d) None of above
99. The bovine colostrum lipid profile is characterized by around 24-48% of
   a) Monounsaturated fatty acids
   b) Polyunsaturated fatty acids
   c) Saturated fatty acids
   d) None of above
100. The bovine colostrum lipid profile is characterized by around 4–5% of
   a) Monounsaturated fatty acids
   b) Polyunsaturated fatty acids
   c) Saturated fatty acids
   d) None of above

Answer Key

1	a	2	d	3	b	4	a	5	d	6	a	7	c
8	a	9	d	10	c	11	b	12	a	13	a	14	a
15	a	16	a	17	b	18	a	19	a	20	a	21	c
22	a	23	b	24	c	25	d	26	b	27	a	28	a
29	b	30	d	31	a	32	c	33	c	34	a	35	c
36	a	37	a	38	b	39	a	40	c	41	d	42	a
43	a	44	b	45	c	46	d	47	c	48	c	49	d
50	d	51	b	52	c	53	c	54	a	55	a	56	d
57	d	58	d	59	d	60	c	61	d	62	a	63	d
64	a	65	b	66	a	67	d	68	c	69	b	70	a
71	b	72	d	73	a	74	a	75	b	76	b	77	d
78	d	79	b	80	d	81	c	82	a	83	d	84	b
85	a	86	d	87	d	88	c	89	b	90	c	91	c
92	d	93	d	94	a	95	b	96	a	97	a	98	c
99	a	100	b										

26

Transportation and Health Management Status

Jessy Bagh[1], Annada Das[2], and Kaushik Satyaprakash[3]

[1]Department of Livestock Production and Management, CVSc and AH, OUAT Bhubaneswar, Odisha

[2]Department of Livestock Products Technology, Faculty of Veterinary and Animal Sciences, WBUAFS, Kolkata, West Bengal

[3]Department of Veterinary Public Health and Epidemiology, Faculty of Veterinary and Animal Sciences, RGSC, BHU, Mirzapur, Uttar Pradesh

Introduction

Livestock transportation is a process of carrying animal from one place to another by different means of transportation. It is a stressful, threating and not familiar event of domestic animals. Livestock is transported for many reasons like marketing, slaughter, changing of owner, re-stocking and desirable grazing area)Animals who are transported for slaughter are stressful due to various component like loading, unloading, restraining, unfavorable weather condition, thrist, hunger. During transportation there are many rules and regulation by different countries which should be strictly implemented) Cattle and other animal species should be transported with partition. Birds and lab animals are transported in cages or any airy cartridge or basket. During transportation food and water should be withheld for 24 hours. if the transportation is more than 24 hours animal should be watered and fed in transit.

Different mode of transportation is mainly depending upon number of animal, distance covered, and economic value of animal and economic status of owners.

By walking: Animal are transported on foot for a shorter distance like 5-10 km. Provide animal adequate grazing and watering during journey. Animal should be moved in early hours of the day.

By road: Distance upto 500 km for 12-16 hrs of journey may be preferred by road vehicle Animals are loaded in trucks, tractor, trolley and other available road vehicle for a longer distance. There should be provision of loading ramp at the start and end point for easy handling. Feeding should be done in regular interval . No rough driving.

By rail: Animals are transported by this means above 500km**.** Transported in wagons . Wagons should be airy and should be spacious. Floor of wagons should be anti-slippery. Horns of horned animals are secured to wagon side in head to tail position. For military horses/race horses special variety of wagons are used)Attendants should accompany them during journey. Ad libitum food and water should be provided before start of journey.

By ship: When the animal are transported for longer distance i.e from one country to another or within same country. Ships/boats should be designed and constructed as per the species, size and weight of the animal.

By air

Mostly precious animals are transported through air to longer distance by well-designed planes in this mode animal is of least stress and done by very short time.

Welfare wrap both physiological and mental wellbeing of animals. Five freedom of welfare, i.e. freedom from physical discomfort, pain and suffering, hunger, fear and distress and obstacles. Factors in which animal welfare depends during transportation is: Handling of animal, species, Breed, Sex, Age, size and physiological condition of animal, Means of transportation, weather condition, Human- animal interaction

Multiple Choice Question

1. Which factor is essential to consider when designing a livestock transport vehicle?
   a) Colour of the vehicle b) Size of the vehicle
   c) Number of seats in the vehicle d) Adequate ventilation and space
2. During long livestock transportation journeys what is the primary purpose of providing rest stops:
   a) To feed the animals b) To clean the vehicle
   c) To provide rest and reduce stress d) To change the vehicle
3. Type of flooring recommended for livestock transport tom prevent slips and falls:
   a) Fmooth surface b) wet surface
   c) Flooring with good traction d) Elevated surface
4. Prevention of disease spread within livestock herds or flocks is followed by what biosecurity measure:
   a) Mixing animals from different sources b) Regular vaccination
   c) Quarantine of sick animals d) Overcrowding animals
5. Document essential for recording details of animal transportation:
   a) Birth certificate b) Vriver's license
   c) Livestock transportation record d) Vehicle insurance
6. Provision for livestock during transportation to maintain their welfare is
   a) Overcrowded space b) Inadequate ventilation
   c) Access to food and water d) Extended travel time
7. Practices helps in monitoring and surveillance of livestock diseases is
   a) Ignoring signs of illness b) Regular veterinary check –ups
   c) Mixing sick and healthy animals d) providing contaminated feed
8. What does a comprehensive herd health management plan include?
   a) Ignoring animal welfare b) Disease control strategies
   c) Overcrowding animals d) Inadequate ventilation
9. During livestock transportation which is the sign of distress?
   a) Normal breathing b) Aggressive behavior
   c) Eating food regularly d) Sleeping comfortably

10. What is the role of a veterinarian in livestock health management?
    a) Overcrowding animals
    b) Providing inadequate nutrition
    c) Disease diagnosis and treatment
    d) Avoiding vaccination
11. When transporting livestock what is the crucial factor for ensuring their welfare?
    a) Speed of vehicle, comfort of the driver
    b) Adequate ventilation and space
    c) Vehicle colour
12. What is the factor that to be avoided during livestock transportation to minimize stress?
    a) Overcrowding,
    b) Adequate rest stops
    c) Providing access to water
    d) Following a planned route
13. What is required when transporting poultry to maintain their health and well – being?
    a) Exposing them to direct sunlight
    b) Keeping them in a crowded environment
    c) providing proper ventilation and temperature control
    d) Using noisy vehicle
14. During poultry transportation which practice should be followed to prevent injuries?
    a) Handling them roughly
    b) Using appropriate crates or containers
    c) Exposing them to extreme temperatures
    d) Mixing different poultry species
15. What is a biosecurity measure followed during poultry transportation to prevent disease spread?
    a) Mixing healthy and sick birds,
    b) Providing contaminated feed,
    c) Using clean and disinfected vehicles and equipement,
    d) Exposing poultry to wild birds
16. Which is the preventing measure required for maintaining the health of livestock and poultry ?
    a) Avoiding vaccination,
    b) Providing a balanced diet,
    c) Overcrowding in shelters,
    d) Ignorning signs of illness
17. What is a sign of distress indicating health issues in poultry?
    a) Normal behavior,
    b) Iethargy and droopiness,
    c) Active movement and vocalization,
    d) Balanced feed intake
18. Which is the important factor of a comprehensive livestock and poultry health management plan?
    a) Ignoring biosecurity measures,
    b) Regular veterinary check-ups and vaccinations,
    c) Avoiding quarantine procedures,
    d) Providing contaminated water

19. In order to maintain good health of livestock and poultry what role does a proper nutrition play?
    a) Overfeeding to increase weight
    b) Providing inadequate feed
    c) Offering a balanced diet based on nutritional requirements
    d) Ignorning feed quality
20. Which type of vehicle is essential for livestock transportation?
    a) Small and compact
    b) High speed racing
    c) Designed for animal welfare
    d) Loud and noisy
21. Which among the following is the primary purpose for providing rest and recovery areas during livestock transportation?
    a) Entertainment for animals
    b) To avoid traffic jams
    c) To allow animals to rest and reduce fatigue
    d) Storage of equipement
22. Which component helps to minimize the risk of injuries during livestock transportation?
    a) Rough handling
    b) Providing spacious crates or containers
    c) Excessive noise
    d) Long travel durations
23. Which kind of container is suitable for poultry birds transportation?
    a) Transparent plastic bags
    b) Open cardboard boxes
    c) Ventilated crates or cages
    d) Sealed metal containers
24. Why do we maintain proper ventilation during poultry transportation?
    a) To increase humidity levels
    b) To reduce odors
    c) To ensure adequate oxygen supply and prevent suffocation
    d) To limit external noise
25. Which factor to be avoided while transporting poultry to prevent stress and injuries?
    a) Regular monitoring
    b) Rough handling and overcrowding
    c) Providing clean water
    d) Short travel distances
26. Which practice is followed during livestock and poultry transportation for maintaining hygiene and sanitation?
    a) Using dirty equipment
    b) Avoiding cleaning and disinfection
    c) Regularly cleaning and disinfecting vehicles and equipements
    d) Mixing different species

27. Which among the following is the primary purpose for regular health checks of livestock and poultry during transportation?
    a) To ensure profitability
    b) To monitor welfare and detect early signs of disease
    c) To increase travel speed
    d) To minimize noise levels
28. Which of the following is essential for disease prevention during transportation for poultry health management?
    a) Ignoring vaccination schedules
    b) Exposing birds to contaminated environments
    c) Implementing biosecurity protocols
    d) Overcrowding in transport vehicles
29. Why is it essential for providing appropriate bedding material for livestock and poultry during transportation?
    a) To increase vehicle weight
    b) To improve comfort and reduce injuries
    c) To promote cleanliness
    d) To increase travel duration
30. Which component determines the stocking density for transporting pigs:
    a) Weight of the pigs b) Age of the pigs
    c) Breed of the pigs d) Colour of the pigs
31. What is the standard height requirement for partitions in livestock transport vehicles?
    a) 1 meter b) 1.5 meters
    c) 2 meters d) 2.5 meters
32. Which flooring material is considered standard for livestock transportation?
    a) Metal bars b) Smooth concrete
    c) Rubber mats d) Wooden planks
33. What is the standard ventilation need for livestock transport vehicle?
    a) Natural ventilation
    b) Mechanical ventilation with fans
    c) Both natural and mechanical ventilation
    d) No ventilation required
34. Recommended floor space required per layer chicken during transportation?
    a) 200 sq cm b) 400 sq cm
    c) 600 sq cm d) 800 sq cm
35. Which component determines the stocking density during transporting broiler chickens?
    a) Weight of the broilers b) Age of the broilers
    c) Breed of the broilers d) Feather color of the broilers

36. What is the partition standard height requirement done in poultry transport crates?
    a) 20 cm b) 30 cm
    c) 40 cm d) 50 cm
37. What is the recommended floor type for poultry transport crates to meet standards?
    a) Solid plastic b) Wire mesh
    c) Perforated metal d) Rubberized surface
38. What is the recommended standard temperature range for poultry transport vehicles?
    a) 10-15 ºC b) 15-20 ºC
    c) 20-25 ºC d) 25-30 ºC
39. Which factor is important in both livestock and poultry while determining stocking density?
    a) Visual appeal b) Safety and Welfare
    c) Noise level d) Vehicle speed
40. To prevent injuries during transportation what is the recommended partition design?
    a) Sharp edges b) Smooth and rounded edges
    c) No partitions required d) Perforated partitions
41. Which disease commonly affects during transportation of livestock due to stress and overcrowding?
    a) Foot mouth disease b) Bovine respiratory disease
    c) Avian influenza, d) Marek's disease
42. What is the initial symptoms in transported cattle due to heat stress?
    a) Increased appetite, b) Excessive salivation,
    c) Rapid breathing and panting, d) Feather ruffling
43. How should livestock be managed with suspected respiratory diseases during transportation?
    a) Increase stocking density,
    b) Provide adequate ventilation and minimize stress,
    c) Limit access to water,
    d) Ignore signs of illness
44. Which of the following condition occur due to poor ventilation and hygiene during transporting sheep?
    a) Foot rot b) Salmonellosis
    c) Wooden breast d) Coccidiosis
45. Which of the following management practice helps to prevent dehydration in transported pigs?
    a) Restricting access to water
    b) providing clean and fresh water regularly
    c) Overcrowding in transport crates
    d) Using non- ventilated transport vehicles

46. Which disease is a concern for poultry affecting respiratory health during transportation?
    a) Fowl cholera
    b) Infectious bronchitis
    c) Bumble foot
    d) Mycoplasma gallisepticum

47. Which among the following is a common sign of stress in transported broiler chickens?
    a) Increased vocalization
    b) Reduced feed intake
    c) Elevated body temperature
    d) Shiny feathers

48. During transportation Which disease can affect egg – laying poultry due to stress and poor handling?
    a) New castle disease
    b) Egg drop syndrome
    c) Marek's disease
    d) Avian pox

49. How should poultry during transportation with suspected infectious diseases be managed?
    a) Mix with healthy birds
    b) Provide adequate space and ventilation
    c) Restrict feed access
    d) Use contaminated equipment

50. What management strategy helps to prevent leg injuries in transported layer hens?
    a) Rough handling and rapid movements
    b) Providing appropriate flooring and partitions
    c) Exposing to extreme temperatures
    d) Overcrowding in crates

51. Which steps should be taken when encountering animals showing signs of illness during transportation?
    a) Quarantine and seek veterinary advice
    b) Ignore and continue transportation
    c) Mix with healthy animals
    d) Reduce ventilation

52. What is an important factor of managing livestock and poultry health during transportation?
    a) Overcrowding and neglecting bio security
    b) Regular monitoring and providing appropriate care
    c) Ignoring vaccination schedules,
    d) Using contaminated feed and water

53. During road transportation which factor is essential in a livestock transport truck?
    a) Wide open roof
    b) Smooth metal floor
    c) Adequate ventilation and space
    d) Low ceiling height

54. What is the standard features required during livestock transportation for vehicle suspension?
    a) Soft and bouncy
    b) Firm and rigid
    c) Adjustable and shock- absorbent
    d) Unstable and shaky
55. In livestock transport vehicles why are anti- slip floors is essential?
    a) To reduce cleaning efforts
    b) To increase vehicle speed
    c) To prevent injuries and stress
    d) To improve vehicle appearance
56. During long distance transportation of livestock which gauge of railway wagon is suitable?
    a) Broad gauge
    b) Narrow gauge
    c) Medium gauge
    d) Double gauge
57. Which is the standard feature required for ventilation in railway wagons during livestock transportation?
    a) Limited ventilation
    b) Natural ventilation & air circulation
    c) No ventilation
    d) Mechanical ventilation only
58. Why do secure partition important min railway wagons during livestock transportation?
    a) To increase noise levels
    b) To minimize space
    c) To prevent injuries and maintain separation
    d) To reduce cleaning efforts
59. To ensure the safety of livestock during transit which feature is crucial in a railway wagon?
    a) Unpadded walls
    b) Slippery flooring
    c) Secure latching and locking mechanisms
    d) Limited access doors
60. Which is the standard feature for railway wagons floor for livestock transportation?
    a) Bare metal surface
    b) Wooden planks or rubber mats with good traction
    c) Smooth and slippery surface
    d) Elevated and perforated surface
61. What is standard requirement for both trucks and railway wagons for loading and unloading facilities?
    a) Steep inclines and narrow pathways
    b) Smooth and even surfaces with proper ramps and facilities
    c) Limited access and high barriers
    d) Wet and muddy conditions

62. During transportation which type of vehicle or wagon design is suitable for reducing stress and injuries?
    a) Overcrowded and tight spaces
    b) Adequate space and partitions with padding
    c) Unstable and shaky platforms
    d) Limited access and high barriers?
63. For transportation of poultry birds by road which type of vehicle is suitable?
    a) Open flatbed truck b) Closed insulated van
    c) Double –decker bus d) Motorized scooter
64. Transportation is done in what time of a day:
    a) Evening/night b) Cooler morning
    c) Afternoon d) Both a & b
65. A combination of high humidity and high environmental temperature is especially deadly for which species:
    a) Pig b) Cattle
    c) Cat d) Poultry
66. Maximum distance covered per day in cow is :
    a) 30 km/day b) 25 km/day
    c) 16 km/day d) 34 km/day
67. Maximum distance covered per day in buffalo is :
    a) 30 km/day b) 25 km/day
    c) 16 km/day d) 34 km/day
68. Maximum distance covered per day in buffalo calf is :
    a) 30 km/day b) 25 km/day
    c) 16 km/day d) 34 km/day
69. Maximum distance covered per day in sheep is :
    a) 30 km/day b) 25 km/day
    c) 16 km/day d) 34 km/day
70. Maximum distance covered per day in goat is :
    a) 30 km/day b) 25 m/day
    c) 16 km/day d) 34 km/day
71. Maximum distance covered per day in pig is :
    a) 30 km/day b) 15 km/day
    c) 16 km/day d) 34 km/day
72. Maximum distance covered per day in piglet is :
    a) 30 km/day b) 10 km/day
    c) 16 km/day d) 34 km/day
73. Maximum distance covered per day in Kid is :
    a) 30 km/day b) 16 km/day
    c) 16 km/day d) 34 km/day

74. Maximum Number of Hours of walking in one day for cow:
    a) 8 hours b) 6 hours
    c) 4 hours d) 12 hours
75. Maximum Number of Hours of walking in one day for calf:
    a) 8 hours b) 6 hours
    c) 4 hours d) 12 hours
76. Maximum Number of Hours of walking in one day for goat &sheep:
    a) 8 hours b) 6 hours
    c) 4 hours d) 12 hours
77. Maximum Number of Hours of walking in one day for Pig:
    a) 8 hours b) 6 hours
    c) 4 hours d) 12 hours
78. Period of rest (Interval) for water in cow & Buffalo:
    a) Every 2 hours b) Every one hours
    c) Every 3 hours d) Every half an hour
79. Period of rest (Interval) for water in calf:
    a) Every 2 hours b) Every one hours
    c) Every 3 hours d) Every half an hour
80. Period of rest (Interval) for water in sheep:
    a) Every 2 hours b) Every one hours
    c) Every 3 hours d) Every half an hour
81. Period of rest (Interval) for water in Goat:
    a) Every 2 hours b) Every one hours
    c) Every 3 hours d) Every half an hour
82. Period of rest (Interval) for water in Pig:
    a) Every 2 hours b) Every one hours
    c) Every 3 hours d) Every half an hour
83. Period of rest (Interval) for food in cow & Buffalo:
    a) Every 2 hours b) Every one hours
    c) Every 3 hours d) Every four hour
84. Period of rest (Interval) for food in Sheep & goat:
    a) Every 2 hours b) Every one hours
    c) Every 3 hours d) Every four hour
85. Period of rest (Interval) for food in calf:
    a) Every 2 hours b) Every one hours
    c) Every 3 hours d) Every four hour
86. Period of rest (Interval) for food in pig:
    a) Every 2 hours b) Every one hours
    c) Every 3 hours d) Every four hour

87. Period of rest (Interval) for food in kid & lamb:
 a) Every 2 hours b) Every one hours
 c) Every 3 hours d) Every four hour

88. Temperature range Minimum/ Maximum during transport in cow & Buffalo is:
 a) 12°C to 30 °C b) 15°C to 25 °C
 c) 30°C to 40 °C d) None

89. Temperature range Minimum/ Maximum during transport in calf & Buffalo is:
 a) 12°C to 30 °C b) 15°C to 25 °C
 c) 30°C to 40 °C d) None

90. Temperature range Minimum/ Maximum during transport in Sheep & Goat is:
 a) 12°C to 30 °C b) 15°C to 25 °C
 c) 30°C to 40 °C d) None

91. Temperature range Minimum/ Maximum during transport in cow & Buffalo is:
 a) 12°C to 30 °C b) 15°C to 25 °C
 c) 30°C to 40 °C d) None

92. Temperature range Minimum/ Maximum during transport in pig is:
 a) 12°C to 25°C b) 15°C to 25 °C
 c) 30°C to 40 °C d) None

93. Number of adult cattle can be carried out per small truck is:
 a) 1 b) 2
 c) 3 d) 4

94. Number of calves can be carried out per small truck is:
 a) 1 b) 2
 c) 4 d) 6

95. Number of sheep/goat can be carried out per truck is:
 a) 10 b) 20
 c) 40 d) 60

96. Floor space required for wooled sheep weighing more than 20 kg in truck is :
 a) 0.18 m^2 b) 0.16 m^2
 c) 0.28 m^2 d) 0.23m^2

97. Floor space required for shorn sheep weighing more than 20 kg in truck is :
 a) 0.18 m^2 b) 0.16 m^2
 c) 0.28 m^2 d) 0.23m^2

98. Floor space required for wooled sheep weighing more than 30 kg in truck is :
 a) 0.18 m^2 b) 0.16 m^2
 c) 0.28 m^2 d) 0.23m^2

99. Floor space required for shorn sheep weighing more than 30 kg in truck is :
 a) 0.18 m^2 b) 0.16 m^2
 c) 0.28 m^2 d) 0.26m^2

100. Rail transport is advocated for distance above:
   a) 500 km b) 300 km
   c) 600 km d) 1000 km

101. What percent of railway transport cause losses due to shrinkage and death:
   a) 5% b) 10%
   c) 1% d) 8%?

102. Average space provided per cattle in Railway wagon should not be less than:
   a) 2 sq meters b) 4 sq meters
   c) 6 sq meters d) 8 sq meters

103. What no of Cattle should be transported by ordinary goods wagon in broad gauge :
   a) <20 b) <15
   c) <25 d) <10

104. What no of calves should be transported by ordinary goods wagon in broad gauge :
   a) <20 b) <15
   c) <25 d) <10

105. What no of Cattle should be transported by ordinary goods wagon in meter gauge :
   a) <6 b) <20
   c) <25 d) <10

106. What no of calves should be transported by ordinary goods wagon in broad gauge :
   a) <20 b) <15
   c) <25 d) <10

107. What no of adult cattle & calves should be transported by ordinary goods wagon in narrow gauge :
   a) < 4 & <6 respectively b) < 8 & <10 respectively
   c) < 10 & <12 respectively d) < 1 & <2 respectively

108. Minimum floor space required for pig while transporting in ship/boat is:
   a) $4^{1/2}$ sq ft b) $2^{3/4}$ Sq ft
   c) $3^{1/2}$ sq ft d) 8 sq ft

109. Minimum floor space required for sheep & goat while transporting in ship/boat is:
   a) $4^{1/2}$ sq ft b) $2^{3/4}$ Sq ft
   c) $3^{1/2}$ sq ft d) 8 sq ft

110. Minimum floor space required for calves while transporting in ship/boat is:
   a) $4^{1/2}$ sq ft b) $2^{3/4}$ Sq ft
   c) $3^{1/2}$ sq ft d) 8 sq ft

111. A condition seen in transport animal (cattle) due to acute stress pH fatigue where meat looks darker known as:
   a) DFD b) PSE
   c) Both d) None

112. A condition seen in pig due to stress and causes abnormal condition of meat fatigue known as:
   a) DFD b) PSE
   c) Both d) None
113. Animal brought for slaughter is kept for how many days in lairage:
   a) 2-3 days b) 4-5 days
   c) 5-6 days d) 10 days
114. Space requirement for stallion being transported by road/rail is :
   a) 2.25 Sq mtr b) 2 sq mtre
   c) 1 sq mtr d) 3 sq mtr
115. Space requirement for mare being transported by road/rail is :
   a) 2.25 Sq mtr b) 2 sq mtre
   c) 1 sq mtr d) 3 sq mtr
116. Space requirement for mares with foal at foot being transported by road/rail is :
   a) 2.25 Sq mtr b) 2 sq mtre
   c) 1 sq mtr d) 3 sq mtr
117. Number of horses should be transported by rail on broad gauge is:
   a) 8-10 b) 15
   c) 20 d) 1
118. Number of horses should be transported by rail on meter gauge is:
   a) 6 b) 15
   c) 20 d) 1
119. While transporting by sea horse are kept in :
   a) Stall b) Pen
   c) Both d) None
120. Floor space requirement for mice while transportation in a box:
   a) 25 sq.cm b) 135 sq.cm
   c) 52 sq.cm d) 160 sq.cm
121. Floor space requirement for hamster while transportation in box is :
   a) 25 sq.cm b) 135 sq.cm
   c) 52 sq.cm d) 160 sq.cm
122. Floor space requirement for rat while transportation in box is :
   a) 25 sq.cm b) 135 sq.cm
   c) 52 sq.cm d) 160 sq.cm
123. Floor space requirement for Guinea pig while transportation in box is :
   a) 25 sq.cm b) 135 sq.cm
   c) 52 sq.cm d) 160 sq.cm

124. Floor space requirement for Rabbit while transportation in box is:
a) 1100 sq.cm b) 135 sq.cm
c) 52 sq.cm d) 160 sq.cm

125. Number of mice to be kept per box during transportation:
a) 25 b) 12
c) 1 d) 2

126. Number of Hamster to be kept per box during transportation:
a) 25 b) 12
c) 1 d) 2

127. Number of Rat to be kept per box during transportation:
a) 25 b) 12
c) 1 d) 2

128. Number of Guinea pig to be kept per box during transportation:
a) 25 b) 12
c) 1 d) 2

129. Number of Rabbit to be kept per box during transportation:
a) 25 b) 12
c) 1or 2 d) None

130. Precious and high value animals are transported by which mode of transport
a) Rail b) Air
c) Road d) Ship

131. Rabbit are transported in:
a) Metallic cages b) Vessels

132. Which animal should not be fed before transport?
a) Pigs b) Buffalo
c) Horse d) Sheep

133. Which animal should not be transported?
a) Diseased b) Heavily pregnant
c) Emaciated d) All of the above

134. Under the Prevention of Cruelty to Animals Act, what is the maximum load limit for transporting a bullock by any vehicle?
a) 400 kg b) 500 kg
c) 600 kg d) 700 kg

135. What is the primary objective of the 'Transport of Animals Rules' in India?
a) Promote livestock sales
b) Ensure animal welfare during transportation
c) Reduce transportation costs
d) Facilitate international trade

136. Which section of the Prevention of Cruelty to Animals Act deals specifically with the transportation of animals?
 a) Section 11 b) Section 22
 c) Section 33 d) Section 44

137. Which Indian legislation lays down the guidelines for transporting animals to prevent unnecessary suffering?
 a) Wildlife Protection Act b) Forest Conservation Act
 c) Prevention of Cruelty to Animals Act d) Indian Penal Code

138. In which year was the 'Transport of Animals Rules' under the Prevention of Cruelty to Animals Act introduced in India?
 a) 1978 b) 1980
 c) 1990 d) 2000

139. In India, which authority has the power to inspect vehicles transporting livestock to ensure compliance with animal welfare regulations?
 a) Local police
 b) Animal Husbandry Department
 c) Transport Department
 d) Food Safety and Standards Authority of India

140. According to Indian regulations, what should be the maximum permissible height of crates for transporting poultry?
 a) 20 cm b) 30 cm
 c) 40 cm d) 50 cm

141. In poultry transportation, what is the recommended temperature range for broilers?
 a) 15-25°C b) 25-35°C
 c) 35-45°C d) Below 15°C

142. What flooring material is often recommended for livestock transport to prevent slippage?
 a) Concrete b) Metal
 c) Rubber d) Wood

143. Which factor is crucial for transporting poultry to minimize stress and injuries?
 a) High humidity b) Bright light
 c) Proper ventilation d) Loud noise

144. Which mode of transportation provides the most controlled environment for livestock?
 a) Open trucks b) Ventilated trucks
 c) Railways d) Ships

145. Which Indian authority oversees the transportation of animals to ensure they are treated humanely?
 a) Ministry of Agriculture b) Animal Welfare Board of India
 c) Indian Veterinary Council d) Ministry of Environment

Answer Key

1	d	2	c	3	c	4	c	5	c	6	c	7	b
8	b	9	b	10	c	11	b	12	a	13	c	14	b
15	c	16	b	17	b	18	b	19	c	20	c	21	c
22	b	23	c	24	c	25	b	26	c	27	b	28	c
29	b	30	a	31	b	32	c	33	c	34	c	35	a
36	c	37	a	38	b	39	b	40	b	41	b	42	c
43	b	44	a	45	b	46	c	47	b	48	b	49	b
50	b	51	a	52	b	53	c	54	c	55	c	56	a
57	b	58	c	59	c	60	b	61	b	62	b	63	b
64	d	65	a	66	a	67	b	68	c	69	d	70	b
71	b	72	b	73	b	74	a	75	b	76	b	77	aa
78	a	79	b	80	b	81	b	82	b	83	d	84	d
85	c	86	c	87	c	88	a	89	b	90	a	91	a
92	a	93	d	94	d	95	c	96	a	97	b	98	c
99	d	100	a	101	a	102	a	103	d	104	b	105	a
106	d	107	a	108	a	109	b	110	c	111	a	112	b
113	a	114	a	115	b	116	a	117	a	118	a	119	a
120	a	121	b	122	c	123	d	124	a	125	a	126	b
127	a	128	b	129	c	130	b	131	a	132	a	133	d
134	b	135	b	136	a	137	c	138	b	139	b	140	c
141	b	142	c	143	c	144	c	145	b				

27

Manure Production and Management

Jessy Bagh[1], Annada Das[2], and Kaushik Satyaprakash[3]

[1]Department of Livestock Production and Management, CVSc and AH, OUAT Bhubaneswar, Odisha

[2]Department of Livestock Products Technology, Faculty of Veterinary and Animal Sciences, WBUAFS, Kolkata, West Bengal

[3]Department of Veterinary Public Health and Epidemiology, Faculty of Veterinary and Animal Sciences, RGSC, BHU, Mirzapur, Uttar Pradesh

Introduction

Manure can be a) solid manure, feed waste, soiled bedding, etc. and b) liquid – urine and detergent

Water. Ideally, solid manure is usually collected and removed twice daily.

India has about 535.78 million livestock and the amount of production of animal waste amounts to about 3 million tons per year. Together farm-level livestock waste includes manure, urine, placenta, bedding,Feed waste, milk house waste etc. These animal wastes are the biggest source of harmful gases, harmful pathogens and odors and therefore public health and environmental concerns.

Livestock waste contains many useful substances components that, if recycled effectively, can be used as fertilizer for crops, food for animals. Economic savings are the biggest benefit of waste management achieved through improvements in human health and the environment, leading to higher productivity, lower medical costs, etc ultimate increase in farmers' income. The animal waste is a major source of harmful gases, harmful pathogens, etc Odor;

Therefore, it has public health and environmental concerns. Thus, animal waste must be disposed of properly to reduce its generation pollutants to protect the environment. About 40% of the world's methane is from agricultural and livestock by-products, followed by 18% waste disposal worldwide (Sorathiya *et al.*, 2014).

Waste generated from dairy farms are: fresh manure, bedding from gutters, manure, etc. Litter from free stalls, rinsing and dilution waste, milking center waste.

Poultry Management: Poultry produces two types of waste: Whole waste poultry manure and used litter. Whole manure is available in cages.Used litter from the deep litter system

Manure production/AU (adult unit) = 40 kg

1 AU = 1 adult cattle and buffalo aged 3 years or >3 years

1/2 AU = heifer about 2 years

1/3 AU = 1 calf (<1 year)/1 adult sheep and goat/1 adult pig

Methods for disposing of agricultural waste

1. Manure pits: Manure excreted by livestock (mainly cattle) is removed and removed thrown into pits. Waste may be dumped and converted Manure used as organic fertilizer.
2. Livestock waste used for energy production – dried dung cakes are used as a fuel for cooking
3. Biogas production: Biogas can be defined as a mixer of gases are formed by the decomposition of organic substances in the absence of oxygen. It consists mainly of methane and carbon dioxide. Somewhat methanogenic Bacteria are responsible for the production of biogas by some biochemical process. Since it comes from a biochemical process, it is is called biogas. Up to 60 liters of biogas can be produced from one kilogram of cow dung, which is sufficient cooking food for a day for a family (4-6 people).

BIOGAS PRODUCTION PROCESS

Biogas production is anaerobic and occurs in two parts stages. They are the acid formation stage and the methane formation stage. In the acid formation stage, biodegradable complex organic compound present in a group of acid-producing bacteria acts on the waste materials present in manure. Organic acids are the main product of this stage. In the second stage, a group of methanogenic bacteria act on the organic acids to produce methane gas (Vikaspedia.in).

Part of the biogas plant

1. Mixing tanks: The feed (manure) is collected in the mixing tank. Sufficient water is added and the material is mixed thoroughly. A homogeneous slurry is created.
2. Inlet pipe: The substrate is fed into the fermenter through the inlet Pipe/Tank.
3. Fermenter: Manure is fermented in the fermenter and biogas is produced through bacterial action.
4. Gas container or gas storage dome: Biogas is collected in the gas container which holds the gas until it is used up.

Advantages of waste disposal from animal husbandry

- Prevents dangerous environmental impacts on air, water, soil, wildlife,and the sea.
- Protects human health in communities and waste disposal facilities.
- Minimizes the risks associated with waste.
- Increases business opportunities.
- Achieves economic savings through improvements in human health and environment, resulting in higher productivity and lower medical costs.
- Creates jobs including low, medium and high skilled jobs.
- Waste to Wealth is a lucrative option for the environmentally conscious and cost-efficient
- Waste management. Achieving sustainable development goals is impossible without dealing with waste management, since each objective is direct or direct indirectly related to waste management

Multiple Choice Questions

1. How much percent of moisture percentage cattle dung have?:
   a) 45-50% b) 55-60%
   c) 30-40% d) 75-80%
2. Nitrogen content in cattle dung:
   a) 0.11% b) 7%
   c) 0.34% d) 4%
3. Dairy farm drainage channel should be:
   a) Closed Type b) Open Type
   c) Pipe System d) None
4. Manure pit walls height shouldn't be more than:
   a) 3-4 meter b) 1.5 -2 meter
   c) 0.5-1 meter d) 4-5 meter
5. Manure pit in term of per cow unit space requirement is:
   a) 1.1 m^3 b) 1.6 m^3
   c) 2.2 m^3 d) 2.8 m^3
6. Stored and decomposed manure has volumetric density of:
   a) 100-200 kg/m^3 b) 1000-3000 kg/m^3
   c) 200-300 kg/m^3 d) 500 kg/m^3
7. Fresh manure has volumetric density of :
   a) 700- 1000 kg/m^3 b) 100-200 kg/m^3
   c) 200-300 kg/m^3 d) 500 kg/m^3
8. Manure produced per day per livestock unit is:
   a) 5-10 kg b) 10-20 kg
   c) 30-40 kg d) 60-70 kg
9. Lime percencent of cattle dung is :
   a) 4-5 % b) 0.31%
   c) 1% d) 4%
10. Flushing out solid and liquid waste together will be preferred in case of :
    a) Buffalo b) Goat
    c) Sheep d) Cattle
11. Process of biogas production is :
    a) Aerobic b) Anaerobic
    c) Active d) Passive
12. Which of the following bacteria is present in rumen of cattle:
    a) Rhizobium b) Azotobacter
    c) Methanobacterium d) Azospirillum
13. Which among the following is methanogens:
    a) Methanobacterium b) Methanobrevibacter
    c) Methanococcus d) All of these

14. Biogas is produced by :
    a) Anaerobic breakdown of biomass
    b) AEROBIC breakdown of biomass
    c) With the help of methanogenic bacteria
    d) Both a and c
15. Liquid waste produced in one year by an ALU in a dairy farm is?
    a) 2500 litres b) 3500 litres
    c) 4500 litres d) 5500 litres
16. Solid manure produced by an ALU/day is ?
    a) 10-20 kg b) 20-30 kg
    c) 30-40 kg d) 40-50 kg
17. What should be the minimum distance of manure pit from wells rivers tanks etc of?
    a) 10 m b) 20 m
    c) 30 m d) 40 m
18. Allnutt's manure pit was described by?
    a) R.G linton b) C.K.Thomas
    c) N.S.R Shastry d) Linnaneus
19. How much percent of organic matter content is present in cow dung:
    a) 20% b) 10%
    c) 5% d) 1-2%
20. Which gas does biogas plant mainly produces?
    a) CO b) CH4
    c) H2S d) N2
21. Percentage of gases approximately present in biogas:
    a) 60% methane & 40% Co2
    b) 80%o2 & 20%CH4
    c) 80% N2 &20% CH4
    d) 90% carbon disulphide and 10% oxygen
22. Why are double gully traps installed to :
    a) Check emittance of foul air
    b) Allow the waste into the drains
    c) Check/ retain entry of solid waste in to the drains
    d) None of the above
23. How much dung is required daily for operating 1 cubic meter capacity biogas plant?
    a) 10 kg b) 25 kg
    c) 50 kg d) 100 kg
24. Biological method of treating manure is:
    a) Close packing b) Activated sludge
    c) Putrefaction d) Conservancy method

25. What should be the width of the drains?
   a) 30-40 cm b) 50-60 cm
   c) 10-20 cm d) 100 cm
26. What should be the slope provided to the drains towards storage tank so that liquid flow down easily?
   a) 1 in 40 b) 1 in 50
   c) 1 in 60 d) 1in 100
27. What should be the shape of the gutter/drain?
   a) Shallow V–shape b) Shallow U–shape
   c) Round shape d) None
28. Which among the following is a method of accelerating bio-oxidation of organic matter passing through a thermophilic stage?
   a) Composting b) Burial
   c) Rendering d) None
29. What is combustible heaps called in incineration method?
   a) Pyres b) Span
   c) Bunds d) Bins
30. Which method is most used method for dead animal composting:
   a) Passive composting pile b) Windrow
   c) Bin d) FYM
31. What is the recommended temperature in composting method?
   a) 55°C b) 25°C
   c) 90°C d) 15°C
32. How much percent of water is present in cattle dung?
   a) 77.5% b) 20.3%
   c) 0.34% d) 0.16%
33. How much percent of organic matter is present in cattle dung?
   a) 77.5% b) 20.3%
   c) 0.34% d) 0.16%
34. Which is the method used as a measure of the effectiveness of wastewater treatment plants?
   a) BOD b) Composting
   c) Biogas d) Bin
35. How much amount of dung is yield by a buffalo per day ?
   a) 4.5 kg b) 10.2 kg
   c) 15.8 kg d) 20 kg
36. How much percent of live weight of a cattle slaughter generate solid waste?
   a) 17 % b) 10%
   c) 27.5% d) 40.8%

37. How much percent of live weight of a sheep/goat slaughter generate solid waste?
    a) 17 % b) 10%
    c) 27.5% d) 40.8%
38. What is the average daily fresh manure production for broilers?
    a) 87 kg/1000 kg live weight b) 73 kg/1000 kg live weight
    c) 200 kg/1000 kg live weight d) 323 kg/1000 kg live weight
39. What is the average daily fresh manure production for broilers?
    a) 87 kg/1000 kg live weight b) 73 kg/1000 kg live weight
    c) 200 kg/1000 kg live weight d) 323 kg/1000 kg live weight
40. Which is the method of bio-oxidation and stabilization process of organic method involving earthworms and microorganism?
    a) Vermi-composting b) Windrow composting
    c) Biogas d) In-vessel composting
41. Which is the most common method of carcass disposal?
    a) Burial b) Incineration
    c) Rendering d) Composting
42. What is the factor that influence the production of bio –gas (methane) from a plant?
    a) Ambient temperature b) pH level
    c) C: N ratio d) All of above
43. What are the two phases in a bio gas plant for gas formation?
    a) Acid phase and Methane phase b) Alkaline phase & Co2 phase
    c) Acid phase and Nitrogen phase d) Alkaline phase & methane phase
44. Which gas is mainly responsible for Green House Gas ?
    a) CH_4 b) N_2
    c) SO_2 d) Co_2
45. What should be the Carbon and Nitrogen ratio in a dung plus urine slurry for bio gas production?
    a) 25 to 30:1 b) 40:2
    c) 50:5 d) 30: 5
46. What happens by direct usage of bio-digested slurry to soil?
    a) Increased soil fertility b) Decreased soil fertility
    c) Soil erosion d) Nothing happen
47. The bio – digested slurry used directly for cultivation of ______ as livestock feed?
    a) Neem b) Azolla
    c) Castor d) Guinea grass
48. Which among the following is not an advantage of Vermi -compost?
    a) Nitrogen Mineralization b) Rapid treatment
    c) High economic value of soil d) High technology

49. Which of the following is not a part of bio gas production process?
   a) Hydrolysis b) Anaerobic production
   c) Aerobic production d) Acetate production

50. What is the optimum temperature for bio gas production ?
   a) 32-35°C b) 40-45°C
   c) 70°C d) 10-15°C

51. What is the optimum solid content for bio gas production?
   a) 8-10% b) 20-22%
   c) 30-35% d) 40%

52. What is the optimum pH requirement for bio gas production?
   a) 6.8-8 b) 8-9
   c) 1-2 d) 4-5

53. What is the size of a bio gas plant to dispose 25 kg of dung?
   a) 1 m^3 b) 2 m^3
   c) 3 m^3 d) 4 m^3

54. What is the size of a bio gas plant to dispose 50 kg of dung?
   a) 1 m^3 b) 2 m^3
   c) 3 m^3 d) 4 m^3

55. What is the size of a bio gas plant to dispose 100 kg of dung?
   a) 1 m^3 b) 2 m^3
   c) 3 m^3 d) 4 m^3

56. One kg of cow dung can produce upto how many litres of biogas?
   a) 30 L b) 60 L
   c) 100 L d) 150 L

57. What is the duration to complete digestion process of cow dung for bio gas production?
   a) 2 month b) 4 month
   c) 1 month d) 15 days

58. How much amount of dung is produced by a buffaloes per day?
   a) 25-40 kg b) 60-70 kg
   c) 10-15 kg d) 5 kg

59. How much amount of dung is produced by sheep and goat per day?
   a) 25-40 kg b) 6-7 kg
   c) 10-15 kg d) 1-2.5 kg

60. How much amount of dung is produced by pig per day?
   a) 15-18 kg b) 8-10 kg
   c) 1-1.5 kg d) 3-5 kg

61. How much amount of dung is produced by horse per day?
   a) 9-18 kg b) 30 kg
   c) 1-1.5 kg d) 5 kg

62. How much amount of urine cattle produced ?
    a) 17-45 ml/kg live wt
    b) 60 ml/kg live wt
    c) 80 ml/kg live wt
    d) 10 ml/ kg live wt
63. How much amount of urine pigs produced?
    a) 5-30 ml/kg live wt
    b) 60 ml/kg live wt
    c) 80 ml/kg live wt
    d) 50 ml/ kg live wt
64. Compost manure is formed from :
    a) Farm and house hold refuse
    b) Animal refuse and rotten vegetables
    c) Organic waste
    d) Green and farmyard manure
65. Which chemical is used for protecting vermi-bed from ant?
    a) Chlorpyrophosphate
    b) DDT
    c) Potasium bisulfate
    d) Bicarbonate
66. Which earthworms species is commonly used for vermi –compost?
    a) Eisenia fetida
    b) Perionix excavates
    c) Both a & b
    d) None
67. Which of the following is not raw material for compost?
    a) Cow dung
    b) Dry leaves
    c) Straws
    d) All of the above
68. What is the maximum temperature required for vermi composting?
    a) 30-35°C
    b) 20-25°C
    c) 25-30°C
    d) 10-15°C
69. Which of the following steps used by farmers helps in multiplying earthworm?
    a) By adding plant materials
    b) By adding cow dung
    c) By mixing biodegradable
    d) All of the above
70. Which of the products cannot be used for vermicompost?
    a) Cow dung
    b) Animal waste
    c) Plant materials
    d) All of the above
71. How much moisture level is required for vermicomposting?
    a) <30
    b) 40-50%
    c) 70-80%
    d) >90%
72. What is the colour of vermicomposting?
    a) Red
    b) Brown
    c) Green
    d) Black
73. Which of the following is not correct regarding vermicompost?
    a) Worms population doubles in 90 days
    b) Worms eat double their body weight
    c) The wooden bin is best for vermicomposting
    d) Red worms are the best for vermicomposting

74. What is rich in vermicompost which makes them to use as biofertilizer?
   a) Calcium
   b) Nitrogen
   c) Phosphorous
   d) All of the above
75. Which of the following is incorrect pair?
   a) Vermicompost-earthworms
   b) Farm compost-farm waste
   c) Farmyard manure- cattle dung urine and litter
   d) Green manure- Chemical compound
76. What is the process of collecting the manure?
   a) By scrapping with shovels
   b) Vacumming using vacumm trucks
   c) Flushing
   d) All of the above
77. What is manure?
   a) Co-product
   b) By-product
   c) Waste
   d) None
78. Which gas does not emit from bio gas?
   a) CH_4
   b) CO_2
   c) H_2S
   d) O_2
79. Which of the following is not an advantage of bio –gas?
   a) Eco-friendly
   b) Reduces soil pollution
   c) Encourages circular economy
   d) Collecting cow manure volume from multiple sites
80. Which of the following is not disadvantage of bio gas?
   a) Time consuming
   b) High cost
   c) To collect cow dung from multiple sites
   d) Reduces water pollution
81. How much percent of nitrogen contain in cow manure compost (NPK)?
   a) 3%
   b) 2%
   c) 1%
   d) 4%
82. Which of the following factors hinders poultry dung to utilise for bio gas production?
   a) C/N
   b) Solid content
   c) Water
   d) pH
83. How much litres of biogas is approximately produced by 1 kg of chicken manure?
   a) 70 litres
   b) 30 litres
   c) 100 litres
   d) 5 litres
84. Bio gas production is :
   a) Cost-effective
   b) Reduces carbon footprint
   c) Reduces methane footprint
   d) All of the above

85. Which country is known for cow dung –based products?
   a) India b) China
   c) Japan d) USA
86. Which of the cow dung product is used for making eco-friendly packaging material?
   a) Cow dung Soap b) Cow dung incense sticks
   c) Cow dung paper d) Cow dung candles
87. Which cow dung product is used as a natural fertilizer?
   a) Cow dung Cakes b) Cow dung ash
   c) Cow dung paper d) Cow dung candles
88. Which country has developed a cow dung- based biofuel?
   a) India b) China
   c) USA d) Japan
89. What is the heating value of gobar gas?
   a) 800 BTU/ 200 kcal b) 500 BTU/ 100 kcal
   c) 100 BTU/ 50 kcal d) 1000BTU/ 300 kcal
90. What is the primary source of manure in a livestock farm?
   a) Animal waste b) Chemical fertilizers
   c) Soil d) Water
91. Which of the following nutrients is the most abundant in nature?
   a) Phosphorus b) Potassium
   c) Nitrogen d) Sodium
92. What is the primary objective of manure management in a livestock farm?
   a) Soil and fertility improvement b) Environmental protection
   c) Water purification d) Livestock feed supplementation
93. What is the process of collection and storage of manure called?
   a) Manure handling b) Manure management
   c) Manure digestion d) Manure excretion
94. Which of these species typically produces the most manure per animal or bird in a farm?
   a) Poultry b) Pig
   c) Cattle d) Sheep
95. What is the potential environmental issue associated with improper livestock manure management?
   a) Air pollution b) Noise pollution
   c) Soil erosion d) Water pollution
96. Which of the following is an advantage of using livestock manure as fertilizer?
   a) Enhancement of soil structure b) Reduction in soil acidity
   c) Decrease in soil organic matter d) Increase in soil compaction

97. What is the recommended way of farmland manure application to minimize nutrient loss?
   a) Surface broadcasting
   b) Open air storage
   c) Landfill deposition
   d) Injection into the soil

98. Which of these abundant nutrients in manure is essential for plant growth?
   a) Calcium
   b) Iron
   c) Nitrogen
   d) Magnesium

99. Which of the following process is commonly used for converting manure into biogas?
   a) Aerobic digestion
   b) Fermentation
   c) Anaerobic digestion
   d) Thermal treatment

100. In which state is the manure most effective as a fertilizer?
   a) Fresh
   b) Decomposed
   c) Dried
   d) Solid

101. What is the main goal of composting manure?
   a) To reduce odours
   b) To improve nutrient availability
   c) To increase manure storage time
   d) To enhance water content

102. What is the purpose of adding bulking agents during manure composting?
   a) Increase moisture content
   b) Increase odour emission
   c) Speed up the composting process
   d) Improve aeration and reduce compaction

103. Which manure management technique involves stacking manure in piles and allowing it to decompose naturally?
   a) Static pile composting
   b) In-vessel composting
   c) Windrow composting
   d) Anaerobic digestion

104. What is the common environmental concern related to manure lagoons?
   a) Leakage and groundwater contamination
   b) Greenhouse gas emission
   c) Soil erosion
   d) Soil compaction

105. What is the primary purpose of manure treatment systems?
   a) Increase manure production
   b) Reduce environmental impact
   c) Enhance animal health
   d) Improve manure texture

106. Which of the following methods can help reduce odour from stored manure?
   a) Increasing the manure pile size
   b) Adding water to the manure
   c) Aerating the manure
   d) Storing manure in closed containers

107. What is the nutrient content in manure influenced by?
a) Animal breed
b) Animal diet
c) Soil type
d) Manure storage temperature

108. What is the most common method of manure storage on farms?
a) Liquid storage tanks
b) Solid stacking
c) Open-air pits
d) Composting piles

109. Which of the following is a benefit of using dried manure as bedding for livestock?
a) Promotes bacterial growth
b) Increases greenhouse gas emissions
c) Enhances nutrient content in manure
d) Absorbs moisture and reduces odour

110. Which type of manure is high in nitrogen content but low in phosphorus and potassium?
a) Poultry manure
b) Cattle manure
c) Swine manure
d) Sheep manure

111. What is the potential risk of storing large amounts of manure in open-air pits?
a) Runoff into water bodies
b) Excessive nutrient absorption by plants
c) Soil alkalinity
d) Increased soil aeration

112. What is the recommended method for transporting manure to farmland for application?
a) Open-air trucks
b) Covered trucks or trailers
c) Dumping directly on fields
d) Spreading manually

113. Which of the following is a negative environmental impact of manure storage?
a) Algal blooms in water bodies
b) Water conservation
c) Soil enrichment
d) Methane production

114. How does manure contribute to greenhouse gas emission?
a) Through methane and nitrous oxide production
b) By absorbing carbon dioxide
c) Through carbon sequestration
d) By reducing nitrogen levels in the atmosphere

115. What is the primary purpose of using manure management systems on a livestock farm?
a) Enhance animal growth rates
b) Maximize manure production
c) Minimize environmental impact
d) Reduce feed costs

116. What is the term for the application of liquid manure directly onto the soil surface?
a) Aerobic composting
b) Anaerobic digestion
c) Lagoon storage
d) Windrow composting

117. What is the term for the application of liquid manure directly onto the soil surface?
   a) Slurry spreading b) Solid stacking
   c) Windrow composting d) Anaerobic digestion
118. Which nutrient is critical for plant photosynthesis and is found in manure?
   a) Carbon b) Nitrogen
   c) Phosphorus d) Sodium
119. What is the purpose of adding straw or hay to manure before composting?
   a) Reduce odour b) Increase water content
   c) Decrease nutrient levels d) Enhance aeration
120. Which of the following is a common environmental concern associated with manure spreading?
   a) Decreased plant growth b) Soil compaction
   c) Nutrient runoff into water bodies d) Increased soil alkalinity
121. In which form is manure most commonly applied to fields for fertilizer use?
   a) Solid b) Liquid
   c) Gas d) Powder
122. What is the purpose of using manure lagoons on a livestock farm?
   a) Temporary storage of manure b) Immediate disposal of manure
   c) Aerobic decomposition of manure d) Enhanced nutrient content in manure
123. What is a potential risk of excess phosphorus in manure spreading?
   a) Increased crop yields b) Soil acidification
   c) Water contamination & eutrophication d) Reduced plant growth
124. What is the primary advantage of using composted manure as a fertilizer?
   a) Reduced odour b) Increased nutrient content
   c) Longer storage time d) Enhanced moisture content
125. Which method of manure management helps reduce greenhouse gas emission and odour while producing energy?
   a) Lagoon storage b) Aerobic composting
   c) Windrow composting d) Anaerobic digestion
126. What is the primary purpose of adding manure to biogas digestors?
   a) Greenhouse gas reduction b) Odour reduction
   c) Soil enrichment d) Energy production
127 What is the potential consequence of inadequate manure management on aquatic ecosystem?
   a) Algal bloom and water pollution b) Soil erosion
   c) Increased fish populations d) Enhanced water clarity
128. What is the term for the process of converting organic matter in manure into a stable, humus-like material?
   a) Composting b) Fermentation
   c) Anerobic digestion d) Gasification

129. What is the ideal moisture content for effective composting of manure?
a) 10-20% b) 40-60%
c) 70-80% d) 90-100%

130. Which method of manure management involves using insects to consume and break down organic waste?
a) Entomophagy b) Insect composting
c) Vermicomposting d) Aquaponics

131. What is the potential challenge associated with using manure as a fertilizer?
a) Variability in nutrient content b) Long shelf life
c) High cost d) Low availability

132. Which of the following is a potential environmental benefit of properly managed manure application?
a) Over-fertilization of crops b) Alkalinity increase
c) Air pollution d) Soil erosion reduction

133. Which manure management system involves storing manure in a pit and allowing solids to settle, creating a liquid layer for spreading?
a) Solid stacking b) Composting
c) Liquid storage and pit storage d) Anerobic digestion

134. What is the primary nutrient concern with manure runoff into water bodies?
a) Nitrogen b) Phosphorus
c) Potassium d) Carbon

135. What is the potential advantage of using manure as a renewable energy source?
a) Decreasing nutrient content in manure
b) Increasing greenhouse gas emissions
c) Reducing dependency on fossil fuels
d) Promoting soil compaction

136. What is the term for the application of composted manure in a controlled environment?
a) Slide-dressing b) Top-dressing
c) Undercutting d) Overlaying

137. What is the potential challenge of using manure lagoons for storage?
a) Risk of leakage and groundwater contamination
b) High nutrient content
c) Efficient odour control
d) Minimal space requirement

138. Which of the following is a potential environmental concern related to manure storage facilities?
a) Soil compaction b) Leakage into groundwater
c) Increased soil acidity d) Enhanced nutrient availability

139. What is the potential advantage of incorporating manure into the soil immediately after application?
   a) Reducing manure volume
   b) Reducing greenhouse gas emission
   c) Enhancing nutrient content in manure
   d) Minimizing nutrient runoff
140. What is the potential challenge of using composted manure as a fertilizer?
   a) Nutrient loss during storage
   b) Increased odour
   c) Difficulty in application
   d) High transportation cost
141. Which of the following is a potential environmental benefit of using manure as a soil conditioner?
   a) Increased greenhouse gas emission
   b) Reduced soil fertility
   c) Decreased soil erosion
   d) Enhanced water pollution
142. What is the potential risk associated with improper storage of manure?
   a) Groundwater contamination
   b) Enhanced nutrient content
   c) Increased soil alkalinity
   d) Reduced soil compaction
143. Which of the following is a potential advantage of using manure for biogas production?
   a) Enhanced soil structure
   b) Reduced nutrient content
   c) Decreased greenhouse gas emission
   d) Renewable energy generation
144. What is the primary purpose of applying manure to farmland?
   a) Soil compaction reduction
   b) Soil enrichment and fertility improvement
   c) Greenhouse gas reduction
   d) Water purification
145. Which nutrient is primarily responsible for algal bloom when manure runoff enters water bodies?
   a) Nitrogen
   b) Phosphorus
   c) Potassium
   d) Calcium
146. What is the process of converting organic material in manure into a more stable form called?
   a) Composting
   b) Fermentation
   c) Anerobic digestion
   d) Aerobic respiration
147. Which manure management method helps control pests and reduce weed growth?
   a) Aerobic composting
   b) Anerobic digestion
   c) Lagoon storage
   d) Windrow composting
148. What is the potential risk of using untreated manure as a fertilizer?
   a) Pathogen contamination
   b) Enhanced nutrient availability
   c) Reduced soil pH
   d) Increased plant growth

149. Which of the following is a potential challenge of using manure as a renewable energy source?
   a) Increased cost of energy production
   b) High nutrient content
   c) Reduced greenhouse gas emission
   d) Inconsistent energy production

150. What is the recommended approach to mitigate the environmental impact of manure application?
   a) Open-air storage
   b) Proper timing and rate of application
   c) Use of untreated manure
   d) Irregular application schedules Food Waste?

Answer Key

1	d	2	c	3	b	4	b	5	c	6	b	7	a
8	c	9	b	10	a	11	b	12	c	13	d	14	d
15	c	16	c	17	a	18	a	19	a	20	b	21	a
22	c	23	b	24	a	25	a	26	a	27	b	28	a
29	a	30	c	31	a	32	a	33	b	34	a	35	b
36	c	37	a	38	a	39	b	40	b	41	a	42	d
43	a	44	a	45	a	46	a	47	b	48	d	49	c
50	a	51	a	52	a	53	a	54	b	55	a	56	b
57	a	58	a	59	d	60	d	61	a	62	a	63	a
64	a	65	a	66	c	67	d	68	a	69	d	70	b
71	c	72	b	73	b	74	d	75	d	76	d	77	a
78	d	79	d	80	d	81	a	82	a	83	a	84	d
85	a	86	c	87	a	88	c	89	a	90	a	91	c
92	b	93	b	94	c	95	a	96	a	97	d	98	c
99	c	100	b	101	b	102	d	103	c	104	a	105	b
106	c	107	b	108	a	109	d	110	a	111	a	112	b
113	d	114	a	115	c	116	b	117	a	118	b	119	d
120	c	121	b	122	a	123	c	124	b	125	d	126	d
127	a	128	a	129	b	130	c	131	a	132	d	133	c
134	b	135	c	136	a	137	a	138	b	139	c	140	c
141	c	142	a	143	d	144	b	145	b	146	a	147	d
148	a	149	d	150	b								

28

Food Waste and Sanitation Management

Monoshree Sarma[1*], Mrinmoyee Sarma[2], Vidya M.K.[3], Safeeda Sultana Begum[4], and Farida Rahman[5]

[1]Department of Veterinary Pharmacology and Toxicology, Institute of Veterinary Science and Animal Husbandry, Siksha 'O' Anusandhan, Bhubaneswar, Odisha

[2]Department of Veterinary Public Health and Epidemiology, Institute of Veterinary Science and Animal Husbandry, Siksha 'O' Anusandhan, Bhubaneswar, Odisha

[3]Department of Physiology and Biochemistry, Veterinary College Hassan, KVAFSU, Karnataka, West Bengal

[4]Department of Veterinary Medicine, COVAS, Kishanjganj, BASU, Patna, Bihar

[5]Department of Veterinary Pharmacology and Toxicology, College of Veterinary Science, Khanapara, Guwahati, Assam

Introuction

Food is defined as any substance, whether processed, semi processed or raw, that is intended for human consumption as well as the inedible parts associated with food that are not intended to be consumed by humans. Food waste is defined as any food and inedible parts of food, removed from the food supply chain that can be recovered or disposed, whereas, food loss is defined as food that unintentionally undergoes deterioration in quality or quantity as a result of food spills, spoils, bruising, wilting or other damages alike owing to infrastructure limitations at the production, storage, processing and distribution stages of food lifecycle. Global food waste management is an issue of concern that requires attention from various stakeholders having diverse expertise. According to statistics, about one third of the food produced for human consumption is either lost or wasted. Globally, the cost of food waste accounts for USD 2.6 trillion, of that USD 1trillion is incurred from greenhouse gas (GHG) emissions, water scarcity, biodiversity loss, increased conflicts and loss of livelihood owing to issues like soil erosion, nutrient loss, reduced yields, wind erosion and pesticide exposure.

Food waste has impacted the global scenario and the major areas of concern are : Green house gas emissions and climate change, water footprint, nutrient loss, sanitation, ecological impacts and economic impacts. Food waste management is related with stages of prevention of food waste, recovery, recycling etc. This includes food waste tracking and prevention, food banks, using food as animal feed, creating renewable energy through anaerobic digestion. To solve issues related to hunger, every stakeholder should join hand to dramatically dwindle the amount of food we waste in our day to day life.

Sanitation

Sanitizer is an agent that reduced the number of bacterial contamination to a safe level. And the process used is known as sanitisation. They are required in partial aerosole cleaning of atmosphere in buildings with high stocking density. Agents or compounds used in sanitary programmes that destroy animal parasites are called as disinfectant. It is a process of converting a place or object from potentially infective state into one which is free from infection. Sanitisation is done to reduce the number of pathogenic bacteria to a safer level. But presence of organic matter on the surface or object impedes their action by inactivating them. Hence, sanitation should be follow after proper cleaning of the surface or the object. Substance used in the sanitisation process can be categorised into non chemical and chemical. Non chemical group includes sunlight, direct flame, heat from different sources, free air access. Chemical group includes gaseous compounds like sulphur dioxide, Chlorine gas, Formaldehyde; liquid compounds like phenol, formalin, Cresol and phenyl; and solid compounds like Bleaching powder, quick lime etc)Sanitisation is a gradual process and not an instantaneous one. There is initial lag phase which is followed by a rapid process of destruction of microorganism. The process will eventually kill the microbes and will make the surface a safer one. Dynamic of sanitisation depends upon concentration of substance, Temperature of the substance, Velocity of the substance per degree rise in temperature and effect of dilution, time of exposure, cleansing of materials prior to use and prior removal of organic matter. Sanitisation can occur both by natural and artificial means. The factors which contribute towards natural destruction of pathogens are sunlight, heat, cold, desiccation, agitation air temperature etc)High temperatures enhance the destruction of exposed bacteria while cold temperatures preserve them especially under freezing temperature. Application of heat is an effective method for destructing pathogenic bacteri a)Both dry as well as moist heats are used in the process of sanitisation. Steam (moist heat) are effective than dry heat and becomes more powerful on addition of disinfectant and detergent in steam or hot water. Artificial sanitation is carried out by chemical substances. The lethal action of the chemical sanitizer is due to its ability to react with protein especially essential enzymes of micro organism. In nut shell, sanitisation by chemical substance is carried out by destruction of bacterial cell, disruption of its organisation, interfering with synthesis and growth of bacteria, interfering with utilisation of energy by bacteria)Germicidal action is due to its hydrolytic and burning action on cells, oxidative action on protoplasm, protein coagulation in protoplasm and disruption of cell wall and membrane. Substances used in the sanitisation process should be highly effective, non- toxic to man, cost effective, easily available, should be non-staining in nature, free of pungent odour, etc)sanitisation creates an environment that is conducive to the health of man and animal. It nullifies all the factors liable for health deterioration; dwindle in production, mortality and morbidity and dramatic economic loss.

MCQs

1. Food waste management accounts for__________ total municipal solid was

   a) 50-60% b) 30-40%

   c) 70% d) 10-20%

2. Most common methods for disposal of food waste

   a) Landfills b) Incinerations

   c) Composting d) All of the above

3. Incineration of food waste contribute___ %
   a) 6 b) 8
   c) 1 d) 5
4. Pre-consumption food waste means, waste from
   a) Farm lands b) Storage & manufacturing
   c) Supply d) All of the above
5. Post-consumption food waste means waste from
   a) Food leftovers in households b) Food leftovers in restaurants
   c) Both a and b d) None of the above
6. Annual food waste in India_____ (m tonnes/year)
   a) 35 b) 40
   c) 25 d) 50
7. Common methods of food waste management
   a) Disposal b) Recycling
   c) Incineration d) Both a & b
8. Methods disposal in food waste management
   a) Animal food b) Landfill
   c) Donation d) All of the above
9. Methods of food waste management in food waste management
   a) Thermochemical convention b) Biological convention
   c) Chemical convention d) All of the above
10. ___________ is one of the most promising options for food waste recycling to bio diesel
    a) Trasification b) Trans esterification
    c) Composition d) Anaerobic digestion
11. Fermentation process mainly produces which chemical
    a) Esters b) CO_2
    c) Ethanol d) Methanol
12. Most common ferment organism
    a) Saccharomyces cerevisiae b) Streptococcus
    c) Zymommas d) Bacillus
13. Which method of disposal of food waste produces most CO_2
    a) Incineration b) Composting
    c) Landfills d) Pyrolysis
14. Sources of food wastes
    a) Agricultural waste b) Residential
    c) Food industries d) All of the above
15. Total solid content in household food waste
    a) 10% b) 20%
    c) 50% d) 5%

16. Ideal moisture concentration for biological conversation of food waste
    a) 40-70% b) 20%
    c) 80% d) 10%
17. Most common methods of food waste disposal in India
    a) Landfill b) Composting
    c) Animal feeding d) All of the above
18. _______ & _______ are the two major natural food waste disposal technologies
    a) Anaerobic digestion b) In-vessel composting
    c) Both a & b d) Incineration
19. Sustainable approaches for food waste management
    a) Animal feeding b) Organic fertilizers
    c) Biofuel d) All of the above
20. Landfills accounts for __________% of foodwaste treatment
    a) 30% b) 60%
    c) 10% d) 90%
21. China minister of food in India
    a) Piyush Goyal b) Ravi Singh
    c) Manoj Shinde d) Samkit Shah
22. Which country ranks 1st in wastage of food ?
    a) India b) USA
    c) China d) Japan
23. Food waste produces which of these greenhouse gas ?
    a) Methane b) Nitrogen
    c) CO_2 d) All of the above
24. Which of these organisations related to food?
    a) UNESCO b) WHO
    c) FAO d) WWF
25. Main cause of food wastage
    a) Supermarkets b) Restaurants
    c) Consumers d) All of the above
26. Which dustbin is used for food waste?
    a) Yellow b) Green
    c) Red d) Blue
27. Food waste bags are called as
    a) Biobags b) Compost bags
    c) Biodegradable liners d) All of the above
28. Who is the Director General of FAO?
    a) Xi-Zinping b) Fa-Huen
    c) Qu-Dongyu d) None of the above

29. Headquarters of FAO located in
    a) Berlin b) Rome
    c) Quetta d) Pune
30. Food waste is
    a) Biodegradable b) Non biodegradable
    c) Both a and b d) Only b
31. Food waste finally ends in
    a) Landfills b) Sewer system
    c) Combustion facilities d) All of the above
32. Example of food waste
    a) Stale food b) Preservable food
    c) Fresh food d) Grains
33. Which country is first in low food waste
    a) Thailand b) Singapore
    c) Pakistan d) Russia
34. Compostable bags are made of
    a) Polyvinyl Chloride b) Plant Starch
    c) Jute d) Both a and b
35. Household kitchen bind are of which size?
    a) 1-2 liters b) 5-10 liters
    c) 10-15 liters d) 50-100 liters
36. India ranks _______ in Global Hunger index
    a) 63 b) 83
    c) 53 d) 73
37. Concequences of food wastage
    a) Loss of soil fertility b) Wastage of resources
    c) Greenhouse gas effect d) All the above
38. Which of the following is done on an individual level?
    a) Burning b) Disposal
    c) Recycling d) Source reduction
39. Which of the following is Municipal solid waste?
    a) Food waste b) Wood waste
    c) Plastic cans d) All of the above
40. Disposible waste contains
    a) Solid b) Liquids
    c) Slurries d) All of the above
41. Which of the following techniques of food waste management helps in production of organic fertilizers?
    a) Anaerobic digestion b) Composting
    c) Use of chemicals d) Both a and b

42. Which of the following helps in the sustainability of the food?
   a) Processing b) Packaging
   c) Consumption d) All of the above
43. Failure in food waste management leads to
   a) Environmental loss b) Social loss
   c) Financial loss d) All of the above
44. Food waste diverted to landfills if not properly managed
   a) Hydrogen b) Nitrogen
   c) Methane d) None of the above
45. Food loss and food waste leads to which of the following affect
   a) Green house effect b) Global warming
   c) Both d) None
46. Which of the following helps in reducing food waste management
   a) Preventing undesirable food surplus b) Preventing over production
   c) Preventing over supply of food d) All of the above
47. What are the gases produced by means of anaerobic digestion?
   a) Biohydrogen b) Biomethane
   c) Both d) None
48. Which is the least used technique of food waste management?
   a) Anaerobic digestion b) Composting
   c) Land filling d) Both a and b
49. HACCP stands for
   a) Hazard activity critical control plan
   b) Hazard analysis critical control points
   c) Hygiene analysis critical control points
   d) Hygiene analysis contamination control plan
50. Most cases of food poisoning are caused by
   a) Bacteria b) Chemicals in food
   c) Eating too much d) All of the above
51. Frozen storage is generally operated at
   a) -0°C b) -18°C
   c) -50°C d) -60°C
52. FAO stands for
   a) Food and animal organization b) Farm activity organization
   c) Food and agricultural organization d) None of the above
53. Food should be cooked to which temperature to prevent microorganisms intervention
   a) 5°C b) 75°C
   c) 100°C d) 60°C

54. ___________ are code of good practices that comprises fundamental principles, procedures and means needed for safe food production

a) GMP
b) PRP (pre-requisite programmes)
c) HACCP
d) None of these

55. _______________provides information on hazard in food to be linked to data on the risk to human health and to improve food safety decision

a) Biological hazard
b) Risk analysis
c) Foscoris
d) Chemical hazard

56. Which of the following is recommended for the managing of risk in the food production process?

a) Food recall procedure
b) Food analysis and testing
c) Risk analysis approach
d) None of these

57. Benefits of implementing HACCP

a) A preventive approach to food safety
b) Reduces the need for and the cost of end product testing
c) Can help and identify process improvements and reduced customer complaints
d) All of the above

58. Which of the following will help in food security and safety and sanitation of food?

a) FAO
b) HACCP
c) Both
d) None

59. Headquarters of FAO is at

a) Australia
b) America
c) India
d) Italy

60. Sustainable method of food waste management

a) Animal feed
b) Landfill
c) Chemical digestion
d) Anaerobic digestion

61. Disinfectant is

a) A chemical agent applied to living organisms
b) A chemical agent applied to in animate objects
c) A physical agent applied to living organisms
d) A physical agent applied to in animate objects

62. Antiseptic is

a) A chemical agent applied to living organisms
b) A chemical agent applied to in animate objects
c) A physical agent applied to living organisms
d) A physical agent applied to in animate objects

63. Which of the following has little role to play when it comes to absolute elimination of micro-organisms?

a) Bactericide
b) Disinfectant
c) Antiseptic
d) Sanitizer

64. Which of the following term means complete destruction of all forms of life in the cleaning of animal accommodation?
   a) Sanitization b) Sterilization
   c) Disinfection d) Cleansing
65. Which of the following is a preliminary process to disinfection?
   a) Sterilization b) Sanitization
   c) Cleansing d) None of the above
66. Which of the following checks that the organic matters for not reduce the power of disinfectants?
   a) Cleanser b) Antiseptic
   c) Sanitizer d) Germicide
67. Which of the following prevents the growth of bacteria?
   a) Bactericide b) Bacteriostat
   c) Both a and b d) None of the above
6 8. Which of the following kills bacteria?
   a) Bactericide b) Bacteriostat
   c) Both a and b d) None of the above
69. What is the suffix applied to any agent that kills microorganisms?
   a) Cide b) Stat
   c) Ing d) None of the above
70. What is the suffix applied to any agent that simply prevents the growth?
   a) Cide b) Stat
   c) Ing d) None of the above
71. Disinfectant destroy
   a) Pathogenic organisms b) Their spores
   c) Both a and b d) None of the above
72. Phenol is a
   a) Disinfectant b) Sanitizer
   c) Germicide d) None of the above
73. Formaldehyde is
   a) Liquid disinfectant b) Gaseous disinfectant
   c) Solid disinfectant d) All of the above
74. Formalin is a
   a) Liquid disinfectant b) Gaseous disinfectant
   c) Solid disinfectant d) All of the above
75. Cresol is a
   a) Liquid disinfectant b) Gaseous disinfectant
   c) Solid disinfectant d) All of the above

76. With reference to disinfectant, the time survivor curve of bacteria is usually
    a) Straight ascending b) Straight descending
    c) Sigmoid d) Parallel to x -axis
77. The time survivor curve of bacteria is usually influenced by?
    a) Concentration b) Temperature
    c) Presence of organic matters d) All of the above
78. In which of the following disinfectant, the lethal activity is owing to oxidising effect?
    a) Mercury salt b) Hydrogen peroxide
    c) Phenol d) Cresol
79. In which of the following disinfectant, the lethal activity is due to cationic nature?
    a) Quaternary compounds b) Formaldehyde
    c) Silver salt d) Mercury salt
80. Formaldehyde exhibit its lethal activity by reacting with which of the following?
    a) Sulphur b) Amino
    c) Nucleic acid d) All of the above
81. Which of the following is NOT true pertaining to disinfectant?
    a) Metallic salts are protein precipitants
    b) Phenol denatures protein
    c) Alkali are more effective than acids
    d) Potassium permanganate is an oxidising agent
82. Action of disinfectant is by?
    a) Destruction of bacterial cell
    b) Interference with synthesis and growth of bacteria
    c) Interference with utilisation of energy by bacteria
    d) All of the above
83. Germicidal action of acid and alkali is due to
    a) Hydrolytic and burning action on cell
    b) Oxidation reaction on protoplasm of cell
    c) Protein coagulation in protoplasm of cell
    d) Disruption of cell wall and cell membrane
84. Germicidal action of phenol cresol and polymixin is due to
    a) Hydrolytic and burning action on cell
    b) Oxidation reaction on protoplasm of cell
    c) Protein coagulation in protoplasm of cell
    d) Disruption of cell wall and cell membrane
85. Germicidal action of hydrogen peroxide and permanganate is due to
    a) Hydrolytic and burning action on cell
    b) Oxidation reaction on protoplasm of cell
    c) Protein coagulation in protoplasm of cell
    d) Disruption of cell wall and cell membrane

86. Germicidal action of alcohol and formaldehyde is due to
    a) Hydrolytic and burning action on cell
    b) Oxidation reaction on protoplasm of cell
    c) Protein coagulation in protoplasm of cell
    d) Disruption of cell wall and cell membrane
87. Which of the following is the basic phenomenon of disinfecting action by chemical means?
    a) Absorption of compound by cell wall
    b) Penetration into cell protoplasm
    c) Reaction of compound with one or more of the cell constituents
    d) All of the above
88. Which of the following factor influences the absorption and penetration of the substance?
    a) Surface tension b) Physiochemical properties
    c) Type of solvent d) All of the above
89. Effect of oils, fats and alcohol on the activity of phenol is
    a) It is reduced b) It is increased
    c) It remains unchanged d) None of the above
90. What happens to the activity of phenol when it is emulsified in soap solution
    a) It is reduced b) It is increased
    c) It remains unchanged d) None of the above
91. What is the relationship between surface tension and activity of disinfectant?
    a) Remain unchanged b) Inversely proportional
    c) Directly proportional d) None of the above
92. Which of the following factor influences germicidal action?
    a) Concentration b) Temperature
    c) Time of use d) All of the above
93. Presence of organic matter on the farm interferes with the activities of disinfectant by?
    a) Protecting the cell by forming a coating on it
    b) Preventing the easy and ready access of the disinfectants
    c) Reacting chemically with disinfectants
    d) All of the above
94. Sanitation is aimed at which of the following?
    a) Creating conditions conducive to the health of animal
    b) Assuring product of good quality
    c) Nullifying factors that deteriorate health
    d) All of the above

95. Which of the following is sporocidal?
    a) 1% mineral acids
    b) 10% amyl-m-cresol
    c) Both a and b
    d) None of the above
96. Ethy alcohol at what concentration is effective against bacterial flora?
    a) 50%
    b) 60%
    c) 70%
    d) 80%
97. At what strength, formaldehyde is effective as general disinfectant in aqueous solution?
    a) 5%
    b) 10%
    c) 15%
    d) 20%
98. Which of the following is an ideal terminal disinfectant for earth floor livestock buildings?
    a) Lysol D
    b) Hydol 72
    c) Dettol
    d) Ibcol
99. Which is more germicidal between Lysol and phenol
    a) Lysol
    b) Phenol
    c) Equipotent
    d) None of the above
100. Chlorine should be used in what concentration in poultry processing plant for their water supply
    a) 1-5 ppm
    b) 5-10 ppm
    c) 10-20 ppm
    d) 20-30 ppm
101. San-o-Fee popular in hatcheries is chemically
    a) Acid
    b) Alkali
    c) Quaternary ammonium compound
    d) Alcohol
102. San-o-Fee is used in hatcheries for
    a) Aerial disinfection
    b) Egg dipping
    c) Incubator and equipment in general
    d) All of the above
103. Chemical name of slaked lime is
    a) Calcium hydroxide
    b) Calcium oxide
    c) Calcium carbonate
    d) Calcium bicarbonate
104. Chemical name of washing soda is
    a) Calcium hydroxide
    b) Calcium oxide
    c) Calcium carbonate
    d) Calcium bicarbonate
105. Chemical name of quick lime is
    a) Calcium hydroxide
    b) Calcium oxide
    c) Calcium carbonate
    d) Calcium bicarbonate
106. Germicidal filtration can be carried out by
    a) Physical filters
    b) Electrostatic precipitation
    c) Both a and b
    d) None of the above

107. Which of the following is effective against air borne bacteria?
a) Chloroxylenol
b) Sulphur dioxide
c) Quick lime
d) Iodophore

108. Which of the following is a basic measure pertaining to sanitation
a) Proper cleaning of the habitation
b) Adequate drainage
c) Proper ventilation
d) All of the above

109. Which of the following is a method of disposal of excreta?
a) Burial process
b) Incineration or burning
c) Drying or spreading
d) All of the above

110. What should be the depth of the trench for disposal of diseased animal excreta?
a) 3 inch
b) 5 inch
c) 6 inch
d) 10 inch

111. What should be the length of a ordinary manure pit?
a) 20 inch
b) 10 inch
c) 15 inch
d) 6 inch

112. What should be the width of ordinary manure pit?
a) 20 inch
b) 10 inch
c) 15 inch
d) 6 inch

113. A ton of manure contains how much nitrogen?
a) 2 kg
b) 2.5 kg
c) 4 kg
d) 4.5 kg

114. A ton of manure contains how much potash?
a) 2 kg
b) 2.5 kg
c) 4 kg
d) 4.5 kg

115. Liquid system for disposal of manure is of which type?
a) Conventional type
b) Lagoon system
c) Both a and b
d) None of the above

116. Lagoons may be
a) Aerobic
b) Anaerobic
c) Both
d) All of the above

117. Aerobic lagoons are best suited for disposal of milking parlour because of
a) Need of large surface area
b) Need for provision of additional aeration
c) Relative inactivity of aerobic organism in cold temperature
d) All of the above

118. Which of the following is impact of food waste?
a) GHG emission and climate change
b) Water footprint
c) Sanitation
d) All of the above

119. Which of the following is NOT a green house gas?
a) Methane b) Ethane
c) Carbon dioxide d) Nitrous oxide

120. How many SDG (Sustainable Development Goals) according to United Nations?
a) 15 b) 16
c) 17 d) 18

121. Which SDG is aimed at efficient use of water?
a) SDG 6 b) SDG 12
c) SDG 15 d) SDG 17

122. Which SDG aims at reducing global food waste at the retail and consumer levels in half by 2030?
a) SDG 6 b) SDG 12
c) SDG 15 d) SDG 17

123. The Food Recovery Challenge is run annually by which organisation?
a) World Health Organisation b) FSSAI
c) FAO d) US Environment Protection Agency

124. Which of the following is a regulatory initiative to check food waste?
a) Good Samaritan Law b) Food Date Labelling
c) Banning of Organic waste to labelling d) All of the above

125. The EU Landfill Directive obliges member states to reduce biodegradable waste going to landfill by what percentage by 2020 compared to 1995?
a) 35% b) 25%
c) 15% d) 5%

126. Heating of an organic matter in the absence of oxyge, resulting in the decomposition of organic matter into gases and charcoal is called as
a) Pyrolysis b) Mechanical Biological Treatment
c) Landfill with gas collection d) Gasification

127. Which of the following is a benefit of Anaerobic Digestion of Food Waste?
a) Renewable Energy Production b) Climate Change Mitigation
c) Improving Urban Air Quality d) All of the above

128. How many steps are there in risk assessment?
a) Four b) Five
c) Six d) Seven

129. Recording the findings' is which step of 'Risk Assessment'?
a) First b) Second
c) Third d) Fourth

130. Studying 'Who may be harmed and how' is which step of 'Risk Assessment'?
a) First b) Second
c) Third d) Fourth

131. 'Identification of Potential Hazards' is which step of 'Risk Assessment'?
   a) First b) Second
   c) Third d) Fourth
132. Evaluation of the risk of incident taken and suggestion of precautions' is which step of 'Risk Assessment'?
   a) First b) Second
   c) Third d) Fourth
133. Reviewing and Updating Risk Assessment' is which step of 'Risk Assessment'?
   a) Fifth b) Second
   c) Third d) Fourth
134. Which of the following is a product of anaerobic digestion?
   a) Biogas for cooking b) Biogas broiler
   c) Electricity d) All of the above
135. What is the full form of PSA?
   a) Pressure Swing Adsorption b) Pressure Swing Absorption
   c) Both a and b d) None of the above
136. Purity of methane in Pressure Swing Adsorption (PSa) technology?
   a) Above 95% b) Above 96%
   c) Above 98% d) Above 99%
137. Purity of methane in water wash technology?
   a) Above 95% b) Above 96%
   c) Above 98% d) Above 99%
138. Purity of methane in Amine Scrubbing technology?
   a) Above 95% b) Above 96%
   c) Above 98% d) Above 99%
139. Purity of methane in membrane technology?
   a) Above 95% b) Above 96%
   c) Above 98% d) Above 99%
140. Purity of methane in cryogenic technology?
   a) Above 95% b) Above 96%
   c) Above 98% d) Above 99%
141. The total cost of biogas upgradation depends on which of the factor?
   a) The quality of raw biogas and biomethane required
   b) Scale of operation
   c) Location of the plant
   d) All of the above
142. Which of the following is an advantage of vehicle running on biomethane?
   a) Above 95% b) Above 96%
   c) Above 98% d) Above 99%

143. Boiling point of methane is

a) -164°C b) -154°C
c) -144°C d) -134°C

144. Fresh Food Waste has a pH of

a) 6.3 b) 7.3
c) 8.3 d) 9.3

145. Which of the following is NOT true for Sulphur dioxide as fumigant?

a) Tarnishes materials b) Less easily eliminated
c) Diffuses promptly d) Bleaches fabric

146. Which of the following is a reason to use gases and vapours for disinfection?

a) Do not harm construction materials of the house
b) Comparative inexpensive
c) Can be applied at normal temperature
d) All of the above

147. Which of the following is an advantage of biogas slurry?

a) The mix fed to the animal is readily accepted in 3 to 4 days of feeding
b) Adult bovine consume it adequately
c) Ad-libitum feeding suffice to meet the maintenance requirement
d) All of the above

148. Boiling point of methane is

a) -164°C b) -154°C
c) -144°C d) -134°C

149. Which SDG is aimed at efficient use of water?

a) SDG 6 b) SDG 12
c) SDG 15 d) SDG 17

150. Chemical composition of ruminal waste depends on

a) Source of feeding b) Level of feeding
c) Dietary level of concentrate d) All of the above

Answer Key

1	a	2	d	3	b	4	d	5	c	6	a	7	d
8	d	9	d	10	b	11	c	12	a	13	d	14	d
15	b	16	a	17	d	18	c	19	d	20	d	21	a
22	c	23	a	24	c	25	d	26	b	27	a	28	c
29	b	30	a	31	d	32	a	33	b	34	b	35	c
36	d	37	d	38	d	39	d	40	d	41	d	42	d
43	d	44	c	45	a	46	d	47	c	48	c	49	b
50	a	51	b	52	c	53	b	54	b	55	b	56	c
57	d	58	c	59	d	60	a	61	b	62	a	63	d

64	b	65	c	66	a	67	b	68	a	69	a	70	b
71	c	72	a	73	b	74	a	75	a	76	c	77	d
78	b	79	a	80	b	81	c	82	d	83	a	84	d
85	b	86	c	87	d	88	d	89	a	90	b	91	b
92	d	93	d	94	d	95	c	96	c	97	a	98	a
99	a	100	c	101	c	102	d	103	a	104	c	105	b
106	c	107	a	108	d	109	d	110	c	111	a	112	c
113	d	114	d	115	c	116	d	117	d	118	d	119	b
120	c	121	a	122	b	123	d	124	d	125	a	126	a
127	d	128	b	129	d	130	b	131	a	132	c	133	a
134	d	135	a	136	b	137	b	138	d	139	d	140	d
141	d	142	d	143	a	144	c	145	c	146	d	147	d
148	a	149	a	150	d								

29

Animal Mortality and Its Disposal

***Ganesh K. Sawaled*[1], *and P. Patil*[2]**

[1]*Department of Veterinary Pathology, Mumbai Veterinary College, Parel, Mumbai Maharashtra*

[2]*Department of Veterinary Pharmacology and Toxicology, College of Veterinary & Animal Sciences, Parbhani, Maharashtra*

Introducrtion

Livestock plays a vital role in any country's economy as animals are a source of livelihood for people, providing milk, meat, and fur, and are used for agricultural work. Hence, the loss of animals due to disease or any other reason results in loss of wealth, livelihood, and nutrition.

In view of this, management of mortality on farms is of utmost importance. There are different ways to manage and dispose of dead animals. The acceptable methods to manage mortality include composting, rendering, incineration, landfills, burial, and disposal pits.

Composting is one of the options for managing mortality on farms. Composting is the decomposing of carcasses by natural processes, viz the use of bacteria, fungi, and other microorganisms to convert organic matter into a stable product called compost. Composting involves the degradation of the carcass by anaerobic bacteria to convert it into liquid material with odor and gases such as hydrogen sulfide and ammonia)The anaerobic process produces heat that kills many viruses and bacteria and allows the growth of only heat-tolerant bacteria)The temperature continues to rise and peaks between 130 to 160 0F. Composting requires a source of energy and nutrients, moisture, oxygen, and pH in the range of 6 to 8.

Rendering is another method of managing mortality on farms. *Rendering* is a process that uses heat to convert animal carcasses into safe, pathogen-free protein and other valuable end products. In this process, dead animals must be preserved quickly and transported promptly. Rendering can be a low-temperature or high-temperature rendering process. The carcass is exposed to high temperatures (130 ^{0}C or 265 ^{0}F) rendering using pressurized steam to ensure the destruction of pathogens. However, there is a chance of transmission of diseases like Bovine transmissible spongiopathy.

Incineration is the thermal destruction of the carcass by using fuel or an electric heater. Generally, small carcasses (Poultry, pig, cat and dog) are disposed of by incineration.

Burial is another method of carcass disposal. However, it poses risk of underground water contamination.

Landfills are sites where waste is isolated from the environment until it is safe. The carcass is degraded biologically, chemically or physically. However, it may results in draining or leakage of contaminated liquid (Leachates) into surrounding area and potable water.

Disposal pits are least preferred method of managing mortality. This method differs from burial because animals are placed in lined pits.

1. The following are the methods of carcass disposal except
   a) Incineration b) Necropsy
   c) Rendering d) Composting
2. The most common method used for disposal of small size animals is
   a) Composting b) Necropsy
   c) Incineration d) All of these
3. The one of the given below method involve decomposition of carcass by natural process like bacteria and microorganism
   a) Composting b) Incineration
   c) Rendering d) None of these
4. The peak temperature maintained in composting is around
   a) < 50 0F b) 50^0F to 100 ^{0}F
   c) 130^0F to 160 ^{0}F d) > 300 ^{0}F
5. The following are the essential factor required in composting except.
   a) Temperature of 130^0F to 160 ^{0}F b) pH of 6-8
   c) Dryness d) Oxygen
6. The dead animal is converted in small particle i.e organic matter by organism is.
   a) Incineration b) Composting
   c) Rendering d) All of these
7. One of the following is most efficient and low cost method of large animal disposal
   a) Composting b) Rendering
   c) Harvesting d) Incineration
8. The one of the following carcass disposal method involve treatment and recycling of organic waste.
   a) Incineration b) Burial
   c) Disposal pits d) Composting
9. The following statement are true for composting except
   a) It is related to involve treatment and recycling of organic waste
   b) It reduces the generation of waste at source
   c) It manages waste that has already generated)
   d) Generated waste can be used as fertilizer
10. The process of converting animal carcass into manure is called.
    a) Composting b) Incineration
    c) Necropsy d) Rendering
11. The converting animal carcass into safe, pathogen-free protein and other valuable end products which can be fed to animal as feed involve one of the following.
    a) Composting b) Incineration
    c) Rendering d) Necropsy

12. The leachates is term related to one the following
    a) Incineration b) Necropsy
    c) Rendering d) Landfills
13. The contaminated liquid that drain from landfill is called as
    a) Compost b) Leachates
    c) Sanitary waste d) All of these
14. The odour produced during composting of animal carcass results due to
    a) Release of Hydrogen sulphide gas b) Release of Ammonia gas
    c) Release of oxygen gas d) Both a and b
15. The process of composting involves the following except
    a) Energy b) Microorganism
    c) pH of 6-8 d) Dry condition in compost
16. The microorganism involved in animal carcass composting are
    a) Psychrophilic microbes b) Mesophilic microbes
    c) Thermophilic microbes d) Psychrotrophic microbes
17. The desired pH range for animal carcass composting is
    a) 3-5 b) 6-8
    c) 9-12 d) Below 3
18. The following statements are true for composting except…
    a) Its low cost compared to other carcass disposal method
    b) Yiled manure
    c) Easy to prepare piles
    d) Yield a byproduct which can be used as animal feed
19. The small animal carcass composting able to kill the pathogenic organism in between
    a) 6 to 12 hours b) 1 to 4 days
    c) 4 to 6 days d) 10-14 days
20. The animal carcass composting should be carried out at distance from potable water source.i.e .
    a) 10 meter away b) 30 meter away
    c) 50 meter away d) 100 meter away
21. The expected land areas for large animal carcass composting is
    a) 2 square meter b) 5 square meter
    c) 8 square meter d) 17 square meter
22. The expected land areas for small animal carcass (pig, sheep, etc.) composting is
    a) 1 square meter b) 2 square meter
    c) 3.5 square meter d) 15.5 square meter
23. The expected land areas for 100 chicken composting is
    a) 1 square meter b) 2 square meter
    c) 3.5 square meter d) 8.7 square meter

24. The *graves, Trenches or open bottom containers* are associated with one of the given below disposal method
    a) Rendering b) Burial method
    c) Incineration d) All of these
25. The chances of contamination of ground and surface water due to microorganism is linked to ..
    a) Rendering b) Incineration
    c) Burial method) d) All of these
26. In Burial method, the contamination of ground and surface water occur due to ..
    a) *E. coli* b) *Cryptosporidium*
    c) Lyssa virus d) Both a and b
27. The organism that can be seen even after decomposition is/ aret..
    a) Prions b) Anthrax spore
    c) Rabies (Lyssa) virus d) Both a and b
28. The diseases which can be transmitted even after composting carcass include.
    a) BSE b) Scrapie
    c) Anthrax d) All of these
29. The animals infected with Anthrax or Foot and Mouth disease are desirable to dispose of by..
    a) Rendering b) Burning/ Incineration
    c) Disposal pits d) All of these
30. The zoonotic as well as pathogenic organism including anthrax spore are destroyed by one of given below method
    a) Rendering b) Incineration
    c) Disposal pits d) Burial
31. The temperature maintained in incineration method of disposal of animal carcass is..
    a) 50 ^{0}c) b) 100 ^{0}C
    c) 200 ^{0}c) d) >850 ^{0}C
32. The incineration method of animal carcass disposal is used in all except
    a) Dog b) Cat
    c) Sheep d) Adult buffalo
33. The prion protein are completely destroyed in one of the disposal method
    a) Rendering b) Incineration
    c) Disposal pits d) Burial
34. The rendering process (High temperature) is particularly discouraged in animal affected with
    a) *Clostridium perfringens.* b) BSE
    c) TSE d) Only b and c
35. The tallow, bone meal, meat meal are byproducts of
    a) Composting b) Burial
    c) Rendering d) Incineration

36. The rendering process of animal carcass give the following as a byproduct except

a) Tallow b) Bone meal

c) Meat meal d) Ash

37. The method of rendering process are

a) Dry process b) Wet process

c) Both a and b are true d) Only b is true

38. Which one of the method of rendering is more efficient (>20 % higher yield)

a) Dry process b) Wet process

c) Composting d) All of these

39. The rendering process involve

a) Compostingof animal carcass b) Cooking of animal carcass

c) Burning of animal carcass d) All of these

40. In high temperature rendering process, the carcass is exposed to

a) 40ºC b) 80ºC

c) 130ºC d) None of these

41. The studies found that the high temperature rendering process is unable to completely destroy

a) *Enterobacter spp.* b) Prion proteins

c) *Clostridium perfringens* d) Both a & b

42. The studies found that the high temperature rendering process is able to completely destroy the following except

a) *Enterobacter spp.* b) *Campylobacter spp.*

c) *Clostridium perfringens* d) *Listeria spp.*

43. The rendering process (High temperature) is particularly discouraged in animal affected with

a) Scrapie b) Mad cow disease

c) Black quarter d) Only a and b

44. The Composting method of animal carcass disposal requires moisture of…

a) <10 % b) 10-30 %

c) 30-40 % d) 40-60%

45. The following statements are true with regards to benefit of animal carcass disposal except

a) Reduced problems with flies and odors

b) Reduce the chance of the spread of disease

c) Increases risk of spread of diseases

d) Yield fertilizer

46. The Risk of ground water contamination is highest in one of method carcass disposal…

a) Burial b) Incineration

c) Burning d) All of these

47. The burial of animal carcass should be avoided in
    a) Flooding
    b) Summer
    c) Water source distance at >200 meters
    d) Availability 5 acres of land
48. The method of disposal of carcass in which animal carcass is placed in lined pit is…
    a) Incineration
    b) Composting
    c) Burning
    d) Disposal pits
49. The ground water contamination is biggest issue in…
    a) Incineration
    b) Rendering
    c) Burning
    d) Disposal pits
50. The following statements are true in case of disposal pits except …
    a) *High chances of ground water contamination*
    b) *Dead animal take longer time to decompose*
    c) *Most common method of carcass disposal.*
    d) Sites should be located on sites with 5% or greater slopes

Answer Key

1	b	2	c	3	a	4	c	5	c	6	b	7	a
8	d	9	b	10	a	11	c	12	d	13	b	14	d
15	d	16	c	17	b	18	d	19	d	20	d	21	d
22	c	23	d	24	b	25	c	26	d	27	d	28	d
29	b	30	b	31	d	32	d	33	b	34	b	35	c
36	d	37	c	38	a	39	b	40	c	41	d	42	a
43	d	44	d	45	c	46	a	47	a	48	d	49	d
50	c												

30

Livestock Economics and Marketing

Anuradha Kumari*, *Utkarsh Kumar Tripathi, Manish Kumar, and Jayant Goyal*

Faculty of Veterinary and Animal Sciences, IAS, RGSC, Banaras Hindu University Varanasi, Uttar PRadesh

Introduction

The term "Economics" is derived from the Greek words 'OIKOS' and 'NOMAS' or 'NEMEIN'. 'Oikos' means house hold and 'Nomas' or 'Nemein' means management. So, in its original sense-economics means house hold management; i.e. satisfying as many wants of the house hold or family as possible by allocating the limited resources at the disposal of the family wisely among different wants. In the modern and practical sense Economics means management of day-to-day problems arising from unlimited wants and limited resources by wisely allocating limited resources to satisfy maximum wants.

Divisions or approach of Economics

There are two approaches a) Traditional approach and Modern approach.

Traditional approach is divided into six main divisions, viz., (i) Production, (ii) Distribution, (iii) Exchange, (iv) Consumption, (v) public finance and (vi) economic planning.

Modern approach studied under (i) Income Theory or Macro Economics; and (ii) Price Theory or Micro Economics, deals with the study of the determination of prices.

Nature of economics: Economics is both an art and science, and is both positive and normative science. Positive science describes while normative science evaluates.

Basic concepts- Basic Terms

Want: "Man is a bundle of desires. Human wants refer to person desire for commodities or goods and services.

Goods: Anything that can satisfy a human want is called a 'goods' in Economics. It has both physical existence and also includes services.

Consumption: It is defined as the destruction or using up of the utility contained in the matter or the commodities and service to satisfy human wants.

Utility: This want-satisfying quality in a good is called Utility. There are three forms of utility i.e. place, form and time utility.

Value: The value of a commodity, thus, means the commodities or services that we can get in return for it; it is, in short, its purchasing power in terms of other commodities and services.

Price: Value is not the same thing as price. When value is expressed in terms of money, it is called price.

Wealth: In Economics anything which has value is called wealth or the term 'Wealth' is synonymous with economic goods.

Assets: Any item of economic value owned by an individual or corporation, especially that which could be converted to cash is considered as assets.

Demand: Demand means desire backed by willingness and ability to pay. Demand varies inversely with price.

Supply: Supply means the quantities that a seller is willing and able to sell at different prices.

Factor of production and their reward:

Production is defined as the creation or addition of value or on wealth. Land, labour, capital and organisation (enterprise) are the four factors of production. Land is rewarded by rent, labour is rewarded by wages, capital is rewarded by interest and organisation is rewarded by profits.

Marketing: Market is a derivative of Latin word 'marcatus' meaning merchandise, wares, traffic, trade or place where business is conducted)

Livestock marketing: Livestock marketing is the marketing of livestock and livestock products that is procuring raw materials (milk, sheep/goat, and eggs), processing them (milk products, mutton/meat, and egg powder), packaging, storing, transporting and distributing to the ultimate consumers.

Marketing functions: The process of marketing involves a number of marketing functions, which may be grouped under:

A. Functions of exchange which include

1. Buying and assembling and
2. Selling.

B. Functions of physical supply which include

1. Transportation and
2. Storage or warehousing.

C. Functions of facilitation which include

1. Standardization and grading
2. Financing
3. Risk bearing
4. Market information and intelligence.

Book-keeping and accounting

Book Keeping

Book Keeping is the art of recording business transactions (pecuniary transactions) in a regulator and systematic manner. Recording is done in the book journal.

Systems of book keeping

Business transactions can be recorded in any system which provides to the businessman, the necessary financial position of his business and the result of his transactions. The following systems of book keeping are followed.

1. **Single entry system:** This type of book keeping involves recording only one side of the transaction or activity. It maintains only the purchases, cash receipts and payments and sales. It is incomplete, inaccurate and unscientific.
2. **Double entry system**: (i) It is most scientific, (ii) It recognizes both the aspects of each transaction and records each aspect, (iii) It is complete, accurate and scientific.

Accounting

Accounting is the science of recording and classifying business transactions and events primarily of a financial character and then of making significant summaries, analysis and interpretations of those transactions and events and communicating the results to decision making persons.

Systems of accounting

Accounting system is a basis for designing polices for accounting business transactions. There are three systems.

a) Cash system or cash receipt and cash payment system.
b) Mercantile system or accrual system.
c) Mixed or hybrid system

1. The term economics means?
   a) Farm management b) House hold management
   c) Resource management d) Wants management
2. Father of economics is?
   a) F.A.Walker b) J.S. Mill
   c) J.B.Say d) Adam Smith
3. Price under a perfect market condition depends primarily upon.
   a) Demand b) Supply
   c) Only on supply d) Both a & b
4. All are part of traditional approach of economics except …
   a) Production b) Micro economics
   c) Distribution d) Economic planning
5. Study of the behaviour of economic system is
   a) Price theory b) Micro economics
   c) Macro economics d) Modern theory
6. Economics is considered as
   a) Positive science b) Normative science
   c) Both d) None
7. Regarding the wants which one is incorrect
   a) Wants are complementary b) Wants are non-recurring
   c) Wants are alternative d) Most of wants are recurring
8. An example of economic good is
   a) Air b) Sunshine
   c) Milk d) Water

9. The art of recording of business transactions in a regular and systematic manner is known as....
   a) Accounting
   b) Book keeping
   c) Auditing
   d) Reporting
10. The consumption involving goods and service that are used to produce other goods
    a) Final consumption
    b) Indirect consumption
    c) Destructive consumption
    d) Direct consumption
11. Want satisfying power in a commodity or service is
    a) Consumption
    b) Satisfaction
    c) Utility
    d) Value
12. Law of diminishing marginal utility is given by.......
    a) J.R.Hicks
    b) R.G.D.Allen
    c) Prof. Alfred Marshall
    d) Adam Smith
13. The additional benefit gained from an increase in consumption decreases with an increase in the level of consumption is ....
    a) Law of demand
    b) Law of diminishing marginal utility
    c) Laws of supply
    d) Law of production
14. The purchasing power of a things in terms of other things is called as
    a) Utility
    b) Price
    c) Value
    d) Demand
15. Not a characteristic of wealth
    a) Utility
    b) Scarcity
    c) Transferability
    d) Internal to man
16. In relation to wealth which statement is incorrect
    a) All money is wealth
    b) All wealth is not be money
    c) All types of capital wealth
    d) All wealth is capital
17. When the marginal product (MP) is constant then the total product (TP) is
    a) Increasing at increasing rate
    b) Increasing at decreasing rate
    c) Increasing at constant rate
    d) Constant
18. Which of the following is not a factor of production
    a) Capital
    b) Entrepreneurship management
    c) Labour
    d) Rent
19. The average cost per unit of production will go on decreasing with every additional unit of increase in output is......
    a) Law of increasing returns or law of decreasing costs
    b) Laws of constant returns or laws of constant costs
    c) Laws of decreasing returns or law of increasing costs
    d) Law of supply

20. Wage paid or received in terms of money is
    a) Money wages b) Nominal wages
    c) Both a and b d) Real wages
21. The shift of supply curve to the right-side means...
    a) Increase in supply b) Decrease supply
    c) No change in supply d) None of the above
22. The output of an organization is
    a) Interest b) Wage
    c) Rent d) Profit
23. The person who put money in a firm in the hope of getting profit are
    a) Investor b) Creditors
    c) Tax authorities d) Debitors
24. The sum of total variable costs and total fixed costs equal to
    a) Marginal cost b) Total cost
    c) Average total cost d) Sunk cost
25. Process of satisfying human want by the use of goods and services is known as
    a) Desire b) Consumption
    c) Utility d) None of these
26. Payment of causal labour comes under
    a) Variable cost b) Fixed cost
    c) Sunk cost d) Overhead cost
27. When cross elasticity of demand for two goods is negative, they are
    a) Substitute goods b) Complementary goods
    c) Competitive goods d) None of these
28. The decline of value of equipment due to wear and tear is called...
    a) Depreciation b) Degradation
    c) Appreciation d) Up gradation
29. When a negligible fall in the prices of a commodity leads to an infinite extension in its demand, then its demand is said to be
    a) Perfectly inelastic b) Imperfectly elastic
    c) Perfectly elastic d) Imperfectly inelastic
30. The cost which has to be incurred even when the production is not undertaken
    a) Marginal cost b) Implicit cost
    c) Explicit cost d) Fixed cost
31. Scarcity definition of economics given by
    a) Adam Smith b) Lionel Robbins
    c) Alfed Marshall d) J.S.Mill
32. Cost incurred for purchase of resource is called
    a) Sunk cost b) Implicit cost
    c) Explicit cost d) All of the above

33. The person who organises business is called ……
   a) Investor b) Creditors
   c) An entrepreneur d) Debitors
34. Methods of forecasting demand
   a) Survey methods b) Market studies and experiments
   c) Statistical or analytical methods d) All of these
35. Method generally adopted in estimating short-term demand is
   a) Survey methods b) Market studies
   c) Statistical methods d) Analytical methods
36. The ration of change in product as related to change in input is called
   a) Total product b) Average product
   c) Marginal product d) Complementary product
37. In principle of substitution price ratio is equal to……
   a) No of units of replaced resources /no of units of added resource
   b) No of units of added resource/ No of units of replaced resources
   c) Cost per unit of added resource/Cost per unit of replaced resource
   d) Cost per unit of replaced resource/ Cost per unit of added resource
38. Not a fixed cost in dairy farming
   a) Depreciation on building b) Wages of permanent labour
   c) Interest of working capital d) Livestock insurance charges
39. Goods that make easy living is called
   a) Necessaries b) Comforts
   c) Luxuries d) None of the above
40. Depreciation rate on equipment's and machineries per annum is …….
   a) 2% b) 5%
   c) 10% d) 15%
41. Desire for something plus the willingness and ability to pay a certain price in order to possess it.
   a) Utility b) Wealth
   c) Price d) Demand
42. Reasons for demand curve slopes downwards
   a) Income effect b) Substitution effect
   c) Price effect d) All of these
43. Demand of a good or service in reference to changes in price of other related goods is
   a) Joint demand b) Composite demand
   c) Cross demand d) Derived demand
44. Goods that are essential for human existence….
   a) Necessaries b) Comforts
   c) Luxuries d) None of the above

45. Exceptional demand curve was developed by
    a) J.R. Hicks
    b) Sir Robert Giffen
    c) Allen
    d) Alfred Marshall
46. Tabular expression of different combinations of two commodities yielding the same level of satisfaction is
    a) Demand curve
    b) Exceptional demand curve
    c) Indifference curve
    d) Indifference schedule
47. Rational zone in classical production curve
    a) Zone I
    b) Zone II
    c) Zone III
    d) All the above
48. Zone of increasing return in classical production curve
    a) Zone I
    b) Zone II
    c) Zone III
    d) All the above
49. The zone of negative return in classical production curve
    a) Zone I
    b) Zone II
    c) Zone III
    d) All the above
50. Necessary condition for the optimum production is
    a) AP>MP
    b) AP and MP decreasing
    c) MP >0
    d) All the above
51. Which of the following production function exists in almost every practical situation in livestock production?
    a) Increasing Returns to Scale
    b) Constant Returns to Scale
    c) Decreasing Returns to Scale
    d) All the above
52. Production function can be expressed in
    a) Tabular form
    b) Algebraic form
    c) Graphical form
    d) All the above
53. A price at which quantity demanded and quantity supplied in a given time and in a given market is equal is referred as
    a) Shadow price
    b) Equilibrium price
    c) Normal price
    d) Market price
54. Difference between total utility and total price is called
    a) Consumers demand)
    b) Market price
    c) Consumer surplus
    d) Equilibrium price
55. Time required for a resource to be completely transformed into product is referred as
    a) Marketing period
    b) Purchasing period
    c) Production period
    d) All the above
56. Marginal factor cost is nothing but
    a) Variable cost
    b) Fixed cost
    c) Price of output
    d) Unit price of input

57. Produced above this point is the profit
   a) Shut down point   b) Break-even point
   c) Both of the above   d) None of the above
58. Shutdown point is the minimum point of
   a) Marginal cost curve   b) Average variable cost curve
   c) Average fixed cost curve   d) Average total cost curve
59. The aggregate demand of all the consumers combined for the commodity or services is called
   a) Individual Seller's demand)   b) Cross demand
   c) Industry demand   d) None of the above
60. Cash costs are
   a) Marginal cost   b) Implicit cost
   c) Explicit cost   d) All the above
61. Non cash costs are otherwise called as
   a) Marginal cost   b) Implicit cost
   c) Explicit cost   d) All the above
62. Income earned from the next best alternative is known as
   a) Sunk cost   b) Opportunity cost
   c) Out of Pocket cost   d) All the above
63. Which of the following shows the results of buying and selling of goods?
   a) Profit and loss account   b) Trading account
   c) Balance sheet   d) Nominal Account
64. Percentage change in output in relation to percentage change in input is known as
   a) Average Product   b) Elasticity of production
   c) Marginal product   d) All the above
65. Fixed cost also known as
   a) Opportunity cost   b) Out of Pocket cost
   c) Sunk cost   d) All the above
66. Cost function is the relationship between
   a) Price and input   b) Cost and output
   c) Input and output   d) None of the above
67. Line connecting the least cost combination of inputs for all output level is
   a) Iso-cost line   b) Iso-cline
   c) Iso-revenue line   d) None of the above
68. A curve showing all possible combinations of two inputs that would produce the same level of output is
   a) Indifference curve   b) Iso-quant
   c) Iso-cost line   d) Production possibility curve

69. In perfect complements, the isoquant is
   a) Convex to the origin
   b) L-shaped
   c) Concave to the origin
   d) None of the above
70. The slope of isoquant is
   a) Price ratio
   b) Marginal rate of product transformation
   c) Marginal rate of factor substitution
   d) All the above
71. Depreciation is decrease in value of
   a) Raw materials
   b) Assets
   c) Output
   d) All the above
72. Increase in value of asset is known as
   a) Net worth
   b) Appreciation
   c) Depreciation
   d) None of the above
73. Among the following an undiscounted measure of investment analysis is
   a) Pay-back period
   b) BCR
   c) NPW
   d) All the above
74. A discounted measure of investment analysis
   a) BCR
   b) IRR
   c) NPW
   d)All the above
75. Balance sheet is otherwise called as
   a) Income statement
   b) Net worth statement
   c) Profit and loss statement
   d) All the above
76. In case of sound investment, the benefit cost ratio should be
   a) Less than one
   b) Zero
   c) Greater than one
   d) None of the above
77. In case of sound investment, the NPW should be
   a) Negative
   b) Zero
   c) Positive
   d) All the above
78. A statement indicating the financial position of the livestock farm
   a) Income statement
   b) Repayment schedule
   c) Balance sheet
   d) All the above
79. A constant amount of principle and corresponding interest is paid up every year in the following method of repayment.
   a) Lump sum
   b) Amortized decreasing
   c) Amortized even
   d) Partial repayment

80. An equal amount of instalments comprising larger proportion of principle and corresponding interest is paid up every year in case of one of the following method of repayment.
a) Lump sum b) Amortized decreasing
c) Amortized even d) Partial repayment

81. A part of principle along with interest is paid up every year in the following method of repayment
a) Lump sum b) Amortized decreasing
c) Amortized even d) Partial repayment

82. The entire amount of principle is paid up on the expiry of the term in the following method of repayment
a) Lump sum b) Amortized decreasing
c) Amortized even d) Partial repayment

83. The loan, given for a maximum period of 7 years to 20 years is coming under the category of
a) Short term loan b) Semi-Medium-term loan
c) Medium term loan d) Long term loan

84. The loan, given for a maximum period of 18 months years to 7 years is coming under the category of
a) Short term loan b) Semi-Medium-term loan
c) Medium term loan d) Long term loan

85. The loan, given for a maximum period of 18 months is coming under the category of
a) Short term loan b) Semi-Medium-term loan
c) Medium term loan d) Long term loan

86. Short term loans are called as
a) Production loan b) Investment loan
c) Seasonal loan d) Both a and c

87. Medium term loans are otherwise known as
a) Production loan b) Investment loan
c) Seasonal loan d) None of the above

88. R's of credit are
a) Returns b) Repayment capacity
c) Risk Bearing ability d) All the above

89. C's of credit are
a) Character b) Capital
c) Capacity d) All the above

90. Budgeting type, typically used for making decisions about adopting a new technology.
a) Partial Budgeting b) Complete Budgeting
c) Both of the above d) None of the above

91. Scarce commodities sold at very high price but in a secret manner
    a) Retail market   b) Seasonal market
    c) Black market   d) All the above
92. Ratio of market output to marketing input in percentage is referred as
    a) Market surplus   b) Market demand
    c) Marketing efficiency   d) None of the above
93. Market for egg and meat are classified under
    a) Very short period market   b) Short period market
    c) Long period market   d) None of the above
94. Markets which are located in big village or town is called
    a) Family Market   b) Local market
    c) National Market   d) World Market
95. Markets where the goods are bought and sold in bulk is called
    a) Retail market   b) Seasonal market
    c) Wholesale market   d) National Market
96. Agent middlemen are
    a) Retailers   b) Brokers
    c) Commission agents   d) Both b and c
97. Merchant middlemen are
    a) Wholesaler   b) Retailer
    c) Both a and b   d) None of the above
98. Market with single seller and few numbers of buyers
    a) Monopoly   b) Monopsony
    c) Oligopoly   d) Oligopsony
99. Market with few numbers of sellers
    a) Monopsony   b) Oligopsony
    c) Monopoly   d) Oligopoly
100 Market with few numbers of buyers
    a) Monopsony   b) Oligopsony
    c) Monopoly   d) Oligopoly
101. In the market structure, when there is only one buyer and many sellers is called
    a) Monopoly   b) Oligopoly
    c) Monopsony   d) Oligopsony
102. Co-operative marketing is example for
    a) Monopoly   b) Monopsony
    c) Oligopoly   d) Oligopsony
103. In a market structure, when there is only one single seller and single buyer it is called.
    a) Monopoly   b) Bilateral monopoly
    c) Monosony   d) Bilateral monopsony

104. MKIS stand for
   a) Marketing Knowledge Information System
   b) Marketing Information System
   c) Middleman Knowledge Information System
   d) Middleman Information System
105. Processing creates
   a) Form utility b) Place utility
   c) Time utility d) Possession utility
106. The word 'Market 'is derived from the latin word Marcatus which means
   a) Merchandise b) Trade
   c) Place d) All of above
107. A producer sells his produce and receive income from
   a) Produce market b) Factor market
   c) Consumer market d) All the above
108. He is the owner of the business....
   a) Creditor b) Proprietor
   c) Debtor d) Merchandiser
109. Which of the fallowing is intangible assets
   a) Cash b) Land
   c) Building d) Goodwill
110. Where is National Institute for Agricultural Marketing (NIAM) located in India?
   a) Jaipur b) New Delhi
   c) Pune d) Bhopal
111. The quality of product is graded based on
   a) PFA b) ICA
   c) ICMR d) BIS
112. NECC fix the price for
   a) Eggs b) Broilers
   c) layers d) Chicks
113. Organisation at national level to fix the price of egg is
   a) APMC b) NECC
   c) NFID d) BIS
114. Macro Economics is also known as
   a) Income theory b) Price theory
   c) Demand theory d) Theory of consumption
115. Which of these is not a function of marketing
   a) Buying b) Selling
   c) Consumption d) Production

116. Sorting of eggs on the basis of their weight is called as....
a) Grading b) Standardization
c) Distribution d) Transportation

117. On the basis of volume of business, market is classified as
a) Bullion market b) Regional market
c) Village market d) Wholesale market

118. The cost that varies with output is
a) Total cost b) Marginal cost
c) Variable cost d) Average cost

119. On the basis of subject matter of sale market may be
a) National market b) Primary market
c) Retail market d) Service market

120. Modern marketing concept is
a) Sales oriented b) Consumer oriented
c) Public welfare is main motto d) All of these

121. Hand to mouth buying means....
a) Buying more than quantity of goods than immediately required
b) Buying goods only as much minimal as possible
c) Buying from single source
d) Buying from large number of sources

122. The process by which the ownership of goods and service is transferred is
a) Selling b) Buying
c) Consumption d) Production

123. Storage creates
a) Form utility b) Place utility
c) Time utility d) Possession utility

124. Marketing function of facilitation include....
a) Storage b) Assembling
c) Standardization and grading d) Transportation

125. The job of collecting, interpreting and disseminating large variety of data for smooth operation of market is
a) Market information b) Market intelligence
c) Market opportunities d) All of these

126. Determinants of consumer behaviour are....
a) Economic factor b) Psychological factor
c) Sociological factor d) All of these

127. Which of the following is the correct accounting equation?
a) Assets = Liabilities + Equity b) Assets = Liabilities - Equity
c) Assets = Equities d) Liabilities = Assets + Equity

128. Which book records all farm transactions in chronological order?
   a) Ledger b) Balance Sheet
   c) Journal d) Cash Book
129. Factor – factor relationship explains
   a) How to produce b) How much to produce
   c) What to produce d) All the above
130. Factor – Product relationship explains
   a) How to produce b) How much to produce
   c) What to produce d) All the above
131. Product – Product relationship explains
   a) How to produce b) How much to produce
   c) What to produce d) All the above
132. All the input variables are allowed to vary and none is fixed in case of
   a) Production function b) Short run production function
   c) Long run production d) All the above
133. Exceptional process of the demand curve sloping upward is known as
   a) Normal demand) b) Giffen paradox
   c) Engel's law d) None of the above
134. Coefficient of elasticity in case of elastic demand is
   a) Zero b) Less than one
   c) Equal to one d) More than one
135. Coefficient of elasticity in case of unitary elastic demand is
   a) Zero b) Less than one
   c) Equal to one d) More than one
136. Coefficient of elasticity in case of inelastic demand is
   a) Zero b) Less than one
   c) Equal to one d) More than one
137. Market risks are due to
   a) Loss of Product b) Destruction of product
   c) Both a and b d) Change in the price of product
138. Demand change with the change in
   a) Price b) Income
   c) Taste and preference d) All the above
139. Higher indifference curve indicates
   a) No relation to utility b) Higher utility
   c) Lower utility d) None of the above
140. When marginal utility is zero, total utility is
   a) Minimum b) Maximum
   c) Zero d) Negative

141. An organisation having the motto of each for all and all for each
   a) Sole proprietor　　b) Joint stock company
   c) Public Sector enterprise　　d) Co-operative societies
142. Economic system that lacks the government control and central economic planning is
   a) Capitalist economy　　b) Socialist economy
   c) Mixed economy　　d) All the above
143. The process of utilities and values are created by the process
   a) Production　　b) Consumption
   c) Distribution　　d) Exchange
144. The purchasing power of the commodity expressed in terms of money is called
   a) Price　　b) Value
   c) Cost　　d) Utility
145. Income expressed in terms of commodities is called
   a) Money income　　b) Real income
   c) Total income　　d) None of the above
146. Resources can be stored are called
   a) Stock resources　　b) Flow resources
   c) Fixed resources　　d) None of the above
147. Resources or services, cannot be stored are called
   a) Stock resources　　b) Flow resources
   c) Fixed resources　　d) None of the above
148. Overhead charges are also known as
   a) Marginal cost　　b) Implicit cost
   c) Sunk cost　　d) All the above
149. Total assets - total liabilities is
   a) Net worth　　b) Net profit
   c) Gross Income　　d) None of the above
150. The price below which the seller will refuse to sell a product is called as
   a) Market Price　　b) Normal Price
   c) Secular Price　　d) Reserve Price

Answer Key

1	b	2	d	3	c	4	b	5	c	6	c	7	b
8	c	9	b	10	b	11	c	12	c	13	b	14	c
15	d	16	d	17	c	18	d	19	a	20	c	21	a
22	d	23	a	24	b	25	b	26	a	27	b	28	a
29	c	30	d	31	b	32	c	33	c	34	d	35	a
36	a	37	c	38	c	39	b	40	c	41	d	42	d

43	c	44	a	45	b	46	d	47	b	48	a	49	c
50	d	51	c	52	d	53	b	54	c	55	c	56	d
57	b	58	b	59	c	60	c	61	b	62	b	63	b
64	b	65	c	66	b	67	b	68	b	69	b	70	c
71	b	72	b	73	a	74	d	75	b	76	c	77	c
78	c	79	b	80	c	81	d	82	a	83	d	84	c
85	a	86	d	87	b	88	d	89	d	90	a	91	c
92	c	93	a	94	b	95	c	96	d	97	c	98	a
99	d	100	b	101	c	102	b	103	b	104	b	105	a
106	d	107	a	108	b	109	d	110	a	111	d	112	a
113	b	114	a	115	c	116	a	117	d	118	b	119	d
120	b	121	b	122	a	123	c	124	c	125	a	126	d
127	a	128	c	129	a	130	b	131	c	132	c	133	b
134	d	135	c	136	b	137	d	138	d	139	b	140	b
141	d	142	a	143	a	144	a	145	b	146	a	147	b
148	c	149	a	150	d								

31

Cattle and Buffalo Production

Cherryl Dimphna Miranda[1]*, and Tanmoy Rana*[2]

[1]*Department of LPM, C.V.Sc, Sri Venkateswara Veterinary University, Tirupati, Andhra Pradesh*

[2]*Department of Veterinary Clinical Complex, West Bengal University of Animal & Fishery Sciences, Kolkata, West Bengal*

Introduction

It appears that cattle were domesticated prior to 4000b)c)From 1961 to 2021, the amount of milk produced worldwide has almost tripled, reaching 918 million tonnes. Production of milk is carried out by about 150 million households worldwide. Smallholders produce the majority of the milk in developing nations, and milk production supports nutrition, food security, and household livelihoods. For small-scale farmers, milk offers comparatively quick returns and is a significant source of revenue. Small-scale farmers using native or local cattle breeds produce the majority of the milk in developing nations; however, to meet the growing demand for milk and milk products in peri-urban areas, more improved or cross-bred cattle are being used)

India is an agricultural country that contributes significantly to the economy. Animal husbandry is an adjunct to agriculture and has vital livestock resources, with cattle and buffalo playing an important role in improving the socio-economic status through contributions to milk, meat, hides, and draft power for agricultural operations. India is one of the world's top milk producers contributing 24 percent of global milk production and having a large number of indigenous germplasm with 53 cattle and 20 buffaloes spread across the country.

Indigenous breeds though have low productivity and typically need to be milked with the calf at foot, indigenous breeds are well suited to the local conditions. The majority of native breeds found in tropical areas belong to the zebu (Bos indicus) type, which is distinguished by its dewlap and hump. The dairy breeds of zebu cattle that are most commonly found are Sahiwal, Red Sindhi, Tharparkar, Kankrej, Gir, Deoni. Native Bos taurus cattle, such as the N'Dama and Criollo breeds, are found in the tropical regions of West Africa and Latin Americ)a)Although specialized dairy breeds like Jersey and Friesian produce large amounts of milk, they are less suited to harsh climates and need a lot of care from veterinarians and managers.

The domestic water buffalo, or Bubalus bubalis, is the primary milk-producing animal in a number of nations and contributes significantly to the world's milk production. In developing nations, small-scale farmers primarily raise one or two buffaloes in mixed crop-livestock systems. The river buffalo and the swamp buffalo are the two subspecies of water buffaloes. Approximately 70 percent of water buffaloes worldwide are river buffaloes. Milk from river buffaloes makes up a significant portion of the milk produced in Pakistan, India, and the Near East. Comparing swamp buffaloes to river buffaloes, the former are smaller and produce less milk. They are mostly raised for draught power and are found mostly in Eastern Asia.

During a lactation, river buffaloes typically yield 1500–4500 liters of milk. They can provide milk and calves for up to 20 years of age, which is a considerably more productive life than cattle. The late age of the animals at first calving, the seasonal nature of oestrus, the long calving interval, and the dry period are just a few of the numerous factors that limit the production of commercial buffalo milk. The goal of breeding programs in the past few decades has been to increase the milk yield of river buffalo, particularly in China, Egypt, India, Pakistan, and Bulgaria)Several well-known breeds of specialized dairy buffalo are Jaffarabadi, Bhadawari, Kundi, Surti, Nili-Ravi, Murrah, and Mehsana.

The 1962 national policy for cattle and buffalo breeding in India emphasized the importance of increasing milk production by incorporating selected dairy breeds of cattle and buffaloes. The NDDB dairy co-operative network provided much-needed market stimulus and pricing incentives, promoting the selection of exotic dairy breeds for cattle crossbreeding. We must increase milk production in order to meet the demands, as dairy animals are raised and bred for their milk. The lactation period is the time after a cow gives birth to a calf when she begins to produce milk. By extending this lactation period, we can improve milk yiel d) However, milk quality needs to match milk output. The administration of dairy farms aims to improve the amount and caliber of milk produced by the milch animals. Breeds that are resistant to disease and have high yields are created as a result.

Small-scale farming systems produce 80–90% of the milk produced in developing nations. Due to the low input requirements of these operations, there is very little production per dairy animal. One of the following production systems provides the majority of the milk produced by smallholders in developing nations:

- Rural smallholder dairying
- Pastoral/agropastoral dairying
- Landless peri-urban dairying

Furthermore, some developing nations have large-scale dairy enterprises in addition to these conventional small-scale milk production systems. Large-scale farmers typically don't produce a significant portion of the country's milk.

Objectives

1. The adaptive changes in response to a single climatic variable in cattle is called
   a) Adaptation b) Acclimation
   c) Acclimatization d) Habituation
2. Thermo neutral zone for exotic cattle in India
   a) 15-30ºC b) 20-25°C
   c) 10-18ºC d) 0-5°C
3. Disease that is responsible for huge economic loss in dairy industry is
   a) Metritis b) Milk fever
   c) Mastitis d) Teat block

4. Measurement of solar radiation in cattle is done by
   a) Pyranometer b) Net radiometer
   c) Vernon globe d) All
5. Ketosis in dairy cattle is due to
   a) Protein deficiency b) Mineral deficiency
   c) Fatty acid deficiency d) Energy deficiency
6. Which of the following region of India is most suitable for livestock production
   a) North-west region b) Coastal region
   c) Eastern region d) Southern region
7. All are non-infectious diseases in cattle except
   a) Milk fever b) Ketosis
   c) Metabolic acidosis d) Wooden tongue
8. Herd average is the total milk production of herd in a day divided by
   a) Total animals in herd b) Total lactating animals in herd
   c) Total breedable females in herd d) Total pregnant animals in herd
9. Calf meat is called
   a) Chevon b) Karabeef
   c) Vension d) Veal
10. Which one is true for water turnover
    a) Amount of water passing through an animal in unit time
    b) Water turnover is more for cattle than sheep and goat
    c) Restricted range of grazing in cattle is due to more water turnover
    d) All
11. Inverse age resistance in cattle is seen for the following disease
    a) FMd b) Anthrax
    c) Babesiosis d) Theileriosis
12. _________ Strength of tincture iodine used for navel cord dip.
    a) 7% b) 17%
    c) 1% d) 10%
13. White heifer disease is categorized as
    a) Congenital disease b) Infectious disease
    c) Skin disease d) Metabolic disease
14. Most prevalent strain of FMD virus in India is
    a) 'A' strain b) 'O' strain
    c) 'Asia-1" strain d) All equally present
15. Blood volume in cattle is roughly ________ % of live body weight
    a) 7 b) 7.7
    c) 8 d) 9.7

16. Major foetal development in cattle takes place in a __________ trimester
 a) First b) Second
 c) Third d) All the above
17. _________ Disease causes severe straining and diarrhoea with mucus and blood in cattle
 a) Calf scour b) Salmonellosis
 c) Giardiasis d) Coccidiosis
18. The best site of hot branding in buffalo
 a) Neck b) Hind quarter
 c) Ear d) Flank
19. The water intake of adult cattle for every kg of dry matter intake is (in litres)
 a) 2-3 b) 3-5
 c) 6-7 d) >7
20. A common method of administering medicines to cattle during respiratory problems.
 a) Pessaries b) Poultices
 c) Electuaries d) Drenches
21. __________ is the lime content in cattle dung
 a) 0.11% b) 0.2%
 c) 0.31% d) 4%
22. Pitch angle in housing of livestock refers to
 a) Slope of roof b) Slope of floor
 c) Slope of drainage d) All
23. Ideal air space requirement per cow is ________
 a) 15 m^3 b) 25 m^3
 c) 22.5 m^3 d) 33.3 m^3
24. Solid manure produced by an ALU/ day is
 a) 10-20 kg b) 20-30 kg
 c) 30-40 kg d) 40-50 kg
25. How many litres of methane can be emitted by a single cow/day
 a) 50-100 b) 100-200
 c) 200-300 d) 300-400
26. In loose houses, extra accommodation can be provided for a short period of time
 a) 5% b) 10-15%
 c) 30-35% d) Cannot be accommodated
27. Under loose housing system, the feeding space (cm) to be provided per calf is
 a) 40-50 b) 20-30
 c) 30-40 d) 50-60
28. Standing space in tail-tail system should be
 a) 1.2 mts b) 1.5 mts
 c) 2 mts d) 2.5 mts

29. Service time for dairy cattle should be
    a) 60 days post-parturient
    b) 70 days post-parturient
    c) 85 days post-parturient
    d) 120 days post-parturient

30. Organized segment of behavior having special function in livestock is known as______
    a) Behavior pattern
    b) Foraging pattern
    c) Both
    d) None

31. In a natural pasture method, the male maintains close body contact with the female and grazes near her before mating. This behavior referred to
    a) Tending
    b) Teasing
    c) Treading
    d) Waltzing

32. Area just behind the cattle head and body which is out of visual field is called as
    a) Blind spot
    b) Flight zone
    c) Flight distance
    d) All

33. Advantages of tail-to-tail system of housing as compare to head-to-head system
    a) Milking supervision easy
    b) Danger of disease spread is less
    c) Easy clearance operation
    d) All of the above

34. Milking before parturition is
    a) Stripping
    b) Prenating
    c) Steaming
    d) Knuckling

35. Population depart from perfect genetic constitution in livestock is known as ___
    a) Mutation
    b) Genetic load
    c) Variation
    d) Adaption

36. The Prevention of Cruelty to Animals was first enacted in
    a) 1960
    b) 1982
    c) 1965
    d) 1999

37. In mixed farming, the contribution of livestock to gross income is
    a) At least 10 %
    b) At least 20%
    c) At least 40%
    d) At least 50%

38. Dairy cattle are _____ type of animal according to their behavior
    a) Solitary
    b) Social
    c) Unsocial
    d) All

39. The number of well-defined Indian breeds of Buffalo as per NBAGR, June 2016 is
    a) 13
    b) 10
    c) 15
    d) 14

40. The open area space requirement in loose housing system for bull is ___________ Sq.ft
    a) 100-120
    b) 180-200
    c) 200-250
    d) 120-140

41. In an open range condition, ________ is the maximum inter-animal distance in cattle herd.

a) 3-5m b) 1-3m

c) 11-12m d) 25-30m

42. Characteristic Cobra hood like horn pattern is seen in which of the following

a) Hallikar b) Kangayam

c) Amrithmahal d) Siri

43. In loose housing system ____________% additional stock can be accommodated.

a) 5% b) 10%

c) 20% d) 25%

44. CIRC is located at

a) Karnataka b) Rajasthan

c) Haryana d) Uttar Pradesh

45. Milk fat (%) in Murrah buffalo

a) 3% b) 5%

c) 7% d) 9%

46. AGMARK indicates

a) Quality and Purity b) Quality

c) Purity d) Quantity

47. The ratio of additive genetic variance to total phenotypic variance in cattle is known as

a) Fertility b) Repeatability

c) Heritability d) None

48. If cow get excited or disturbed at milking time, it holds the milk due to release of

a) Oxytocin b) Renin

c) Adrenaline d) Prolactin

49. Handsome cattle breed

a) Deoni b) Kankrej

c) Krishna valley d) Tharpakar

50. Sawaichal" is the characteristic gait of which cattle breed

a) Ongole b) Pulikulam

c) Kankrej d) Tharparkar

51. Most distinctive breed of zebu cattle

a) Red sindhi b) Sahiwal

c) Gir d) Ongole

52. _____ buffalo breed has wedge shaped body

a) Jaffarabadi b) Mehasana

c) Badhawari d) Surti

53. Percentage of cows countribution in world milk production
    a) 77 b) 68
    c) 83 d) 59
54. Percentage of buffaloes contribution in world milk production
    a) 77 b) 68
    c) 83 d) 59
55. Critical temperature of H.F. and Jersy
    a) 70-80 °F b) 80-90°F
    c) 90-95°F d) 60-75°F
56. Humidity above ______ causes detrimental effects in cattle?
    a) 80% b) 70%
    c) 60% d) 90%
57. Female animal with its offspring is known as
    a) Heifer b) Calf at foot
    c) Springer d) Downcalver
58. Skin temperature of cattle
    a) 25ºC b) 30°C
    c) 27ºC d) 33°C
59. Upper limit for comfort zone for zebu cattle
    a) 30ºC b) 22°C
    c) 28ºC d) 25°C
60. Average consumption of water by adult cattle per day(liters)
    a) 150-160 b) 80-90
    c) 100-110 d) 75-90
61. Each ICDP includes ___________ breedable females
    a) 1 lakh b) 10,000
    c) 1 million d) 10 million
62. ICDP exotic cattle breeding farm for HF cattle was established at
    a) Andeshnagar (UP) b) Nessargahta (Karnataka)
    c) Both d) None of the above
63. AICRP on cattle was launched in
    a) 1970 b) 1968
    c) 1971 d) 1983
64. In hilly areas, _______ exotic breed was used in cattle development programme
    a) Brown swiss b) H.F
    c) Jerssey d) None of the above
65. AICRP on buffalo was launched in
    a) 1970 b) 1968
    c) 1971 d) 1983

66. ICDP exotic cattle breeding farm for jersey was established at
   a) Andesh Nagar (UP)
   b) Hesaraghatta (Karnataka)
   c) Orissa
   d) None of the above
67. ICDP exotic cattle breeding farm for surti was established at
   a) Rajasthan
   b) Orissa
   c) Gujrat
   d) Tamilnadu
68. ICDP exotic cattle breeding farm for murrah was established at
   a) Rajasthan
   b) Orissa
   c) Gujrat
   d) Tamilnadu
69. Central council of Gosamvardhanam set up by the government of India in the year_____
   a) 1952
   b) 1928
   c) 1955
   d) 1965
70. Sunandini is a product of __________ project
   a) Indo-danish
   b) AICRP
   c) Indo-swiss
   d) Indo-german
71. Feeding management of cattle in hot environment
   a) Low protein low fiber
   b) High protein low fiber
   c) High protein high fiber
   d) Low protein low fiber
72. Optimum number of services per conception
   a) 2.50
   b) 2.25
   c) 1.50
   d) 1.75
73. Ideal Calving Interval in buffaloes
   a) 18-19 months
   b) 13-14 months
   c) 19-20 months
   d) 10-11 months
74. Which of the following is a recently recognized buffalo breed
   a) Kosali
   b) Banni
   c) Belahi
   d) Motto
75. Progeny testing of Sahiwal utilizes how many bulls per cycle
   a) 4
   b) 10
   c) 2
   d) 8
76. The breed developed in and around Patna during1875, by crossbreeding Short Horn male X Native cow
   a) Taylor
   b) Sunandini
   c) Frieswal
   d) Brahman
77. Quantity of blood required in the udder to produce one ml of milk is
   a) 40-50 ml
   b) 150-200 ml
   c) 240-260 ml
   d) 400-500 ml

78. Space requirement for manure storage is
    a) 4 tonnes/m^3 b) 4.5 quintal/m^3
    c) 0.45 quintals/m^3 d) None
79. Muzzle printing is scientifically known as
    a) Muzzleglyphics b) Muzzlegraphy
    c) Dermatoglyphics d) None
80. Pulsation ratio for slow and fast milking is __________ & __________, respectively.
    a) 1:1, 2.5:1 b) 3.5:1, 4:1
    c) 4.5:1, 1:3 d) 0.5:1, 1:4
81. Most reliable sign of estrus in buffalo is
    a) Mucus discharge b) Swollen vulva
    c) Standing to be mounted by male d) Frequent urination
82. As compared to beef, karabeef is rich in
    a) Protein b) Lysine
    c) Both d) None
83. Corrective measures for seasonal breeding in buffaloes
    a) Utero-ovarian massage b) Hormone injection
    c) Summer protection d) All of the above
84. Buffalo can pull a weight of 1 ton and having a draught ability of
    a) 2 H.P b) 3.5 H.P
    c) 0.75 H.P d) 1.5 H.P
85. Urea may be fed to ruminants at the rate of
    a) 3% of concentrate b) 1% of body weight
    c) Both a & b d) None
86. Duration of rumination in cattle is about ______hrs
    a) 15-20 b) 4-9
    c) 10-12 d) 20-22
87. Cattle domesticated at
    a) 5000 B.C. b) 3000 B.C
    c) 4000 B.C. d) 3500 B.C
88. Indian wild buffalo
    a) Mehasana b) Arni
    c) Jaffarbadi d) Surti
89. Heaviest among the milch cattle breed
    a) Tharpakar b) Red sindhi
    c) Gir d) Sahiwal
90. Average milk yield of Sahiwal (in kgs)
    a) 2150 b) 1675
    c) 1725 d) 1400

91. Which breed of cattle contain highest fat content in milk
   a) Gir b) Tharpakar
   c) Sahiwal d) Red sindhi
92. Best dairy breed of cattle in India
   a) Gir b) Tharpakar
   c) Sahiwal d) Red sindhi
93. Average milk yield of Gir (in kgs)
   a) 2150 b) 1675
   c) 1725 d) 1400
94. Average milk yield of Murrah buffalo (in kgs)
   a) 600-800 b) 1360-2270
   c) 2500-2700 d) 800-1000
95. Which breed of buffalo contain highest fat content in milk
   a) Murrah b) Nili Ravi
   c) Jaffarbadi d) Surti
96. Average milk yield of Tharparkar (in kgs)
   a) 2150 b) 1675
   c) 1725 d) 1400
97. Average milk yield of Red sindhi (in kgs)
   a) 2150 b) 1675
   c) 1725 d) 1400
98. Chemical used in milk tester
   a) Phenyl alcohol b) HCl
   c) Sulfuric acid d) Caustic soda
99. Average amount of man hours per cow per annum as per cow shed system is
   a) 180 b) 250
   c) 150 d) 90
100. Volumetric density of fresh manure is (in kg m^3)
   a) 300-500 b) 700-1000
   c) 500-700 d) 400-600
101. The first embryo transfer cattle calf born in India during____ year
   a) 1986 b) 1997
   c) 1988 d) 1996
102. When was the first embryo transfer buffalo calf born in India
   a) 1986 b) 1997
   c) 1987 d) 1996
103. In cattle, ovulation occurs after ________ hours of LH surge
   a) 24 hrs b) 48 hrs
   c) 32 hrs d) 12 hrs

104. If pregnancy does not occur which hormone is secreted on 17-18th day by uterus
a) Progesterone b) Estrogen
c) PGF2- alpha d) All the above

105. Progesterone can be given as
a) Pessaries b) PRID
c) S/C implant d) All the above

106. Longest lactation period in world
a) Jersey b) Brown swiss
c) Ayurshire d) None of the above

107. Average lactation period of Gir cattle breed (in days)
a) 325 b) 305
c) 315 d) 335

108. Average lactation period of jersey cattle breed (in days)
a) 325 b) 305
c) 315 d) 365

109. Native place of Guernsey cattle
a) Holland b) Scottland
c) France d) Netherland

110. _____ breed has the double dished head
a) Jersey b) HF
c) Brown Swiss d) None of the above

111. _____ buffalo breed has the longest lactation period
a) Murrah b) Mehasana
c) Surti d) Jaffarbadi

112. Naval flap is absent in _______ buffalo breed
a) Murrah b) Nagpuri
c) Surti d) Jaffarbadi

113. Naval flap is absent in _________ cattle breed
a) Sahiwal b) Gir
c) Haryana d) Ongole

114. Crossing between animals having one common ancestor
a) Out crossing b) In crossing
c) Line breeding d) Cross breeding

115. Crossing between two different species
a) Out crossing b) In crossing
c) Species hybridization d) Cross breeding

116. Crossing between animals of 2, 3 or more breed
a) Line breeding b) Cross breeding
c) Rotational crossing d) Criss crossing

117. Crossing between pure bred sire with ND dam
    a) Grading up b) Rotational crossing
    c) Species hybridization d) Cross breeding
118. Out crossing is preferred for
    a) Outstanding herd) b) Less than average herd
    c) All the above d) None of the above
119. Sunandhini is cross between
    a) Brown swissXNd b) JersseyXND
    c) HFXNd) d) None of the above
120. Which is most suitable exotic breed for cross breeding
    a) Jersey b) HF
    c) Brown Swiss d) None of the above
121. Dewlap is found in ______ buffalo breed
    a) Surti b) Mehasana
    c) Jaffarabadi d) Murrah
122. Dwarf breed of buffalo
    a) Jaffarabadi b) Mehasa
    c) Jerangi d) Surti
123. Minimal age of animal for entry in central herd register
    a) 6 M b) 12M
    c) 8M d) 14M
124. Herd registration centres were established in
    a) 1962-63 b) 1950-51
    c) 1982-83 d) 1941-42
125. Buffalo could be maintained in herd upto
    a) 5th lactation b) 6th lactation
    c) 3rd lactation d) 9th lactation
126. Peak yield in buffalo observed in ______
    a) 1st lactation b) 2nd lactation
    c) 4th lactation d) 6th lactation
127. CIRB is located at
    a) Hissar b) Guntur
    c) Haryana d) Goa
128. Number of semen freezing centers in India
    a) 70 b) 80
    c) 90 d) 60
129. In ruminants ______ percentage of dietary protein are degraded to ammonia in the rumen
    a) 30 b) 40
    c) 70 d) 60

130. The number of calving pens required at livestock farm is equal to
   a) 10 % of total flock
   b) 10% of total breedable female flock
   c) 20% of total breedable female flock
   d) 30% of total breedable female flock

131. Buffalo breed with sword shape horn is
   a) Jaffarabadi b) Nagpuri
   c) Surti d) Murrah

132. Energy requirement for cattle and buffaloes are expressed in terms of
   a) TDN b) SE
   c) DE d) ME

133. The wallowing is a feature of
   a) Swine b) Buffalo
   c) Both d) None of the above

134. The lower utilization of leaves protein in rumen is due to the presence of
   a) Condensed tannins b) Phytates
   c) Lignins d) Cellulose

135. When a female calf is twin with male calf, the condition is known as
   a) Buller b) Free martin
   c) Nymphomanic d) None

136. Lifespan of cattle
   a) 15-20 yrs b) 25-30 yrs
   c) 30-35 yrs d) 35-40 yrs

137. Nagori is _____
   a) Milch breed b) Dual purpose breed
   c) Draught breed d) None

138. A cow always in heat is known as
   a) Buller b) Free martin
   c) Anestrous d) None

139. Copper colour body coat is a characteristic feature of ___________ buffalo breed
   a) Nili-ravi b) Bhadawari
   c) Kundi d) Murrah

140. Colostrum feeding based on body weight of
   a) 1/10 b) 1/15
   c) 1/20 d) 1/25

141. Vechur is a
   a) Small breed b) Intermediate breed
   c) Large breed d) None

142. Major cause of calf mortality
 a) FMd b) Calf scour
 c) Pneumonia d) None
143. Best milk producer breed of buffalo in India
 a) Jaffarabadi b) Murrah
 c) Bhadawari d) Mehasana
144. Average number of days between two successive calvings for cows in the herd is known as
 a) Calving interval b) Generation interval
 c) Calving index d) Herd average
145. Buffalo breed of Southeast countries and China belongs to
 a) Mediterranean type b) Riverine type
 c) Swamp type d) All
146. Which of the following phase of lactation has negative energy balance
 a) Early phase b) Mid phase
 c) Last phase d) None
147. The covered area (m^2) for a cow in loose housing
 a) 3.5 b) 2.5
 c) 5.0 d) 7.0
148. The maximum heat tolerance exotic breed of cattle is
 a) HF b) Brown swiss
 c) Jersey d) Guernsey
149. The pH of fresh milk is
 a) 6.4-6.6 b) 6.7-6.8
 c) 6.8-7.0 d) None
150. The body weight range of calves (kgs)
 a) 25-30 b) 28-35
 c) 33-39 d) 38-45

Answer Key

1	b	2	c	3	c	4	d	5	d	6	a	7	d
8	a	9	c	10	d	11	c	12	b	13	a	14	b
15	b	16	c	17	d	18	b	19	b	20	c	21	c
22	a	23	c	24	c	25	b	26	b	27	a	28	b
29	c	30	a	31	a	32	a	33	a	34	b	35	b
36	a	37	a	38	b	39	a	40	c	41	c	42	b
43	b	44	d	45	c	46	a	47	c	48	c	49	d
50	c	51	a	52	c	53	a	54	b	55	a	56	c
57	b	58	d	59	a	60	c	61	a	62	c	63	b

64	c	65	a	66	c	67	c	68	d	69	a	70	c
71	b	72	d	73	b	74	b	75	d	76	a	77	d
78	b	79	c	80	a	81	c	82	c	83	d	84	c
85	c	86	b	87	c	88	b	89	d	90	a	91	d
92	c	93	b	94	b	95	c	96	c	97	c	98	a
99	c	100	b	101	a	102	c	103	a	104	c	105	d
106	a	107	a	108	d	109	c	110	a	111	b	112	b
113	c	114	c	115	c	116	c	117	a	118	b	119	a
120	a	121	c	122	c	123	a	124	a	125	d	126	c
127	a	128	b	129	d	130	b	131	b	132	a	133	c
134	a	135	b	136	a	137	c	138	a	139	b	140	a
141	a	142	c	143	b	144	c	145	c	146	a	147	a
148	b	149	a	150	a								

32

Sheep and Goat Production and Management

A.K. Srivastava, K.J. Ankuya, H.A. Patel, and D.A. Patel

Department of Livestock Production Management
College of Veterinary Science and Animal Husbandry
Kamdhenu University, Sardarkrushinagar, Gujarat

Introduction

There are many migratory, semi-migratory and sedentary shepherd communities in India with sheep rearing along with goats as the main livelihood)Besides scores of land less wages-earning families keep small numbers of goats for crucial supplementary income. Sheep and goat farming, due to its quicker and better returns on investment provides an additional source of income to farmers who normally depend on crops for their livelihood) Thus these animals fit in ideally in a mixed farming system. In India, goats and sheep are mostly maintained under extensive system which includes migratory, transhumance, free range, grazing community pastures, stubbles of cropped lands supplemented with crop residues and tree-lopping. Although a number of management systems are in practices varying from region to region these may be conveniently divided in to extensive, Semi-intensive and Intensive systems.

Breeds of Sheep

Total sheep population in the country is 74.26 Million during the year 2019. Sheep population has increased by 14.13% over previous Livestock Census (2012). 45 Indigenous breeds of sheep are classified into four groups based on agro-ecological regions.

Classification of sheep breeds based on agro-ecological regions in India

Northern temperate region	North-western, central arid and semi-arid region	Southern region semi-arid central peninsular area and hot and humid along the coast	Eastern region
Bhakarwal (CW) Changthangi (CW) Gaddi (CW) Gurez (CW) Karnah (AW) Kashmir Merino(AW) Poonchi (CW) Rampur Bushair(CW)	Chokla (CW) Hissardale (AW) Jaisalmeri (MCW) Jalauni (MCW) Kheri (MCW) Magra (CW) Malpura (MCW) Marwari (MCW) Muzaffarnagari (MCW) Nali (CW) Patanwadi (CW) Pugal (MCW) Sonadi (MCW) Munjal(M)	Bellary (MCW) Coimbatore (MCW) Daccani (M) Hassan (M) Kanguri (M) Kilakarsal (M) Madras Red (M) Mandya (M) Mecheri (M) Nellore (M) Nilgiri (AW) Rammand White (M) Tiruchy Black (M) Vembur (M)	Balangir (MCW) Bonpala (MCW) Chottanagpuri (MCW) Ganjam (MCW) Garole (M) Tibetan (CW) Shahbadi
Within parenthesis is the major product of the bree d) (AW), Apparel wool; (CW), Carpet wool; (MCW), Mutton and Carpet wool; (M), Mutton.			

Classification of Indigenous sheep breeds based on utility

Apparel wool breeds	Superior carpet Wool breeds	Coarse carpet Wool breeds	Hairy Meat breeds
Hissardale Niligiri Kashmir merino Avivastra Bharat Merino	Chokla Nali Marwari Magra Jaisalmeri Pugal Patanwadi Tibetan Bonpala Gaddi Rampur Bushair Poonchi Karnah Gurez Changthangi	Malpura Sonadi Muzzafarnagri Jalauni Deccani Bellary Coimbatore Chottanagpuri Balangir Ganjam Bhakarwal Sh0ahabadi	Nellore Hassan Mecheri Kilakarsal Madras Red Trichy Black Kenguri Mandya Vembur

Description and peculiar characters of some Indian sheep breeds

S.N.	Breed	Home tract	Characters
1.	Chokla (Shekhavati)	Sikar, Churu & Jhun-jhunu (Rajasthan)	Roman nose, medium size compact body, also known as "Indian Merino"
2.	Nali	Ganganagar, Churu & Jhunjhunu (Rajasthan)	Canary coloration of wool (Yellow wool)
3.	Marwari	Marwar region (Rajas-than)	most disease resistant breed, Triple purpose sheep breed
4.	Pugal	Bikaner (Rajasthan)	Yellow streak above eyebrow
5.	Jaisalmeri	Jaisalmer (Rajasthan)	Roman nose
6.	Sonadi	Udaipur (Rajasthan)	--
7.	Nellore	Nellore (AP)	The tallest breed of sheep in India, Best mutton breed of India, Also known as "Goat like sheep" (No wool)
8.	Mandya (Bannur)	Karnataka	The smallest sheep breed
9.	Garole	Sundarban (WB)	Most prolific sheep breed of India
10.	Ganjam	Ganjam (Orissa)	
11.	Gaddi	Kullu & Kangra Valleys (HP) (nomadic tribe Gad-dis rear this breed)	Very sturdy & very good climber Polled ewes & horned rams, Undercoat used for making "Kullu shawls" & blankets
12.	Bhakarwal	Lower hills of Himalaya (Nomadic tribe Bhakarw-al rear this breed)	Rams are horned but ewes hornless,
13.	Gurez	Kashmir	Biggest among Kashmir breeds

Crossbreds of sheep

S.N.	Crossbred	Origin	Cross
1.	**Hissardale**	**Govt. Livestock Farm, Hisar**	**Bikaneri ewe (Magra) × Australian Merino ram**
2.	Avikalin	CSWRI, Avikanagar	Rambouillet ram × Malpura ewe
3.	Avivastra	CSWRI, Avikanagar	Rambouillet ram × Chokla ewe
4.	Avimans	CSWRI, Avikanagar	Malpura & Sonadi × Dorset & Suffolk
5.	Bharat Merino	CSWRI, Avikanagar	Chokla & Nali × Merino & Rambouillet
6.	Kashmir Merino	--	Gaddi, Bhakarwal & Poonchi × Merino & Rambouillet
7.	Indian Karakul	Bikaner	Marwari, Malpura & Sonadi × Karakul
8.	Nilgiri Synthetic	Tamilnadu	Nilgiri × Merino & Rambouillet
9.	Patanwadi Synthetic	GAU, Dantiwada	Patanwadi × Merino & Rambouillet

Classification of Exotic sheep breeds based on productivity

Fine wool breeds	Mutton breeds	Dual purpose	Fur breeds	Long coarse wool breeds
Merino Rambouillet Polworth	Suffolk Southdown Dorset	Corriedale	Karakul	Lincoln Leicester

Description of exotic sheep breeds

S.N.	Breed	Origin	Characters
1.	**Merino**	Spain	**Best fine wool breed in the world, Ewes polled & rams have spiral horns**
2.	**Rambouillet**	**Rambouillet (France)**	Developed from Spanish Merino
3.	Lincoln	England	**Largest & heaviest breed in the world**
4.	Leicester	England	Purest English breed
5.	Southdown	England	**Mousey grey face, Oldest English breed**
6.	Karakul	Bukhara province of Uzbekistan (Central Asia)	**Best Pelt (good quality fur) producing breed in the world**
7.	Suffolk	England	**Best mutton breed**
8.	Dorset	England	--

Breeds of Goat

Total goat population in the country is 148.88 Million during the year 2019. The goat population has increased by 10.14% over previous Livestock Census (2012). Total registered breeds of Indian goat are 39 and out of them, 6 goat breeds have been recognized in Gujarat. It includes Gohilwadi, Kutchi, Kahmi, Mahesana, Surti and Zalawadi. Indigenous breeds of goat are classified in four groups based upon geographical region which is mentioned in below table:

Classification of goat breeds based on Geographical region

North temperate Region breed	North western arid & semi-arid region breed	Southern region breed	Eastern region breed
Chegu Changthangi Gaddi Bhakarwali	Jamunapari Barbari Jhakrana Beetal Sirohi Kutchi Marwari Mehasana Gohilwadi Zalawadi Surti Kahmi Rohilkhandi	Malabari Osmanabadi Sangamneri Kanni-Adu Attapady Black Berari Bidri Kodi Adu Kankan Kalyan Nandidurga Salem black	Black-Bengal Ganjam Asam hill

Classification of goat breeds on the basis of their body size

Classification of goat breeds on the basis of utility

Milk	Meat		Fibre
Beetal Jamunapari Jakharana Surti	Barbari Bengal Gaddi Ganjam Gohilwadi Kannai Adu Kutchi	Malabari Marwadi Mehsana Osmanabadi Snagamneri Sirohi Zalawadi	Chegu Chsngthangi

Description and peculiar characters of some Indian goat breeds

S.N.	Breed	Home tract	Characters
1.	Jamunapari	Etawah, Agra (UP)	**Biggest & most majestic breed of Indian goat,** **"Roman nose" (parrot mouth appearance)** **Most beautiful Indian goat,** **Creamy white body colour with shining hair,** Thick growth of hairs on buttocks known as **"Feathers"**

2.	Barbari **(City breed)**	Etawah, Agra (UP), Bharatpur (Rajasthan)	**Origin: Barbera city (East Africa)** **Dwarf breed highly suitable for stall feeding &** generally found in cities so it is also known as **"city breed"** **Indian goat with maximum milk fat (5%)**
3.	Beetal	Punjab, Haryana	**Buck possesses marked beard but females are beardless, roman nose**
4.	Jhakrana	Alwar (Rajasthan)	Skin popular for **tanning purpose**
5.	Kutchi	Kutch (Gujarat)	**Corkscrew shaped horns**
6.	Black-Bengal	Nadia (WB)	**Best chevon breed of India,** **Highly prolific goat breed of India**
7.	Chegu	Lahul & Spiti Valleys (HP)	Pashmina producing breed
8.	Changthangi (Pashmin a)	Changthang (Ladakh)	Pashmina producing breed, Pashmina used for making high- quality **Kashmiri "Rug or Shawl"**
9.	Malabari	Malabar (Kerala)	-
10.	Osmanabadi	Osmanabad (Maharashtra)	The breed is known for **early maturity, prolificacy and good dressing percentage**
11.	Ganjam	Odisha	**"Big size horns"** are a characteristic feature of Ganjam goats.
12.	Kahmi	Gujarat	Excellent migratory capacity

Description of exotic goat breeds

S.N.	Breed	Origin	Characters
1.	Sannen	Switzerland	Also known as **"Milk queen"**
2.	Alpine	Africa	Milch purpose breed
3.	Angora	Turkey	**"Mohair"** (white soft silky hairs) producing breed of goat, Also known as **"sheep like goat"**
4.	Anglo-Nubian	England	**Roman nose,** also known as **"Jersey of goat"** **Most outstanding dual- purpose goat breed** widely used for the upgrading of desi stock
5.	Toggenburg	Switzerland	**Horn absent,** maximum adaptability in exotic breeds
6.	Boer	Southern Africa	**Meat type breed used for cross-breeding for meat**
7.	Orenberg	Kazakhstan	-

Questions

1. Scientific name of domestic goat is

   a) *Ovis aries*   b) *Capra hircus*

   c) *Bos indicus*   d) *Bubalus bubalis*

2. Scientific name of domestic sheep is
   a) *Ovis aries*
   b) *Capra hircus*
   c) *Bos indicus*
   d) *Bubalus bubalis*
3. Which of the following is not a member of suborder Artiodactylia (Even toed/ cloven footed animals)
   a) Cattle
   b) Buffalo
   c) Sheep
   d) Horse
4. Sheep and goat belong to which order?
   a) Cetacea
   b) Rodentia
   c) Ungulata
   d) Logomorpha
5. Sheep and goat belong to which family?
   a) Cervidae
   b) Bovidae
   c) Suidae
   d) Phocidae
6. As per 20th Livestock Census (2019), sheep population in India is
   a) 65.07 Million
   b) 74.26 Million
   c) 109.85 Million
   d) 148.88 Million
7. As per 20th Livestock Census (2019), goat population in India is
   a) 65.07 Million
   b) 74.26 Million
   c) 135.17 Million
   d) 148.88 Million
8. What is percentage change in sheep population of India in 20th Livestock Census (2019) over 19th Livestock Census (2012)?
   a) 14.13 increase
   b) 16.13 increase
   c) 18.13 increase
   d) 20.13 increase
9. What is percentage change in goat population of India in 20th Livestock Census (2019) over 19th Livestock Census (2012)?
   a) 10.14 increase
   b) 12.14 increase
   c) 14.14 increase
   d) 16.14 increase
10. As per 20th Livestock Census, which of the following state ranks first in sheep population?
    a) Rajasthan
    b) Telangana
    c) Tamil Nadu
    d) Karnataka
11. What is contribution of sheep in total livestock population of India in 20th Livestock Census?
    a) 13.8 %
    b) 12.8 %
    c) 17.7 %
    d) 21.7 %
12. As per 20th Livestock Census, which of the following state ranks first in goat population?
    a) Uttar Pradesh
    b) West Bengal
    c) Bihar
    d) Rajasthan

13. What is contribution of goat in total livestock population of India in 20th Livestock Census?
    a) 14.1 % b) 20.1 %
    c) 27.7 % d) 33.7 %
14. As per 20th Livestock Census, which of the following state ranks first in sheep and goat population?
    a) Uttar Pradesh b) Rajasthan
    c) West Bengal d) Bihar
15. What is contribution of sheep and goat in total livestock population of India?
    a) 31.4 % b) 37.5 %
    c) 41.5 % d) 43.7 %
16. Which of the following animal was first domesticated by the ancient human?
    a) Cattle b) Sheep
    c) Horse d) Goat
17. During which period the goat was domesticated?
    a) 14000-12000 B.C. b) 12000-10000 B.C.
    c) 9000-7000 B.C. d) 4000-6000 B.C.
18. What is "Bezoar"?
    a) It is a wild goat breed of hill mountain of Iran and Asia Minor
    b) It is a wild goat of Sindh
    c) It is a wild sheep from Arab
    d) It is a wild sheep from Agfganistan
19. Two seals from Mohenjo- daro show a wild animal with enormous curled side spreading horns. The wild animal is identified as
    a) Buffalo b) Goat
    c) Sheep d) Deer
20. It is assumed that the Markhor and Bezoar gave rise to majority of Indian and Central Asian breeds of ___________.
    a) Buffalo b) Sheep
    c) Goat d) Deer
21. As per 20th Livestock Census, what is the rank of India in goat population in the world?
    a) First b) Second
    c) Third d) Fourth
22. Which of the following animal is termed as "Poor man's cow?
    a) Buffalo b) Sheep
    c) Brahma d) Goat
23. The "Poor man's cow" term was given by which great leader?
    a) Jawahar Lal Nehru b) Lala Lajpat Rai
    c) Bal Gangadhar Tilak d) Mohandas K. Gandhi

24. Which of the following animal is termed as "Wet nurse of infant" in Europe?
   a) Buffalo b) Cattle
   c) Goat d) Sheep

25. Present day breeds of which domestic animal have been originated from two remote species namely Musimon and Vignes?
   a) Buffalo b) Sheep
   c) Goat d) Deer

26. Sheep is known as "golden hoofed animal" because of its:
   a) Wool b) Hoof
   c) Waste and manure d) Grazing habit

27. Sheep is known as "Poor man's mobile bank" because it produces
   a) Wool and skin b) Meat
   c) Waste and manure d) All the above

28. What was the total meat production of India during the year 2021-22?
   a) 6.69 million tonnes b) 7.43 million tonnes
   c) 8.13 million tonnes d) 9.29 million tonnes

29. What was the total wool production of India during the year 2021-22?
   a) 33.04 million Kg b) 38.14 million Kg
   c) 46.05 million Kg d) 48.14 million Kg

30. What was the contribution of goat in total milk production of India during the year 2021-22?
   a) 1.23 % b) 2.24 %
   c) 2.93 % d) 3.37 %

31. What is diploid chromosome number in the sheep?
   a) 44 b) 48
   c) 52 d) 54

32. What is diploid chromosome number in the goat?
   a) 44 b) 52
   c) 54 d) 60

33. While comparing doe and cow, generally 1 cow is equivalent to how many does?
   a) 4 doe b) 5 doe
   c) 6 doe d) 8 doe

34. A sheep breed having Roman nose, medium size compact body, also known as "Indian Merino"
   a) Nali b) Deccani
   c) Marwari d) Chokla

35. Which of the following is the tallest breed of sheep in India and also considered as best mutton breed of India?
   a) Mecheri b) Nellore
   c) Marwari d) Chokla

36. Which of the following is also known as goat like sheep (no wool)?
   a) Mecheri b) Nellore
   c) Marwari d) Chokla
37. Which of the following is the smallest sheep breed of India?
   a) Mandya b) Malpura
   c) Patanwadi d) Marwari
38. Which of the following is the most prolific sheep breed of India
   a) Garole b) Mandya
   c) Malpura d) Patanwadi
39. Which of the following is the heaviest sheep breed found in Kashmir?
   a) Bhakharwal b) Gaddi
   c) Gurej d) Poonchi
40. Which of the following breeds have been used to develop cross bred Hissardale at Govt. Livestock Farm, Hisar
   a) Bikaneri ewe (Magra)× Australian Merino ram
   b) Rambouillet ram × Malpura ewe
   c) Rambouillet ram × Chokla ewe
   d) Patanwadi × Merino & Rambouillet
41. Which of the following breed(s) have been used to develop cross bred Avikalin at ICAR-CSWRI, Avikanagar
   a) Bikaneri ewe (Magra)× Australian Merino ram
   b) Rambouillet ram × Malpura ewe
   c) Malpura & Sonadi × Dorset & Suffolk
   d) Patanwadi × Merino & Rambouillet
42. Which of the following breeds have been used to develop cross bred Avivastra at ICAR-CSWRI, Avikanagar
   sa) Bikaneri ewe (Magra)× Australian Merino ram
   b) Rambouillet ram × Malpura ewe
   c) Rambouillet ram × Chokla ewe
   d) Patanwadi × Merino & Rambouillet
43. Which of the following breeds have been used to develop cross bred Avimans at ICAR-CSWRI, Avikanagar
   a) Malpura & Sonadi × Dorset & Suffolk
   b) Rambouillet ram × Malpura ewe
   c) Rambouillet ram × Chokla ewe
   d) Patanwadi × Merino & Rambouillet
44. Which of the following breeds have been used to develop cross bred Bharat Merino at ICAR-CSWRI, Avikanagar
   a) Malpura & Sonadi × Dorset & Suffolk
   b) Rambouillet ram × Malpura ewe
   c) Chokla & Nali × Merino & Rambouillet
   d) Patanwadi × Merino & Rambouillet

45. Which of the following breeds have been used to develop cross bred Nilgiri synthetic by TANUVAS Tamil Nadu
   a) Bikaneri ewe (Magra)× Australian Merino ram
   b) Rambouillet ram × Nilgiri ewe
   c) Nilgiri × Merino & Rambouillet
   d) Nilgiri × Merino

46. Kathiawari sheep breed which is famous for 'Joria wool' is native of
   a) Kutch, Gujarat b) Marwar, Rajasthan
   c) Coastal Maharashtra d) Himalayan region

47. Which of the following is the best carpet and heaviest wool producing breed in India?
   a) Chokla b) Magra
   c) Jaisalmeri d) Pugal

48. Nali is a breed of _____________region.
   a) Northern temperate region
   b) North-western, central arid and semi-arid region
   c) Southern region semi-arid, central peninsular, hot & humid along coast
   d) Eastern region

49. Corriedale is a breed of which category?
   a) Fine wool breeds b) Mutton breeds
   c) Pelt breeds d) Dual purpose

50. Which of the following breed is also known as 'Guinea goat"
   a) Beetal b) Malbari
   c) Barbari d) Jamunapari

51. According to the classification of goat breeds based on agro-ecological regions in India which breed belong to Eastern region.
   a) Ganjam b) Beetal
   c) Changthangi d) Kannaiadu

52. Breed of goat famous for common ring shawl from 'Pashmina' is
   a) Ganjam b) Beetal
   c) Changthangi d) Barbari

53. Breed of goat having excellent meat and skin quality with multiple birth is
   a) Ganjam b) Beetal
   c) Jamunapari d) Black Bengal

54. Which of the following breed is the biggest and most majestic breed of goat with roman nose and feathers?
   a) Beetal b) Malbari
   c) Barbari d) Jamunapari

55. Which of the following goat breed is globally famous as "Milk Queen"?
   a) Saanen b) Alpine
   c) Anglo-Nubian d) Toggenburg

56. Which of the following goat breed is globally famous as "Jersey cow"?
    a) Saanen b) Alpine
    c) Anglo-Nubian d) Toggenburg
57. White breed of goat with compact body, milch purpose and native of Gujarat is
    a) Kutchi b) Mehsani
    c) Surti d) Kahmi
58. The tallest sheep breed of India is
    a) Nellore b) Magra
    c) Mandya d) Madras Red
59. The shortest sheep breed of India is
    a) Nellore b) Magra
    c) Mandya d) Madras Red
60. Which of the following sheep breed is globally famous for pelt production?
    a) Dorset b) Rambouillet
    c) Suffolk d) Karakul
61. What is the total number of sheep breeds registered in NABAGR at the end of year 2023?
    a) 35 b) 40
    c) 45 d) 48
62. What is the total number of goat breeds registered in NABAGR at the end of year 2023?
    a) 35 b) 39
    c) 42 d) 45
63. Macherla sheep breed which is registered recently at NBAGR, is native of?
    a) Tamil Nadu b) Andhra Pradesh and Telangana
    c) Maharashtra d) Odhisha
64. Recently identified Anjori goat breed is native of
    a) Chhatisgadh b) Tamil Nadu
    c) Andhra Pradesh and Telangana d) Maharashtra
65. What is the name of sheep breed of temperate and Himalayan region of India, which has been named after the nomadic tribe which rear them?
    a) Muzaffarnagari b) Nali
    c) Patanwadi d) Bhakarwal
66. Which of the following pair correctly represent the best mutton breeds of India and the world respectively
    a) Rambouillet and Nellore b) Corrridale and Mandya
    c) Southdown and Nellore d) Southdown and Mandya
67. Which of the following sheep breed can thrive on salty water?
    a) Nellore b) Mandya
    c) Garole d) Chokla

68. Which of the following goat breed looks like sheep?
 a) Kutchi b) Gohilwadi
 c) Beetal d) Angora

69. Which of the following sheep breed looks like goat?
 a) Nellore b) Mandya
 c) Garole d) Chokla

70. The Anglo Nubian breed is cross of Nubian (Egypt) and __________, which is also known as Jersey cow of goat worl d)
 a) Sirohi b) Beetal
 c) Jamunapari d) Surti

71. Which of the following is the most beautiful Indian goat and also known as the best dairy goat of South East Asia?
 a) Sirohi b) Beetal
 c) Jamunapari d) Zalawadi

72. Which of the following is the tallest goat breed of the country?
 a) Sirohi b) Beetal
 c) Jamunapari d) Zalawadi

73. Sumi-Ne a native of Nagaland is breed of which species?
 a) Goat b) Sheep
 c) Pig d) Chicken

74. Identify the meat type goat breed frequently used for cross-breeding and is native of Southern Africa.
 a) Toggenberg b) Saanen
 c) Boer d) Orenberg

75. Origin of Saanen breed is:
 a) Switerzer land b) Turkey
 c) USa) d) Scotland

76. Although a number of management systems are in practices for sheep and goat rearing varying from region to region these can be conveniently divided in to
 a) Two groups. b) Three groups
 c) Four groups d) Five groups

77. Which of the following system includes migratory, transhumance, free range, pasture and range grazing management of goats and sheep?
 a) Extensive, b) Semi-intensive
 c) Intensive systems d) None of the above

78. Which of the following system is characterized by low input – low return system?
 a) Extensive, b) Semi-intensive
 c) Intensive systems d) Integrated system

79. Which of the following is not an important features of extensive system of rearing goats and sheep-
    a) The system allows use of land unsuitable for agriculture crop production
    b) Involves minimum utilization of family labour
    c) Low input – low return system
    d) Minimum safety from predators and inclement weather
80. Which of the following is not an important economic features of extensive system of rearing goats and sheep-
    a) The adult body weight are lower
    b) The reproduction rates are lower
    c) The mortality rates are lower
    d) The milk production are lower
81. Which of the following is not an important features of Semi – intensive system of rearing
    a) Limited use of agriculture and industrial by products
    b) Relatively higher requirement of labour and capital than intensive system
    c) Risk for protection from predators and inclement weather is reduced
    d) Possibility of optimum production through adequate supplementation of diet
82. The extensive system is described as ____________ because the family labour is the main input.
    a) Integrated Farming system
    b) Mixed farming system
    c) Zero gazing system
    d) Zero input system
83. Which of the following system is also known as zero grazing systems?
    a) Extensive
    b) Semi-intensive
    c) Intensive systems
    d) None of the above
84. Which of the following system is characterized by high input – high output system?
    a) Extensive
    b) Semi-intensive
    c) Intensive systems
    d) Integrated system
85. Which of the following is not an important features of Intensive system of sheep and goat rearing?
    a) Maximum use of agriculture and industrial by products.
    b) Relatively low return per unit of land)
    c) Complete protection of animals from predators and inclement weather.
    d) Possibility of maximum production through adequate management.
86. When the sheep and goats are housed intensively, which system of housing is suitable?
    a) Only run space should be provided
    b) Only pen or covered space should be provided.
    c) Only paddock should be provided
    d) Both Run space and covered space should be provided

87. When the sheep and goats are taken for grazing during the day time, which system of house is suitable?
   a) Only run space should be provided
   b) Only pen or covered space should be provided.
   c) Only paddock should be provided
   d) Both Run space and covered space should be provided
88. Optimum breadth of shed for small ruminants should be ___ and it should not exceed ___.
   a) 8 meter and 12 meter   b) 10 meter and 14 meter
   c) 12 meter and 16 meter   d) 16 meter and 20 meter
89. The height of chain link used for open space should be 4 feet
   a) 4 Feet   b) 4 Meter
   c) 6 Feet   d) 6 Meter
90. What should be the height of eave and height at ridge in the small ruminants' house?
   a) Height of eave 1.5 meter and height at ridge should be 2.5 meter
   b) Height of eave 2.5 meter and height at ridge should be 3.5 meter
   c) Height of eave 3.0 meter and height at ridge should be 4.0 meter
   d) Height of eave 3.5 meter and height at ridge should be 4.5 meter
91. What is the minimum floor space requirement for the adult sheep and goat?
   a) Covered space 1.0 square meter and Open space 2.0 square meterr
   b) Covered space 2.0 square meter and Open space 4.0 square mete
   c) Covered space 2.5 square meter and Open space 5.0 square meter
   d) Covered space 3.0 square meter and Open space 6.0 square meter
92. What is the minimum floor space requirement for the Breeding bucks and rams?
   a) Covered space 1.0 square meter and Open space 2.0 square meter
   b) Covered space 1.5-2.0 square meter and Open space 3.0-4.0 square meter
   c) Covered space 2.5-3.0 square meter and Open space 5.0-6.0 square meter
   d) Covered space 3.0 square meter and Open space 6.0 square meter
93. What is feeding and watering space requirements of sheep and goats under Indian conditions?
   a) 10-15 cm per animal   b) 20-25 cm per animal
   c) 30-35 cm per animal   d) 40-50 cm per animal
94. The flock shed used for housing ewes or does kept for breeding purpose should be 15m (l) x 4m (w) x 3 m (h) and it should not accommodate more than
   a) More than 30 animals in a shed,
   b) More than 40 animals in a shed
   c) More than 60 animals in a shed
   d) More than 80 animals in a shed

95. Rams or bucks kept for breeding purpose should be housed
   a) Individually
   b) In groups with other Rams or bucks
   c) In groups with other does or ewes
   d) In groups with other lambs or kids

96. In areas where the rainfall is quite heavy; which type of flooring is preferred
   a) Moorum flooring. b) Kutcha flooring
   c) Wooden /slatted flooring d) Concrete flooring

97. Which type of the housing system is preferred in temperate regions to protect the animals from severe cold?
   a) Houses without covered space
   b) Houses with provision of covered and open space
   c) Slatted floor houses
   d) Underground houses

98. The slatted floor is prepared
   a) 1.0 meter below the ground level b) 1.0 meter above the ground level
   c) 2.0 meter below the ground level d) 2.0 meter above the ground level

99. Which of the following is not an important features of slatted floor housed
   a) These are suitable for the regions where humidity and rainfall period is of long duration.
   b) Wooden stripes of 2.5 cm thickness and 5.0 cm breadth are placed parallel to each other to prepare a slate.
   c) A gap of 2.5 cm between two stripes is kept.
   d) The slatted floor is prepared 1.0 meter above the ground level.

100. For a comfortable house for sheep and goat the orientation of the house should be -
   a) East-west direction
   b) North south direction
   c) In the circular shape with paddock all sides
   d) In any direction as per belief of the farmer.

101. What is dry matter requirement of milch type goat?
   a) 1.5-2.5 % of body weight b) 2.5-3.0 % of body weight
   c) 5.0-7.0 % of body weight d) 10.0-12.0 % of body weight

102. Identify the incorrect statement from the following
   a) Goats have higher basal metabolic rate than cattle.
   b) Maintenance requirements of goats are higher than those of cattle
   c) For its size the goat can consume substantially more feed than sheep
   d) Maintenance requirements of meat type goats are higher than those of dairy type goats.

103. Feeding pattern in goat is
   a) Grazing less selective b) Grazing more selective
   c) Browsing less selective d) Browsing more selective

104. Feeding pattern in sheep is

a) Grazing less selective
b) Grazing more selective
c) Browsing less selective
d) Browsing more selective

105. Feeding extra concentrate over maintenance ration 3-4 weeks prior to the breeding season is called as

a) Flushing
b) Steaming up
c) Challenge feeding
d) Ringing

106. Feeding extra concentrate over maintenance ration prior to the parturition is called as

a) Flushing
b) Steaming up
c) Challenge feeding
d) Ringing

107. An allowance of 300g concentrate mixture having 12-15 5 DCP and 65-70 % TDN per head /day during last ___________ of pregnancy over and above good grazing is recommended for steaming up.

a) 4 weeks
b) 6 weeks
c) 8 weeks
d) 10 weeks

108. What is the weaning age in the sheep and goats?

a) One month
b) Two month
c) Three month
d) Four months

109. What is the weaning weight in the sheep and goats?

a) 8 kg
b) 10 kg
c) 12 kg
d) 18 kg

110. Which of the following statement is incorrect regarding weaning?

a) Sheep and goats are weaned at 12 kg body weight
b) Sheep and goats should be weaned around six months of age
c) While weaning weight of kid/lamb is more important than age
d) The weaning should be abrupt

111. Headquarter of ICAR-Central Sheep and Wool Research Institute (ICAR-CSWRI) is located at

a) Avikanagar, Rajasthan
b) Karnal, Haryana
c) Makhdoom, U.P.
d) Hissar, HJaryana

112. Which year the Central Sheep and Wool Research Institute (ICAR-CSWRI) was established?

a) 1952
b) 1962
c) 1972
d) 1973

113. Headquarter of ICAR-Central Institute for Research on Goat (ICAR-CIRG) is located at

a) Avikanagar, Rajasthan
b) Karnal, Haryana
c) Makhdoom, U.P.
d) Hissar, HJaryana

114. Which year the ICAR-Central Institute for Research on Goat (ICAR-CIRG) was established?

a) 1959 b) 1969

c) 1979 d) 1989

115. In which year the All India Co-ordinated Research Project on Goats (AICRPG) was launched at five centres by the Indian Council of Agricultural Research (ICAR)?

a) 1971 b) 1975

c) 1979 d) 1981

116. An old broken mouthed ewe which has been retained in a breeding flock because of her excellent breeding performance is known as.

a) Hog b) Gimmer

c) Seggy d) Crone

117. What is broken mouth in sheep and goats?

a) All the teeth are broken

b) One or more incisors are missing/ worn out

c) Upper jaw is broken

d) Lower jaw is broken

118. What is (are) the advantages of Flushing in the sheep and goats?

a) More eggs (ova)are shed, and this results in more offspring

b) The females come in heat more promptly

c) Conception is more certain.

d) All the above

119. Act of mating in sheep is called as

a) Serving b) Foaling

c) Tupping d) Ringing

120. Act of mating in goat is called as

a) Serving b) Foaling

c) Tupping d) Ringing

121. Terminology for act of parturition in sheep and goat

a) It is lambing in goat and kidding in sheep

b) It is tupping in sheep and serving in goats

c) It is serving in sheep and tupping in goats

d) It is lambing in sheep and kidding in goats

122. What is sound produced by the goat?

a) Bellowing b) Bleating

c) Croaks d) Howls

123. What is temporary dental formula for sheep and goat?

a) 2 (I 0/4, C 0/0, PM 3/3, M 0/0) b) 2 (I 1/3, C 0/0, PM 3/3, M 0/0)

c) 2 (I 0/4, C 1/1, PM 2/2, M 0/0) d) 2 (I 0/4, C 0/0, PM 3/3, M 3/3)

124. What is permanent dental formula for sheep and goat?
a) 2 (I 0/4, C 2/2, PM 2/2, M 2/2)
b) 2 (I 1/4, C 1/1, PM 3/3, M 3/3)
c) 2 (I 0/4, C 0/0, PM 3/3, M 3/3)
d) 2 (I 0/4, C 1/1, PM 3/3, M 2/2)

125. At what age the first (Central) pair of incisor erupts in sheep and goats?
a) 12-15 months
b) 21-24 months
c) 27-30 months
d) 33-36 months

126. At what age the second (Medial) pair of incisors erupts in sheep and goats?
a) 12-15 months
b) 21-24 months
c) 27-30 months
d) 33-36 months

127. At what age the third (Lateral) pair of incisor erupts in sheep and goats?
a) 12-15 months
b) 21-24 months
c) 27-30 months
d) 33-36 months

128. At what age the fourth (Corner) pair of incisor erupts in sheep and goats?
a) 12-15 months
b) 21-24 months
c) 27-30 months
d) 33-36 months

129. What is the age of full mouth in sheep and goats?
a) 1 year
b) 2 years
c) 3 years
d) 4 years

130. What is full mouth?
a) Animal possess 2 pair of incisors and 2 pairs of Molars
b) Animal possess 3 pair of incisors, 3 pairs of Pre-molars and Molars
c) Animal possess 4 pair of incisors, 3 pairs of Pre-molars and Molars
d) Animal possess 4 pair of incisors, 4 pairs of Pre-molars and Molars

131. Which of the following method of identification is usually not used in sheep and goats?
a) Ear tagging
b) Ear notching
c) Colour marking
d) Hot Branding

132. What is the purpose of dipping in sheep?
a) To control internal parasites
b) To control external parasites
c) To control Protozoan diseases
d) To make the shearing easier

133. Identify the incorrect statement
a) Dipping should be done in late evening
b) Dipping should be done in early morning
c) Dipping frequency depends on the season
d) Dipping should be preferably performed when it rains

134. What precaution one should take during the dipping of sheep?
a) Dip the animals only in early evening
b) Provide sufficient drinking water before dipping.
c) Prolong drying is preferred
d) Dipping should be performed when it rains

135. Which one of the following is not an objective of castration in sheep and goat?
   a) Castrated animals are more docile and easy to handl
   b) A small number of male animals are required for breeding
   c) Castration avoids indiscriminate breeding
   d) Castrated animal produce inferior quality of meat

136. Optimum age for castration in goat and sheep is
   a) 1 month b) 3 month
   c) 6 months d) 12 months

137. Castration by Burdizzo's method is
   a) Open method b) Closed and bloodless method
   c) Surgical method d) Rubber elastrator method

138. What is a Teaser animal?
   a) Castrated male sheep or goat
   b) A vasectomized sheep or goat
   c) Used for selective breeding programmes
   d) They are produced by burdizzo's castrators.

139. What is a docking?
   a) It is removal of testis
   b) It is rendering gonads non-functional
   c) It is cutting of tail
   d) It is removal of wool around eye and head region

140. Optimum age for docking in sheep is
   a) 7- 11 days b) 28-30 days
   c) 6 weeks d) 12 Weeks

141. What is minimum floor space required by the sheep and goats during transportation?
   a) 0.1 to 0.2 square meter/ animal b) 0.3 to 0.4 square meter/ animal
   c) 0.5 to 0.6 square meter/ animal d) 1.0 to 1.2 square meter/ animal

142. In case of transportation of small ruminants necessary vaccination shall be done:
   a) 07 days in advance b) 14 days in advance
   c) 21 days in advance d) Before 1 month

143. What is maximum speed of the truck while transportation of sheep and goats to avoid jerks and jolts?
   a) Not exceeding 40 km per hour b) Not exceeding 50 km per hour
   c) Not exceeding 60 km per hour d) Not exceeding 70 km per hour

144. Flushing increases the lambing rate by
   a) 5 to 10 per cent b) 10 to 20 per cent
   c) 15 to 20 per cent d) No effect on lambing

145. The natural space in between incisor and first premolar is known as
   a) Diastema b) Dental pad
   c) Felt d) Medulla

146. Ewe or doe in groups require minimum floors space ____ sq. meter / animal.
   a) 1.0 sq. meter / animal
   b) 1.5 sq. meter / animal
   c) 2.0 sq. meter / animal
   d) 3.0 sq. meter / animal.

147. Ewe or doe ewe with lamb require minimum floors space _______ sq. meter / animal.
   a) 1.0 sq. meter / animal
   b) 1.5 sq. meter / animal
   c) 2.0 sq. meter / animal
   d) 3.0 sq. meter / animal.

148. Lacrimal pouches are found in which of the following animals?
   a) Sheep
   b) Horses
   c) Pigs
   d) Camels

149. Wool is the thick, wavy and fibrous protective covering of the sheep, which is mainly consists of insoluble protein called ________.
   a) Globulin
   b) Albumin
   c) Chitin
   d) Keratin

150. Wool protein keratin is mainly synthesized from which sulphur containing amino acid?
   a) Arginine
   b) Glutamine
   c) Glycine
   d) Cysteine

151. What is optimum weaning age of goat?
   a) 2 Months
   b) 3 Months
   c) 4 Months
   d) 6 Months

152. The nutritional requirements of a goat weighing 50 kg and yielding 2 litres of milk with 4 per cent fat may be met by feeding of
   a) 200 g of concentrate mixture and 2 kg of berseem or lucerne
   b) 300 g of concentrate mixture and 3 kg of berseem or lucerne
   c) 400 g of concentrate mixture and 5 kg of berseem or lucerne
   d) 500 g of concentrate mixture and 6 kg of berseem or lucerne

153. In goats milk feeding is continued upto the _______ kg of body weight obtained by the kids
   a) 5 kg
   b) 10 kg
   c) 15 kg
   d) 25 kg

154. Upto what extent salt of may be mixed with the daily grain ration of goats?
   a) 1%
   b) 2 %
   c) 5 %
   d) 7.5 %

155. Wool is made up of a protein known as ________________.
   a) Albumin
   b) Keratin
   c) Lanolin
   d) Chitin

156. Average estrous cycle of goat is
   a) 14 days
   b) 19 days
   c) 22 days
   d) 28 days

157. A castrated male sheep called as

a) Ram b) Sire

c) Wedder d) Runt

158. What is meaning of *Bomb Lamb*?

a) Owning of lamb for suckling b) Disowned lamb

c) Stealing of lamb d) Selling of lambs

159. Steely wool is caused by deficiency of which mineral in the diet?

a) Iron b) Selenium

c) Copper d) Manganese

160. Feeding behavior of sheep is

a) Browsing b) Soiling

c) Grazing d) Plucking

161. The breed of goat having high ovulation and kidding percent is

a) Barbari b) Jamnapari

c) Garole d) Black Bengal

162. The prehensile organ of goat is

a) Lower lip b) Tongue

c) Teeth d) Muzzle

163. Wool is described as ________ protein and is classified as an insoluble.

a) 100 % b) 60%

c) 80 % d) 25%

164. In very dense fleeced fine wool sheep, there may be more than ______fibers per square inch of skin area:

a) 50,000 b) 20000

c) 30000 d) 10000

165. Sonadi is a breed of _____________region.

a) Northern temperate region

b) North-western, central arid and semi-arid region

c) Southern region semi-arid, central peninsular, hot & humid along coast

d) Eastern region

166. Which of the following is considered as most disease resistant breed of sheep in India?

a) Patanwadi b) Garole

c) Gurez d) Marwari

167. Wool is an excellent insulator and:

a) It protect sheep against heat in summer

b) It protect sheep against cold in winter

c) Both a and b

d) None of the above

168. The loss of weight of wool after removal of yolk, dirt, water, vegetable, animal and mineral matter when the wool is scoured is known as

a) Shrinkage
b) Sorting
c) Cleanliness
d) Scouring

169. Which of the following chemical is used in the chemical shearing of sheep?

a) Glutaraldehyde @ 12 mg per kg wt
b) Hexachlorophene @ 20 mg per kg wt
c) Quaternary ammonium @ 50 mg per kg wt
d) Cyclophosphamide @ 24 mg per kg wt

170. Sudden introduction of ram in the ewes flock after prolonged separation bring more number of ewes into oestrous which is known as

a) Doe effect
b) Buck Effect
c) Ram Effect
d) Ewe Effect

171. Feeding schedule for kids should be such that a weekly growth rate of ____is obtained.

a) 0.4 kg
b) 0.6 kg
c) 0.8 kg
d) 1.0 kg

172. How much wool can absorb moisture

a) About 5% of its weight
b) About 25% of its weight
c) About 35% of its weight
d) About 50% of its weight

173. Spinning system for grading of wool has been originated in which country

a) U.K.
b) U.S.A
c) Australia
d) Newzealand

174. What is diamond ram?

a) Castrated after first service
b) Vasectomized ram
c) Uncastrated Ram
d) Castrated lamb at early age

175. The process of removal of wool fibre from sheep skin through use of chemical application(Sodium sulphide) or administration (10-14 mg of thallium) for artificial moult in sheep is known as

a) Fellomongering
b) Felting
c) Carbonization
d) Skirting

176. Which of the following breed is dwarf breed, highly suitable for stall feeding and generally found in cities so it is also known as 'City breed' of goat?

a) Surti
b) Barbari
c) Jamunapari
d) Beetal

177. What is dressing percentage in sheep?

a) 35-40 %
b) 48-52 %
c) 60-64 %
d) 70-75 %

178. For rotational grazing pasture should be divided into compartments and it should be managed to support ________ ewes and their lambs, per acre.
a) 5 to 6 b) 15 to 20
c) 10 to 12 d) 20 to 25

179. Which of the following is famous as the largest and the heaviest sheep breed of the world?
a) Lincoln b) Suffolk
c) Karakul d) South down

180. Which of the following is famous as best mutton breed of the world?
a) Suffolk b) Karakul
c) Lincoln d) South down

181. What is optimum breeding age in sheep and goat?
a) 6-7 months b) 10-12 months
c) 18-20 months d) 24-30 months

182. What is optimum breeding weight in sheep and goat?
a) 10-12 kg b) 16-18 kg
c) 20-22 kg d) 30-32 kg

183. What is length of gestation period in Sheep?
a) 95-98 days b) 127-132 days
c) 147-153 days d) 275-280 days

184. Ideally kidding or lambing interval should be
a) 5 – 6 months b) 7 – 8 months
c) 11-12 months d) 14-16 months

185. Which of the following is main breeding season for sheep and goats
a) September 15 to October 31 b) December 15 to January 31
c) March 15 to April 30 d) May 15 to June 30

186. Which of the following is minor breeding season for sheep and goats
a) September 15 to October 31 b) December 15 to January 31
c) March 15 to April 30 d) May 15 to June 30

187. To prevent wool blindness in some breeds, the excess wool around the eyes are clipped away regularly, the process is referred to as.
a) Tagging b) Eyeing
c) Ringing d) Crutching

188. Shearing the lock of wool and dirt from the dock is called as.
a) Tagging b) Eyeing
c) Ringing d) Crutching

189. The process which facilitate easy and proper mating for the ram, clipping of wool around the penis is referred as
a) Eyeing b) Tagging
c) Ringing d) Crutching

190. Removal of wool around the perennial region and base of the tail of an ewe is known as

a) Tagging
b) Eyeing
c) Ringing
d) Crutching

191. What is Raddling?

a) The process of allowing the ram to run along with a ram harness containing crayon, which is rubbed on the ewe's rump when mating takes place.
b) Clipping the lock of wool and dirt from the dock
c) The process which facilitate easy and proper mating for the ram, clipping of wool around the penis.
d) Removal of wool around the perennial region and base of the tail of an ewe.

192. As a guideline, ewes and does should be mated only when they reach

a) 50 per cent of the average adult body weight
b) 60 per cent of the average adult body weight
c) 70 per cent of the average adult body weight
d) 90 per cent of the average adult body weight

193. In which of the following mating system teaser ram or buck detects the ewes or does in heat, which are mated and separated out for breeding with desired ram or buck?

a) Hand mating
b) Flock mating
c) Pen mating
d) Oestrous synchronization

194. Which of the following is not an advantage of oestrous synchronization?

a) Oestrous cycle of the ewe is synchronized so that large numbers of them come in heat at one time.
b) This would help in reducing the cost of artificial insemination or natural breeding and subsequent care at lambing
c) It gives a uniform flock of lambs, which will facilitate their disposal and fetch more prices.
d) It is a very complex and costly process which cannot be employed in breeding by small farmers.

195. Which one of the following is not a type of natural mating systems in sheep and goat?

a) Hand mating
b) Flock mating
c) Pen mating
d) E.T.T.

196. Which one of the following is a type of Artificial mating system in sheep and goat?

a) Pen mating
b) A.I.
c) Hand mating
d) Monogamous mating system

197. What is optimum male female ratio in sheep and goat in tropical climatic region?

a) 1 : 10
b) 1 : 20
c) 1 : 30
d) 1 : 40

198. What is optimum male female ratio in sheep and goat in temperate climatic conditions?
   a) 1 : 10 b) 1 : 20
   c) 1 : 40 d) 1 : 50
199. The mating system practiced normally by the farmers, in which males are allowed to run along with the females throughout the day and night is termed as
   a) Hand mating b) Flock mating
   c) Pen mating d) Oestrous synchronization
200. The mating system in which the ewes / does are divided in to batches varying from 20-25 ewes/does and males are turned into the flock only during the night time and separated during day time is referred as
   a) Hand mating b) Flock mating
   c) Pen mating d) Oestrous synchronization
201. Identify periodic operation at sheep and goat farm
   a) Grazing b) Suckling to lambs by ewes
   c) Cleaning of shed d) Shearing
202. How many times shearing is done in India?
   a) One time in a year b) Two time in a year
   c) Three time in a year d) Not specific, depends on farmers wish
203. In a true wool fiber which of the following layer is absent in its structure?
   a) Cuticle b) Cortex
   c) Medulla d) Squamous cells
204. Wool fiber can be stretched upto____ of its original shape
   a) 50% b) 60%
   c) 70% d) 80%
205. Due to irregular surface of the wool fiber, which of the following property of wool is exploited
   a) Elasticity b) Softness
   c) Felting d) Non-conductivity of heat
206. Wool is the thick, wavy and fibrous protective covering of sheep which is mainly consist of
   a) Insoluble protein, keratin b) Soluble protein, keratin
   c) Insoluble protein, chitin d) Insoluble carbohydrate, keratin
207. Structure of wool consists of how many morphological components?
   a) 1 b) 2
   c) 3 d) 4
208. Identify corrects statement
   a) Wool has more diameter than hair
   b) In hair medulla is almost absent; whereas in wool it is present
   c) Cuticle of wool is irregular while in hair it is regular and smooth
   d) Wool has more elasticity than hair

209. Which country has first rank in wool production?
   a) China
   b) New Zealand
   c) Australia
   d) India

210. Wool clothing provides superior comfort in
   a) Hot weather only
   b) Cold weather only
   c) During rainy season
   d) Both hot and cold weather

211. The wools grown on which part of body considered as the best in the fleece
   a) Head
   b) Belly
   c) Shoulders
   d) Limbs

212. Identify incorrect physical property of wool
   a) Wool is fire resistant
   b) Wool is inelastic
   c) Wool is easy to sew
   d) Wool insulates against noise

213. Identify incorrect chemical property of wool
   a) Wool is easily and extremely vulnerable attacked by alkalis.
   b) Wool absorbs moisture (hygroscopic)
   c) Wool is only damaged by hot sulphuric acid and nitric acid)
   d) Bleaches that contain chlorine compounds will not damage wool

214. A bag, sack, square or oblong package into which fiber is compressed, is known as
   a) Bale
   b) Ball
   c) Bellies
   d) Bold

215. The removal of vegetable matter, such as burrs and seeds, from wool and wool fabrics by chemical treatment and the usual agent for converting the fault to carbon is sulphuric acid.
   a) Skirting
   b) Carbonization
   c) Carding
   d) Combing

216. What is fast colour in wool industry?
   a) A dye which acts very fast on wool fiber
   b) A dye which is stable to colour destroying agents
   c) A dye which is unstable to colour destroying agents
   d) None of the above

217. Which of the following product is obtained from wool grease, which is a secretion from the sebaceous glands of the sheep?
   a) Poplin
   b) Nep
   c) Tartan
   d) Lanolin

218. What is Scouring?
   a) A reduction in length or width of a material caused by certain treatments, especially washing
   b) Removing the stained, unusable, or undesirable portions of a fleece
   c) Separating a fleece or fiber into groups of comparable character and quality
   d) It is actual separation of dirt, grease, and foreign matter from grease wool this is usually done in a lukewarm, mildly alkaline solution.

219. Identify incorrect statement regarding Mohair
   a) Mohair is obtained from the Angora rabbit
   b) Mohair is obtained from the Angora goat
   c) Mohair is highly resilient and strong.
   d) Mohair's luster, not softness, determines its value

220. Pashmina is obtained from which of the following animal(s)
   a) Chegu and Changthangi breeds of Goat
   b) Chegu and Changthangi breeds of Sheep
   c) Merino breed of sheep
   d) Nilgiri breed of sheep

221. The total length of a wool fibre after removing the crimps or waviness by straightening it, is called as
   a) Staple length
   b) Fibre length
   c) Medullation length
   d) Cortical length

222. Process in yarn manufacture in which the fibres are brushed up, made more or less parallel, have considerable portions of foreign matter removed and are put into a manageable form is known as
   a) Carbonization
   b) Skirting
   c) Carding
   d) Felting

223. For the 70S and 90S wool fibers
   a) 70S is having more diameter than 90S
   b) 70S is having less diameter than 90S
   c) Diameter for both 70S and 90S is same
   d) Diameter cannot be ascertained from the spinning count.

224. Traditionally, the standard method of measuring wool fibers is by a micro projection technique in which short longitudinal sections of the fibers are projected onto a screen at.
   a) 100-fold magnification
   b) 500-fold magnification
   c) 1000-fold magnification
   d) 5000-fold magnification

225. Keratin is the wool protein which has high proportion of
   a) Cobalt containing amino acid Iodine containing amino acid
   b) Chlorine containing amino acid
   c) Sulphur containing amino acid
   d) Cobalt containing amino acid

Answer Key

1	b	2	a	3	d	4	c	5	b	6	b	7	d
8	a	9	a	10	b	11	a	12	d	13	c	14	b
15	c	16	d	17	c	18	a	19	b	20	c	21	a
22	d	23	d	24	c	25	b	26	c	27	d	28	d

29	a	30	c	31	d	32	d	33	b	34	d	35	b
36	b	37	a	38	a	39	c	40	a	41	b	42	c
43	a	44	c	45	c	46	a	47	b	48	b	49	d
50	c	51	a	52	c	53	d	54	d	55	a	56	c
57	c	58	a	59	c	60	d	61	c	62	b	63	b
64	a	65	a	66	c	67	c	68	d	69	a	70	c
71	c	72	c	73	a	74	c	75	a	76	b	77	a
78	a	79	b	80	c	81	b	82	d	83	c	84	c
85	b	86	d	87	b	88	a	89	a	90	b	91	a
92	b	93	d	94	c	95	a	96	c	97	d	98	b
99	c	100	a	101	c	102	d	103	d	104	a	105	a
106	b	107	b	108	c	109	c	110	b	111	a	112	b
113	c	114	c	115	a	116	d	117	b	118	d	119	c
120	a	121	d	122	d	123	a	124	c	125	a	126	b
127	c	128	d	129	c	130	c	131	d	132	b	133	a
134	b	135	d	136	a	137	b	138	b	139	c	140	a
141	b	142	b	143	a	144	b	145	a	146	a	147	b
148	a	149	d	150	d	151	b	152	c	153	c	154	b
155	b	156	b	157	c	158	b	159	c	160	c	161	d
162	b	163	a	164	a	165	b	166	d	167	c	168	a
169	d	170	c	171	b	172	b	173	a	174	c	175	a
176	b	177	b	178	c	179	a	180	b	181	b	182	c
183	c	184	b	185	a	186	c	187	b	188	a	189	c
190	d	191	a	192	c	193	a	194	d	195	d	196	b
197	c	198	c	199	b	200	c	201	d	202	b	203	c
204	c	205	c	206	a	207	c	208	d	209	c	210	c
211	c	212	b	213	d	214	a	215	b	216	b	217	d
218	d	219	a	220	a	221	b	222	c	223	a	224	b
225	c												

33

Swine Production Management

Anuradha Kumari, *Utkarsh Kumar Tripathi, Manish Kumar, and Anshuman Kumar*

Faculty of Veterinary and animal Sciences, IAS, RGSC, Banaras Hindu University Varanasi, Uttar Pradesh

Introduction

India enjoys one of the largest livestock wealth in the world India has continued to experience an increasing growth in its livestock sector. Between 2010-11 and 2019-20, gross value-added (GVa) from livestock sector grew at an extraordinary rate of 7.6% annually. Among the livestock species, pig finds an important place as it being reared by socio-economically weaker sections of the rural India) Pig as compared to other livestock species has a great potential to contribute to faster economic return, because of certain important inherent traits like high fecundity, better-feed conversion efficiency, early maturity and short generation interval. Pig farming requires small investment on its housing and equipment. It has immense potential to ensure nutritional and economic security for the weaker sections of the society.The pig grows fast and is a prolific breeder, farrowing 10-12 piglets at a time. It is capable of producing two litters per year under good management conditions. The carcase yield is high (65 -80% of live weight). Pigs convert inedible feeds, forages, and certain grain by products into valuable nutrition's mean. The faeces of pigs are useful in maintaining soil fertility.

Pig population

According to the 20th Livestock census of India pigs comprises 1.7 % to the total livestock population (http://dahd.nic.in). The total Pigs in the country are 9.06 million in the current Census, declined by 12.03% over the previous Census. Out of the total pigs 20.98% are either exotic or crossbred and rest indigenous 79.02 % of the total pigs. The exotic breed mainly comprises Hampshire, Large White York Shire, Duroc, Landrace, and Tamworth. Total number of indigenous pig breeds has been reported to be 13 by NBAGR (http://www.nbagr.res.in). Distribution of overall pig population in country indicates Assam is having highest pig population (23.17%) followed by Jharkhand (14.12%) and Meghalaya (07.83%).Pig farming is adapted to both diversified and intensified agriculture.

Drawback of Pig Farming

In India, 70% of the pig population is reared under traditional smallholder, low-input demand driven production system, except forlimited number of semi-commercial pig farms in Kerala, Punjab and Goa) The most of pig are reared in a zero or low cost input system, a feeding system based on locally available grains, vegetables and agriculturalby-products along with kitchen waste.Farmers in the rural areas keep these pigs as scavengers which make them more susceptible to disease and skin infections. This practice of rearing makes them less appealing to the consumers who prefer a clean and hygienic production of pork. So, a clean, hygienic and scientific approach will not only help in healthy development of animals but also helps in increasing the appeal for pork production and consumption, thereby increasing the overall profit. Lack of Support from the development and financial bodies to establish pork based industries is hindering the growth of pig farming.

Contribution in Meat production

Pork supplies nearly one – half of the meat production from domestic animals in the world It is high in phosphorus, potassium, iron, zinc, manganese and magnesium and lower in calcium and sodium. Pork production in India is growing steadily in a slow pace and the share of pork in total meat production of the country has remained almost static over a decade. Pork contributes 4.06%, of production of meat in country (2020-21). Average yield of pigs in India is 35 kg/animals, which is about 55 % less than the corresponding value of world average.

Distribution of pig in India

Distribution of pig population across the country is not uniform, forinstance, thick population of pigs is recorded mainly in the states of Uttar Pradesh (30 percent), followed by north-eastern states (25 percent), Bihar (15 percent), West Bengal (6 percent), Karnataka (4 percent), Jharkhand (4 percent), and Kerala (3 percent).

Breeding of Pig

Over 20% of the pigs kept in India are crossed withexotic breeds, but with a large population of inbreeding because of non-systematic breeding and selection. In nutshell, the pig rearing is still not a recognize venture, requires science and technology drivensupport to make it a vibrant enterprise for weaker section of India

Status of Pig husbandry in India

Pig husbandry and pork production in India has been gaining slow but steady momentum since from VIth Five Year Plan. There is a deficit of 50% in terms of production-demand of pork. In order to full fill this gap in country, ICAR launched an All India Coordinated Research Project on Pig. All India Coordinated Research were established in different location of the country in the year 1970-71 in order to generate location specific information on pig breeding, feeding and health covered measures. However due to limited number of pig population and infrastructural facilities, the centres could not multiply and the distribute number of recommended pig variety. In the absence of commercialization of the pig industry, private entrepreneurs have not taken up large scale breeding and production of the recommended pig variety. Hence the mid termappraisal committee on AICRP on pigs in 1990 has therefore recommended, establishment of one National Research Centre on Pig to carry out the research and development studies on pigs. There after National Research Centre on pig has established at Guwahati in 2002. Currently, ICAR-NRC on Pig, located in Rani, Kamrup district of Assam is coordinating 15 All India Coordinated

Research Project on Pig.

1. Group of pig is known as:

a) Litter b) Runt

c) Drove d) Farrow

2. As per 20th livestock census-2020which statehas highest pig population in India?

a) Uttar Pradesh b) Jharkhand

c) Meghalaya d) Assam

3. Feed cost represents approximately .... % of overall costs in raising pigs.

a) 55-60 b) 60-65

c) 60-70 d) 70-80

4. As per BIS standard which of the following is the floor space requirement for farrowing a sow in covered area?

a) 7.0-9.0 m^2 b) 9.5-10.5 m^2

c) 12-14 m^2 d) 11-11.5 m^2

5. The feed conversion ratio in pig is.

a) 5:1 b) 4:1

c) 3:1 d) 2:1

6. A young female pig kept for breeding purpose which has not conceived yet is termed as.

a) Gilt b) Sow

c) Barren d) Barrow

7. Which of the following is the dominance hierarchy among the members of the litter in which they come to a general agreement that particular nipple will be suck by particular piglet?

a) Cross fostering b) Teat order

c) Split suckling d) Self suckling

8. Castrated male pig is known as

a) Barrow b) Gelding

c) Steer d) Wether

9. Which one is not a component of pig sties

a) Guard rail b) Pig board

c) Farrowing crates d) Creep area

10. Boar taint is an objectionable odour found in meat of?

a) Barrow b) Gilt

c) Boar d) Stag

11. NRC Pigis situated at which of the following state of India?

a) Dirang, Arunachal b) Jharnapani, Nalaland

c) Rani, Assam d) Bikaner, Rajasthan

12. A popular English breed of swine that has a good mothering ability is?

a) Large White Yorkshire b) Landrace,

c) Tamworth d) Berkshire

13. Scientific name of Indian wild boar is?
    a) *Sus. vittatus*
    b) *Sus. scrofa*
    c) *Sus. meridionalis*
    d) *Sus algira*
14. Smallest piglet in a litter is called as?
    a) Crit
    b) Card
    c) Runt
    d) All the above
15. New born piglets have eight tusks like teeth known as?
    a) Needle teeth
    b) Eye teeth
    c) Wolf teeth
    d) All of these
16. In organized farming practice of increasing the energy content in feed of gilts and dry sows two weeks before breeding is known as?
    a) Creep feeding
    b) Steaming up
    c) Flushing up
    d) None of these
17. Minium floor space requirement under covered area for a boar should (m^2) be?
    a) 0.9-1.8
    b) 1.8-2.7
    c) 6.0-7.0
    d) None of these
18. Length of gestation period for sow is .... days?
    a) 104
    b) 114
    c) 124
    d) 134
19. The practice of self-feeding concentrates to baby pigs in a separate area away from the dam is known as
    a) Creep feeding
    b) Flushing
    c) Steaming up
    d) None of these
20. Which of the following country has the highest number of pigs?
    a) USA
    b) China
    c) France
    d) India
21. Among the nutritional disease which is the most common in piglets?
    a) Hog cholera
    b) Piglet diarrhea
    c) Piglet anemia
    d) Swine pox
22. Dressing % of swine is
    a) 40-45
    b) 45-50
    c) 60-65
    d) 65-70
23. Rooting behaviourseen mostlyin which of the following animals?
    a) Rabbit
    b) Swine
    c) Equine
    d) Camel
24. Which of the following traits are severely affected by inbreeding in pigs?
    a) Pre weaning gain in piglets
    b) Litter size in pig
    c) Fat % in sow milk
    d) Mature body weight of sow
25. The length of estrus cycle in sow is
    a) 14 days
    b) 17 days
    c) 21 days
    d) 28 days

26. Swine breed with 'golden red' pigmentation on skin is famous for best quality bacon is
    a) Hampshire b) Tamworth
    c) Landrace d) Berkshire
27. Five minutes of daily contact with mature boar is sufficient to stimulate early puberty in gilts is known as......
    a) Bruce effect b) Lee boot effect
    c) Boar effect d) Whitten effect
28. Starter ration for pigs should contain ....CP
    a) 12-14 % b) 16-18%
    c) 20-22% d) 22- 24%
29. Height of guard rails above the floor of the farrowing pen should be
    a) 15 cm b) 25 cm
    c) 35 cm d) 45 cm
30. Medium size black colour English breed with a white belt entirely encircles the body including both front leg and feet is characteristics of which of the following?
    a) Hampshire b) Landrace
    c) Berkshire d) Large White Yorkshire
31. Normally duration of suckling period in piglets is ...
    a) 26 days b) 36 days
    c) 46 days d) 56 days
32. Black coloured indigenous pigs breed with large heart shaped ears and typical bull dog face appearance is
    a) Niang Megha b) Ghoongroo
    c) Agonda Goan d) Tenyi Vo
33. Maximum number of sows in a farrowing per pen is
    a) One b) Two
    c) Ten d) Any number
34. Flushing in sow causes
    a) Increased ovulation rate b) Increased growth rate
    c) Increased fertility d) Increased birth weight of piglets
35. The potential for production of more no of piglets in each farrowing is known as
    a) Fertility b) Fecundity
    c) Reproduction rate d) Prolificacy
36. Boar Taint is a strong smell and taste on the meat from a boar can be prevented by
    a) Proper heating of pork to an internal temperature of 77°C
    b) Castrating male pigs at an early stage
    c) Providing proper rest before slaughter
    d) Proper feeding of finishing boar

37. Length of gestation period for pig is
    a) 1 months, 1 week, 1 days b) 2 months, 2 week, 2 days
    c) 3 months, 3 week, 3 days d) 4 months, 4 week, 4 days
38. Average birth weight of piglets is....
    a) 1 kg b) 2 kg
    c) 3 kg d) 4 kg
39. Indian pig population is .... % of world pig population
    a) 1.33 b) 2.18
    c) 3.56 d) 5.0
40. Pig population density is maximum in
    a) Meghalaya b) Nagaland
    c) Manipur d) Tripura
41. Meat of pig
    a) Lard b) Beef
    c) Mutton d) Pork
42. AICRP on Pigs was initiated in
    a) 1951 b) 1961
    c) 1971 d) 1981
43. Teat order after farrowing established in ....
    a) 24 hours b) 3 days
    c) 15 days d) 30 days
44. Highest per capita pork consumption in India is in
    a) Himachal Pradesh b) Uttar Pradesh
    c) Nagaland d) Assam
45. Objective of castration in pig is
    a) To maintained good appetite b) To keep pig fit
    c) To ensure proper feeding d) To prevent boar odour in cooked meat
46. Chromosome no in pig
    a) 18 pairs b) 19 pairs
    c) 20 pairs d) 21 pairs
47. Carcass traits have
    a) Low heritability b) Moderate heritability
    c) High heritability d) All of these
48. Which is not economically important carcass traits of pig
    a) Back fat thickness b) Loin eye area
    c) Fertility d) Meat to bone ratio
49. Piglets weaned at the age of .... Week in India
    a) 3 weeks b) 5 weeks
    c) 6 weeks d) 8 weeks

50. Piglets should be given iron injection by .... after birth
   a) 3 days b) 3 week
   c) 3 months d) Immediately after birth
51. New born pig mortality is mainly due to....
   a) Piglets'anemia b) Cannibalism
   c) Enteritis d) Crushing by mother
52. Wallowing is needed for
   a) Sheep's b) Pigs
   c) Goats d) Cattle
53. Birth of hairless piglets is due to
   a) Copper deficiency b) Vit A deficiency
   c) Iodine deficiency d) Zinc deficiency
54. Meaty hogs should have a loin-eye area ......
   a) 1.5 square inches or more b) 4.5 square inches or more
   c) 7.5 square inches or more d) 15.5 square inches or more
55. Best method of identification in pig is
   a) Tagging b) Ear notching
   c) Tattooing d) Flesh marking
56. Breeding age of gilts/pigs
   a) 8-10 months b) 11-12 months
   c) 14-15 months d) 16-17 months
57. Out crossing is
   a) Brother sister mating
   b) Mating of sow of one breed and boar of another breed
   c) Mating of unrelated animals within breed
   d) Mating of offspring with either of the parents
58. Value of the crossbred offspring exceed the average of the parent is known as
   a) Inbreeding depression b) Heterosis
   c) Epistasis d) Heritability
59. Finishrefers to the ....
   a) Conformation of the hog's body b) Fat on the hog body
   c) Muscling on the hog body d) Yield of lean cuts
60. Mating of crossbred back to parental purebreds is
   a) Rotational crossing b) Criss -crossing
   c) Terminal crossing d) Roto- terminal crossing
61. Not a system of farrowing
   a) One litter a year system b) Two litter a year system
   c) Three litter a year system d) Multiple furrowing system

62. Diamond skin disease in pig caused by
    a) Mites b) Tick
    c) Bacteria d) Lice
63. Breeding age of boars
    a) 8-10 months b) 10-12 months
    c) 14-15 months d) 16-17 months
64. During which phase of oestrous cycle sow allow mounting by boar
    a) Pro-oestrus b) Oestrus
    c) Dioestrus d) Metoestrus
65. Standing heat reflex consists of
    a) Immobilization b) Arching of the back
    c) Cocking of ear d) All of these
66. Vasectomised boar is
    a) Rider b) Stag
    c) Runt d) Teaser
67. For higher conception rate gilts are bred twice at .... hours interval during heat
    a) 12 b) 24
    c) 36 d) 48
68. For higher conception rate sows are bred twice at ......hours interval during heat
    a) 12 b) 24
    c) 36 d) 48
69. In which mating method sow in heat is brought to individual boar for service .....
    a) Hand mating b) Pen mating
    c) Flock mating d) Herd mating
70. Recommended floor space for creep area is
    a) 5-10 sft b) 15-20 sft
    c) 25-30 sft d) 35-40 sft
71. Average volume of ejaculate in boar is considered as normal?
    a) 50 ml b) 100 ml
    c) 150 ml d) 200 ml
72. Average age of castration in boar is
    a) 1-2 weeks b) 2-3 weeks
    c) 5-6 weeks d) 8 weeks
73. The back fat thickness of the carcass is normally being measured at all of the following places except one?
    a) At the level of first rib b) At the level of last rib
    c) At first lumbar vertebra d) At last lumbar vertebra
74. Stage II of farrowing is
    a) Dilation of cervix b) Phase of foetus expulsion
    c) Phase of placenta expulsion d) Vulvar swelling & discharge

75. Phenomenon in which the absorption of large molecules of colostrum ceases following ingestion of feed is known as?

a) Lactation failure
b) Gut closure
c) Lactation anestrous
d) Piglets scour

76. Early weaning age of pig is

a) Immediately after birth
b) 3 to 6 weeks
c) 8-9 weeks
d) 10-12 weeks

77. Not a advantage of early weaning

a) Sows rebred early
b) Reduced feed cost
c) Piglets are more uniform at weaning
d) Losses due to crushing are avoided

78. Permanent removal of part of litter before complete weaning is known as....

a) Early weaning
b) Fractional weaning
c) Pre-weaning
d) Split suckling

79. Split weaning not leads to

a) Uniform crop of piglets
b) Overcome post weaning growth lag
c) Body weight loss of sow
d) Reduced weaning to oestrus interval in sows

80. Inter farrowing interval comprised of

a) Lactation length + Gestation length
b) Gestation length +weaning to oestrous interval
c) Lactation length + weaning to oestrous interval
d) Gestation length +Lactation length+ weaning to oestrous interval

81. Pigs fall in which of the following categories?

a) Omnivorous polygastric
b) Omnivorous monogastric
c) Carnivorous polygastric
d) Carnivorous monogastric

82. As per nutritional requirement the body weight of starter pig is....

a) 2-5 kg
b) 5-15 kg
c) 15-35 kg
d) 35-90 kg

83. Thumps represents which of the following in case of the pigs?

a) Anaemia
b) Laboured breathing
c) Dyspnoea
d) Anorexia

84. Supplementation of which of the following is required in pig ration for vitamin B_{12} supply?

a) Fresh green forage
b) Animal protein concentrate
c) Plenty of soil exposure
d) Plant protein concentrate

85. First limiting amino acid in swine ration is....

a) Methionine
b) Tryptophan
c) Lysine
d) Threonine

86. Tryptophan is pro-vitamin for
   a) Cysteine b) Nicotinamide
   c) Threonine d) Methionine
87. Parakeratosis occurs due
   a) Copper deficiency b) Vit A deficiency
   c) Iodine deficiency d) Zinc deficiency
88. Essential fatty acids in pig ration includes ....
   a) Linoleic acid b) Arachidonic acid
   c) Linolenic acid d) All of these
89. Which essential fatty acids is on top priority among three E.F.A in pig ration
   a) Linoleic acid b) Arachidonic acid
   c) Linolenic acid d) Stearic acid
90. Added to feeds in micro quantities to improve productivity, are known as
   a) Pre-mix b) Feed additives
   c) Essential amino acids d) Essential fatty acids
91. Beneficial effect of antibiotics may be due to
   a) Sparing action of antibiotics b) Thinning of mucosa
   c) Action on micro-organisms d) All of these

Large Size	**Medium Size**		**Small Size**
Beetal Jamunapari Jakharana	Barbari Chegu Chsngthangi Gaddi Ganjam GOhilwadi Kannai Adu Kutchi	Malabari Marwadi Mehsana Osmanabadi Snagamneri Sirohi Surti Zalawadi	Black Bengal

92. Birth of blind, dead and mummified pigs occur due to deficiency of?
   a) Copper b) Vit A
   c) Iodine d) Zinc
93. Anaemia in pigs occurs due to
   a) Copper deficiency b) B -Vitamin deficiency
   c) Iron deficiency d) All of these
94. Body weight for economic slaughter of pig in India?
   a) 60 kg b) 70 kg
   c) 80 kg d) 90 kg
95. Body weight for economic slaughter of pigs in U.S.A?
   a) 60 kg b) 70 kg
   c) 80 kg d) 90 kg

96. The optimum level of fibre in swine rations is ………

a) 2-4% b) 6-8%

c) 8-10% d) 10-12%

97. Pre-Starter ration for pigs should contain ….Crude Protein (CP).

a) 12-14 % b) 16-18%

c) 20-22% d) 22- 24%

98. Dry pre starter feeds also known as

a) Milk replacer b) Creep feed

c) Mash feed d) Grower feed

99. MMA stands for

a) Mastits Metritis Anemia b) Mastits Metritis Agalactia

c) Mastits Metabolic Agalactia d) Metabolic Metritis Agalactia

100 Pigs are given a measure amount of food once, twice or thrice a day is known as

a) Ad lib feeding system b) Restricted feeding system

c) Appetite feeding system d) Self-feeding system

101. As per ICAR-NBAGR no of registered pig breed in India

a) 10 b) 11

c) 12 d) 13

102. Home tract of Ghurrah pig breed is……

a) Uttar Pradesh b) Bihar

c) Jharkhand d) Assam

103. Which of the following pig breed is of Denmark Origin, noted for their prolificacy and better feed utilization efficiency?

a) Hampshire b) Tamworth

c) Landrace d) Berkshire

104. One of the newer breeds of swine with two-thirds of body is red colour, with constant white face

a) Hereford b) Tamworth

c) Chester white d) Duroc

105. One of the largest black colour American breed, having drooping ear is ….

a) Berkshire b) Poland China

c) Hampshire d) Landrace

106. Which of the following is a bacterial disease of swine?

a) Foot and Mouth Disease b) Swine Eryseplas

c) Swine Influenza d) Classical Swine Fever (CSF)

107. Which of the following animals' functional ovary give the appearance of a cluster of grapes or lobulated.

a) Sow b) Mare

c) Deer d) Goat

108. In sow which of the following type's uterus are found?
a) Bipartite uterus b) Bicornuate uterus
c) Duplex uterus d) Simplex uterus

109. In the sow the rings of cervix are which of the following?
a) Interlocking rings b) Annular rings
c) Cork screw shaped d) None of the above

110. The sow is coming under which of the following type's breeders?
a) Non-seasonally polyestrus b) Seasonally polyestrous
c) Seasonally monoestrous d) Long-day breeders

111. Which of the following is the time of ovulation in sow?
a) 12-24 hours before end of estrus b) 35-45 hours after onset of estrus
c) 12-24 hours after onset of estrus d) 10-15 hours after end of estrus

112. Which of the following is the optimum time for service in Sow?
a) 30-36 hours after onset of estrus b) 18-24 hours after onset of estrus
c) 12-30 hours after onset of estrus d) None of the above

113. Application of pressure on which of the following body areas exhibit rigidity reflex by sow that occurs during natural mating with a boar?
a) Sow's back b) Sow's Neck
c) Sow's Hump d) Sow's Head

114. Boar odour or boar taint is caused by which of the following pheromone?
a) Methyl-p-hydroxy benzoate b) 17-alpha hydroxylase
c) C-16 unsaturated androgens d) None of the above

115. Spermatozoa retain their fertilizing capacity in the female reproductive tract of sow for
a) 24-48 Hours b) 36-48 Hours
c) 48-72 Hours d) 72-96 Hours

116. Which of the following is the shape of boar glans penis?
a) 'S'- shape b) Corkscrew
c) Straight d) Curved upward

117. Which of the following accessory sex glands is absent in boar
a) Vesicular gland b) Bulbourethral gland
c) Prostate gland d) Ampullae

118. As per BIS standard which of the following is the floor space requirement for a weaner/fattening pigs in open area?
a) $0.9 – 1.8\ m^2$ b) $1.8 – 2.7\ m^2$
c) $1.4\text{-}1.8\ m^2$ d) $6.25\text{-}7.5\ m^2$

119. Standard feeding space requirement for a sow with litter is?
a) 20-30 cm b) 30-40 cm
c) 60-75 cm d) 75-100 cm

120. Which of the following is the maximum recommended number of dry sow/gilts can be kept per pen?
   a) 1 b) 10
   c) 30 d) 50

121. Which of the following is the watering space required as compared to that of feeding space for pigs?
   a) 1/2 b) 1/5
   c) 1/10 d) 1/15

122. A dwelling place consists of one or more pen for pigs is known as
   a) Sties b) Barn
   c) Creep d) Stable

123. Heat tolerance capacity of pig is very less because of....
   a) Few sweat gland b) Spare coat of hair
   c) Thick layer of fat below the skin d) All of these

124. Which of the following is not a method to reduce heat load in pigs?
   a) Hog wallows b) Internal fogging
   c) Panting of body d) Ventilation fans

125. Exposer of pigs to direct sunlight for more than 2.5 to 3 hours will lead?
   a) Pale soft exudates (PSE)
   b) Porcine stress syndrome (PSS)
   c) Dark firm and dry (DFD)
   d) Mastitis Metritis Agalactia complex (MMa)

126. Malignant hyperthermia condition in pigs due to direct sunlight exposer for more than 2.5 to 3 hours can be detected by?
   a) Halothane sensitivity test b) Riding test
   c) Back pressure test d) Cocking test

127. Scientific name of modern pig is
   a) Sus scrofa b) Sus Cristatus
   c) Sus domestica d) Sus philipinesis

128. Not a component of farrowing pen
   a) Pig fenders b) Creep area
   c) Infrared lamp d) Hog wallow

129. An effective means of preventing the piglets to be crushed by sow is?
   a) Pig fenders b) Creep area
   c) Nipple drinker d) Wallow

130. Which of the following is not a vice of pigs?
   a) Snout biting b) Wallowing
   c) Navel suckling d) Savaging

131. Which one is not pig restraining device
a) Pig board b) Snare
c) Guard rail d) Hurdle

132. A boar castrated after used for service is ....
a) Stag b) Barrow
c) Teaser d) Runt

133. A steel crate used in the farrowing pen to reduce overlaying piglet mortality by restricting lateral movements of sow is......
a) Guard rail b) Farrowing crate
c) Pig fenders d) Pig board

134. Male pig castrated before reaching sexual maturity.
a) Barrow b) Boar
c) Stag d) Runt

135. A male with one or both testes undescended know as ......
a) Runt b) Ridgling
c) Ring d) Render

136. Act of mating in pig known as....
a) Farrowing b) Coupling
c) Covering d) Serving

137. Sound produced by pig is......
a) Squealing b) Drove
c) Chitterlings d) Pigling

138. Which traits shows good response to hybrid vigour
a) Back fat thickness b) Loin eye area
c) Litter size d) Carcass length

139. Thigh and buttock of hog that is slaughtered for meat is......
a) Bacon b) Chitterlings
c) Ham d) Lard

140. The number of farrowing per sow per year is........
a) Farrowing index b) Farrowing crate
c) Farrowing rate d) Farrowing interval

141. Interval between weaning of sow and re-mating is
a) Service period b) Gestation period
c) Lactation period d) Dry period

142. Defecation of pigs in lying and feeding area is known as
a) Savaging b) Pen fouling
c) Shrinkage d) Powdering

143. As per 20th livestock census-2020 pig population in India...
a) 8.66 million b) 9.06 million
c) 7.16 million d) 10.29 million

144. Advisable time to breed after parturition in sow is……

a) Immediately after farrowing
b) After 45 days of farrowing
c) After 60 days of farrowing
d) First estrus 3-9 days after weaning

145. Boar pace back and forth along the fence often chopping their jaw and salivation, such action called

a) Ram effect
b) Ranting
c) Courtship
d) Ridgling

146. Gestation period of wild pigs is

a) 114 days
b) 124 days
c) 134 days
d) 144 days

147. SMEDI in pigs is

a) A viral disease
b) A nutritional deficiency disease
c) A bacterial disease
d) A parasitic disease

148. A young hog, especially one that has been weaned.

a) Smedi
b) Shoat
c) Boarling
d) Stag

149. Needle teeth are

a) Canine teeth
b) Incisor teeth
c) Both incisor and canine
d) None of the above

150. No of essential amino acid for pig

a) 0
b) 8
c) 10
d) 12

Answer Key

1	c	2	d	3	d	4	a	5	c	6	a	7	b
8	a	9	b	10	c	11	c	12	a	13	b	14	d
15	d	16	c	17	c	18	b	19	a	20	b	21	c
22	d	23	b	24	b	25	c	26	b	27	c	28	c
29	b	30	a	31	d	32	b	33	a	34	a	35	b
36	b	37	c	38	a	39	a	40	b	41	d	42	c
43	b	44	c	45	d	46	b	47	c	48	c	49	d
50	a	51	d	52	b	53	c	54	b	55	b	56	a
57	c	58	b	59	b	60	b	61	c	62	c	63	b
64	b	65	d	66	d	67	a	68	b	69	a	70	b
71	d	72	b	73	c	74	b	75	b	76	b	77	b
78	b	79	c	80	d	81	b	82	b	83	b	84	b
85	c	86	b	87	d	88	d	89	a	90	b	91	d
92	b	93	d	94	b	95	d	96	b	97	d	98	a

99	b	100	b	101	d	102	a	103	c	104	a	105	b
106	b	107	a	108	b	109	c	110	a	111	b	112	c
113	a	114	c	115	a	116	b	117	d	118	a	119	d
120	b	121	c	122	a	123	d	124	c	125	b	126	a
127	c	128	d	129	a	130	b	131	c	132	a	133	b
134	a	135	b	136	b	137	a	138	c	139	c	140	a
141	a	142	b	143	b	144	d	145	b	146	b	147	a
148	b	149	c	150	b	151		152		153		154	

34

Working Animal Production and Management

Jessy Bagh[1], Annada Das[2], and Kaushik Satyaprakash[3]

[1]*Department of Livestock Production and Management, CVSc & AH, OUAT, Bhubaneswar, Odisha*

[2]*Department of Livestock Products Technology, Faculty of Veterinary and Animal Sciences, WBUAFS, Kolkata, West Bengal*

[3]*Department of Veterinary Public Health and Epidemiology, Faculty of Veterinary and Animal Sciences, RGSC, BHU, Mirzapur, Uttar Pradesh*

Introduction

Man have used different animals like cattle, buffaloes, horses, donkeys, mules, yak, camel and elephants for different kinds of work. Draft animals evolved during course of time have advantages of stability, sustainability and environmental friendliness. Different animals have different draught capacities for performing different types of work. The approximate power developed by various animals in terms of horse power are- Horse-1.0: Bullock-0.74: Buffalo-0.75: Cow-0.45: Maule-0.75: Donkey- 0.35. Draught developed by the animal is generally proportional to its body weight.

Draught ability: Work is done when force is exerted to move an object over a distance. Work in the strict sense of "Force exerted x distance through which the force is moved". Work performed by animals can be measured by quantifying their capacity to generate power.

Draught Power (W) = Draught (N) x Speed (m/s)

Management of different working animals

1. Cattle and Buffalo Bullocks: they are used for various operations like ploughing, harrowing, threshing, harvesting, for lifting water and for transporting people and agricultural produce. The average speed of a pair of bullocks pulling a cart is around 4-5 km per hour. If not overdriven, they can travel 25-30 km or even 40 km in favorable condition. Atmospheric temperature played a more prominent role on the onset of fatigue in the bullocks compared to load imposed on them. Farmers generally consider a pair of good bullocks to be sufficient to carry out all the cultivation and transport job during one year on a 2.5 hectare holding.
2. Working buffaloes: Domestic buffalo is the predominant working animal in the rice growing area Buffaloes are extensively used for cultivation and carting. The working swamp buffalo has a short body with a large girth and short thick legs. It is extensively well adapted to hot and humid climate and marshy land

Working capacity of buffaloes is affected by several factors like breed, age, physical condition, health, speed of travel and type of harness and equipment used
Duration of the working day varies from 6 to 8 hours with 4 -5 hours rest periods

3. Horses: Horses, donkeys and mules are common equines that used as work and pack animals both by the army and civilians. Horse is one of the earliest species that man has domesticated.Horses are better draught animals than bullocks, draught developed as well as speed of work, hence horsepower developed is higher in them
4. Camels: Camels are best used either for riding or carrying baggage during nighttime when it is cool. Camels used for draught work like ploughing, water lifting etc should not be worked for more than 5-6 hours a day. Camels should be housed in suitable and simple sheds consisting of an open space with an enclosure for shelter against sun, rain and drought. Camels are troublesome during the rutting season, and therefore the males and females should be kept separate during this season
5. Yak: Yak used as pack animal for carrying goods on the high altitude and also for riding on the rough and sloppy hills. Hybrids are good draught bullock for ploughing and other agricultural operations
6. Elephant : Elephant, the largest present day terrestrial mammals. Elephants are used for riding purpose in forest areas. Also used for removing individual tress and transportation of timber in the forest Elephants are allowed to work for 6 hours in a day morning in 3 hrs and evening 3 hrs for 6 days in a week with a total of 8 to 9 months in a year. A fully grown elephant can lift and carry a load of up to 500 to 550 kg for short distance. The average walking speed of an elephant is about 4 km per hour.

Multiple choice question

1. How much distance can a buffalo bullock can travel in a normal day:
   a) 10 km b) 50 km
   c) 5 km d) 25 km
2. Draught developed by animal is generally proportional to its :
   a) Body weight b) Body temperature
   c) Body height d) metabolic rate
3. Tractive power is measured in :
   a) Watt b) kWh
   c) kw^2 d) All of the above
4. Rate at which work is performed is known as :
   a) Draft b) Tractive power
   c) Power d) all of the above
5. Approximate power developed by a bullock is about :
   a) 1 HP. b) 0.25 HP.
   c) 0.74 HP. d) 0.45 HP
6. Approximate power developed by a Buffalo is about :
   a) 1 HP b) 0.25 HP
   c) 0.75 HP d) 0.45 HP

7. Approximate power developed by a cow is about :
   a) 1 HP, b) 0.25 HP
   c) 0.74 H d) 0.45 HP
8. Approximate power developed by a Mule is about :
   a) 1 HP, 0 b) .25 HP
   c) 0.75 HP d) 0.45 HP
9. Approximate power developed by a Donkey is about :
   a) 1 HP b) 0.35 HP
   c) 0.74 HP d) 0.45 HP
10. Normal speed of a bullock is :
   a) 3.4 Km/h b) 6 Km/h
   c) 3 Km/h d) 1 Km/h
11. Bullock required how much energy to carry one kg load over one meter:
   a) 1J b) 2J
   c) 3J d) 6J
12. Training of a bullock for work should start at the age of:
   a) 1-2 year b) 2-3 year
   c) 3-4 year d) 4-5 year
13. Ten bullocks can replace how many tractor:
   a) 1 b) 2
   c) 3 d) 4
14. Average draught developed by a bullock is in proportion of :
   a) 1/2 of bwt, b) $1/10^{th}$ of bwt,
   c) $1/5^{th}$ of bwt, d) $1/3^{rd}$ of bwt
15. A camel under load should not be required to work how many hour per day at a stretch:
   a) 10 b) 6
   c) 4 d) 2
16. Sources of power used in agriculture include:
   a) Human b) Animal
   c) Mechanical d) All of the above
17. Which country is known for Great Run of Bulls:
   a) India b) England
   c) Spain d) Srilanka
18. An ideal draught bullock should have:
   a) Good carriage and disposition b) Low carriage and disposition
   c) No carriage and disposition d) All of the above
19. Traditional bullock carts can carry a how much maximum load:
   a) 1 tonne b) 2 tonne
   c) 3 tonne d) 4 tonne

20. Working bullocks use for agriculture operation work for how many days in a year:
    a) 100 days b) 200 days
    c) 300 days d) 400 days
21. Draught animal power is a :
    a) Non renewable energy b) Renewable energy
    c) Both d) None of the above
22. Traditionally draught animals are harnessed using :
    a) Yoke b) Yolk
    c) Rope d) Cart
23. One adult worker and a pair of oxen will be sufficient for :
    a) 3-4 ha land b) 10-12 ha land
    c) 12-15 ha land d) 20 ha land
24. Speed of bullock cart is :
    a) 10-12 km/hr b) 8-9 km/hr
    c) 5-6 km/hr d) 3 km/hr
25. How much time should be spent by camel for grazing and browing to meet the requirement:
    a) 6-8 hrs b) 9-10 hrs
    c) 2-3 hrs d) 4-5 hrs
26. Camel used for draught purpose should not be worked for more than how many hours:
    a) 5-6 hrs b) 6-8 hrs
    c) 1-2 hrs d) 9 hrs
27. At what age elephant calves are first trained in timber logging:
    a) 5 years b) 6, years
    c) 2 years d) 3 years
28. How many hours a day elephant are allowed to work:
    a) 6 hours b) 10 hours
    c) 12 hours d) 2 hours
29. How many days in a week elephant are allowed to work:
    a) 6 days b) 4 days
    c) 3 days d) 7 days
30. How many month in a year elephant are allowed to work:
    a) 8-9 month b) 10 month
    c) 12 month d) none
31. A adult elephant is allowed to carry what weight of load for short distance:
    a) 500-550 kg b) 600 kg
    c) 700 kg d) None
32. Average walking speed of an elephant is about:
    a) 4k m/hr b) 6 km/hr
    c) 8 km/hr d) 10 km/hr

33. Working hours for bullocks recommended for normal (Carting) is:
    a) 6 hours b) 8 hrs
    c) 10 hrs d) 4 hrs
34. Working hours for bullocks recommended for heavy (Carting) is:
    a) 6 hours b) 8 hrs
    c) 10 hrs d) 4 hrs
35. Working hours for bullocks recommended for normal (ploughing) is:
    a) 6 hours b) 8 hrs
    c) 10 hrs d) 4 hrs
36. Working hours for bullocks recommended for heavy (ploughing) is:
    a) 6 hours b) 8 hrs
    c) 10 hrs d) 4 hrs
37. Average speed of a good riding camel is :
    a) 8-11 km/hr b) 3-4 km/ hr
    c) 20km/ hr d) 30 km/hr
38. Average birth weight of an elephant is:
    a) 90-120 kg b) 50-60 kg
    c) 150 kg d) 200 kg
39. What kind of training do elephant get:
    a) To carry heavy load b) Act in circus
    c) Both d) None
40. Fastest speed at which elephant can run:
    a) 25 mph b) 15 mph
    c) 35 mph d) None
41. Group of elephant is known as:
    a) Caravan b) Pack
    c) Colony d) Herd
42. Average lifespan of elephant:
    a) 20-30 years b) 50-70 years
    c) 100 years d) 10 years
43. Age at maturity in female elephant:
    a) 12-14 years b) 5-6 years
    c) 20 years d) 25 years
44. Gestational period of of elephant is :
    a) 22 month b) 10 month
    c) 32 month d) 12 month
45. When elephant compete for female there is high rise of testosterone called as:
    a) Musth b) Hustle
    c) Bust d) None

46. At what age musth phenomenon start in healthy male elephant:
 a) 20-25 years b) 10-15 years
 c) 35-40 years d) None
47. Formula for weighing elephant is :
 a) W= 12.8 (Cg + Ng) – 4281 b) 4152.4 + 14.76Cg + 8.84 Ng
 c) Both d) None
48. Ivory is obtained from teeth of:
 a) Tiger b) Elephant
 c) Lion d) Snake
49. Unit of measuring Horse length is:
 a) Leg b) Hand
 c) Finger d) None
50. One hand is equal to:
 a) 10 cm b) 50 cm
 c) 20 inch d) 10 inch
51. Tampering of cups of teeth is also known as:
 a) Winking b) Bishoping
 c) Chewing d) Lordosis
52. Young one of horse is known as:
 a) Foal b) Poult
 c) Kid d) Calf
53. Act of mating in horse is known as:
 a) Calving b) Serving
 c) Covering d) Foaling
54. Act of Parturition is known as:
 a) Calving b) Serving
 c) Covering d) Foaling
55. Number of chromosomes in horse:
 a) 64 b) 62
 c) 60 d) 54
56. Male horse known as:
 a) Stallion b) Tordia
 c) Boar d) Jack
57. Female horse is called as:
 a) Mare b) Jenny
 c) Sow d) Doe
58. Mule is cross between :
 a) Jack & Jenny b) Stallion & Mare
 c) Jack and Mare d) Jack & Mare

59. For which disease mallein test is used for diagnosis:
 a) Tetanus b) Glanders
 c) Strangles d) Anthrax
60. Test used for pregnancy diagnosis in horse is :
 a) Cuboni's test b) Mallein test
 c) Both d) None
61. Which disease has symptoms of protrusion of third eye- lid and wooden horse:
 a) Anthrax b) Strangles
 c) Glanders d) Tetanus
62. Sickle shape ear in horse indicates:
 a) Indian blood b) Arabian blood
 c) American blood d) English blood
63. Group of horse is known as :
 a) Pack b) Flock
 c) Band d) Caravan
64. Method of casting used in horse:
 a) Reuffs method b) Alternative method
 c) Sideline method d) None
65. Mare use caslick's operation for :
 a) Prevention of prolapsed vulva b) Colostrum feeding to calf
 c) Restraining d) Rumenotomy
66. Which country use mare's milk for human consumption:
 a) India b) Mongolia
 c) America d) Russia
67. Galvaynes's groove disappear in horse completely at the age of :
 a) 15 years b) 30 years
 c) 20 years d) 25 years
68. Season affects horse reproduction because they are :
 a) Non seasonal breeder b) Short day breeder
 c) Long day breeder d) None
69. Female mule is called as:
 a) Hinny b) Zony
 c) Molly d) Hule
70. Difference between ponies and horses is :
 a) Chromosomes b) Age
 c) Colour d) Height
71. Gestation period in horse:
 a) 330-345 days b) 280-290 days
 c) 14 -120 days d) 500-700 days

72. Galvayne's groove appears in which teeth of horse:
   a) Upper corner incisor   b) Lower middle incisor
   c) Upper first molar   d) Lower middle incisor
73. Wolf teeth found in some of the horses are :
   a) Incisor   b) Molar
   c) Premolar   d) Canine
74. Gall bladder is absent in :
   a) Horse   b) Buffalo
   c) Sheep   d) Cow
75. In which place horse are kept:
   a) Stable   b) Shed
   c) Kennel   d) None
76. Which species has dental star:
   a) Horse   b) Cattle
   c) Pig   d) Poultry
77. Sound produced by Ass is called as:
   a) Braying   b) Neigh
   c) Whinny   d) Grunting
78. Sound produced by horse is known as:
   a) Neigh   b) Grunting
   c) Whinny   d) Braying
79. Horse refusing habit to move forward is known as:
   a) Jibbing   b) Whinny
   c) Braying   d) Grunting
80. Formula for calculating body weight of horse is :
   a) $GL^2/300$ b) $GL^2/330$
   c) Both   d) None
81. Single hoof is the characteristics of :
   a) Goat   b) Horse
   c) Pig   d) cattle
82. Colic is very common in which animal:
   a) Goat   b) Horse
   c) Pig   d) Cattle
83. Types of gait in horse is:
   a) Trot   b) Gallop
   c) Canter   d) All of the these
84. Animal commonly used in polo game:
   a) Goat   b) Horse
   c) Pig   d) Cattle

85. Gestational Period of she camel is :

a) 390 days
b) 490 days
c) 290 days
d) None of the above

86. Camel belongs to order:

a) Camelidae,
b) Tylopoda
c) Artiodactyla
d) Mammalia

87. Camel capable of pulling load equivalent to _______ percent of body weight

a) 40%
b) 80%
c) 90%
d) 100%

88. Borders of Arabia domesticated Dromedary by:

a) 500 BC
b) 1800 Bc
c) 200 BC
d) 300 BC

89. Llama and Alpaca living in south America is:

a) Single humped
b) Doubled humped
c) Humpless
d) Triple hump

90. A fermented product prepared from camel milk is :

a) Sour milk
b) Sweet curd
c) Kumiss
d) Shreekhand

91. Total number of teeth present in camel:

a) 32-38
b) 30
c) 25
d) 26

92. Maturity of cow camels is at:

a) 3 years
b) 2 years
c) 8 years
d) 5 years

93. Maturity of male camels is at:

a) 3 years
b) 2 years
c) 8 years
d) 5 years

94. Average life of camels is :

a) 40 years
b) 20 years
c) 80 years
d) 50 years

95. Rutting period in male camel:

a) Flaccid Testis
b) Dry flaccid testis
c) Turgid testis
d) None of the above

96. Female camel ovulation is induced by:

a) Spontaneous
b) Coitus
c) Human touch stimulus
d) One of the above

97. Average length of estrous cycle in camel is:

a) 3-5 days
b) 30 days
c) 7-15 days
d) 23 days

98. Shape of uterus in female camel is :
   a) Y-shape   b) A shape
   c) T-shape   d) Intermediate between Y and T
99. Number of mammary gland in camel is :
   a) 2   b) 4
   c) 8   d) 6
100. Organ in camel acts as prehensile organ is:
   a) Teeth   b) Tongue
   c) Lip   d) Both b & c
101. A black pigment is secreted from which gland in male camel during rut:
   a) Carpal gland   b) Orbital gland
   c) Cowper's gland   d) Pole gland
102. Duration of mating process in camel takes about :
   a) 20-25 hrs   b) 20-25 mint
   c) 1-2 hrs   d) 1-2 min
103. Sexual excitement period in camel is known as :
   a) Rut   b) Thoot
   c) Musth   d) All of the above
104. Average birth weight in camel is around:
   a) 35- 40 kg   b) 20-25 kg
   c) 10-15 kg   d) 50-60 kg
105. Typical sign of pregnancy in camel is :
   a) Cocking of tail   b) Winking of clitoris
   c) Waxing of teat   d) All the above
106. What does hump of camel store:
   a) Water   b) Fat
   c) Protein   d) Vitamins
107. At position do camel mate:
   a) Sitting   b) Standing
   c) sleeping   d) Walking
108. Number of hump present in Bactrian camel:
   a) Single   b) Double
   c) Both   d) None
109. The Arabian camel is commonly known as :
   a) Italian   b) Bactrian
   c) Dromedary   d) Australia
110. What kind of placenta present in camel:
   a) Intact type   b) Diffuse (Horse) type
   c) cotyledonary   d) Zonary

111. Most of pregnancy in camel is present in :
   a) Left horn of uterus
   b) Right horn of uterus
   c) Both
   d) None

112. Number of toes in each foot of camel:
   a) One
   b) Two
   c) Three
   d) None

113. Salivary glands secretes :
   a) 50-60 litres
   b) 30-40 litres
   c) 10 litres
   d) 100-70 litres

114. A group of camel is known as:
   a) Caravan
   b) Flock
   c) Pack
   d) Colony

115. Which disease in camel is commonly known as "sool" in camel:
   a) Anthrax
   b) Malaria
   c) Trypanosomiasis
   d) Black quarter

116. Features of Adaption in desert for camel:
   a) Fat stored in hump
   b) Slit like nostrils closes during sand stroms
   c) Tough and horny pad on feet
   d) All of the above

117. Best age for breaking or training camel is :
   a) 4-6 years
   b) 1-2 years
   c) 7-8 years
   d) None

118. Age of castration in camel is :
   a) 0-1 years
   b) 1-2 years
   c) 3-4 years
   d) 4-5 years

119. Baby camel is known as:
   a) Foal
   b) Calf
   c) Kid
   d) Lamb

120. Rectal temperature of camel is taken when the camel is:
   a) Sitting
   b) Sleeping
   c) Standing
   d) Eating

121. Colon acts as major site for _________ reabsorbtion
   a) Salt
   b) Water
   c) Minerals
   d) Fat

122. Feeding habits of camel is:
   a) Grazing
   b) Browsing
   c) Rooting
   d) Pecking

123. Pulse rate of camel is:

a) 10-20/min b) 20-25/min

c) 30-50/min d) 50-70/min

124. RBC of camel swell up to :

a) 240% b) 300%

c) 440% d) 380%

125. Dry matter requirement for camel is :

a) 1.8 to 2%, b) 2.8 to 4%

c) 4-5% d) 5-6.2%

126. Who among the following is known as ship of the desert:

a) Camel b) Yak

c) Horse d) Mithun

127. Life span of camel is :

a) 10-15 years b) 20-40 years

c) 50-60 years d) 70-80 years

128. Dressing percent of camel is :

a) 55-65% b) 70%- 75%

c) 30-45% d) 80%

129. Canine teeth in camel also known as:

a) Wolf teeth b) Tushes

c) None d) Both

130. Sex ratio of camel (Male: Female):

a) 1: 20 b) 1: 30-35

c) 1: 40-45 d) 1: 5

131. Camels breed mostly in which month :

a) Summer b) Winter

c) Rainy d) Autumn

132. A camel can pull _____ percent of its weight:

a) 90% b) 40%

c) 80% d) 100%

133. Slaughter age of camel:

a) 1-2 years b) 2-3 years

c) 3-4 years d) 5-6 years

134. Calving interval in camel is :

a) 500 days b) 775 days

c) 330 days d) 290 days

135. In local language of Rajasthan act of mating is called as:

a) Lakhana b) Makhana

c) Rithana d) None of the above

136. A Specialized inflatable diverticulum of the soft palate called as:
   a) Preen b) Hob
   c) Bulb d) Gula
137. Which animal 's male and female comes to heat:
   a) Mithun b) Yak
   c) Camel d) Horse
138. Glans penis of camel is of what shape:
   a) Hook shape b) Crochet needle
   c) Both d) None
139. Trypanosomiasis in camel is commonly known as:
   a) Surra b) Tibersa
   c) Sool d) Both a and b
140. Breaking and training of camel is done at an age of :
   a) 2-3 years b) 4-6
   c) 7-8 d) 1-2
141. Camel of RBcs are:
   a) Enucleated b) Nucleated
   c) Having Large Nucleus d) All of the above
142. Which of the following is known as "ceremonial ox" or mountain cattle:
   a) Gaur b) Yak
   c) Mithun d) Bison
143. Highest population of yak is present in :
   a) India b) Nepal
   c) USA d) China
144. Monday morning sickness is also known as:
   a) Tryps b) Tetanus
   c) Azoturia/Tying up d) None
145. Horse saddle, headcollar, bridle is put on which side:
   a) Right b) Left
   c) Either d) None
146. Activities done while breaking horse:
   a) Tie one leg up
   b) Make it lie down
   c) Make it around in the round pen until he comes to you
   d) None
147. What is the name for cleaning a horse teeth:
   a) Cleaning b) Loping
   c) Floating d) Brushing

148. Frequency of cleaning horse teeth:

a) Every 1-2 months
b) 1-2 times in a year
c) Every 2nd year
d) Every 7-9 week

149. Where is cannon bone of horse:

a) Between knee and hoof
b) Between ear
c) Top of the tail
d) None

150. Horse just started under saddle training:

a) Green Broke
b) Red Broke
c) Pacer
d) All of these

Answer Key

1	d	2	a	3	a	4	c	5	c	6	c	7	d
8	c	9	c	10	a	11	c	12	b	13	a	14	c
15	b	16	d	17	c	18	a	19	a	20	a	21	b
22	a	23	a	24	c	25	a	26	a	27	a	28	a
29	a	30	a	31	a	32	a	33	a	34	b	35	d
36	a	37	a	38	a	39	c	40	a	41	d	42	b
43	a	44	a	45	a	46	a	47	c	48	b	49	b
50	c	51	b	52	d	53	c	54	d	55	d	56	A
57	A	58	D	59	B	60	A	61	d	62	b	63	a
64	c	65	a	66	b	67	d	68	c	69	c	70	d
71	a	72	a	73	c	74	a	75	a	76	a	77	a
78	a	79	a	80	b	81	b	82	b	83	d	84	b
85		86		87		88		89		90		91	
92		93		94		95		96		97		98	
99		100	c	101	d	102	b	103	d	104	a	105	b
106	b	107	a	108	b	109		110		111		112	
113		114		115		116		117		118		119	
120	a	121		122	b	123	c	124	a	125	a	126	
127	b	128	a	129	b	130	b	131	b	132	b	133	b
134	b	135		136		137		138		139		140	a
141	a	142	c	143	d	144	c	145	b	146	c	147	c
148	b	149	a	150	a	151		152		153		154	

35

Camel and Equine Production Management

Jessy Bagh[1], Annada Das[2], and Kaushik Satyaprakash[3]

[1]Department of Livestock Production and Management, CVSc & AH, OUAT Bhubaneswar, Odisha

[2]Department of Livestock Products Technology, Faculty of Veterinary and Animal Sciences, WBUAFS, Kolkata, West Bengal

[3]Department of Veterinary Public Health and Epidemiology, Faculty of Veterinary and Animal Sciences, RGSC, BHU, Mirzapur, Uttar Pradesh

Introduction

Camel Nomenclature

Family: Camelidae

Order: artiodactyla (even –toed ungulates)

Suborder: Tylopoda (Pad on foot)

The family Camelidae includes two genera: Camelus and Lama The genus Camelus consists of two species namely. Camelus dromedarius (unicorn or dromedary) with habitat in dry, hot, arid areas of Africa, Asia and Australia and Camelus bactrianus Double-humped or Bactrian) habitat in cold, dry areas of the central Palearctic Ecozone. These two species are commonly called Old World camels. The Species belonging to the genus Lama are Lama vicugna Vicunaand Lama guanaco guanaco, Lama glama (llamaand Lama pacos alpaca . These four Species are called New World camels and have their habitat in South America Camels are considered a "ship of the desert" as a means of transport and Towing ability in the desert. The camel also played an important role in civil law and order, defense and battles from antiquity to the present day. Suitable for camels for transport to hot, dry and sandy regions.

Special features of camels

- Camel is considered a mysterious animal due to its extraordinary strength, resist thirst and hunger. They are herbivores by nature
- Fine hairs on the camel's body serve as insulation and help it turn away from heights ambient temperature.
- They owe a greater thickness to their skin, which is why water is lost through evaporation consider less for camels.
- Its hump acts as a storehouse of fatty acids that allow the camel to thrive long under drought conditions.

- The above factors contribute to camels going without drinking water for long periods of time.
- They use more and more water whenever they are available preserved in their body for longer.
- The skin fold hangs from the supraorbital region over the eyes of camels and long eyelashes prevent sand from getting into the eyes during sand flows.
- The bushy hairs present in the ears prevent sand from blowing into the camel's ears.
- Camels can also voluntarily close their nostrils during dust storms.
- Camels have a specific breeding season, the so-called rutting season, which is particularly pronounced in males. It begins in early winter and lasts until spring. Female camels show signs of Heat. During the rutting season, blood androgen levels rise. Male during this time camels make gurgling noises, become violent, chase female camels, grind his teeth, lashes his tail, wags his head and neck, foams at the mouth and urinate, spray urine everywhere. Male camel in rut protruding his palate Valve (DULa Arabic name that occurs in both sexes, but is more developed in men and tongue so that it hangs like a blister, usually on the left side Mouth. Puberty begins in females at the age of 5, and rutting begins in males prominent in 8-15 years. Sex ratio 1: 15-30 (stallion: mare). Pregnancy period 365-410 days. An average adult resting camel consumes about 2 kg; growing, working and lactating animals of 2.5 to 3.00 kg dry matter per 100 kg body weight.

Water management for camels

- Camels each have a drinking capacity of 200 liters. They can withstand dehydration even for a month. A dehydration loss of up to 30% of the body fluctuations in weight and body temperature of up to 6 °C are tolerated without tolerance any inconvenience. A camel's daily water intake is 25 to 35 liters, depending on its needs age, gender, climate and composition of the feed.
- Common diseases of camelsura or trypnosomiasis. This disease is caused by *Trypnosoma evansi*. We can prevent this disease by controlling vectors are flies named Tobanus and Stomoxis. For his treatment, Any antiprotozoal drugs can be used, but most often suramin is used along with the dose
- Rate of 4 mg/kg body weight. Camel milk is characterized by a low fat content (1.5-1.5%). 3% and low protein content (2.5%) have a longer shelf life, a higher ratio of ß-casein to k- Casein, absence of lysozyme C and ß-lactoglobulin and presence of whey acidic protein and peptidoglycan recognition protein. There are reports about it antibacterial and other therapeutic properties.

Horses

Horses include horses, ponies, donkeys, donkeys and their crosses between different species(mules and jennets) and zebras. All these species belong to the family Equidae. The horse is one of the earliest domesticated animal species.Horses are herbivorous monogastric animals.

They have simple stomachs and can digest significant amounts of fiber feeds on the appendix

They have even toes, a gap-free hoof and are quick-footed.

Horse characteristics

Puberty age: 15-24 months

Breeding period: 18 years ± 2 years

Gestation period: 336 ±5 days (average 340 days)

Duration of the estrous cycle: 21 days ± 5 days

Feeding horses:

Horses consume about 1.2 percent dry matter of their body weight when resting condition. At medium load it increases to 2 percent and at heavy load it increases to 3 percent work. Fiber is fed at a rate of 1% of body weight.

Water Requirements: Horses typically consume 20-55 liters of water depending on horse type, age, gender, work intensity, physiology Condition of animals, physical and chemical composition of food and Environmental conditions.

Multiple choice Question

1. Gestational Period of she camel is :
   a) 390 days　　b) 490 days
   c) 290 days　　d) None of the above
2. Camel belongs to order:
   a) Camelidae　　b) Tylopoda
   c) Artiodactyla　　d) Mammalia
3. Camel capable of pulling load equivalent to ________ percent of body weight
   a) 40%　　b) 80%
   c) 90%　　d) 100%
4. Borders of Arabia domesticated Dromedary by:
   a) 500 BC　　b) 1800 BC
   c) 200 BC　　d) 300 BC
5. Llama and Alpaca living in south America is:
   a) Single humped　　b) Doubled humped
   c) Humpless　　d) Triple hump
6. A fermented product prepared from camel milk is :
   a) Sour milk　　b) Sweet curd
   c) Kumiss　　d) Shreekhand
7. Total number of teeth present in camel:
   a) 32-38　　b) 34
   c) 2　　d) 26
8. Maturity of cow camels is at:
   a) 3 years　　b) 2 years
   c) 8 years　　d) 5 years
9. Maturity of male camels is at:
   a) 3 years　　b) 2 years
   c) 8 years　　d) 5 years

10. Average life of camels is :
    a) 10 years
    b) 20-40 years
    c) 80 years
    d) 50 years
11. Rutting period in male camel:
    a) Flaccid Testis
    b) Dry flaccid testis
    c) Turgid testis
    d) None of the above
12. Female camel ovulation is induced by:
    a) Spontaneous
    b) Coitus
    c) Human touch stimulus
    d) None of the above
13. Average length of estrous cycle in camel is:
    a) 3-5 days
    b) 30 days
    c) 7-15 days
    d) 23 days
14. Shape of uterus in female camel is :
    a) Y- shape
    b) A shape
    c) T- shape
    d) Intermediate between Y and T
15. Number of mammary gland in camel is :
    a) 2
    b) 4
    c) 8
    d) 6
16. Organ in camel acts as prehensile organ is:
    a) Teeth
    b) Tongue
    c) Lip
    d) Both B & C
17. A black pigment is secreted from which gland in male camel during rut:
    a) Carpal gland
    b) Orbital gland
    c) Cowper's gland
    d) Pole gland
18. Duration of mating process in camel takes about :
    a) 20-25 hrs
    b) 20-25 mint
    c) 1-2 hrs
    d) 1-2 min
19. Sexual excitement period in camel is known as :
    a) Rut
    b) Thoot
    c) Musth
    d) All of the above
20. Average birth weight in camel is around:
    a) 35- 40 kg
    b) 20-25 kg
    c) 10-15 kg
    d) 50-60 kg
21. Typical sign of pregnancy in camel is :
    a) Cocking of tail
    b) Winking of clitoris
    c) Waxing of teat
    d) All the above
22. What does hump of camel store:
    a) Water
    b) Fat
    c) Protein
    d) Vitamins

23. At position do camel mate:
    a) Sitting
    b) Standing
    c) sleeping
    d) Walking
24. Number of hump present in Bactrian camel:
    a) Single
    b) Double
    c) Both
    d) None
25. The Arabian camel is commonly known as :
    a) Italian
    b) Bactrian
    c) Dromedary
    d) Australia
26. What kind of placenta present in camel:
    a) Intact type
    b) Diffuse (Horse) type
    c) Cotyledonary
    d) Zonary
27. Most of pregnancy in camel is present in :
    a) Left horn of uterus
    b) Right horn of uterus
    c) Both
    d) None
28. Number of toes in each foot of camel:
    a) One
    b) Two
    c) Three
    d) None
29. Salivary glands secretes :
    a) 50-60 litres
    b) 30-40 litres
    c) 10 litres
    d) 100-70 litres
30. A group of camel is known as:
    a) Caravan
    b) Flock
    c) Pack
    d) Colony
31. Which disease in camel is commonly known as "sool" in camel:
    a) Anthrax
    b) Malaria
    c) Trypanosomiasis
    d) Black quarter
32. Features of Adaption in desert for camel:
    a) Fat stored in hump
    b) Slit like nostrils closes during sand stroms
    c) Tough and horny pad on feet
    d) All of the above
33. Best age for breaking or training camel is :
    a) 4-6 years
    b) 1-2 years
    c) 7-8 years
    d) None
34. Age of castration in camel is :
    a) 0-1 years
    b) 1-2 years
    c) 3-4 years
    d) 4-5 years

35. Baby camel is known as:
   a) Foal b) Calf
   c) Kid d) Lamb
36. Rectal temperature of camel is taken when the camel is:
   a) Sitting b) Sleeping
   c) Standing d) Eating
37. Colon acts as major site for ________ reabsorbtion
   a) Salt b) Water
   c) Minerals d) Fat
38. Feeding habits of camel is:
   a) Grazing b) Browsing
   c) Rooting d) Pecking
39. Pulse rate of camel is:
   a) 10-20/min b) 20-25/min
   c) 30-50/min d) 50-70/min
40. RBC of camel swell up to :
   a) 240% b) 300%,
   c) 440% d) 380%
41. Dry matter requirement for camel is :
   a) 1.8 to 2% b) 2.8 to 4%
   c) 4-5% d) 5-6.2%
42. Who among the following is known as ship of the desert:
   a) Camel b) Yak
   c) Horse d) Mithun
43. Life span of camel is :
   a) 10-15 years b) 20-40 years
   c) 50-60 years d) 70-80 years
44. Dressing percent of camel is :
   a) 55-65% b) 70%- 75%
   c) 30-45% d) 80%
45. Canine teeth in camel also known as:
   a) Wolf teeth b) Tushes
   c) None d) Both
46. Sex ratio of camel (Male: Female):
   a) 1: 20 b) 1: 30-35
   c) 1: 40-45 d) 1: 5
47. Camels breed mostly in which month :
   a) Summer b) Winter
   c) Rainy d) Autumn

48. A camel can pull _____percent of its weight:
    a) 90% b) 40%
    c) 80% d) 100%
49. Slaughter age of camel:
    a) 1-2 years b) 2-3 years
    c) 3-4 years d) 5-6 years
50. Calving interval in camel is :
    a) 500 days b) 775 days
    c) 330 days d) 290 days
51. In local language of Rajasthan act of mating is called as:
    a) Lakhana b) Makhana
    c) Rithana d) None of the above
52. A Specialized inflatable diverticulum of the soft palate called as:
    a) Preen b) Hob
    c) Bulb d) Gula
53. Which animal 's male and female comes to heat:
    a) Mithun b) Yak
    c) Camel d) Horse
54. Glans penis of camel is of what shape:
    a) Hook shape b) Crochet needle
    c) Both d) None
55. Trypanosomiasis in camel is commonly known as:
    a) Surra b) Tibersa
    c) Sool d) Both a and b
56. Breaking and training of camel is done at an age of :
    a) 2-3 years b) 4-6
    c) 7-8 d) 1-2
57. Camel of RBcs are:
    a) Enucleated, b) Nucleated
    c) Having Large Nucleus d) All of the above
58. Order of horse belongs:
    a) Perisodactyla b) Tylopoda
    c) Mammalia d) Artiodactyla
59. Methods of identification in horse is :
    a) Ear notching b) Branding
    c) Tagging d) None
60. Branding done for identification of horse is also known as :
    a) Square system of branding, b) Circle system of branding,
    c) Angle system of branding, d) Triangle system of branding

61. Riding test is related to:
    a) Heat detection b) Training of horses
    c) Pregnancy d) None
62. Breeding procedure of horse include:
    a) Hand mating, b) Pasture Mating,
    c) coral mating d) All of the above
63. Galvanye's groove in teeth appear at the age of:
    a) 10-25 years b) 50 years
    c) 60 years d) 70 years
64. Unit of measuring Horse length is:
    a) Leg b) Hand
    c) Finger d) None
65. One hand is equal to:
    a) 10 cm b) 50 cm
    c) 20 inch d) 10 inch
66. Tampering of cups of teeth is also known as:
    a) Winking b) Bishoping
    c) Chewing d) Lordosis
67. Young one of horse is known as:
    a) Foal b) Poult
    c) Kid d) calf
68. Act of mating in horse is known as:
    a) Calving b) Serving
    c) Covering d) Foaling
69. Act of Parturition is known as:
    a) Calving b) Serving
    c) Covering d) Foaling
70. Number of chromosomes in horse:
    a) 64 b) 62
    c) 60 d) 54
71. Male horse known as:
    a) Stallion b) Tordia
    c) Boar d) Jack
72. Female horse is called as:
    a) Mare b) Jenny
    c) Sow d) Doe
73. Mule is cross between :
    a) Jack & Jenny b) Stallion & Mare
    c) Jack and Mare d) Jack & Mare

74. For which disease mallein test is used for diagnosis:
    a) Tetanus b) Glanders
    c) Strangles d) Anthrax
75. Test used for pregnancy diagnosis in horse is :
    a) Cuboni's test b) Mallein test
    c) Both d) None
76. Which disease has symptoms of protrusion of third eye- lid and wooden horse:
    a) Anthrax b) Strangles
    c) Glanders d) Tetanus
77. Sickle shape ear in horse indicates:
    a) Indian blood b) Arabian blood
    c) American blood d) English blood
78. Group of horse is known as :
    a) Pack b) Flock
    c) Band d) Caravan
79. Method of casting used in horse:
    a) Reuffs method b) Alternative method
    c) Sideline method d) None
80. Mare use caslick's operation for :
    a) Prevention of prolapsed vulva b) Colostrum feeding to calf
    c) Restraining d) Rumenotomy
81. Which country use mare's milk for human consumption:
    a) India b) Mongolia
    c) America d) Russia
82. Galvaynes's groove disappear in horse completely at the age of :
    a) 15 years b) 30 years
    c) 20 years d) 25 years
83. Season affects horse reproduction because they are :
    a) Non seasonal breeder b) Short day breeder
    c) Long day breeder d) None
84. Female mule is called as:
    a) Hinny b) Zony
    c) Molly d) Hule
85. Difference between ponies and horses is :
    a) Chromosomes b) Age
    c) Colour d) Height
86. Gestation period in horse:
    a) 330-345 days b) 280-290 days
    c) 14 -120 days d) 500-700 days

87. Galvayne's groove appears in which teeth of horse:
    a) Upper corner incisor b) Lower middle incisor
    c) Upper first molar d) Lower middle incisor
88. Wolf teeth found in some of the horses are :
    a) Incisor b) Molar
    c) Premolar d) Canine
89. Gall bladder is absent in :
    a) Horse b) Buffalo
    c) Sheep d) Cow
90. In which place horse are kept:
    a) Stable b) Shed
    c) Kennel d) None
91. Which species has dental star:
    a) Horse b) Cattle
    c) Pig d) Poultry
92. Sound produced by Ass is called as:
    a) Braying b) Neigh
    c) Whinny d) Grunting
93. Sound produced by horse is known as:
    a) Neigh b) Grunting
    c) Whinny d) Braying
94. Horse refusing habit to move forward is known as:
    a) Jibbing b) Whinny
    c) Braying d) Grunting
95. Formula for calculating body weight of horse is :
    a) $GL^2/300$ b) $GL^2/330$
    c) Both d) None
96. Single hoof is the characteristics of :
    a) Goat b) Horse
    c) Pig d) Cattle
97. Colic is very common in which animal:
    a) Goat b) Horse
    c) Pig d) Cattle
98. Types of gait in horse is:
    a) Trot b) Gallop
    c) Canter d) All of the these
99. Animal commonly used in polo game:
    a) Goat b) Horse
    c) Pig d) Cattle

100. Monday morning sickness is also known as:
   a) Tryps b) Tetanus
   c) Azoturia/Tying up d) All of these
101. Horse saddle, headcollar, bridle is put on which side:
   a) Right b) Left
   c) Either d) None
102. Activities done while breaking horse:
   a) Tie one leg up
   b) Make it lie down
   c) Make it around in the round pen until he comes to you
   d) None
103. What is the name for cleaning horse teeth:
   a) Cleaning b) Loping
   c) Floating d) Brushing
104. Frequency of cleaning horse teeth:
   a) Every 1-2 months b) 1-2 times in a year
   c) Every 2nd year d) Every 7-9 week
105. Where is cannon bone of horse:
   a) Between knee and hoof b) Between ear
   c) Top of the tail d) None
106. Castrated male horse is called as:
   a) Geld b) Stallion
   c) Jack d) Gimmer
107. Horse just started under saddle training:
   a) Green Broke b) Red Broke
   c) Pacer d) All of These
108. Young horse less than four years of age is called as:
   a) Filly b) Foal
   c) Hinny d) Mare
109. Person who trims horse feet is known as:
   a) Farrier b) Shoer
   c) Smith d) All the above
110. Term used for a horseback rider or any person involved with horses:
   a) Equestrian b) Farrier
   c) Either d) None
111. Where are the horse's two blind spots:
   a) Directly in front of nose b) Directly behind his tail
   c) Both d) None

112. Spongy Triangular pad at the bottom of a horse's hoof is called as:
 a) Frog b) Sole
 c) Wall d) None

113. To what range a horse rotate its ears:
 a) 180° b) 360 °
 c) 90 ° d) None

114. Number of eyelids present in horses:
 a) 3 b) 5
 c) 7 d) 1

115. What is the response called as when horse pulls his lips back to sniff:
 a) The flehmen response b) Butting
 c) Rooting d) Mounting

116. What kind of stomach horse have:
 a) Simple b) Ruminant
 c) Pseudoruminant d) All of the above

117. Age at which horse is considered fully developed is :
 a) 6 years b) 3 years
 c) 4 years d) 8 years

118. Body part most commonly cause Lameness:
 a) Hoof b) Knee
 c) Cannon d) Pelvic

119. In advance pregnancy and lactation the protein requirement in mare should be :
 a) Increase b) Decrease
 c) First increase then decreases d) None

120. What type of retina is present in horse:
 a) Ramp b) Flat
 c) Round d) All of the above

121. Estrus cycle length in mare:
 a) 21 days b) 40 days
 c) 35 days d) 52 days

122. Duration of heat in mare:
 a) 1-2 hrs b) 21 hrs
 c) 1-2 days d) 7-9 days

123. Mare with normal ovary function but showing no sign of heat is known as:
 a) Silent heat b) Aggressive heat
 c) Buller heat d) None

124. Age of puberty in horse:
 a) 1-2 years b) 5 years
 c) 7 years d) 4 years

125. Which horse's foot structure got nature of anti-concussion and anti slipping is:
 a) Hock b) Frog
 c) Hoof d) Knee

126. Which of following qualities help horse to tolerate urea like ruminants:
 a) Caecum well developed
 b) Rumen absent
 c) Stomach and diaphragm very close
 d) All of the above

127. Adult un- castrated horse which is not used for breeding purposes is known as:
 a) Entire b) Jenny
 c) Filly d) Cob

128. Young mature male horse known as:
 a) Colt b) Jack
 c) Filly d) Buck

129. Horse is native of which country:
 a) North America b) Scotland
 c) Russia d) Australia

130. Horse pulse is measured from:
 a) Maxillary artery b) Jugular vein
 c) femoral artery d) Abdominal artery

131. Normal pulse rate of horse:
 a) 36-42 b) 10-15
 c) 15-22 d) 60-76

132. Guttural pouch in race horse acts as: Heart cooler,
 a) Brain cooler b) Lung cooler
 c) None d) Both

133. Guttural pouch in horse is:
 a) Small valve in heart b) Out- pocketing of stomach
 c) Out –pocketing of lung d) Out-pocketing of Eustachian tube

134. Grooming in horse improves: Cleanliness,
 a) Appearance b) Blood circulation
 c) Both a and b d) Itching

135. Saddling commonly done in which species:
 a) Horse b) Elephant
 c) Racing dog d) Bull

136. Hogging means :
 a) Clipping of tail b) Clipping of mane
 c) Shaving of hind quarter d) Clipping of nose

137. Hair of horse mane projected on forehead is known as:
a) Forelock b) Hock
c) Chestnut d) Frog

138. Stud is :
a) Castrated male b) Female below one year of age
c) Stallion used for breeding, d) Female horse above 3 years of age

139. Movement of horse head is known as :
a) Nodding b) Wagging
c) Both, N d) One

140. Chestnut in horse is :
a) Horny irregular growth b) Covering
c) Long tail d) Spot in nostril

141. One stallion usually kept with :
a) 80-100 mares b) 100-120 mares
c) 30-40 mares d) 60-70 mares

142. Which test detects "Equine infectious anaemia":
a) Coggins test b) Mallein's test
c) Cuboni's test d) All of the above

143. A white patch on forehead of horse is known as:
a) Snip b) Blaze
c) Star d) Stripe

144. White marking covering whole forehead up to muzzle in horse is called as:
a) Blaze b) Snip
c) Star d) Strip

145. Fodder best for horse as it is rich in protein and calcium is :
a) Barley b) Maize
c) Lucerne d) Oat

146. Number of beats heard in walk, trot, canter, and gallop is :
a) 4,2,3, and 4 respectively b) 1,2,3 and 4 respectively
c) 2,2,3 and 4 respectively d) 4,3,2,1 respectively

147. Common vices of horse are:
a) Crib bitting b) Wind sucking
c) Both d) None

148. Centre of gravity in horse resides in:
a) Centre of barrel b) Centre of rib cage
c) At head between ear d) Centre of Rump

149. Arabian horse is usually what colour:
a) Bay b) Grey
c) Chestnut d) All of the above

150. Life span of horse:

a) 25-30 years

b) 50-60 years

c) 10 years

d) 80 years

Answer Key

1	a	2	c	3	a	4	c	5	c	6	c	7	b
8	a	9	d	10	b	11	b	12	d	13	a	14	c
15	b	16	c	17	d	18	b	19	d	20	a	21	a
22	b	23	a	24	b	25	c	26	b	27	a	28	b
29	a	30	a	31	a	32	d	33	b	34	b	35	b
36	a	37	b	38	b	39	c	40	a	41	a	42	a
43	b	44	a	45	b	46	b	47	b	48	b	49	b
50	b	51	a	52	d	53	c	54	a	55	d	56	a
57	a	58	b	59	c	60	c	61	a	62	d	63	a
64	b	65	a	66	b	67	a	68	c	69	d	70	
71	a	72	a	73	d	74	b	75	a	76	d	77	b
78	a	79	c	80	a	81	b	82	c	83	c	84	c
85	d	86	a	87	a	88	c	89	a	90	a	91	a
92	a	93	a	94	a	95	b	96	b	97	b	98	d
99	b	100	d	101	b	102	c	103	c	104	b	105	a
106	a	107	a	108	a	109	d	110	a	111	c	112	a
113	a	114	a	115	a	116	a	117	a	118	a	119	a
120	a	121	a	122	a	123	a	124	a	125	c	126	a
127	a	128	a	129	a	130	a	131	a	132	a	133	d
134	c	135	a	136	b	137	a	138	c	139	a	140	a
141	c	142	a	143	c	144	a	145		146	a	147	c
148	b	149	d	150	a								

36

Wildlife and Zoo Animal Management

***Sindhu K.*[1] *and Tanmoy Rana*[2]**

[1]*Department of AHVS, Government of Karnataka, Karnataka*

[2]*Department of Veterinary Clinical Complex, West Bengal University of Animal & Fishery Sciences, Kolkata, West Bengal*

Introduction

This chapters covers wide range of topics like taxonomy of wild animals, difference criteria among the species identification, feeding and nutritional requirements of wild and captive zoo animals, housing standards in zoo, habitats and behavioral changes and its management, environmental impact on captive animals, acts and zoo regulations governing wild and captive animals, handling and restraining of wild/captive animals, Purpose of restraining, techniques of immobilization and complications associated with the immobilization. Various national and international organizations working on wildlife conservation. In-situ/ ex-situ conservation projects undertaken by government of India

The MCQ on Wildlife and Zoo animal management

1. The Father of Taxonomy
   a) De Candolle b) Louis Pasteur
   c) Carl Linnaeus d) Paul Ehrlich
2. Taxonomic classification sequence
   a) Kingdom, Phylum, Class, Order, Family, Genus & Species
   b) Phylum, Kingdom, Class, Family, Order, Genus & Species
   c) Species, Family, Kingdom, Order, Phylum, Class & Genus
   d) Class, Order, Genus, Kingdom, Phylum, Family & Species
3. Which Phylum contains all animals with backbones
   a) Phylum – Echinodermata b) Phylum – Arthropoda
   c) Phylum – Chordata d) Phylum – Annelida
4. The Scientific name of Cheetah is
   a) Acinonyx b) Panthera
   c) Neofelis d) Felis
5. *Panthera onca* is the scientific name of
   a) Lion b) Tiger
   c) Leopard d) Jaguar

6. The odd-toed ungulates belongs to order
   a) Artiodactyla b) Marsupialia
   c) Perissodactyla d) Proboscidea
7. The largest primate existing on earth is
   a) Gibbons b) African Gorilla
   c) Chimpanzee d) Orangutan
8. The scientific name of the national animal of India is
   a) Felis domesticus b) Panthera leo
   c) Felis tigris d) Acinonyx jubatus
9. The National bird of India is
   a) Pea-hen b) Pea-cock
   c) Indian roller d) The great Indian bustard
10. The national aquatic animal of India is
   a) Rohu b) Olive riddle turtles
   c) Malabar gliding frog d) The gangetic river dolphin
11. Recognition of Zoo Rules, 2008 was enacted as per
   a) The Wildlife (Protection) Act 1972 b) PCA act 1960
   c) The constitution of India article 51 d) ABC rules 2023
12. India belongs to which zoogeographical regions of the world
   a) Palaearctic b) Neotropical
   c) Afrotropic or Ethiopian d) Indo-Malayan or Oriental
13. ________ works to prevent the global trade of wildlife
   a) UNO b) UNICEF
   c) CITES d) ZOO
14. The 4 categories of the Protected Areas in India are
   a) National Parks, Sanctuaries,
   b) Conservation Reserves and Community Reserves.
   c) Both A & B
   d) None of the above
15. IUCN stands for
   a) Indian Union for Conservation of Nature
   b) International Union for Common Nations
   c) Intercontinental Union for Conservation of Nature
   d) International Union for Conservation of Nature and Natural Resources
16. A National Board for Wildlife was established and chaired by ________________ of India to provide policy framework for wildlife conservation
   a) The President
   b) The Prime Minister
   c) The MoEF&CC Ministry
   d) The Chief Minister of concerned state

17. The Indian Constitution entails the subject of forests and wildlife in……...
    a) The Concurrent list
    b) The central list
    c) The state list
    d) All of the above
18. India's first National Park
    a) Keoladeo National Park
    b) Bandipur National Park
    c) Kaziranga National park
    d) Jim Corbett National Park
19. The total number of Wildlife Sanctuaries in India are
    a) 537
    b) 490
    c) 990
    d) 250
20. A Biosphere Reserve contains
    a) Transition zone
    b) Buffer zone
    c) Core zone
    d) All of the above
21. ____ number of Biosphere Reserves are present in India
    a) 20
    b) 15
    c) 18
    d) 25
22. A type of habitat in biosphere where the organisms live deep inside the oceans
    a) Pelagic
    b) Benthic
    c) Lentic
    d) Lotic
23. A type of habitat in biosphere where the organisms/ animals living at junction of sea and rivers
    a) Terrestrial habitat
    b) Estuarine habitat
    c) Marine habitat
    d) Freshwater habitat
24. Minimum size of outdoor enclosure (per pair) required for Tigers is
    a) 1000 sq mtr
    b) 500 sq mtr
    c) 750 sq mtr
    d) 1500 sq mtr
25. Minimum size of outdoor enclosure required for Indian Brow antlered deer is
    a) 2000 sq mtr
    b) 500 sq mtr
    c) 4000 sq mtr
    d) 1500 sq mtr
26. Minimum size of outdoor enclosure required for Himalayan black bear,
    a) 1000 sq mtr
    b) 2500 sq mtr
    c) 750 sq mtr
    d) 1500 sq mtr
27. Minimum size of outdoor enclosure required for One-horned Indian Rhinoceros
    a) 2000 sq mtr
    b) 500 sq mtr
    c) 4000 sq mtr
    d) 1500 sq mtr
28. Minimum size of outdoor enclosure required for Jackal, Wolf and Wild dog
    a) 200 sq mtr
    b) 500 sq mtr
    c) 400 sq mtr
    d) 750 sq mtr
29. Minimum size of the Aviary required for Flying birds (mixed species enclosure)
    a) 200 sq mtr
    b) 500 sq mtr
    c) 400 sq mtr
    d) 300 sq mtr

30. Minimum size of outdoor enclosure required for Crocodile/ Gharial
    a) 800 sq mtr
    b) 500 sq mtr
    c) 400 sq mtr
    d) 750 sq mtr
31. Minimum size of enclosure required for phyton
    a) 80 sq mtr
    b) 50 sq mtr
    c) 40 sq mtr
    d) 75 sq mtr
32. Area of the zoo (hectares) required for the large zoo is
    a) 75
    b) 35
    c) 10
    d) 10 or less
33. No. of visitors in a year (in lakhs) for the medium sized zoo is
    a) 7.5
    b) 3.5
    c) 1.0
    d) Less than 1
34. No. of endangered species to be kept in small zoo are
    a) 5
    b) 4
    c) 3
    d) 2
35. The total land area under moat should not exceed _____ of the land area of the enclosure
    a) 10%
    b) 20%
    c) 25%
    d) 30%
36. Which among the following is digitigrade carnivora
    a) Otters
    b) Civets
    c) Bears
    d) Wolf
37. Which among the following is plantigrade carnivora
    a) Dogs
    b) Cats
    c) Armadillos
    d) Skunks
38. Porcupine belongs to order
    a) Primates
    b) Carnivora
    c) Rodentia
    d) Omnivore
39. Which among these belongs to order Artiodactyla
    a) Bovidae
    b) Cervidae
    c) Suidae
    d) All of the above
40. Which among these are called barking deer
    a) Muntjack
    b) Barasingha
    c) Cheetal
    d) Chevrotain
41. Which among these deer exhibit nocturnal behavior
    a) Swamp deer
    b) Spotted deer
    c) Mouse deer
    d) Musk deer
42. The order Carnivora can be broken down into Family
    a) Canidae
    b) Hyaenidae
    c) Mustelidae
    d) All of the above

43. The family Felidae, can be broken down into Genus
    a) Genus Acinonyx
    b) Genus Panthera
    c) Genus Neofelis
    d) All of the above
44. The dorsal covering of the tortoise is known as
    a) Hard shell
    b) Crude shell
    c) Carapace
    d) Plastron
45. The complete restriction of muscular activity or immobilization is
    a) Hyperkalemia
    b) Hypocalcemia
    c) Hypercalcemia
    d) Hypokinesia
46. SAZARC stands for
    a) South East Asian Zoos Association
    b) South Asian Zoo Association for Regional Cooperation
    c) South African Association of Zoological Gardens and Aquaria
    d) Canadian Association of Zoos and Aquariums
47. Fasting without access to food for __________ hours in a week are a part of the Lion feeding Management.
    a) 12
    b) 18
    c) 24
    d) 48
48. ________ remains the best model for establishing dietary composition parameters for both cheetahs and tigers
    a) Domestic dogs
    b) Feral pigs
    c) Wild dogs
    d) Domestic cats
49. Fasting of captive felids followed by CZA is _____
    a) Once in a week
    b) Twice a week
    c) Once in a month
    d) Alternate days
50. Wild Asian elephants eat ____ of body weight
    a) 5%
    b) 3%
    c) 10%
    d) 2%
51. Crocodiles are _______ predators
    a) Ambush
    b) Rooster
    c) Loafing
    d) Apex
52. The sub adult crocodiles consume ______ of their body weight a week
    a) 6-7 %
    b) 7-8 %
    c) 8-10 %
    d) 10-12 %
53. the diet of Giraffe should contain less than ____ starch
    a) 10%
    b) 20%
    c) 30%
    d) 40%
54. The process of growing antlers increases a (Male deer) buck's energy requirement by____
    a) 44%
    b) 33%
    c) 22%
    d) .11%

55. ____________ is the herbivore non ruminant animals
 a) Hippopotamus b) Barasingha
 c) Guar d) Sambar deer
56. The protein requirement of captive primates is ______
 a) 15% b) 20%
 c) 25% d) 30%
57. Which among the following are direct method of wild animal census
 a) Sample animal census b) Aerial count method
 c) Wate hole count method d) All of the above
58. Which among the following are indirect method of wild animal census
 a) Kill evidence count method b) Counting of tracks method
 c) Fecal deposit count method d) All of the above
59. Tiger census include __________ following methods
 a) Pug mark & trap camera method b) Pop/Scat identification method
 c) Radio collar method d) All of the above
60. POP cast method is used to extract_______
 a) Pug marks b) Poops / Scat identification
 c) Scratch marks d) None of the above
61. claws in pug marks impression represents _____ species
 a) Felids b) Canids
 c) Probosidae d) Suidae
62. The PML (pug mark length) of full-grown adult tiger is
 a) 10 cms b) 10-12 cms
 c) 15-17 cms d) Less than 10 cms
63. Pelleted scat is observed in ____
 a) Ungulates b) Carnivores
 c) Wild Canids d) Wild Felids
64. Tubular large scat is observed in __________
 a) Wild canids b) Wild felids
 c) Both a & b d) Equids
65. The differentiating feature which separates ivory from bamboo is
 a) Xylem & phloem b) Horizontal lines
 c) Vertical lines d) Cross hatched lines/Schreger lines
66. Which among the following is not a physical method of restraining the wild animals
 a) Dart pistols b) Trap/ squeeze cages
 c) Lassos/ catch pole d) Leather gloves
67. The remote drug delivery system employed in wild animals are
 a) Pole syringes b) Blow pipes
 c) Dart pistols & Dart rifles d) All of the above
68. The dart needle 2.0 mm x 30 mm size is used to dart
 a) Elephants b) Young deers
 c) Lions & Tigers d) Wild dogs

69. The CO_2 Injection pistol covers the distance range of ________
   a) 1 to 20 meters b) 1 to 30 meters
   c) 1 to 40 meters d) 1 to 50 meters

70. The CO_2 Injection rifle covers the distance range of ________
   a) 1 to 50 meters b) 1 to 75 meters
   c) 1 to 100 meters d) 1 to 125 meters

71. The blow pipe projectors covers the distance range of ________
   a) 1 to 10 meters b) 1 to 20 meters
   c) 1 to 30 meters d) 1 to 40 meters

72. In the power loaded rifles; the thumb rule of CO_2 pressure: distance travelled is ___
   a) 2 bars: 5 meters b) 2 bars: 7 meters
   c) 2 bars: 9 meters d) 2 bars: 11 meters

73. Excertional myopathy Capture myopathy condition is commonly encountered in ________
   a) Wild canids b) Wild ungulates
   c) Wild felids d) Wild rodents

74. The antidote used for xylazine reversal is
   a) Desferrioxamine b) Salbutamol
   c) Chlorpromazine d) Yohimbine

75. The potent opioid agonist used in sedation of elephant
   a) Etorpine b) Morphine
   c) Oxymorphone d) Hydromorphone

76. Immobilon LA contents are________
   a) Meditomidine & Ketamine b) Diazepam & Xylazine
   c) Xylazine & Ketamine d) Etorphine hcl & Acepromazine

77. Which among the following is not a Long-Acting Neuroleptics (LAN)
   a) Acepromazine b) Haloperidol
   c) Zuclopenthixol d) Meditomidine

78. The Prevention of Cruelty to Animals Act was implemented in the year
   a) 1947 b) 1950
   c) 1960 d) 1972

79. The Wildlife Act was enacted in the year
   a) 1972 b) 1982
   c) 1960 d) 1990

80. The IUCN stands for
   a) Indian Union for Conservation of nature
   b) International Organization for Natural Conservation
   c) International Understanding for The Conservation of Natural Resources
   d) International Union for the Conservation of Nature and Natural Resources

81. The only living members of which are being kept in captivity or as a naturalized population outside its historic range is termed as
   a) Extinct
   b) Extinct in wild
   c) Critically Endangered
   d) Endangered
82. The international network for monitoring wildlife trade is
   a) WTC
   b) Trade & Commerce chamber
   c) UNESCO
   d) TRAFFIC
83. TRAFFIC stands for
   a) Trade Record Analysis of Flora & Fauna in Commerce International
   b) Trade Record Analysis of Fruits and Fruit Byproducts International
   c) The Trade Assessment of Fauna and Flora in International Commencement
   d) None of the above
84. CITES stands for
   a) Congress on International Trade enforcements
   b) Committee on International Trade in Extinct Species of Wildlife
   c) Convention on International Trade in Endangered Species of Wild Fauna and Flora
   d) All of the above
85. UNESCO's initiative MAB stands for
   a) Mammal Animals Biosphere program
   b) Man and the Animal Biosphere program
   c) Marine and the Biosphere program
   d) Man and the Biosphere program
86. An international treaty adopted at the Earth Summit in Rio de Janeiro
   a) Convention on Biological Diversity
   b) UNESCO's initiative MAB
   c) TRAFFIC
   d) CITES
87. Convention on the Conservation of Migratory Species of Wild Animals is also known as
   a) The Ramsar Convention
   b) The Bonn Convention
   c) Convention on Biological Diversity
   d) International Convention for the Regulation of Whaling
88. The Convention on Wetlands of International Importance is popularly known as
   a) The Ramsar Convention
   b) The Bonn Convention
   c) Convention on Biological Diversity
   d) The Washington convention
89. WWF stands for
   a) World Wrestling Formation
   b) World Wildlife Federation
   c) Wildlife World for Fun
   d) World Wide Fund for Nature

90. An agreement under which industrialized countries will reduce their collective emissions of greenhouse gases
   a) UNESCO's initiative MAB
   b) Agenda 21
   c) Kyoto Protocol
   d) World Summit on Sustainable Development (WSSD)

91. ___________ the apex advisory body in the field of Wildlife Conservation in the country
   a) Animal Welfare Board of India
   b) Indian Board for Wildlife
   c) Friends of the Earth International
   d) All of the above

92. Which among the following are National conservation projects
   a) Project Tiger
   b) Project Elephant
   c) GOI UNDP Sea Turtle Project
   d) All of the above

93. Total number of chapters in The Indian Wildlife (Protection) Act, 1972
   a) III Chapters
   b) V Chapters
   c) VII Chapters
   d) IX Chapters

94. The conservation of genetic resources in natural populations of plant or animal species is
   a) *In-situ conservation*
   b) Ex-situ conservation
   c) State of the art conservation
   d) All of the above

95. The Biosphere reserve which covers forests of Tamil Nadu, Kerala and Karnataka is
   a) Suderbans
   b) Pachmarhi
   c) Agasthyamalai
   d) **Nilgiri**

96. The Kanchanjunga biosphere reserve is present in
   a) Himachal
   b) Assam
   c) Sikkim
   d) Nagaland

97. Which law made teak wood a government property
   a) The Madras Wild Elephant Preservation Act -1873
   b) The Indian Forest Act – 1865
   c) The Environment Protection Act, 1986
   d) The Wildlife (Protection) Act, 1972

98. ___________ the first wildlife legislation in Modern India
   a) The Madras Wild Elephant Preservation Act -1873
   b) The Prevention of Cruelty to Animals Act - 1960
   c) The Environment Protection Act, 1986
   d) The Wildlife (Protection) Act, 1972

99. Total number of biological hot spot in India
   a) 1
   b) 2
   c) 3
   d) 4

100. __________ issued guidelines for tourism and management of tiger reserves in India
   a) The National Tiger Conservation Authority
   b) WII
   c) AWBI
   d) Tourism department

Answer Key

1	c	2	a	3	c	4	d	5	c	6	c	7	b
8	c	9	b	10	d	11	a	12	d	13	c	14	c
15	d	16	b	17	a	18	d	19	a	20	d	21	c
22	b	23	b	24	a	25	d	26	a	27	a	28	c
29	d	30	c	31	a	32	a	33	b	34	c	35	b
36	c	37	a	38	c	39	d	40	a	41	c	42	d
43	d	44	c	45	d	46	b	47	c	48	d	49	a
50	d	51	a	52	c	53	a	54	c	55	a	56	c
57	d	58	d	59	d	60	a	61	b	62	c	63	a
64	c	65	d	66	a	67	d	68	c	69	b	70	d
71	a	72	a	73	b	74	d	75	a	76	d	77	d
78	c	79	a	80	d	81	b	82	d	83	a	84	c
85	d	86	a	87	b	88	a	89	d	90	c	91	b
92	d	93	c	94	a	95	d	96	c	97	b	98	a
99	b	100	a										

37

Poultry Production and Management

***Amitava Roy*[1], *Tanmoy Rana*[2], and *Probhakar Biswas*[3]**

[1]*Department of Livestock Farm Complex, West Bengal University of Animal & Fishery Sciences, Kolkata, West Bengal*

[2]*Department of Veterinary Clinical Complex, West Bengal University of Animal & Fishery Sciences, Kolkata, West Bengal*

[3]*Department of Avian Sciences, West Bengal University of Animal & Fishery Sciences, Kolkata, West Bengal*

Introduction

The review provides an explanation of the Indian poultry market's trend in management. Everything you need to know about diseases, their attacks, processing, production, feeding, and market trends is included in this review. For farmers, raising poultry is a vital source of revenue that allows them to meet their basic necessities. Because of the high consumption rate and current population growth, there is a sharp increase in demand for chicken meat. Meat consumption is required to provide additional nutritious intake. Generally speaking, the poultry sector plays a critical role in creating micro and macrobusiness opportunities and enhancing human nutrition. The Indian economy is dominated by small-scale commercial ventures for women and the delivery of manure for agricultural purposes. Animal health is ensured by the supply of high-quality feed, which maintains nutritional values. The weight and age of the chickens, their rate of development, the quantity of eggs they produce, the climate (cold or rainy weather increases energy consumption), and the amount of nutrition they acquire from foraging all affect how much feed and how much nutrition it contains. This review article includes general information about poultry products as well as details on food grade, diseases that affect poultry, and pest control.

1. Pre-brooding management refers to the several procedures used to raise recently hatched chicks.

   a) Before arriving at farm b) After arriving at farm

   c) At the age of two weeks d) At the age four week

2. The shed chosen for brooding needs to be separated from the other shed by a minimum of

   a) 60 Foot b) 100 Foot

   c) 180 Foot d) 140 Foot

3. To reduce chances of microbial growth in shed, wall should be cemented from ground at a distance of

   a) 2.0-2.5 Foot b) 3.0-3.5 Foot

   c) 2.5-3.0 Foot d) 3.5-4.0 Foot

4. After being removed, the equipment should be cleaned with a brush and then treated with a disinfectant.
   a) $KMnO_4$ b) Formalin
   c) Hot water d) Cold water

5. Shed should preferably be clean and disinfected
   a) One week before arrival of chick
   b) Two weeks before arrival of chicks
   c) Three weeks before arrival of chicks
   d) Four weeks before arrival of chicks

6. In case of cold weather, brooder should be turned on at least
   a) 8 hours before arrival b) 10 hours before arrival
   c) 12 hours before arrival d) 20 hours before arrival

7. Chick guards should stay away from the brooder edge at a distance of
   a) 1-2 Foot b) 2-3 Foot
   c) 3-4 Foot d) 4-5 Foot

8. It is recommended to use antibiotics for early chick mortality in order to
   a) 1-3 days b) 3-5 days
   c) 5-7 days d) 7-9 days

9. When the chicks arrive at the farm, there should be a two-inch layer of litter underneath them.
   a) Single layer of paper b) Double layer of paper
   c) Triple layer of papers d) None of the above

10. Special care and management of baby chicks until they do not require artificial source
    a) Brooding b) Rearing
    c) Laying d) All of the above

11. A brooding system where each individual brooder can hold between 300 and 400 chicks is referred as
    a) Colony brooder system b) Continuous brooder
    c) System Battery brooding d) Tier brooding

12. A large number of chicks are brooded at once in a single house under a practice termed as
    a) Colony brooder system b) Continuous brooder system
    c) Battery brooding d) Tier brooding

13. During first three weeks of chick's life litter should have slight moisture and after that it should contain about
    a) 10% moisture b) 15% moisture
    c) 20% moisture d) 25% moisture

14. Paper is placed on the litter during the first few days of a chick's existence, and it should be taken off after
    a) 1-2 days b) 2-3 days
    c) 3-4 days d) 4-5 days

15. When chicks discover where the extra heat is coming from, the guard needs to be extended to cover a larger region on

a) First day
b) Second day
c) Third day
d) Fourth day

16. During the first week, the temperature should be comfortable at a point that is two inches above the litter's floor and six inches outside the canopy

a) 75 °F
b) 85 °F
c) 95 °F
d) 105 °F

17. The brooder temperature should be reduced by 5 °F weekly according to the age but not beyond

a) 75 °F
b) 85 °F
c) 95 °F
d) 105 °F

18. Male chicks in a breeder flock should be kept at a higher temperature than female chicks when they are being raised

a) 02-05 °F
b) 05-08 °F
c) 08-10 °F
d) 10-11 °F

19. Birds feces contain approximately moisture %

a) 55-60
b) 65-70
c) 75-80
d) 85-90

20. Level of CO at which poisoning can occur in the chicks is

a) 0.01%
b) 0.02%
c) 0.03%
d) 0.04%

21. Genetics is the science devoted to the study of

a) Resemblance
b) Offspring
c) Inheritance
d) Parents

22. Basic constituent of all living material

a) Gene
b) Cell
c) Chromosome
d) Tissue

23. The part of cell which is responsible for transmission of hereditary factors is

a) Cell wall
b) Cytoplasm
c) Nucleus
d) Protoplasm

24. How many types of cells according to their function

a) 02
b) 3
c) 04
d) 05

25. Cell that compose the tissues of the body are

a) Auto cells
b) Sex cells
c) Functional cells
d) Somatic cells

26. Rod like structures within the nucleus are

a) Gene
b) Reticulum
c) Chromosome
d) Chlorophyll

27. Total pairs of chromosomes in chicken are
    a) 38 b) 39
    c) 40 d) 41
28 Evidently the pairs of macro chromosomes are
    a) 04 b) 06
    c) 08 d) 10
29. Number of pairs of micro chromosomes are
    a) 33 b) 34
    c) 35 d) 36
30. Types of chromosomes are
    a) 02 b) 04
    c) 06 d) 08
31. History of birds is as old as
    a) 100 million years ago b) 125 million years ago
    c) 150 million years ago d) 175 million years ago
32. The first bird on earth was
    a) Red Jungle Fowl b) Archaeopteryx
    c) Gallus domesticus d) Gallus gallus
33. The species that modern poultry most likely developed from is
    a) Green jungle fowl b) Grey jungle fowl
    c) Red jungle fowl d) Black jungle fowl
34. Domestication of chicken stated in China
    a) 8000 BC b) 2500 BC
    c) 2000 BC d) None of these
35. Domestication of chicken started in Indus valley
    a) 2500 BC b) 2000 BC
    c) 1500 BC d) 1200 BC
36. Birds were used first not for food purpose but for
    a) Religious purpose b) Cock fighting
    c) Entertainment d) All of the above
37. Cock fighting was banned due to cruelty in
    a) 1800 A.D. b) 1850 A.D.
    c) 1900 A.D. d) 1950 A.D.
38. American Poultry Association started its work in
    a) 1870 b) 1871
    c) 1872 d) 1873
39. A collection of common breeds developed in a certain area are referred to as
    a) Breed b) Strain
    c) Class d) Genus
40. Number of classes of poultry are
    a) Three b) Four
    c) Five d) Six

41. Loss of appetite and weight occur due to Aflatoxin level in feed (ppm) @
 a) 0.055 b) 0.065
 c) 0.075 d) 0.085

42. Aflatoxin levels in feed cause a severe decline in growth and productivity as well as mortality (ppm) @
 a) 10.00 b) 20.00
 c) 30.00 d) 40.00

43. Loss in weight and emaciated flocks occur due to Ochratoxin level in feed (ppm) @
 a) 0.50 b) 1.00
 c) 1.50 d) 2.00

44. Ochratoxin level in feed (ppm) causes mortality to begin, emaciated flocks to become less productive, and output to decline @
 a) 10.00 b) 20.00
 c) 30.00 d) 40.00

45. Loss in weight with liver damage occur due to Citranin level in feed (ppm) @
 a) 10 b) 20
 c) 30 d) 40

46. Pronounced hemorrhages in intestine occur due Citranin level in feed (ppm) @
 a) 100 b) 150
 c) 200 d) 250

47. The amount of trichothecenes in feed (ppm) causes fat on the liver, mouth ulcers, and a decrease in production @
 a) 05 b) 10
 c) 15 d) 20

48. Gizzard ulcers, enlarged kidneys, pale comb, and death are caused by the amount of trichothecenes (ppm) in feed @
 a) 05 b) 10
 c) 15 d) 25

49. Loss in weight and production, anemia and pale comb occur due to Zeralenone level in feed (ppm) @
 a) 050 b) 100
 c) 150 d) 200

50. Ascites means
 a) Mortality due to higher CO_2 level in environment
 b) Belly of bird containing water
 c) Toxicity due to higher NH_3 level in environment
 d) Higher level of citric acid in blood of the bird

51. When the level of NaCl in the laying diet is low, feed intake and egg production decrease
 a) 05% b) 10%
 c) 15% d) 20%

52. Lethal dose of $KMnO_4$ for the chicken body weight is
a) 02 g/kg b) 04 g/kg
c) 06 g/kg d) 08 g/kg

53. Renyl powder is an example of
a) Disinfectant b) Antibacterial
c) Diuretic d) Antiparasitic

54. Causative organism of Pullorum disease is
a) Salmonella galinarum b) Salmonella pullorum
c) Salmonella typhimorium d) Salmonella entridis

55. Causative organism of Typhoid disease is
a) Salmonella galinarum b) Salmonella pullorum
c) Salmonella typhimorium d) Salmonella entridis

56. Causative organism of Omphalistis disease may be
a) Salmonella typhimorium b) Salmonella pullorum
c) Salmonella sporogenes d) Salmonella entridis

57. Causative organism of Infectious Coryza disease is
a) Salmonella galinarum b) Hemophilus para gallinarum
c) Salmonella sporogenes d) Salmonella entridis

58. Causative organism of Chronic Respiratory disease is
a) Salmonella galinarum b) Mycoplasma gallisepticum
c) Mycoplasma synoviae d) Salmonella entridis

59. Causative organism of Newcastle disease is
a) Orthoparamyxovirus b) Paramyxovirus type-1
c) Birna virus d) Adenovirus

60. Causative organism of Rani Khet disease is
a) Orthoparamyxovirus b) Paramyxovirus type-1
c) Birna virus d) Adenovirus

61. Poultry housing enhance bird's production by providing
a) Physical environment b) Hot environment
c) Moderate environment d) Cold environment

62. For construction of poultry shed, soil should be
a) Clay b) Saline
c) Sandy d) Sandy loan

63. In temperate areas the direction of shed should be
a) Towards North South b) Towards East West
c) Both A and b d) Direction is not important

64. In the cold areas length of shod must be
a) Towards North South b) Towards East West
c) Both a & b d) Direction is not important

65. Movement of water flow in the shed should be
a) From young towards old stock b) From old towards young stock
c) Out of the shed d) In the middle of shed

66. Poultry shed should not be close to
a) Hill top
b) Populated area
c) Vaccine market
d) Feed market

67. Poultry shed should be located on
a) Hill top
b) Plane land
c) In the valley
d) Sloping hill side

68. Outer boundary of the farm should be planted with
a) Vegetable
b) Fodder crop
c) Trees
d) Bushes

69. Recommended length of open sided shed is
a) 100 Feet
b) 500 Feet
c) 1000 Feet
d) 2000 Feet

70. Recommended length of environment-controlled house is
a) 300 Feet
b) 50 Feet
c) 100 Feet
d) 1000 Feet

71. Recommended width of an open sided shed is
a) 30 Feet
b) 50 Feet
c) 100 Feet
d) 150 Feet

72. Recommended width of an environmentally controlled shed is
a) 20 Feet
b) 40 Feet
c) 100 Feet
d) 500 Feet

73. Standard height of poultry shed in hot areas
a) 12-14 Feet
b) 13-15 Feet
c) 05-07 Feet
d) 08-10 Feet

74 Standard height of poultry shed in cold area is
a) 07-08 Feet
b) 08-10 Feet
c) 12-13 Feet
d) 13-15 Feet

75. Minimum distance between two poultry sheds should be
a) 5 Feet
b) 20 Feet
c) 50 Feet
d) 100 Feet

76. Minimum distance between two poultry farm should be
a) 01 km
b) 05 km
c) 10 km
d) 20 km

77. Minimum distance of poultry shed from the road should be
a) 25 feet
b) 40 feet
c) 75 feet
d) 100 feet

78. The recommended amount of floor space in traditional style poultry houses for broiler chickens is
a) 05 sq.ft./bird
b) 03 sq.ft./bird
c) 02 sq.ft./bird
d) 01 sq.ft./bird

79. Recommended floor space for layer birds on litter floor system is
a) 1.75 sq.ft./bird
b) 2.50 sq.ft./bird
c) 4.50 sq.ft./bird
d) 5.50 sq.ft./bird

80. Recommended floor space for egg type breeder birds is
a) 1.0 sq.ft./bird
b) 2.0 sq.ft./bird
c) 3.0 sq.ft./bird
d) 4 .0 sq.ft./bird

81. In birds fertilization takes place in
a) Ovary
b) Uterus
c) Infundibulum
d) Vagina

82. In birds fertilization take place in
a) Ovary
b) Uterus
c) Vagina
d) None of these

83. Various components of the digestive tract grow in fowls during their embryonic development from
a) Hypoblast
b) Epiblast
c) Mesoderm
d) None of these

84. In fowls during embryonic development skin is developed from
a) Hypoblast
b) Epiblast
c) Mesoderm
d) None of these

85. In fowls during embryonic development feathers are developed from
a) Hypoblast
b) Epiblast
c) Mesoderm
d) None of these

86. In fowls during embryonic development beak is developed from
a) Hypoblast
b) Epiblast
c) Mesoderm
d) None of these

87. In fowls during embryonic development claws are developed from
a) Hypoblast
b) Epiblast
c) Mesoderm
d) None of these

88. In fowls during embryonic development nervous system is developed from
a) Hypoblast
b) Epiblast
c) Mesoderm
d) None of these

89. The lens and retina of a bird's eye develop during its embryonic stage from
a) Hypoblast
b) Epiblast
c) Mesoderm
d) None of these

90. The mouth and vent cavity linings of fowls grow during embryonic development from
a) Hypoblast
b) Epiblast
c) Mesoderm
d) None of these

91. In fowls during embryonic development respiratory organs are developed from
a) Hypoblast
b) Epiblast
c) Mesoderm
d) None of these

92. In fowls during embryonic development secretary organs are developed from
    a) Hypoblast b) Epiblast
    c) Mesoderm d) None of these
93. In fowls during embryonic development bones are developed from
    a) Hypoblast b) Epiblast
    c) Mesoderm d) None of these
94. In fowls during embryonic development muscles are developed from
    a) Hypoblast b) Epiblast
    c) Mesoderm d) None of these
95. How many types of pox viruses that can cause disease
    a) Two b) Three
    c) Four d) Five
96. The reproductive organs of fowls develop during the embryonic stage from
    a) Hypoblast b) Epiblast
    c) Mesoderm d) None of these
97. In a laying hen, a developing egg remains in magnum for a period of
    a) 1-2 hour b) 3-4 hours
    c) 5-6 hour d) 7-8 hour
98. In a laying hen, a developing egg remains in isthmus for a period of
    a) 1-2 hours b) 5-6 hours
    c) 9-10 hours d) 11-12 hours
99. A developing egg in a laying hen stays in the shell gland for a duration of
    a) 1-3 hour b) 8-10 hours
    c) 18-20 hours d) None of these
100. During a chicken embryonic development, the cleavage starts in
    a) Infundibulum b) Magnum
    c) Isthmus d) Uterus
101. Length of uterus in the reproductive system of a bird is
    a) 05 cm b) 10 cm
    c) 15 cm d) 20 cm
102. Length of infundibulum in the reproductive system of a bird is
    a) 05 cm b) 10 cm
    c) 15 cm d) 20 cm
103. Main function of vagina of a hen is
    a) Fertilization b) Cleavage formation
    c) Albumin secretion d) Sperm storage
104. Somites are blocks of cells that segregate off from the
    a) Ectoderm b) Endoderm
    c) Mesoderm d) Dorsal mesoderm
105. Incubation period of Chicken egg is
    a) 11 days b) 16 days
    c) 21 days d) 26 days

106. Incubation period of Quail egg is
   a) 11 days b) 14 days
   c) 17 days d) 20 days
107. Incubation period of Pheasant egg is
   a) 14 days b) 21 days
   c) 28 days d) 35 days
108. Incubation period of Duck egg is
   a) 14 days b) 28 days
   c) 42 days d) None of these
109. Incubation period of Peacock egg is
   a) 14 days b) 28 days
   c) 42 days d) None of these
110. Incubation period of Ostrich egg is
   a) 11 days b) 21 days
   c) 31 days d) 42 days
111. In the embryonic development, allantois serves as
   a) Nutritive b) Bacteriostatic
   c) Insulatitive d) None of these
112. Hatching eggs are shifted from setter to hatcher at the age of
   a) 16 days b) 17 days
   c) 20 days d) 18 days
113. Throughout the development of the embryo, the chorio-allantoic membrane acts as
   a) Nutritive b) Bacteriostatic
   c) Insulatitive d) Respiratory surface
114. During incubation process the heart of a chicken embryo starts beating at
   a) 2nd day of incubation b) 3rd day of incubation
   c) 4th day of incubation d) 5th day of incubation
115. During incubation process the heart of a chicken embryo starts beating at
   a) 4th day of incubation b) 6th day of incubation
   c) 8th day of incubation d) None of these
116. Follicle stimulating hormone is produced by
   a) Posterior pituitary b) Anterior pituitary
   c) Thymus gland) d) Adrenal gland
117. Follicle stimulating hormone is produced by
   a) Posterior pituitary b) Thymus gland
   c) Adrenal gland d) None of these
118. The days needed for each yolk in a hen's body to fully mature are
   a) 05 days b) 10 days
   c) 15 days d) 20 days
119. In a laying hen an individual yolk matures in
   a) 10 days b) 20 days
   c) 30 days d) 40 days

120. Progesterone hormone is secreted by
a) Shell gland b) Magnum
c) Isthmus d) Ovary

121. Recommended floor space of meat type breeder birds is
a) 3.5 sq.ft./bird b) 4.5 sq.ft./bird
c) 5.5 sq.ft./bird d) 6.5 sq.ft./bird

122. Relative humidity require
a) 60-65% b) 75-80%
c) 85-90% d) 90-100%

123. Temperature required during 1st week of brooding is
a) 95 °F b) 75 °F
c) 85 °F d) 80 °F

124. Temperature required during 2nd week of brooding is
a) 90 °F b) 70 °F
c) 80 °F d) 75°F

125) Temperature required during 3rd week of brooding is
a) 85 °F b) 65 °F
c) 75 °F d) 70 °F

126 Temperature required during 4th week of brooding is
a) 80 °F b) 90 °F
c) 70 °F d) 65 °F

127. Temperature required during 5th week of brooding is
a) 75 °F b) 80 °F
c) 65 °F d) 60 °F

128. Temperature required during 6th week of brooding is
a) 65 °F b) 75 °F
c) 85 °F d) 95 °F

129. Thermo neutral zone for poultry bird is
a) 25-50 °F b) 55-75 °F
c) 75-85 °F d) 85-100 °F

130. Respiration rate of the birds is governed by
a) CO_2 content of the blood b) O_2 content of the blood
c) H_2O content of the blood d) N content of the blood

131. Normal respiration rate of bird ranges between
a) 5-10 cycles/min b) 15-25 cycles/min
c) 60-70 cycles/min d) 80-100 cycles/min.

132. Body temperature of adult poultry bird is
a) 106.5 °F b) 120.5 °F
c) 130.5 °F d) 150.5 °F

133. The process by which a bird loses heat when it comes into contact with chilly air is known as
a) Conduction
b) Convection
c) Radiation
d) Evaporation

134. Mechanisms of heat lost from bird's body through waves of energy is called
a) Conduction
b) Convection
c) Radiation
d) Evaporation

135. When a bird comes into contact with a cold object, its body loses heat througha mechanism known as
a) Conduction
b) Convection
c) Radiation
d) Evaporation

136. Mechanisms of heat test from bird's body through respiration is called
a) Conduction
b) Convection
c) Radiation
d) Evaporative heat lost

137. Thermal stress stated when environmental temperature exceed from
a) 15 ^{0}C
b) 25 ^{0}C
c) 35 ^{0}C
d) 45 ^{0}C

138. When insulating chicken sheds, insulation should be prioritised more
a) Windows
b) Doors
c) Walls
d) Ceiling

139. Minimum R-value of roof for hot climatic conditions should be
a) 02
b) 04
c) 08
d) 12

140. Minimum R-value of walls for hot climatic conditions should be
a) 01
b) 02
c) 04
d) 08

141. Causative organism of Infectious Bursal disease is
a) Orthoparamyxo virus
b) Paramyxovirus type-1
c) Birna virus
d) Adenovirus

142. Causative organism of Gumboro disease is
a) Orthoparamyxo virus
b) Paramyxovirus type-1
c) Birna virus
d) Adenovirus

143. Causative organism of Avian Nephrosis syndrome is
a) Orthoparamyxo virus
b) Paramyxovirus type-1
c) Birna virus
d) Adenovirus

144. Causative organism of Hydropericardium syndrome is
a) Orthoparamyxovirus
b) Paramyxovirus type-1
c) Birna virus
d) Adenovirus

145. Causative organism of Angara disease is
a) Orthoparamyxovirus
b) Paramyxovirus type-1
c) Birna virus
d) Adenovirus

146. Causative organism of Fowl Pox disease is
a) Orthoparamyxovirus
b) Paramyxovirus type-1
c) Pox virus
d) Adenovirus

147. Causative organism of Marek's disease is
a) Orthoparamyxovirus
b) Paramyxovirus type-1
c) Herpes virus
d) Adenovirus

148. Causative organism of Range Paralysis disease is
a) Orthoparamyxovirus
b) Paramyxovirus type-1
c) Herpes virus
d) Adenovirus

149. Causative organism of Avian Leukosis disease is
a) Orthoparamyxovirus
b) Paramyxovirus type-1
c) Herpes virus
d) Oncoronavirus c

150. Causative organism of Coccidiosis disease is
a) Orthoparamyxovirus
b) Paramyxovirus type-1
c) Emeria Tanella
d) Adenovirus

151. Causative organism of Caecal Coccidiosis disease is
a) Orthoparamyxovirus
b) Paramyxovirus type-1
c) Emeria Tanella
d) Adenovirus

152. Causative organism of Intestinal Coccidiosis disease is
a) Emeria Maxima
b) Paramyxovirus type-1
c) Emeria Tanella
d) Adenovirus

153. There are about species that cause Coccidiosis in chicken
a) 08
b) 09
c) 10
d) None of the above

154. Most susceptible age of chicken for coccidiosis attack is
a) 2nd week
b) 3rd week
c) 4th weeks
d) None of the above

155. Specific symptom of Intestinal Coccidiosis that confirms the disease is
a) Bloody diarrhea
b) Blood in droppings
c) Pin point hemorrhages in intestine
d) Birds reluctant to move

156. The drug of choice for Coccidiosis is
a) Amprolium
b) Nocox
c) Coccidak
d) Diasulfina

157. Never give during coccidiosis attack
a) Vitamin A&K
b) Vitamin C
c) Vitamin B complex
d) All of the above

158. Medicine for coccidiosis should be administered in the following way
a) Continuous for 5 days
b) Continuous for 7 days
c) Continuous for 3 days, 2 days rest & then 2 days
d) None of the above

159. Coccidiosis is a disease

a) Viral
b) Bacterial
c) Mycotic
d) Managemental

160. Spores of coccidiosis when seen under microscope are ______ in shape

a) Oval
b) Spherical
c) Round
d) Doubled walled oval

Answer Key

1	a	2	b	3	a	4	a	5	a	6	b	7	b
8	b	9	b	10	a	11	a	12	b	13	d	14	b
15	c	16	c	17	a	18	a	19	c	20	a	21	c
22	b	23	c	24	a	25	d	26	c	27	b	28	b
29	a	30	a	31	c	32	b	33	c	34	d	35	b
36	d	37	b	38	d	39	c	40	b	41	c	42	a
43	a	44	a	45	c	46	b	47	a	48	b	49	b
50	b	51	b	52	b	53	c	54	b	55	a	56	a
57	b	58	b	59	b	60	b	61	a	62	d	63	b
64	a	65	a	66	b	67	d	68	c	69	a	70	a
71	a	72	b	73	a	74	b	75	c	76	a	77	d
78	d	79	a	80	b	81	c	82	d	83	a	84	b
85	b	86	b	87	b	88	b	89	b	90	b	91	a
92	a	93	c	94	c	95	c	96	c	97	b	98	a
99	c	100	c	101	b	102	b	103	d	104	d	105	c
106	c	107	c	108	b	109	b	110	d	111	d	112	d
113	a	114	a	115	d	116	b	117	d	118	b	119	a
120	d	121	a	122	a	123	a	124	a	125	a	126	a
127	a	128	b	129	b	130	a	131	b	132	a	133	b
134	c	135	a	136	d	137	c	138	d	139	b	140	b
141	c	142	c	143	c	144	d	145	c	146	c	147	c
148	c	149	d	150	c	151	c	152	a	153	b	154	b
155	c	156	a	157	c	158	c	159	d	160	d		

38

Laboratory Animal Production and Management

A.K. Srivastava

Department of Livestock Production Management, College of Veterinary Science and Animal Husbandry, Kamdhenu University, Sardarkrushinagar, Gujarat

Introduction

An animal, which has more or less of comparable (similar) physiology and body composition with various biological system as human beings, which are tiny, easy to handle, less expensive and co-operative are called as "Laboratory Animals".

Importance of Laboratory Animal in Bio-Medical Research

Laboratory animals are used in basic biological research, disease diagnosis, immunology, virology, applied medicine and demonstration/teaching. Materials collected from diseased animals need confirmation through microbiological and pathological means of diagnosis. Rats, Beagle dogs and primates are engaged in toxicological research. These are used to study the functions of organs, response of a particular organ or the whole system to drug and the method of evolving surgical techniques and demonstration of experimental surgery need experiment animals. Hamster have cheek pouches which may extend to halfway down the length of the body, are used to temporarily store food and, when full, should not be mistaken for a tumor. An entire shelled peanut can fit in a Syrian hamster cheek pouch. Cats are most commonly used in neurological research. Dogs are widely used in biomedical research, testing, and education — particularly beagles, because they are gentle and easy to handle. Non-human primates are used in toxicology tests, studies of AIDS and hepatitis, studies of neurology, behaviour and cognition, reproduction, genetics and xenotransplantation.

Institutional Animal Ethics Committee (IAE c) : Control and supervises the experiments on animals at institute or organizations and it is working under CCSEA (Committee for control and supervision of experiments on animals) New Delhi. CCSEA was earlier known as CPCSEA (Committee for the purpose of control and supervision of experiments on animals). Committee insist/maintain proper feeding, management and humane treatment to laboratory animals.

Classification of Laboratory Animals

1. **Conventional:** Animals derived and grown in general environment, but free from diseases communicable to human.

2. **Gnotobiotic:** Animal with known / fully defined microflora and microfauna (virus, bacteria, fungi and protozoa)is said to be gnotobiotic animal.
3. **Specific pathogen free animals (S.P.F.):** An animal which is made free from specific or particular microbe is known as specific pathogen free (SPF) animal.
4. **Germ free animals (Axenic)** : An animal which don't have any demonstrable microbes is known as germ free (GF) animal. Objectives of raising germ free animals includes to study the role of microbes in nutrition, to investigate the physiology of animals without infection and to conduct biological, toxicological and microbiological assay.

Why laboratory animal?

- They are smaller in size so they need minimum space and less feed) So that cost of production and maintenance is less.
- Most of the laboratory animals are not a natural host for most of the diseases human or animal so that they can be used in microbiological and virological research. The results so obtained can be applied directly for human or veterinary medicine.
- *Rat and mouse are better adaptable due to omnivores in habit, robust physical constitution, prolific breeding, shorter generation interval and easy to tame.*
- *Guinea pigs are very sensitive to a number of human pathogens, hence used extensively in biomedical research.*
- *Rabbits are prolific breeders and relatively having a huge body size compared to rat, mice and guinea pigs. They are mainly used in therapeutic trials,* raising hyper immune sera and to identify pyrogen in infusion fluids.

IMPORTANT DEFINITIONS

- **Albino:** A pink-eyed, white fur /wool animal having no pigmentation.
- **Bio-assay:** The safety and potency of vaccine, level of toxin and toxoids needed are to be standardized in laboratory animals for use in field condition.
- **Boar:** A male guinea pig
- **Broiler rabbit:** Rabbit which grow very fast for meat purpose.
- **Bruce effect:** This is a particularly interesting phenomenon, in which the pregnancy is very likely to fail in a recently impregnated female mouse when she encounters a normal male mouse other than the one with which she mate d)
- **Buck:** Adult male of rat/mouse/rabbit
- **Bunny:** A young rabbit below 20 weeks of age.
- **Cannibalism:** The practice of a female rabbit eating her own young ones.
- **Clowder:** Group of cat
- **Cobby:** A rabbit term meaning stout and stocky: short legged.
- **Colony:** Group of rat/mouse/guinea pig
- **Coprophagy:** Process of re-ingesting some of the faecal materials.
- **Cuniculture:** Rabbit farming is known as *Cuniculture.*
- **Doe:** Adult female of rat/mouse/rabbit which has produced at least one litter.
- **Dumbo**: Variety of rat that has ears placed more on the side than the top of the head.

- **Fryer:** 10-12 weeks old rabbits ready for market.
- **Inbreeding:** A breeding program involving the mating of closely related rabbit stock, such as brother and sister.
- **Kindle / Kit:** Young one of rabbit
- **Kindling Box:** A box provided to does so that she can make a nest and have young ones in it. Also called as nest box.
- **Kindling:** The process of giving birth to kits in rabbits.
- **Kittens:** Young one of rat/mouse/guinea pig/cat.
- **Lee-Boot effect:** This is the condition where female mice housed together in groups of four or more tend to become pseudopregnant; that is although they are virgins, they develop long lived progesterone secreting corpora lutea as if they were pregnant.
- **Litter:** Young rabbits of a doe born at the same time.
- **Monogamous mating:** 1 male is housed with 1 female
- **Out Breeding:** A breeding program involving the mating of unrelated animals of the same breed.
- **Pelt:** Skin of animal still wool attached to it.
- **Polygamous mating:** 1 male is housed with 4-5 females
- **Pup**: A baby guinea pig
- **Quad:** A group of rabbits that refers to breeding groups.
- **Queen**: Adult female of cat
- **Rabbitry:** A rabbit-raising enterprise or a place where domestic rabbits are kept.
- **Roaster:** Culled rabbits
- **Service:** The mating act of the buck with the doe.
- **Sire:** Male parent of an offspring.
- **Sow:** A female guinea pig
- **Tail carry**: Rats may pick up their tails in their mouths and carry them.
- **Tom:** Adult male of cat
- **Venison:** Meat of rabbit
- **Warren:** Group of rabbit
- **Weaning:** Process by which young one become independent of the doe for their nourishment.
- **Whitten effect:** This is the condition that occurs when mice are housed in larger groups. Their estrous cycle become longer and longer and eventually stops.

Sr. No.	Traits	Rat	Mice	Rabbit	Guinea pig
(1)	Zoological Name	*Rattus novergicus*	*Mus musculus*	*Oryctolagus cuniculus*	*Cavia porcellus*
(2)	Chromosomes no.	42	40	44	64
(3)	Birth Weight (gms)	4.5-6.0	1.0	30-100	75-100
(4)	Litter Size	5-16	5-12	7-10	3-6

(5)	Adult Male B.wt (gms)	300-500	25-40	2.5-5.0 kg	500-1000
(6)	Adult Female bwt (gms)	200-400	25-40	2.0-4.5 kg	500-800
(7)	Maturity age (days)	70-84	36-48	180-210	72-90
(8)	Mating age (days)	80-100	48-60	180-210	72-120
(9)	Gestation period (days)	21-22	19-21	29-32	59-72
(10)	Male: Female Ratio	1:3	1:8	1:10	1:12
(11)	Estrus Cycle (days)	4-5	4-5	Induced	14-16
(12)	Estrus Period (hrs)	10-20	10-20	.....	6-11
(13)	Weaning age (days)	18-21	18-21	28-42	14-16
(14)	Weaning Weight (gms)	25-55	8-12	100-150	160-230
(15)	Mammary gland (pair)	6	3-5	4	2-3
(16)	Body Temperature	37.5 ^{0}C	37.4 ^{0}C	38.5 - 39.5 ^{0}C	38.3-40.0 ^{0}C
(17)	Pulse/minute	120	120	130	120
(18)	Respiration rate	110	110	30-60	42-104

Questions

1. An animal, which has more or less of comparable physiology and body composition with various biological system as human beings, which are tiny, easy to handle, less expensive and co-operative are called as

   a) Pack animal b) Laboratory animal

   c) Livestock d) Meat animal

2. Cats are most commonly used in

   a) Neurological research b) Muscular research

   c) Osteological research d) Digestive system research

3. What is full form of IAEC?

   a) International Animal Ethics Committee

   b) International Animal Ethology Commission

   c) Institutional Animal Entomology Commission

   d) Institutional Animal Ethics Committee

4. Which of the following Committee insist/maintain proper feeding, management and humane treatment to laboratory animals?

   a) IVRI b) CDRI

   c) CCSEA d) NBAGR

5. What is the full form of CCSEA?

   a) Company for Control and Supervision of Experiments on Animals.

   b) Commission for Central Supervision of Exotic Animals.

   c) Council for Central Supervision of Ethology of Animals.

   d) Committee for Control and Supervision of Experiments on Animals.

6. Laboratory animals derived and grown in general environment, but free from diseases communicable to human are known as
   a) Conventional b) Gnotobiotic
   c) Specific pathogen free animals d) Germ free animals
7. Animal with known / fully defined microflora and microfauna (virus, bacteria, fungi and protozoa is said to be
   a) Conventional b) Gnotobiotic
   c) Specific pathogen free animals d) Germ free animals
8. An animal which is made free from specific or particular microbe is known as
   a) Conventional b) Gnotobiotic
   c) Specific pathogen free animals d) Germ free animals
9. A laboratory animals which don't have any demonstrable microbes is known as
   a) Conventional b) Gnotobiotic
   c) Specific pathogen free animals d) Germ free animals
10. What is (are) objective (s) of raising germ free animals or axenic animals
    a) To study the role of microbes in nutrition
    b) To investigate the physiology of animals without infection
    c) To conduct biological, toxicological and microbiological assay
    d) All the above
11. What is (are) the research area (s) in which the laboratory animals are used
    a) Drug assay
    b) To study the function of organs
    c) To conduct biological, toxicological and microbiological assay
    d) All the above
12. The most widely used invertebrate species as laboratory animal is
    a) Fruit fly (Drosophila melanogaster)
    b) Cockroach (Periplanata americana
    c) Frog (Rana tigrina)
    d) Earthworm (Pheretima poshthuma
13. Which breed of dog has been most widely used in biomedical research, testing, and education as laboratory animals?
    a) Great dane b) Beagle
    c) Mastiff d) Doberman
14. Which of the following laboratory animals are used in studies of AIDS and hepatitis, studies of neurology, behaviour and cognition, reproduction, genetics and xenotransplantation
    a) Cat b) Zebra fishes
    c) Non-human primates d) Rabbits

15. Which of the following laboratory animals are mainly used in therapeutic trials, raising hyper immune sera and to identify pyrogen in infusion fluids
    a) Rat b) Mice
    c) Guinea pig d) Rabbit

16. The results of experiments in which __________ animals are used are likely to be more meaningful due to the lack of interference by overt or subclinical disease.
    a) Conventional b) Gnotobiotic
    c) Specific pathogen free animals d) All the above

17. It is proven that fewer animals are required in an experiment where __________ laboratory animals are used, because of the more reliable results obtained
    a) Conventional b) Gnotobiotic
    c) Specific pathogen free animals d) All the above

18. Colloquially the inside of the SPF unit behind the shower is known as the -------- side, and the outside is the ------- side.
    a) Clean and Dirty b) Dirty and Clean
    c) Dirty and Dirty d) Clean and Clean

19. Which of the following is not an effective methods of sterilising diets
    a) Autoclaving b) Fumigation
    c) Homogenization d) Irradiation

20. Diets intended for SPF animals usually receive a dose of
    a) 1.0 megarads (Mrads) b) 2.5 megarads (Mrads)
    c) 5.0 megarads (Mrads) d) 7.5 megarads (Mrads)

21. The SPF building is constructed to a high specification and inside the animal unit is at
    a) Positive pressure to the atmosphere
    b) Negative pressure to the atmosphere
    c) Neutral pressure to the atmosphere
    d) Isobar to the atmosphere

22. Which of the following statement is incorrect?
    a) The building is constructed to a high specification to make it virtually airtight.
    b) Air from the airconditioning plant only is introduced to the animal unit.
    c) Inside the animal unit is at negative pressure to the atmosphere.
    d) Inside the animal unit is at positive pressure to the atmosphere.

23. In a SPF building the shower suite usually consists of how many sections?
    a) Two sections b) Three sections
    c) Four sections d) Five sections

24. The air flow through the shower suite is always from the
    a) Interior to the exterior
    b) Exterior to the interior
    c) Any direction as per the design of the building
    d) Upward to the downward direction

25. What is amount of formalin solution required for the fumigation of the SPF unit?
    a) 1 ml of a 10% formalin solution per cubic foot
    b) 3 ml of a 10% formalin solution per cubic foot
    c) 5 ml of a 10% formalin solution per cubic foot
    d) 10 ml of a 10% formalin solution per cubic foot
26. What is amount of formalin solution required for the fumigation of the SPF unit?
    a) 10 ml of a 10% formalin solution per cubic metre
    b) 25 ml of a 10% formalin solution per cubic metre
    c) 35 ml of a 10% formalin solution per cubic metre
    d) 50 ml of a 10% formalin solution per cubic metre
27. Personnel who have been in contact with conventional laboratory animals should undergo a *'waiting period'* before entering the SPF unit and this period is
    a) 10 days or less b) Two to three weeks
    c) Three to four weeks d) Four to six weeks
28. In the process of fumigation of the SPF building, it should be left for at least _______ before it is purged of fumigant.
    a) Six hours b) Twelve hours
    c) Twenty four hours d) Forty eight hours
29. While sterilising the diets of SPF animals the autoclave is programmed to provide a high temperature, short exposure cycle of
    a) 121° C for 12 min b) 130° C for 12 min
    c) 121° C for 1012 min d) 130° C for 1012 min
30. While sterilising the diets of SPF animals the autoclave is programmed to provide a lower temp., long exposure cycle.
    a) 121° C for 12 min b) 111° C for 12 min
    c) 121° C for 1015 min d) 111° C for 1015 min
31. For sterilising the diets of SPF animals by fumigation method which of the following gas is used?
    a) Ethylene oxide b) Methylene oxide
    c) Carbon di oxide d) Dimethyl Ether
32. For sterilising the diets of SPF animals by the gas fumigation method which of the following is a major disadvantage of the method?
    a) The diet has to be ventilated for up to 1 day before it is free of fumigant.
    b) The diet has to be ventilated for up to 3 days before it is free of fumigant.
    c) It damage the nutrients by destroying vitamins.
    d) It damage the nutrients by denaturing proteins.
33. The most common method of sterilization is irradiation using gamma rays produced by the radioactive isotope is
    a) ^{6}Carbon (^{6}c) b) ^{8}Carbon (^{8}c)
    c) ^{58}Cobalt (^{58}Co) d) ^{60}Cobalt (^{60}Co)

34. Diets intended for axenic animals usually receive a dose of
   a) 1.0 megarads (Mrads) b) 2.5 megarads (Mrads)
   c) 5.0 megarads (Mrads) d) 7.5 megarads (Mrads)

35. Which of the following is not an advantage of irradiation method for sterilization of diet?
   a) These highly penetrating rays are effective for destroying microorganisms.
   b) The nutritional and physical damage to the diet is minimised.
   c) These highly penetrating rays are effective for raising the temperature of diet and diet become easily digestible.
   d) These highly penetrating rays are effective for sterilization without causingthe exposed materials to become radioactive.

36. When a package has received a dose of 2.5 Mrads, previously applied yellow or orange indicator sticker should turned to when the package emerges indicating that it has received a dose of 2.5 Mrads.
   a) Dark red b) Dark Blue
   c) Black d) Dark Yellow

37. Which of the following laboratory animal is the most commonly used experimental animal?
   a) Rat b) Mice
   c) Guinea pig d) Rabbit

38. Laboratory mice are usually bred and housed in cages made of ____________ with solid floors.
   a) Polycarbonate b) Polypropylene
   c) Poly ethylene d) Both A and B

39. A mouse can produce a litter
   a) Every 3 weeks b) Every 4 weeks
   c) Every 5 weeks d) Every 6 weeks

40. How many generations from a mouse may be achieved in one year?
   a) 3 generations b) 5 generations
   c) 7 generations d) 10 generations

41. When the young ones of mice may be weaned?
   a) 1416 days b) 1821 days
   c) 2832 days d) 4042 days

42. What is the scientific name of the mice?
   a) Mus musculus b) Rattus norvegicus
   c) Cavia porcellus d) Mesocricetus auratus

43. What is the duration of gestation period in mice?
   a) 1416 days b) 1921 days
   c) 2628 days d) 3032 days

44. At the time of birth in mice, young ones are
   a) Fully developed
   b) Have fur but blind
   c) Eyes opend but naked
   d) Blind and naked
45. Knock out mouse means that
   a) It has one or more genes inoperable
   b) It has one or more genes operable
   c) It has 3 generations in breeding line simultaneously
   d) It has 5 generations in breeding line simultaneously
46. When the World Laboratory Animal Day is celebrated?
   a) 23 January
   b) 22 February
   c) 15 March
   d) 24 April
47. What should be the minimum cage height for the mice?
   a) 8 cm
   b) 10 cm
   c) 12 cm
   d) 15 cm
48. What is the minimum floor space per animal recommended for the mice (more than 40 gm)?
   a) 80 cm^2
   b) 100 cm^2
   c) 120 cm^2
   d) 200 cm^2
49. Optimal environmental temperature range for mouse rooms is.
   a) 12-16 °C
   b) 16-20 °C
   c) 20-26 °C
   d) 26-30°C
50. Which of the following statement is incorrect regarding housing of mice.
   a) Slightly higher environmental temperatures (22 to 26 °c)should be considered if the mice have to be housed on wire bottom cages
   b) Slightly lower environmental temperatures (18 to 22 °c) should be considered if the mice have to be housed on wire bottom cages
   c) Slightly higher environmental temperatures (22 to 26 °c) should be considered if hairless mice are being housed in cages with limited amounts of bedding.
   d) The preferences of mice for temperature depended upon the type of cage flooring
51. What should be the optimum Relative Humidity for mouse rooms?
   a) It should be kept at 35 ± 10%
   b) It should be kept at 45 ± 10%
   c) It should be kept at 55 ± 10%
   d) It should be kept at 75 ± 10%
52. What is (are) the consequence (s) of the low humidity levels in the mice house?
   a) Mice may suffer from respiratory problems
   b) More dust from bedding and feed,
   c) Excessive drying of mucous membranes
   d) All the above
53. What is (are) the consequence (s) of the high humidity levels in the mice house?
   a) Bedding may fail to evaporate moisture leading to rapid soiling of cages
   b) Increased production of ammonia by urease-producing bacteri a)

c) Infections of the upper airways may occur more easily
d) All the above

54. Mice should be subjected to a regular light: dark cycle, of.
a) 12 hours light, 12 hours dark
b) 6 hours light, 18 hours dark
c) 18 hours light, 6 hours dark
d) Any light regimen

55. Rat and mice are
a) Dirunal
b) Nocturnal
c) Both nocturnal and diurnal
d) Depending upon the availability of food

56. Which colour of light can be used to facilitate daytime husbandry and for observing activity of rodents during the day as most rodents are less sensitive to this than other animals and humans.
a) Red
b) Green
c) Blue
d) Yellow

57. What is reversed lighting schedule in laboratory animal house?
a) With lights on at night and off at day
b) With lights on at day and off at night
c) With lights on at the floor of the animal house at day
d) With lights on at the bottom of each cage as and when required

58. What should be the maximum light intensity in the mice room?
a) It should not exceed 100 lux
b) It should not exceed 250 lux
c) It should not exceed 350 lux
d) It should not exceed 500 lux

59. What should be the maximum permissible level of sound frequency in the mice room?
a) It should not exceed 15 dB
b) It should not exceed 35 dB
c) It should not exceed 45 dB
d) It should not exceed 55 dB

60. Which of the following statement is incorrect regarding environmental enrichment of laboratory animals
a) By providing environmental enrichment the living conditions of laboratory animals improved as they get opportunities to perform a more species-specific behavioural repertoire.
b) Environmental enrichment or modifications to the environments of animals in order to improve their biological functioning.
c) Barren, restrictive and socially deprived housing conditions does not interfere with the development and function of brain and behavioural functions.
d) Environmental enrichment should meet the animal's needs, be practical, inexpensive and pose no risk to humans, the animals and to the experiment.

61. Which of the following is the correct property of bedding material?
a) Absorbent
b) Toxic
c) Dusty
d) Mouldy

62. What is (are) the characteristics of the female mice?
 a) Female mice are poly-estrous.
 b) Female mice are spontaneous ovulators
 c) Female mice have oestrous cycle of 4-5 days duration.
 d) All the above

63. Identify the incorrect statement from the following.
 a) Female mice are poly-estrous and spontaneous ovulators
 b) Female mice have oestrous cycle of 19-21 days duration.
 c) In mice, mating, estrus and ovulation most often occur during the dark phase.
 d) The cyclicity of estrus and ovulation are controlled by the diurnal rhythm of the photoperiod.

64. Female mice housed in groups will become di-estrous, an-estrous or pseudopregnant, while the introduction of a male into such a group will synchronize their estrous cycles, the phenomenon is known as
 a) Bruce effect b) Whitten effect
 c) Lee-boot effect d) Circadian rhythm effect

65. If the female is housed with a second male within 24 hours after a successful mating, implantation of fertile egg cells will be prevented and the female will return to estrus in 4-5 days, the phenomenon is known as
 a) Bruce effect b) Whitten effect
 c) Lee-boot effect d) Circadian rhythm effect

66. What is the scientific name of the rat?
 a) Mus musculus b) *Rattus norvegicus*
 c) *Cavia porcellus* d) *Mesocricetus auratus*

67. Which of the following is not a strain of rat
 a) Wistar b) Sprague-Dawley
 c) Californian d) Hooded Long Evans

68. Weaning age in rat is
 a) 1215 days b) 1821 days
 c) 2427 days d) 30-32 days

69. Ringtail is a disease of rats and causative agent for it is
 a) Virus b) Bacteria
 c) Parasites d) Possibly low humidity

70. Which of the following is organ is not present in the body of rat?
 a) Duodenum b) Teeth
 c) Gall Bladder d) Pancreas

71. What is the duration of gestation period in the rat?
 a) 11-13 days b) 15-16 days
 c) 21-22 days d) 28-30 days

72. What is average litter size in the rats?
   a) 2-4 b) 5-6
   c) 7-8 d) 9-11
73. What is length of oestrus cycle in rats?
   a) 2-4 days b) 4- 5 days
   c) 6-8 days d) 10-12 days
74. What is age at first mating in the rats?
   a) 30 days b) 50 days
   c) 60 days d) 70 days
75. Rats and mice are identified by touching fur in different places with a harmless dye such as Carbofusfuschin and Gentian violet etc. These mark should be renewed once in every _______.
   a) Three weeks. b) Four weeks
   c) Five weeks d) Six weeks
76. What is optimum cage height suitable for housing the rats.
   a) 15 cm b) 30 cm
   c) 45 cm d) 60 cm
77. According to the Council of Europe 2002, Minimum floor area (cm^2) per adult rat weighing more than 400 gm is
   a) 200 cm^2 b) 250 cm^2
   c) 350 cm^2 d) 400 cm^2
78. Polycarbonate or polypropylene cages are better than stainless steel cages, why?
   a) Because these cages are less noisy
   b) Because these cages are light in weight
   c) Because these cages have better heat insulation
   d) All the above
79. In rats and mice the most active periods occur at the
   a) Beginning of the dark period. b) End of the dark period..
   c) Both beginning and end of the dark period d) Active throughout the night period
80. Identify the incorrect statement from the following.
   a) Nesting materials, such as paper towels or wood wool, are highly recommended for rodents, especially for breeding animals.
   b) Pre-weaning mortality can be decreased in rats through the use of proper nesting material.
   c) Rats and mice prefer empty cage than nest box and nesting material.
   d) Provision of nesting material as a method of enrichment is considered to have a more obvious effect on the welfare of rodents than other cage additions, such as toys.
81. What is the the average lifespan of laboratory rats?
   a) Varies between 6 month to 1 year b) Varies between 1-2 years
   c) Varies between 2-4 years d) Varies between 4-6 years

82. Young ones of rat and mice are born
    a) Blind and naked in all strains
    b) With fur and eyes open in all strains
    c) Blind but with fur in some strains
    d) Naked but eyes opened in some strains

83. What is the scientific name of the guinea pig?
    a) Mus musculus
    b) Rattus norvegicus
    c) Cavia porcellus
    d) Mesocricetus auratus

84. Which of the following is not a variety of Guinea pigs?
    a) English smooth hair
    b) Abyssinian rosetted hair
    c) Peruvian very long hair
    d) Sprague-Dawley no hair

85. Weaning age in guinea pig is
    a) 14 days
    b) 21 days
    c) 28 days
    d) 35 days

86. The feeding habit of guineapig is
    a) Strictly herbivore
    b) Omnivore
    c) Carnivore
    d) Detritivore

87. Which of the following is organ is not present in the body of guinea pig?
    a) Duodenum
    b) Pancreas
    c) Tail
    d) Gall bladder

88. What is the duration of gestation period in the guinea pig?
    a) 11-13 days
    b) 21-22 days
    c) 31-32 days
    d) 59-72 days

89. What is average litter size in the guinea pig?
    a) 1-3
    b) 3-6
    c) 7-9
    d) 9-12

90. What is age at sexual maturity in the guinea pig?
    a) 30-40 days
    b) 50-60 days
    c) 60-80 days
    d) 80-100 days

91. Young ones of guinea pigs are born
    a) They are fully furred, their eyes are open and the teeth are fully developed
    b) They are blind but with fur and teeth
    c) They are naked but eyes open and teeth fully developed
    d) They are fully blind and naked

92. New-born guinea pigs look like small-sized adults and they are fully furred, their eyes are open and the teeth are fully developed, hence they are termed as
    a) Precocial
    b) Altricial
    c) Abyssinian
    d) Peruvian

93. Which of the following laboratory animal is precocial?
    a) Rat b) Mice
    c) Guinea pig d) Hamster
94. What is the optimum male: female ratio in the Guinea pigs?
    a) 1: 2-4 b) 1: 5-7
    c) 1: 8-12 d) 1: 18-20
95. For Guinea pigs the diet must be supplemented with
    a) Vitamin A b) Vitamin B
    c) Vitamin C d) Vitamin K
96. Number of mammary glands in the guinea pigs?
    a) 1 pair b) 2 pairs
    c) 3 pairs d) 4 pairs
97. How many toes are present in the fore and hind limbs in guinea pig?
    a) 4 toes in the fore limb and 3 in the hind limb
    b) 3 toes in the fore limb and 4 in the hind limb
    c) 4 toes in the fore limb and 5 in the hind limb
    d) 5 toes in the fore limb and 4 in the hind limb
98. In which of the laboratory animals mammary glands are found in both sexes?
    a) Rat b) Hamster
    c) Rabbit d) Guinea pig
99. On which day after the birth the young guinea pigs start to eat solid food and drink water?
    a) On the day of birth b) 7 days after the birth
    c) 14 days after the birth d) 21 days after the birth
100. What is average weight at adult stage in the guinea pig?
    a) 200-400 gram b) 500-600 gram
    c) 800-1000 gram d) 1200-1500 gram
101. Guinea pigs follow
    a) Diurnal rhythm b) Nocturnal rhythm
    c) Circadian rhythm d) Ultradian rhythm
102. What is Ultradian rhythm
    a) Animal show a day-night cycle of activity
    b) Animals are active in night
    c) Animals are active in day
    d) Activity is not dependent on the light-dark regime
103. Identify the incorrect statement from the following.
    a) Guinea pigs do not show a day-night cycle of activity.
    b) The activity of guinea pig is dependent on the light-dark regime.

c) There is alternating phases of activity and rest that lasting for about 2-3 hours in the guinea pigs.

d) The activity in guinea pig is characterized by an ultradian rhythm.

104. In male guinea pigs the shape of genital opening is

a) Round shape b) Longitudinal slit

c) Y-shape d) Horizontal slit

105. In female guinea pigs the shape of genital opening is

a) Round shape b) Longitudinal slit

c) S-shape d) Horizontal slit

106. Which of the following phenomenon does not appear to occur in guinea pigs:

a) Pseudo pregnancy b) Postpartum oestrus

c) Oestrous d) Copulatory plugs

107. Guinea-pigs are commonly bred in

a) Hand mating system b) Monogamous breeding system

c) Polygamous breeding system d) Harem system

108. Which of the vitamin is not synthesized in the digestive tract of the guinea pig?

a) Vitamin A b) Vitamin C

c) Vitamin D d) Vitamin K

109. Generally Vitamin C is provided in the drinking water as ascorbic acid to the guinea pigs, hence the drinking spouts/ bottles should be made up of

a) Metal b) Plastic

c) Wood d) Glass

110. What is optimum room temperature required by Guineapigs for optimum breeding efficiency?

a) About 15°C b) About 18°C

c) About 21°C d) About 24°C

111. What is the scientific name of the Hamster?

a) Mus musculus *b) Rattus norvegicus*

c) Cavia porcellus *d) Mesocricetus auratus*

112. Weaning age in Hamster is

a) 14 days b) 21 days

c) 28 days d) 35 days

113. What is optimum mating weight in the hamsters?

a) 50 gram b) 100 gram

c) 150 gram d) 200 gram

114. Which laboratory animal possesses cheek pouches in which they gather food for later storage in their nests?

a) Guinea Pig b) Rat

c) Fruit fly d) Hamsters

115. Which of the following is body part of hamsters possess a pouch?
   a) Cheek
   b) Oesophagus
   c) Duodenum
   d) Stomach

116. What is the duration of gestation period in the hamsters?
   a) 12 days
   b) 16 days
   c) 20 days
   d) 24 days

117. What is average litter size in the hamsters?
   a) 1-3
   b) 3-6
   c) 7-9
   d) 9-12

118. What is age at sexual maturity in the hamsters?
   a) 6 weeks
   b) 9 weeks
   c) 12 weeks
   d) 15 weeks

119. At what time the hamster are most active?
   a) In day light
   b) In dark
   c) Irrespective of day
   d) All time with adequate supply of feed

120. What is the optimum male: female ratio in the hamsters?
   a) 1: 2
   b) 1: 5
   c) 1: 8
   d) 1: 10

121. What is length of the oestrous cycle in hamsters?
   a) 4 days
   b) 7 days
   c) 10 days
   d) 14 days

122. Identify the incorrect statement from the following
   a) In artificially controlled illumination hamster do not show any seasonal breeding behaviour.
   b) Hamsters are polyoestrous, and the length of the oestrous cycle is 10 days.
   c) In hamsters, ovulation occurs spontaneously between 6 and 10 hours after the beginning of oestrus.
   d) In hamsters female exhibit 'lordosis' just before and during oestrus.

123. At the time of birth the young ones of hamsters are
   a) Fully develop
   b) With open eyes and no fur
   c) With closed eyes and with fur
   d) With closed eyes and naked

124. Normally hair/ fur start growing on __________ day after parturition in hamsters.
   a) 3rd day
   b) 7th day
   c) 11th day
   d) 14th day

125. In hamsters normally eyes are opened on __________ day after parturition in hamsters.
   a) 3rd day
   b) 7th day
   c) 11th day
   d) 14th day

126. ' Wet tail' disease is commonly seen in which of the following laboratory animal.

a) Rat b) Mice

c) Guinea pig d) Hamster

127. Which of the following is **not** a characteristics of the foundation stock

a) The animals should be healthy, free from any disease, active vigorous and of good quality.

b) They should have good production record with respect to litter size at birth and at weaning.

c) They should have good production record with respect litter weight at birth and at weaning.

d) They should be cross bred.

128. Which of the following is not a criteria for the section of breeding stock of laboratory animals?

a) The female parent should have a breeding record and not be prone to infanticide

b) The animal should be in good health and show no deformities

c) If possible animals should be selected from the fifth or sixth litters.

d) The parent stock should not be aggressive when handled

129. Which of the following is not classified as permanently mated group breeding systems of laboratory animal?

a) Monogamy b) Polygamy

c) Harem system d) Both a and b

130. Which of the following is not classified as temporarily mated group breeding systems of laboratory animal?

a) Hand-mating systems b) Harem system

c) Monogamy d) Both a and b

131. Mating systems, in which the one or more males are housed with several females and female is allowed to litter down in the presence of the male and other members of the groups, is known as

a) Monogamy b) Polygamy

c) Harem system d) Hand mating system

132. Mating systems, in which a single male and female housed together throughout their life, is known as

a) Monogamy b) Polygamy

c) Harem system d) Hand mating system

133. Mating systems, in which males and females are run together, but females are separated from the groups prior to parturition, is known as

a) Monogamy b) Polygamy

c) Harem system d) Hand mating system

134. Mating systems, in which the male and female are left together only for sufficient time for mating to occur, is known as

a) Monogamy b) Polygamy

c) Harem system d) Hand mating system

135. From the stand point of genetics and maintenance of good records in rat and mice breeding management, which mating may be considered as the best system?

a) Monogamy b) Polygamy

c) Harem system d) Hand mating system

136. Which technique is the most reliable method in determining pregnancy in the laboratory animals?

a) Abdominal palpation b) Test Mating

c) Weight gain method d) Rectal Palpation

137. The feed in which purified components such as carbohydrates (starch, sucrose), purified protein sources (casein, lactalbumin), refined oils and synthetic vitamins and refined mineral supplements are used as ingredients are known as

a) Purified diets b) Chemically defined diets

c) Germ free diets d) Hand rearing

138. The feed which are made from the basic nutrients e.g. Glucose, triglycerides, essential fatty acids, individual amino acids, vitamins and minerals which can be obtained in a pure form are known as

a) Purified diets b) Chemically defined diets

c) Germ free diets d) Hand rearing

139. The process of reingesting some of the faecal materials which is practiced by all rodents and logomorphs is known as

a) Paired feeding b) Euthanasia

c) Coprophagy d) All the options are correct

140. Which of the following feeding system has been shown to be beneficial in the long run in terms of reduced morbidity and mortality in rats and mice?

a) Restricted feeding *b) Ad li*b feeding

c) Cafeteria feeding d) Purified diets

141. What is (are) the consequence(s) of ad libitum feeding in rats and mice?

a) Obesity

b) Decreased survival

c) An increased incidence of tumours in older animals

d) All the above

142. What is (are) advantage(s) of restricted feeding in rats.

a) Significantly improves survival

b) Controls adult body weight and obesity

c) Reduces age-related renal, endocrine and cardiac diseases

d) All the above

143. How much feed restriction is recommended in rats?

a) 10% b) 15%

c) 20% d) 25%

144. Which of the following microorganism is subclinical transmitted by the guinea pigs?

a) Bordetella sp. b) Aspicularis sp.

c) Myocoptes sp. d) Myobia sp.

145. Which of the following is measures to prevent disease in laboratory animal house

a) Use of protective cloths and overshoes

b) Provision of barrier at laboratory animal unit with liquid dip, and showering.

c) Waste accumulated in the cages should be washed with hot water (82°c) for at least 3 minutes

d) All the options are correct

146. What is the scientific name of the rabbit?

a) Mus musculus b) *Oryctolagus cuniculus*

c) Cavia porcellus *d) Mesocricetus auratus*

147. Weaning age in rabbit is

a) 14 days b) 21 days

c) 46 weeks d) 78 weeks

148. Leading country in rabbit production is

a) India b) China

c) USA d) France

149. How many Chromosome are found in rabbits?

a) 24 b) 34

c) 44 d) 54

150. What is duration of gestation period in rabbits?

a) 24 days b) 28 days

c) 32 days d) 36 days

151. During March 1978, first batch of 60 New Zealand white rabbits were imported by ICAR-CSWRI from.

a) United Kingdom b) U.S.A.

c) U.S.S.R. d) New Zealand

152. As per the 20th Livestock Census (2019) the total rabbit population in India is.

a) 424000 b) 550000

c) 654000 d) 958000

153. What is the feed conversion efficiency, in rabbits supplemented with high grain diets?

a) 1.7- 1.9 b) 2.0- 2.4

c) 2.5- 3.0 d) 3.5 –4.0

154. The broiler rabbits have a high growth rate reaching market weight of about ------------ at 12 weeks of age

a) 1.0 kg b) 2.0 kg

c) 3.0 kg d) 3.5 kg

155. Where is the Head quarter of ICAR- Central Sheep and Wool Research Institute (CSWRI) located?

a) Hissar, Haryana
b) Makhdoom, Uttar Pradesh
c) Bikaner, Rajasthan
d) Avikanagar, Rajasthan

156. Identify the constraints in rabbit farming

a) Surplus availability of germ plasm
b) Lack of technical know-how
c) Availability of a well-organized market for rabbit meat
d) Organized regular slaughter of rabbits

157. Native of White giant breed of rabbit is

a) Belgium
b) England
c) Russia
d) U.S.A.

158. Identify the fur breed of rabbit from the following

a) Dutch
b) White Giant
c) Angora
d) Soviet Chinchilla

159. Which of the following is not a type of production cycle in rabbit farming

a) Extensive reproduction
b) Semi intensive reproduction
c) Intensive reproduction
d) Composite Reproduction

160. In rabbits, generally the fibre content of diet should be

a) 4 to 6%
b) 10-12 %
c) 14 to 16%
d) 18 to 20%

161. Broiler rabbits can be reared in

a) Deep litter system
b) Cage system
c) Hutches
d) All the options are correct.

162. For calm kindling and better protection of the kits a nest box is essential. What should be the measurement of nest box?

a) 12 inch length, 12 inch width and 12 inch height
b) 22 inch length, 22 inch width and 12 inch height
c) 22 inch length, 12 inch width and 12 inch height
d) 22 inch length, 22 inch width and 22 inch height

163. What is average litter size in the rabbits?

a) 1-3
b) 3-5
c) 6-8
d) 10-12

164. What is the approximate number of young one produced in a year by a female rabbit under intensive system?

a) 6-8
b) 15-20
c) 18-26
d) 30-48

165. What is the total carcass weight (kg) of offspring / year in relation to dam weight is produced by the rabbit in a year?

a) 1-2 b) 10-12
c) 14-20 **d) 18-29**

166. What is the optimum male: female ratio in the rabbits?
a) 1: 2 b) 1: 5
c) 1: 8 d) 1: 10

167. Meat of rabbit is called as
a) Venison b) Beef
c) Veal d) Chevon

168. Protein content of rabbit meat is
a) 20.8 % b) 18.8 %
c) 15.7 % d) 11.9 %

169. Which of the following country is native of Flemish giant breed of rabbit
a) Belgium b) Newzealand
c) Former U.S.S.R d) U.S.A.

170 . Which of the following breed of rabbit is famous for its prolificacy and fast growth?
a) Flemish giant b) White giant
c) Grey giant d) New Zealand White

171. Which of the following country is native of New Zealand White breed of rabbit?
a) Belgium b) Newzealand
c) England d) U.S.A.

172. Which of the following breed of rabbit is a synthetic breed of rabbit?
a) Soviet Chinchilla b) Grey giant
c) Californian d) New Zealand red

173. Which of the following breed of rabbit has a thick fold of skin around the front of chest, which is very obvious when the rabbit is in good condition?
a) Soviet Chinchilla b) Grey giant
c) Californian d) New Zealand red

174. Which of the following breed of rabbit is white in colour with black extremities?
a) Soviet Chinchilla b) White giant
c) Himalayan d) New Zealand White

175. Which of the following country is native of Angora breed of rabbit?
a) Belgium b) New Zealand
c) Turkey d) England

176. In rabbit the testicle descends from the body cavity into the scrotum at around
a) 3 weeks b) 6 weeks
c) 9 weeks d) 12 weeks

177. In rabbits, at the time of mating
a) Female should be taken to male's cage
b) Male should be taken to male's cage

c) Both should be taken to a new cage
d) Both a and bare correct

178. What is the optimum time for determining pregnancy in the rabbits by palpation method?
a) 4th to 6th day after mating
b) 7th to 9th day after mating
c) 10th to 14th day after mating
d) 20th to 24th day after mating

179. At the time of birth the young ones of rabbits are born
a) Fully develop
b) With open eyes and no fur
c) With closed eyes and with fur
d) With eyes closed and naked

180. In rabbits normally eyes are opened on __________ day after parturition.
a) 3rd day
b) 7th day
c) 11th day
d) 14th day

181. Rabbits are primarily.
a) Monogastric herbivorous animal
b) Monogastric omnivorous animal
c) Polygastric herbivorous animals
d) Polygastric herbivorous animals

182. Average dry matter consumption of rabbit, when maintained on dry roughage is
a) About 12 % of their bodyweight
b) About 2.5 – 3.5 % of their bodyweight
c) About 4.05.5 % of their bodyweight
d) About 68 % of their bodyweight

183. Causative agent for Ear canker disease is
a) Eimeria magna
b) Eimeria perforans
c) Psoroptes cuniculi
d) Trichophyton microsporon

184. A female rabbit with its young would produce quantity of manure throughout the year about
a) 50 to 100 kg
b) 75 to 125 kg
c) 150-200 kg
d) 250 to 300 kg

185. What is the dressing percentage in rabbit?
a) 45 %
b) 55 %
c) 65 %
d) 72 %

186. In rabbit shearing should be done how many times a year?
a) 2 times
b) 3 times
c) 4 times
d) 5 times

187. Which of the method of wool harvesting is commonly preferred in most of the countries including India?
a) Shearing
b) Plucking
c) Combing
d) Depilation

188. Who first described the Three Rs (3Rs) guiding principles for more ethical use of animals in product testing and scientific research in the year 1959?
a) W. M. S. Russell and R. L. Burch

b) H.M. Buchanan-Smith and a Rennie
c) A Vitale and S. Pollo
d) M.J. Prescott and DB Morton

189. Which of the following is not a part of the Three Rs (3Rs) guiding principles for more ethical use of animals in product testing and scientific research?
a) Replace the animals with possible alternative
b) Reduce the number of animals
c) Reimbursement of the animal expanses
d) Refine the experiment

190. Which of the following is has been recently added in the Three Rs (3Rs) guiding principles for laboratory animals as fourth R?
a) Replace the animals with possible alternative
b) Rehabilitation of the animals after the experiment
c) Reduce the number of animals
d) Refine the experiment

191. Select appropriate statement
Statement 1: Young one of rabbits are born blind and hairless.
Statement 2: Hares are precocial, generally born with hair and are able to see.
a) Statement 1 is correct while Statement 2 is wrong
b) Statement 2 is correct while Statement 1 is wrong
c) Both Statement 1 and statement 2 are correct
d) Both Statement 1 and statement 2 are wrong

192. Select appropriate statement
Statement 1: In rabbits the incisor teeth grow continuously.
Statement 2: In rabbits both the male and female have nipples, normally four pairs.
a) Statement 1 is correct while Statement 2 is wrong
b) Statement 2 is correct while Statement 1 is wrong
c) Both Statement 1 and statement 2 are correct
d) Both Statement 1 and statement 2 are wrong

193. Select appropriate statement
Statement 1: Protein content of rabbit meat is 20.8 % which is higher than the beef.
Statement 2: Fat content of rabbit meat is 10.2 % which is higher than the pork.
a) Statement 1 is correct while Statement 2 is wrong
b) Statement 2 is correct while Statement 1 is wrong
c) Both Statement 1 and statement 2 are correct
d) Both Statement 1 and statement 2 are wrong

194. Select appropriate statement
Statement 1: New Zealand White breed of rabbit was evolved in England
Statement 2: New Zealand White breed is the one used most widely throughout the world for meat production.

a) Statement 1 is correct while Statement 2 is wrong
b) Statement 2 is correct while Statement 1 is wrong
c) Both Statement 1 and statement 2 are correct
d) Both Statement 1 and statement 2 are wrong

195. Select appropriate statement

Statement 1: Small breeds of rabbits (Polish, Dutch) are first bred at the age of 8 months.

Statement 2: Medium breeds of rabbits are first bred at the age of 12 months.

a) Statement 1 is correct while Statement 2 is wrong
b) Statement 2 is correct while Statement 1 is wrong
c) Both Statement 1 and statement 2 are correct
d) Both Statement 1 and statement 2 are wrong

196. Select appropriate statement

Statement 1: A female rabbit appears to have no definite oestrous cycle.

Statement 2: Rabbits are induced ovulators.

a) Statement 1 is correct while Statement 2 is wrong
b) Statement 2 is correct while Statement 1 is wrong
c) Both Statement 1 and statement 2 are correct
d) Both Statement 1 and statement 2 are wrong

197. Select appropriate statement

Statement 1: At the time of mating the male should be lifted to female's cage to avoid fighting

Statement 2: After successful mating the male usually produce a typical cry and fall down on one side of the doe.

a) Statement 1 is correct while Statement 2 is wrong
b) Statement 2 is correct while Statement 1 is wrong
c) Both Statement 1 and statement 2 are correct
d) Both Statement 1 and statement 2 are wrong

198. Select appropriate statement

Statement 1: A rabbit should be picked up by obtaining a firm grip on the loose skin over the scruff of the neck with one hand and use the other hand to support the hind quarters.

Statement 2: Young rabbits can be lifted by grasping their ears firmly.

a) Statement 1 is correct while Statement 2 is wrong
b) Statement 2 is correct while Statement 1 is wrong
c) Both Statement 1 and statement 2 are correct
d) Both Statement 1 and statement 2 are wrong

199. Select appropriate statement

Statement 1: In rabbits sexing is usually done at weaning along with tattooing.

Statement 2: While sexing in rabbits when the vent area is gently pressed the female will show slightly raised cylindrical round tip.

a) Statement 1 is correct while Statement 2 is wrong
b) Statement 2 is correct while Statement 1 is wrong
c) Both Statement 1 and statement 2 are correct
d) Both Statement 1 and statement 2 are wrong

200. Select appropriate statement

Statement 1: The density of Angora wool is 1.1g per cubic centimeter, whereas Merino sheep wool density is approximately 1.3 g per cubic centimeter.

Statement 2: The softness of Angora wool is produced by the extreme smoothness of the cuticle which confers the fluffiness to other fibres when blended with them.

a) Statement 1 is correct while Statement 2 is wrong
b) Statement 2 is correct while Statement 1 is wrong
c) Both Statement 1 and statement 2 are correct
d) Both Statement 1 and statement 2 are wrong

Answer Key

1	b	2	a	3	d	4	c	5	d	6	a	7	b
8	a	9	d	10	d	11	d	12	a	13	b	14	c
15	d	16	c	17	c	18	a	19	c	20	b	21	a
22	c	23	d	24	a	25	a	26	c	27	b	28	c
29	b	30	c	31	a	32	b	33	d	34	c	35	c
36	a	37	b	38	d	39	a	40	b	41	b	42	a
43	b	44	d	45	a	46	d	47	c	48	b	49	c
50	b	51	c	52	d	53	d	54	a	55	b	56	a
57	a	58	c	59	d	60	c	61	a	62	d	63	b
64	b	65	a	66	b	67	c	68	b	69	d	70	c
71	c	72	d	73	b	74	c	75	d	76	d	77	c
78	d	79	c	80	c	81	c	82	a	83	c	84	d
85	a	86	a	87	c	88	d	89	b	90	c	91	a
92	a	93	c	94	c	95	c	96	c	97	a	98	d
99	a	100	c	101	d	102		103	b	104	a	105	b
106	a	107	d	108	b	109	d	110	b	111	d	112	b
113	b	114	d	115	a	116	b	117	c	118	a	119	d
120	b	121	a	122	b	123	d	124	b	125	b	126	
127	d	128	c	129	c	130	c	131	b	132	a	133	c
134	d	135	a	136	a	137	a	138	b	139	c	140	a
141	d	142	d	143	d	144	a	145	d	146	b	147	c

148	b	149	c	150	c	151	a	152	b	153	c	154	
155	d	156	b	157	c	158	c	159	d	160	d	161	d
162	c	163	c	164	d	165	d	166	d	167	a	168	a
169	a	170	b	171	c	172	c	173	a	174	c	175	c
176	d	177	a	178	c	179		180	c	181	a	182	d
183	c	184	c	185	b	186	c	187	a	188	a	189	c
190	b	191	c	192	c	193	a	194	c	195	d	196	c
198	a	199	a	200	c								

39

Milk

Utkarsh Kumar Tripathi[1], Sakshi[2], Anuradha Kumari[1], and Manish Kumar[1]

[1]*Faculty of Veterinary and animal Sciences, IAS, RGSC, BHU*

[2]*Division of Medicine, ICAR-IVRI, Izzatnagar, Bareilly*

Introduction

The livestock sector, particularly the dairy sector, plays a vital role in India's economy and contributes significantly to the country's milk production. The continuous growth and development of this sector have led to India becoming the world's largest milk producer. It has seen significant growth, with a Compound Annual Growth Rate (CAGR) of 13.36% from 2014-15 to 2021-22. This sector's contribution to the total Gross Value Added GVa in agriculture and allied sectors has risen from 24.38% in 2014-15 to 30.19% in 2021-22, accounting for 5.73% of the total GVA in 2021-22.

The country's livestock population, as per the 20th Livestock Census, includes approximately 303.76 million bovines (cattle, buffalo, mithun, and yak), 74.26 million sheep, 148.88 million goats, 9.06 million pigs, and about 851.81 million poultry.

The dairy sector stands as the single largest agricultural commodity, contributing 5% to the national economy and directly employing more than 8 crore farmers. India leads the world in milk production, contributing 24.64% of global milk production. The milk production has been growing at a CAGR of 5.85% over the past 9 years, increasing from 146.31 million tonnes in 2014-15 to 230.58 million tonnes in 2022-23. In comparison to the previous year, the world milk production grew by 0.51% in 2022. As of 2022-23, the per capita availability of milk in India is 459 grams per day, significantly higher than the world average of 322 grams per day in 2022.

According to the Food Safety and Standards Authority of India (FSSAI), "Milk" is defined as the normal mammary secretion derived from complete milking of a healthy milch animal, without either addition thereto or extraction therefrom. It is the primary source of nutrition for young mammals before they are able to digest other types of food Milk which is adjusted for milk fat or milk SNF content or both, may also be named "milk" provided that the minimum and maximum limits for fat and SNF are as per the standards of milk. Lactation physiology plays a crucial role in milk production from cows. The process of lactation involves the synthesis of milk in the mammary glands of the cow, which is then secreted into the mammary gland1. This process is initiated at the end of pregnancy.

The early lactation period imposes a considerable metabolic stress on the dairy cow, which is accompanied by an increased occurrence of health disorders. The high metabolic priority of the mammary gland during early lactation imposes metabolic stress on the dairy cow. The mammary gland and the immune system compete for the availability of glucose and amino acids, which are major limitations for milk production. The lactation cycle is a fundamental factor significantly affecting a cow's nutritional requirements. As dairy cows progress through various lactation stages, their nutritional needs evolve, demanding tailored diets to support their milk production, body condition, and reproductive performance.

1. What is the functional unit of the mammary glands responsible for milk secretion?
   a) Alveoli
   b) Ducts
   c) Nipples
   d) Cisterns
2. Which embryonic layer gives rise to the mammary alveoli?
   a) Mesoderm
   b) Endoderm
   c) Ectoderm
   d) Epidermis
3. What anatomical structures connect milk formation to distribution in cows?
   a) Alveoli
   b) Ducts
   c) Nipples
   d) Cisterns
4. How many pairs of mammary glands do cows typically have?
   a) 1
   b) 2
   c) 3
   d) 4
5. What specialized structures store large quantities of milk in cows before milking?
   a) Alveoli
   b) Ducts
   c) Nipples
   d) Cisterns
6. Which hormones are responsible for the proliferation of the udder tubular system?
   a) Estrogen and progesterone
   b) Growth hormones and corticosteroids
   c) Insulin and prolactin
   d) Thyroid hormones and oxytocin
7. What is the primary function of the internal suspensory ligament and lateral 7. suspensory ligament in cows?
   a) Milk synthesis
   b) Milk secretion
   c) Udder support
   d) Hormone production
8. Which phase of lactation involves the onset of milk secretion and enzymatic differentiation of mammary alveolar cells?
   a) Mammogenesis
   b) Lactogenesis
   c) Galactopoiesis
   d) Involution
9. What hormone stimulates milk ejection from the mammary gland during suckling?
   a) Estrogen
   b) Progesterone
   c) Prolactin
   d) Oxytocin

11. Which phase of lactation follows a dynamic curve with rapid acceleration, peak yield, and gradual decline?
    a) Mammogenesis b) Lactogenesis
    c) Galactopoiesis d) Involution
12. What process restores the mammary gland to a virgin-like state after milk secretion ceases?
    a) Mammogenesis b) Lactogenesis
    c) Galactopoiesis d) Involution
13. Which hormones play essential roles in each stage of the lactation process?
    a) Thyroid hormones b) Growth factors
    c) Insulin d) Cortisol
14. Which hormone is responsible for maintaining milk production during the later stages of lactation?
    a) Estrogen b) Progesterone
    c) Prolactin d) Somatotropin (GH)
15. What anatomical structure connects the alveoli to the teat cistern in the udder?
    a) Alveolar ducts b) Lactiferous sinus
    c) Udder lobules d) Teat canal
16. Which hormone stimulates milk synthesis and alveolar cell growth during pregnancy?
    a) Estrogen b) Progesterone
    c) Prolactin d) Oxytocin

    What is the primary function of the streak canal in the teat?
    a) Milk synthesis b) Milk secretion
    c) Udder support d) Preventing bacterial entry
17. Which hormone triggers milk ejection during milking?
    a) Estrogen b) Progesterone
    c) Prolactin d) Oxytocin

    What is the role of prolactin in the mammary gland during lactation?
    a) Stimulating milk ejection b) Promoting milk synthesis
    c) Regulating udder blood flow d) Controlling udder temperature
18. Which phase of lactation involves the gradual reduction in milk production after peak yield?
    a) Mammogenesis b) Lactogenesis
    c) Galactopoiesis d) Involution
19. What is the primary source of energy for milk synthesis in cows?
    a) Glucose b) Fatty acids
    c) Amino acids d) Lactose

20. Which of the following statements about cow's milk is incorrect?
    a) Cow's milk contains 80% whey protein, not casein.
    b) Cow milk has less carbohydrate than mother's milk.
    c) Cow's milk has more K+ and Na+ than infant formula feeds.
    d) Cow's milk has more protein than breast milk.
21. What is the approximate moisture content of cow milk?
    a) 30% b) 50%
    c) 83% d) 90%
22. What percentage of fat is typically found in cow milk?
    a) 9% b) 10%
    c) 15% d) 4%
23. Milk is an emulsion of _____ in water.
    a) Oil b) Water
    c) Soap d) Dirt
24. In milk, the whey proteins are in _____ solution, and the casein is in colloidal suspension.
    a) Water b) Colloidal
    c) Fat d) Gas
25. Approximately what size are fat globules in milk solution?
    a) 10^-2 to 10^-3 b) 10^-4 to 10^-5
    c) 10^-5 to 10^-6 d) 10^-6 to 10^-7
26. Which method can be used to compute fat crystallization in cow milk?
    a) JMR b) DMR
    c) NMR d) CMR
27. What does the Iodine Value state regarding fat?
    a) Fractional b) Iodine
    c) Fatty acid d) Distillation
28. Which organic compounds have both amines and carboxyl functional groups?
    a) Amino acids b) Alcohol
    c) Carboxylic acid d) Amine
29. Which of the following cannot be classified as a type of casein?
    a) α-casein b) β-casein
    c) κ-casein d) Delta-casein
30. Which method is NOT used to make caseinate particles flocculate and coagulate?
    a) Precipitation by acid b) Precipitation by enzymes
    c) Precipitation by water d) None of the mentioned
31. Which of the following are whey proteins?
    a) α-lactalbumin b) β-lactoglobulin
    c) κ-lactis d) α-lactalbumin & β-lactoglobulin

32. Which fat-soluble vitamins are present in milk?
    a) A
    b) D
    c) A & D
    d) B

33. Which vitamin is abundant in buffalo milk compared to cow milk?
    a) Vitamin A
    b) Vitamin D
    c) Vitamin E
    d) Vitamin K

34. Which mineral is present in higher amounts in goat milk compared to cow milk?
    a) Calcium
    b) Magnesium
    c) Phosphorus
    d) Potassium

35. Which milk has the highest fat content among cow, buffalo, and goat milk?
    a) Cow milk
    b) Buffalo milk
    c) Goat milk
    d) All have similar fat content

36. What is the standard fat content (minimum) required for cow milk in India?
    a) 2.5%
    b) 3.0%
    c) 4.5%
    d) 5.0%

37. Which milk protein is responsible for the coagulation of milk during cheese-making?
    a) Casein
    b) Whey protein
    c) Lactoferrin
    d) Albumin

38. What is the ideal pH range for milk?
    a) 5.0 - 5.5
    b) 6.0 - 6.5
    c) 6.5 - 6.8
    d) 7.0 - 7.2

39. Which milk component contributes to the white color of milk?
    a) Lactose
    b) Casein
    c) Fat globules
    d) Whey proteins

40. What is the primary sugar found in milk?
    a) Glucose
    b) Sucrose
    c) Lactose
    d) Fructose

41. Which milk product is obtained by fermenting milk with lactic acid bacteria?
    a) Butter
    b) Yogurt
    c) Ghee
    d) Paneer

42. Which milk product is rich in probiotics and aids in gut health?
    a) Cheese
    b) Buttermilk
    c) Condensed milk
    d) Skim milk

43. What is the recommended daily intake of milk and milk products for adults according to ICMR (Indian Council of Medical Research)?
    a) 200 ml
    b) 300 ml
    c) 500 ml
    d) 1 liter

44. Which milk component is responsible for the formation of curd during fermentation?
 a) Lactose b) Casein
 c) Whey proteins d) Fatty acids

45. Which milk product is obtained by churning cream?
 a) Butter b) Cheese
 c) Yogurt d) Ghee

46. What is the primary function of lactoferrin in milk?
 a) Enhancing milk flavor b) Regulating calcium absorption
 c) Binding iron d) Promoting fat digestion

47. Which milk component is responsible for the yellow color of butter?
 a) Lactose b) Casein
 c) Carotenoids d) Fatty acids

48. What is the primary sugar found in buffalo milk?
 a) Glucose b) Sucrose
 c) Lactose d) Fructose

49. Which milk protein is most abundant in goat milk?
 a) α-lactalbumin b) β-lactoglobulin
 c) κ-casein d) α-casein

50. Which milk product is obtained by fermenting milk with specific bacterial strains to produce a thick, creamy consistency?
 a) Paneer b) Yogurt
 c) Ghee d) Buttermilk

51. What is the standard fat content (minimum) required for buffalo milk in India?
 a) 5.0% b) 6.0%
 c) 7.0% d) 8.5%

52. Which milk component is responsible for the formation of curd during fermentation?
 a) Lactose b) Casein
 c) Whey proteins d) Fatty acids

53. Which milk product is obtained by churning cream to separate butterfat from buttermilk?
 a) Butter b) Cheese
 c) Yogurt d) Ghee

54. What is the primary function of lactoferrin in milk?
 a) Enhancing milk flavor b) Regulating calcium absorption
 c) Binding iron d) Promoting fat digestion

55. Which milk component contributes to the white color of milk?
 a) Lactose b) Casein
 c) Fat globules d) Whey proteins

56. Which milk product is rich in probiotics and aids in gut health?

a) Cheese b) Buttermilk

c) Condensed milk d) Skim milk

57. Which milk component contributes to the white color of milk?

a) Lactose b) Casein

c) Fat globules d) Whey proteins

58.. Which milk product is rich in probiotics and aids in gut health?

a) Cheese b) Buttermilk

c) Condensed milk d) Skim milk

59. What is the recommended daily intake of milk and milk products for adults according to ICMR (Indian Council of Medical Research)?

a) 200 ml b) 300 ml

c) 500 ml d) 1 liter

60. Which milk component is responsible for the formation of curd during fermentation?

a) Lactose b) Casein

c) Whey proteins d) Fatty acids

61. Which milk product is obtained by churning cream to separate butterfat from buttermilk?

a) Butter b) Cheese

c) Yogurt d) Ghee

62. What is the primary function of lactoferrin in milk?

a) Enhancing milk flavor b) Regulating calcium absorption

c) Binding iron d) Promoting fat digestion

63. Which milk component is responsible for the yellow color of butter?

a) Lactose b) Casein

c) Carotenoids d) Fatty acids

64. What is the primary sugar found in buffalo milk?

a) Glucose b) Sucrose

c) Lactose d) Fructose

65. Which milk protein is most abundant in goat milk?

a) α-lactalbumin b) β-lactoglobulin

67. c) κ-casein d) α-casein

Which method is NOT used to make caseinate particles flocculate and coagulate?

a) Precipitation by acid b) Precipitation by enzymes

c) Precipitation by water d) None of the mentioned

68. Which milk product is rich in probiotics and aids in gut health?

a) Cheese b) Buttermilk

c) Condensed milk d) Skim milk

69. The term Pasteurization was coined by

a) Louis Pasteur b) Dr. Soxhlet

c) Robert Koch d) Vergese Kurien

60. Pasteurization of milk was first discussed by

a) Louis Pasteur b) Robert Koch

c) Dr. Soxhletd d) Vergese Kurien

71. Pasteurization of milk is done to

a) To render milk safe for human consumption by destroying pathogenic microorganisms

b) Improve keeping quality of milk by destruction of almost all spoilage organisms

c) Reduce cream line of milk

d) Both a and b

72. Pasteurized milk has disadvantages of

a) Reduced nutritive value b) Decreases cream line of milk

c) Not clotting with rennet d) All of the above

73. Which bacteria is considered as index of pasteurization

a) *Mycobacterium tuberculosis* b) *Coxiella burnetti*

c) *Brucella abortus* d) *Bacillus anthracis*

74 Which test is done to detect inadequate pasteurization

a) Catalase test b) Phosphatase test

c) Milk ring test d) Oxidase test

75. During pasteurization cream line of milk and temperature- time are

a) Inversely related b) Directly related

c) Not related at all d) Depending upon type of milk

76. What is the temperature time combination of pasteurization to destroy phosphatase enzyme

a) 61.1°C and 30 minutes b) 71.1°C and 15 seconds

c) 58.9°C and 30 minutes d) Both a and b

77. What is the temperature time combination for bottle pasteurization

a) 71.1°C and 15 seconds b) 58.9°C and 30 minutes

c) 61.1°C and 30 minutes d) 63-66°C for 30 mins

78. Batch pasteurization is done at

a) 71.1°C for 15 seconds b) 58.9°C and 30 minutes

c) 63°C and 30 minutes d) 66°C for 30 minutes

79. Flash pasteurization is done at

a) 72°C for 15 seconds b) 58.9°C and 30 minutes

c) 63°C and 30 minutes d) 66°C for 30 minutes

80. Which of the following is not the advantage of flash pasteurization

a) Less space requirement

b) More milk can be pasteurized in less time

c) Quick & adequate heating and still maintaining product quality
d) Greater milk stones in heating system

81. What is the pressure of pasteurized milk in high temperature short time (HTST) pasteurization system

a) 15 psi
b) 14 psi
c) 13 psi
d) 16 psi

82. For properly pasteurized milk coliform count should be

a) 1 in 1 ml
b) 1 in 100 ml
c) Absent in 1:10 dilution
d) Absent in 1:100 dilution

83. ______________ are used in packaging machine to check contamination of milk

a) Aseptic packs
b) Drip reflectors
c) Bacterial culture media
d) All of the above

84. What is the time temperature combination of ultra high temperature (UHT) pasteurization

a) 72°C for 15 seconds
b) 58.9°C and 30 minutes
c) 63°C and 30 minutes
d) 135-150°C without holding or for a fraction of second

85. The only organism survive in UHT is

a) *Bacillus stearothermophilus*
b) *Mycobacterium tuberculosis*
c) *Coxiella burnetti*
d) *Brucella abortus*

86. What is the shelf life of UHT mik at room temperature

a) 7-10 days
b) 20-30 days
c) 2-6 months
d) 1-2 years

87. The time temperature combination for Stassanization is

a) 58.9°C and 30 minutes
b) 63°C and 30 minutes
c) 135-150°C without holding or for a fraction of second
d) 74°C for 7 seconds

88. The thermization is

a) a method to temporary inhibit bacterial growth
b) Done at 57-68°C/ 63-65°C for 15 secs & cooling to 4 °C to prevent aerobic spore formers from multiplication
c) Both a and b
d) Veg form converts to aerobic spores on thermization and can be destroyed on

89. Subsequent pasteurization Vacreation is

a) Pasteurization of milk/cream under reduced pressure by direct steam
b) First developed in New Zealand by M/s Murray Deodorizers Ltd
c) Removes undesirable odours
d) All of the above

90. Uperisation is

a) Shortened form of the word ultra pasteurization that has been developed in Switzerland

b) Done at 115-130°C for 2-4 seconds

c) Done to extend the shelf life of milk to 15-30 days

d) All of the above

91. Sterilization of milk is done at

a) 58.9°C and 30 minutes b) 63°C and 30 minutes

c) 74°C for 7 seconds d) 115-121°C for 20-30 minutes

92. The temperature time combination for electric pasteurization

a) 161°F to 163°F for 15-20 seconds

b) 161°F to 163°F for 15-20 minutes

c) 161°C to 163°C for 15-20 minutes

d) 161°C to 163°C for 15-20 seconds

93. __________ is the process of removing 99% of bacteria in milk by centrifugal force

a) Vancreation b) Bactofugation

c) Microfugation d) Pasteurization

94. Another name for batch or holding pasteurization is

a) LTST b) LTLT

c) HTST d) HTLT

95. What is the full form of FDV in HTST pasteurization

a) Floating device valve b) Full diversion valve

c) Flow diversion valve d) Floating decimal value

96. Another name for HTST is

a) Vancreation b) Batch pasteurization

c) Holding pasteurization d) Flash pasteurization

97. After pasteurization, the milk should be cooled to temperature below

a) 15°C b) -5°C

c) 5°C d) 0°C

98. What was the growth rate of milk production in India over the past 9 years?

a) 4.85% b) 5.85%

c) 6.85% d) 7.85%

99. What was the per capita availability of milk in India during 2022-23?

a) 359 grams per day b) 459 grams per day

c) 559 grams per day d) 659 grams per day

100. The heating temperature of milk for homogenisation

a) 50-55°C b) 65-70°C

c) 65-70°F d) 50-55°F

101. The size of fat globules in homogenized milk is

a) <5 microns
b) >5 microns
c) >2 microns
d) <2 microns

102. Homogenization was introduced by

a) Louis Pasteur
b) Dr. Soxhlet
c) Buttenberg
d) Robert Koch

103. The micro-filtration process of milk

a) Uses porous membranes with cut off pore size of microns (10^{-6} m)
b) Is used in the separation of selective bacteria from milk and it is capable to remove more than 99% bacteria from skim milk
c) Enhances keeping quality of milk by 3-4 days
d) All of the above

104. dia-filtration is

a) A modification of ultra filtration in which water is added to the feed as ultra filtration proceeds in order to wash-out feed components able to pass through the membrane
b) Uses porous membranes with cut off pore size of microns (10^{-6} m)
c) It is a way of producing milk, rich in protein and fat and very low in lactose and salts content
d) Both a and c

105. Which of the following is not the type of LTLT pasteurization

a) Water jacketed type
b) Water spray type
c) Heat exchanger type
d) Coil vat type

106. Which of the following is the type of HTST

a) Water jacketed type
b) Tubular heat exchanger
c) Plate heat exchanger
d) Both b and c

107. Double stage homogenisation is done when the milk fat percentage is

a) <4%
b) >4%
c) >6%
d) <6%

108. Preservation of evaporated milk is done by

a) Pasteurization
b) Sterilization
c) Vancreation
d) Uperization

109. Which test is done for rapid assessment of stability to processing for sterilisation

a) Phosphatise test
b) Peroxidise test
c) Rosalic acid test
d) Alcohol test

110. Expand the term HACCP

a) Hazards analysis and critical control points
b) Harmful assessment and critical control points
c) Hazard analysis and chemical control procedure
d) Hazard analysis and common control points

111. Total how many principles are there for HACCP
   a) 5 b) 6
   c) 7 d) 8

112. CIP in milk plant stands for
   a) Cleaning in person b) Cleaning in place
   c) Contamination in places d) Correction in population

113. Which of the following is not the advantage of CIP
   a) Ensure that all equipment receives uniform heat treatment day after day by eliminating the human factor
   b) Less damage to equipment
   c) Saving of total clean up costs and in man hours
   d) Increases possibility of contamination

114. How much pressure is needed for one stage homogenisation
   a) 2000-2500 psi b) 1500-2000 psi
   c) 2500-3000 psi d) 1000-1500 psi

115. What is the pressure at both the stages in two stage pasteurization
   a) Stage 1-2000 psi, stage 2- 1000 psi
   b) Stage 1-2000 psi, stage 2- 500 psi
   c) Stage 1-500 psi, stage 2- 2000 psi
   d) Stage 1-1500 psi, stage 2- 1500 psi

116. Which country is the largest milk producer in the world?
   a) India b) United States
   c) China d) New Zealand

117. Which country is the second-largest milk producer in the world?
   a) India b) United States
   c) China d) Pakistan

118. Which country has the highest milk surplus?
   a) India b) United States
   c) China d) New Zealand

119. Which country has the highest milk deficit?
   a) China b) Italy
   c) Mexico d) Algeria

120. Which country is the largest milk producer in Africa?
   a) Egypt b) Kenya
   c) South Africa d) Ethiopia

121. Which country is the largest milk producer in Latin America?
   a) Argentina b) Brazil
   c) Colombia d) Mexico

122. Which country is the largest milk producer in the European Union?
   a) Germany b) France
   c) United Kingdom d) Scotland

123. The permissible limits recommended by FAO(1957) for the use of hydrogen peroxide for milk is
   a) < 600 ppm
   b) >600 ppm
   c) <800 ppm
   d) >800 ppm

124. Lactoperoxidase/ thiocyanate/ hydrogen peroxide (LP) system of milk preservation is ________ for gram negative bacteria and ___________ for gram positive bacteria.
   a) Bacteriostatic, bactericidal
   b) Bactericidal, Bacteriostatic
   c) Bactericidal, Bactericidal
   d) Bacteriostatic, Bacteriostatic

125. Expand the term MMPO
   a) Meat and meat product order
   b) Meat and milk products order
   c) Milk and milk products order
   d) Milk and meat products order

126. The government of India promulgated the MMPO in
   a) June 1962
   b) June 1972
   c) June 1982
   d) June 1992

127. The adulteration of milk is punishable under ________ of IPC
   a) Section 427
   b) Section 420
   c) Section 377
   d) Section 328

128. Adulteration of water in milk cannot be detected by
   a) By determining specific gravity of milk
   b) By detecting nitrate in milk
   c) By determining freezing point of milk
   d) By fucoma test

129. The fat content of milk can be detected by
   a) Gerber method
   b) Fucoma test
   c) Babcock method
   d) All of the above

130. The analytical method for fat detection is
   a) Rose- gottileb method
   b) Gerber method
   c) Babcock method
   d) All of the above

131. Which of the following is not a thickening agent for the milk
   a) Starch
   b) Calcium carbonate
   c) Annatto
   d) Sugar

132. Addition of which adulterant in milk is considered as double fraud
   a) Addition of preservatives
   b) Addition of colouring agents
   c) Addition of neutralizers
   d) Addition of thickening agent

133. Rosalic acid test is done for detection of
   a) Sodium hydroxide
   b) Potassium hydroxide
   c) Calcium hydroxide
   d) All of the above

134. The colouring agent for milk is/are
   a) Coal tar dyes
   b) Gelatine
   c) Annatto
   d) Both a and c

135. The adulteration of buffalo milk with cow milk can be detected by
   a) Valenta test
   b) Fucoma test
   c) HANSA test
   d) Pyne test
136. The adulteration of vegetable fat in ghee is detected by
   a) Valenta test
   b) Fucoma test
   c) HANSA test
   d) Pyne test
137. Baudin test is done for detection of
   a) Vegetable fat in ghee
   b) Adulteration of buffalo milk
   c) Water in milk
   d) Milk protein
138. Adulteration of vegetable fat in ghee is detected by
   a) Valenta test
   b) Baudin test
   c) Bomner's Phyto-Sterol-Test
   d) All of the above
139. Adulteration of cotton seed oil in ghee is detected by
   a) Valenta test
   b) Baudin test
   c) Halphens Test
   d) Bomner's Phyto-Sterol-Test
140. Pyne test is used for detection of
   a) Milk proteins
   b) Animal fat
   c) Cotton seed oil adulteration
   d) Detection of thickening agents
141. Alcohol alizarin test is done for
   a) Milk protein
   b) Alkalinity of milk
   c) Acidity of milk
   d) Physical contamination of milk
142. The natural germicidal activity of milk is destroyed by heating milk to _____
   a) 60-80 - for 30 minutes
   b) 80-100 - for 30 minutes
   c) 80-100 - for 30 seconds
   d) 60-80- for 30 seconds
143. What does "Milk" refer to according to FSSAI?
   a) Mammary secretion
   b) Processed product
   c) Milk substitute
   d) Essential part of a product
144. What is a "Composite milk product" according to FSSAI?
   a) Processed product
   b) Milk substitute
   c) Essential part of a product
   d) Mammary secretion
145. What does "Heat treatment" mean according to FSSAI?
   a) Boiling milk
   b) Pasteurization, etc.
   c) Heating to a certain temperature
   d) Killing bacteria
146. What does "Analogue in the dairy context" mean according to FSSAI?
   a) Processed product
   b) Milk substitute
   c) Mammary secretion
   d) Essential part of a product
147. What was the total milk production in India during 2022-23? a)
   a) 210 million tonnes
   b) 220 million tonnes
   c) 230.58 million tonnes
   d) 240 million tonnes

148. Which state contributed the highest share to India's milk production in 2022-23?

a) Uttar Pradesh b) Rajasthan

c) Madhya Pradesh d) Gujarat

149. What does the term "Integrated Veterinary Health Certificate (VHc)" refer to according to DAHD?

a) A certificate that incorporates the DAHD's sanitary requirements along with those of the Ministry of Health and Family Welfare/Food Safety and Standards Authority of India's (FSSAI) food safety requirements

b) A certificate that is required for the import of Milk and Milk Product into India

c) A certificate that needs to be certified by the exporting country along with the consignments to be exported into India

d) All of the above

150. What was the total milk production in India during 2022-23?

a) 210 million tonnes b) 220 million tonnes

c) 230.58 million tonnes d) 240 million tonnes

Answer Key

1	a	2	c	3	c	4	d	5	d	6	b	7	c
8	b	9	d	10	c	11	d	12	b	13	d	14	b
15	c	16	d	17	d	18	b	19	d	20	a	21	a
22	c	23	d	24	a	25	a	26	c	27	d	28	b
29	a	30	d	31	d	32	d	33	c	34	b	35	c
36	b	37	b	38	a	39	c	40	b	41	c	42	b
43	b	44	b	45	b	46	a	47	c	48	c	49	d
50	d	51	b	52	d	53	b	54	a	55	c	56	b
57	b	58	b	59	b	60	b	61	b	62	a	63	c
64	c	65	c	66	d	67	d	68	b	69	a	70	c
71	d	72	d	73	b	74	b	75	a	76	d	77	d
78	c	79	a	80	d	81	a	82	c	83	b	84	d
85	a	86	c	87	d	88	c	89	d	90	d	91	d
92	a	93	b	94	b	95	c	96	d	97	c	98	b
99	b	100	b	101	d	102	c	103	d	104	d	105	c
106	d	107	c	108	b	109	d	110	a	111	c	112	b
113	d	114	a	115	b	116	a	117	b	118	d	119	a
120	d	121	b	122	a	123	c	124	b	125	c	126	d
127	b	128	d	129	d	130	a	131	c	132	d	133	d
134	d	135	c	136	a	137	a	138	d	139	c	140	a
141	c	142	a	143	a	144	c	145	b	146	b	147	c
148	a	149	d	150	c								